Lens Implantation

Monographs in Ophthalmology 4

Dr. W. JUNK PUBLISHERS THE HAGUE - BOSTON - LONDON

Lens Implantation

30 Years of Progress

P. LEONARD and J. ROMMEL

Departments of Ophthalmology
of the Universities of Leiden and Leuven

Dr. W. JUNK PUBLISHERS THE HAGUE - BOSTON - LONDON

REPRINTED FROM Bull. Soc. belge Ophtal. 194, 1982

Distributors:

for the United States and Canada

Kluwer Boston Inc.
190 Old Derby Street
Hingham, MA 02043
USA

for all other countries

Kluwer Academic Publishing Group
Distribution Center
P.O. Box 322
3300 AH Dordrecht
The Netherlands

ISBN-13: 978-94-009-8020-4 e-ISBN-13: 978-94-009-8018-1
DOI: 10.1007/978-94-009-8018-1

CONTENTS

CHAPTER I
HISTORY

CHAPTER II
THE CLASSIC MODERN LENS

CHAPTER III

MATERIALS, MANUFACTURE, AND STERILIZATION

CHAPTER IV

THE OPTICS OF INTRAOCULAR LENSES

CHAPTER V

PRE-, PER-, AND POSTOPERATIVE MANAGEMENT

CHAPTER VI

THE IRIS SUPPORTED LENSES

CHAPTER VII

IRIDOCAPSULAR AND CAPSULAR SUPPORTED LENSES

CHAPTER VIII

ANGLE SUPPORTED LENSES

CHAPTER IX

MIXED RESULTS AND COMPARATIVE STUDIES

CHAPTER X

SECONDARY LENS IMPLANTATION

CHAPTER XI

LENS IMPLANTATION IN CHILDREN TRAUMATIC AND INFANTILE CATARACTS

CHAPTER XII

LENS IMPLANTATION AND THE ENDOTHELIUM

CHAPTER XIII

LENS IMPLANTATION AND INFLAMMATORY RESPONSE AND GLAUCOMA

CHAPTER XIV

LENS IMPLANTATION AND CYSTOID MACULAR EDEMA

CHAPTER XV

LENS IMPLANTATION AND RETINAL DETACHMENT

CHAPTER XVI
GUIDELINES

FOREWORD

The authors of this book are busy practical men with no particular barrow to push.

The text of the book includes a comprehensive review of all aspects of intraocular lens surgery including details of the design, optics chemistry and sterilization of intraocular lenses. Its value is enhanced by excellent illustrations and extensive tabulated references to the literature.

Accounts of patient acceptability are balanced against candid discussion of complications and their management.

The historical introduction recalls that in the early stages of development of the art, over a period of 10 years, two dozen different lens designs were proposed, most claiming elimination of problems which had arisen with their predecessors. Eventually nearly all disappeared from the scene.

In an age where every cataract surgeon has to determine a personal position on intraocular lens implantation the author's reflections on these matters are timely. Intraocular lenses are neither a miracle nor a menace, provided that personal decisions and preferences are carefully thought through and put into practice upon the basis of known facts and not upon the basis of fickle fashion and fad.

This book provides a background upon which the reader can evaluate in his own mind the validity of information provided by the manufacturers of various lens designs.

In practice it is emphasized that, however helpful videotape and film presentations may be, there is no substitute for proper surgical apprenticeship as with any other kind of operation. The author's background of protracted apprenticeship and subsequent practice in intraocular lens surgery adds weight to their words.

It is my pleasure to comment their objectivity, scholarship and industry, and to express my convection that they have produced an outstanding book of reference.

C.D. Binkhorst, M.D., F.A.C.S.

Terneuzen, 23 October 1981.

INTRODUCTION

In the late seventies, the Belgian Ophthalmological Society honored us with the assignment of constructing a report on the evolution and the current concepts of lens implantation and the rehabilitation of the cataract patient.

Our intention si to give a critical overview of what has happened in the area of lens implantation over the last 30 years and how this evolution has led to the present situation at the beginning of the 1980's. We thus describe the possibilities and the limitations of the classic lens models and the surgical techniques associated with them. We hope this information will form a guide for the evaluation of the full range of existing and future lens types. It is also with this intention that we discuss the materials from which the lenses are manufactured, their optical qualities, and the various sterilization methods. Finally, on the basis of the data at our disposal and our own experience, we discuss the effects of the implant lens on the surrounding eye structures.

We owe a great deal of thanks Cornelius D. Binkhorst, who introduced us in the 1960's to the world of lens implantation. He not only taught us the techniques, but also, and most importantly, gave us the principles of sound surgical judgment. His immediate contribution to the present work consisted of placing all of his photographic materials at our disposal.

Our thanks also go to Professor Emeritus M.C. Colenbrander and Professor J.A. Oosterhuis of Leiden and to Professor L. Missotten of Leuven, who years ago entrusted us with the beginning of lens implantation in their respective services.

We must also express our gratitude to all those who have helped by word and deed in the preparation of this work. They are too numerous to list here.

CHAPTER I

HISTORY

The credit for the idea of replacing the opaque crystallin of the human eye with an implant apparently must go to an itinerant Italian healer called Tadiny, whose idea of lens implantation was mentioned by Casanova in his memoires (Taieb, 1955). In Warsaw in 1766, Tadiny showed Casanova tiny crystal lenses that he said he could insert under the cornea to replace the eye's natural lens. Two years later in Barcelona after a second meeting, Casanova concluded that Tadiny had yet actually to implant a lens. According to R. Marx (1970), Tadiny must have been a rather well-known healer also in our country, since he had placed advertisements in the *Gazette van Gent* in 1788, 1791, and 1792.

DEn Heer Chevalier *de Tadiny*, Paltz-Graeve en Oogmeeſter van Vrankryk, genoegzaem bekend door zyne zeldzaeme Wetenſchappen, woonende tot Bruſſel by Mr. *Beegmans*, Apotheker op den hoek van de Beyerſche Straete, is den 2 dezer binnen deze Stad aengekomen, van waer hy zig heeft begeven nae Ipren by Mr. *van der Ghinſt*, Negoçiant aldaer, om de operatie te doen aen Joff. zyne Moeder, die van twee Cataractes is overvallen; hy zal den 9. van Ipren nae Kortryk vertrekken, alwaer hy acht dagen zal verblyven; en logeren in het Daemberd.

The Chevalier de Tadiny, Count Palatine and oculist from France, who is well known for his rare science and who resides in Brussels at the house of Mr. Beegmans, pharmacist, at the corner of Bavarian Street, came to this city on the second of this month from whence he has gone to Ypres to Mr. van der Ghinst, a merchant there, to perform an operation on his mother, who has two cataracts. He shall leave Ypres for Kortrijk on the 9th where he shall stay for eight days, lodging in the Damier.

MOnſieur le Chevalier *de Tadiny*, Comte Palatin, Oculiſte de la Cour de France, venant de Londres, eſt depuis quelques ſemaines arrivé à Tournai, où il a operé quelques pauvres & autres Habitans de ladite Ville avec un ſuccès qui rarement a failli en preſence de quelques Médécins & Chirurgiens, leſquels ont approuvé ſa nouvelle méthode d'operer & ils ont déclaré, qu'ils n'ont jamais vu aucun Oculiſte qui opére avec une franchiſe & ſans aucun embaras, comme ledit Sr. *Tadiny*; il eſt parti dudit Tournai le 9. de ce mois pour ſe rendre à Courtrai, où il reſtera huit jours à l'Hôtel du Damier; de Courtrai il ira à Bruges, où il reſtera huit jours auſſi; & il ſe rendra de Bruges à Bruxelles, où il reſtera quinze jours à l'Hôtel Rouge chez le Sr. *Stevenar*; & comme cet habile Oculiſte doit paſſer par cette Ville de Gand, il deſcendra chez Milord *Champon* ſur le *Kauter* le 25. ou le 26. de ce mois de Mars: les Perſonnes, tant pauvres qu'autres, qui auront beſoin de ſon talent, pourront ſe rendre au ſusdit Hôtel chez Milord *Champon.*

The Chevalier de Tadiny, Count Palatine and Oculist at the Court of France, arrived a few weeks ago in Tournai from London. In Tournai he operated on some poor people and other inhabitants of the city with only rare failures. This was done in the presence of some physicians and surgeons, who have approved of his new surgical method. They declared that they had never seen any oculist operate with such boldness and without complications as did the Seigneur Tadiny. He left Tournai on the 9th of this month to go to Kortrijk where he will stay eight days at the Hotel Damier. From Kortrijk he will go to Bruges where he will also stay eight days. From Bruges he will go to Brussels where he will stay fourteen days at the Hôtel Rouge with the Seigneur Stevenar. This skillful oculist will come to this city of Ghent and will stay with Milord Champon on the Kauter on the 25th or the 26th of this month of March. Those people, poor or otherwise, who have need of his talents can go to the hotel of Milord Champon.

Fig. I-1. — Originals (and translations) of two announcements placed by Tadiny in the *Gazette van Gent* in 1788 and 1792.

The first person to attempt the actual implantation of an artificial lens was Casaamata, an Italian ophthalmologist who lived in Dresden. According to W. Münchow (1964), R. Shiferli, a Swiss ophthalmologist, described in 1797 the lens implantation he had observed Casaamata doing in Leipzig. He commented on the attempt as follows (Münchow, 1964, p. 774):

> It is known that vision is not restored after surgery to the healthy condition since the lens is missing. To repair this loss, Casaamata attempted to insert a glass lens through the corneal wound into the eye. He observed, however, that this glass lens could not replace the natural lens since the glass lens immediately fell to the bottom of the eye. But there is another method to make up for the loss of the lens, and this is the best and usual method: convex glasses are worn by the patient in front of the eye that has been operated on in the same way as one wears spectacles.

I. Posterior Chamber Lenses

The modern history of lens implantation begins only about thirty years ago. Harold Ridley's first lens implantation was carried out in

1949 at the Thomas Hospital in London. The patient was a woman of about 60 years of age. Ridley performed a straightforward extracapsular extraction, which presumably provided normal aphakic refraction, after which he implanted his posterior chamber lens in a secondary procedure. This seems to be the only secondary implantation of this lens type that he ever performed. An error was made in estimating the refractive power of the implant lens, causing an overcorrection of the eye of some 14 diopters. This problem was resolved for future lenses by considerably reducing the strength of the lens.

The final standard model was a biconvex lens of +24 D (in aqueous) made of fully polymerized methylmethacrylate (Transpex ICI). It measured 8.35 mm in diameter and 2.40 mm in thickness. The radius of the anterior curve was 17.8 mm and that of the posterior curve, 10.7 mm. Its weight in air was 112 mg.

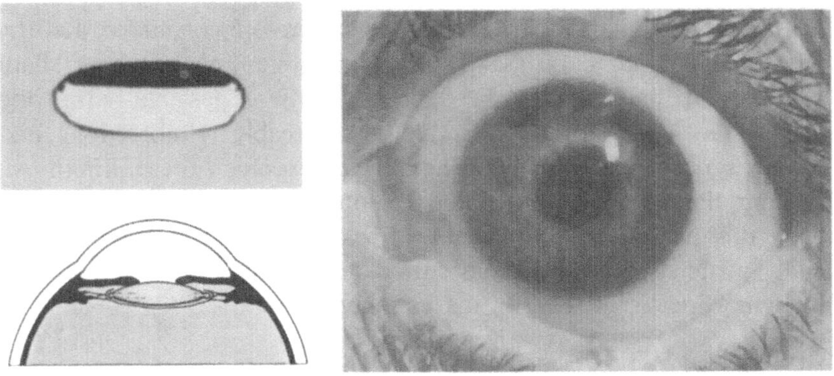

Fig. I-2. — Original Ridley implant manufactured by Rayner (London); schematic representation of the implant in situ, and photograph of an eye containing this lens (Courtesy C. D. Binkhorst.)

All the subsequent implantations Ridley performed with this lens were primary procedures, i.e., the lenticulus was placed in the posterior chamber between the iris and the intact posterior capsule immediately after the extracapsular removal of the cataract. Ridley reported on his initial results in July 1951 on the occasion of an Oxford congress (Ridley, 1952). Impressed with the favorable short term performance of these lenses, other ophthalmic surgeons entered the field of implant surgery, among them A. Arruga, J. Barraquer, C.D. Binkhorst, E. Epstein, J. François, T. Hamdi, L. Paufique, and W. Reese.

For a number of years, this implant technique was applied in various countries with mixed success, to be followed by lenses of other designs and different fixating principles. Ridley himself abandoned the posterior chamber lens in 1960.

Reviewing the first decade of implant surgery, we should like to recall a number of ideas and lessons that emerged. It would be shortsighted to ignore them.

First of all, lens implantation proved to be an effective method of restoring binocular vision in patients with unilateral cataract.

The idea of using polymethylmethacrylate to make the lenses, turned out to be sound. It was expected that the eye would tolerate this material well since it had been observed during World War II that fragments of Perspex windshields of aircraft that had lodged in the eye were well tolerated. The tissue reaction in these injured eyes was insignificant provided no sharp edge came in contact with a sensitive or mobile eye structure. It was therefore concluded that the lens implant had to be as smooth as possible—no rough or sharp edges—and that it had to be fixed as firmly as possible within the eye. Ridley opted for capsular fixation, possibly reinforced by iris-to-lens synechiae. As many authors have observed (Reese, Binkhorst, Epstein, Paufique), this resulted in longstanding stable fixation of even this heavy lens if it was well-positioned. When the lens was badly centered, iris atrophy occurred because of the friction of the overlying iris tissue against the peripheral haptic rim.

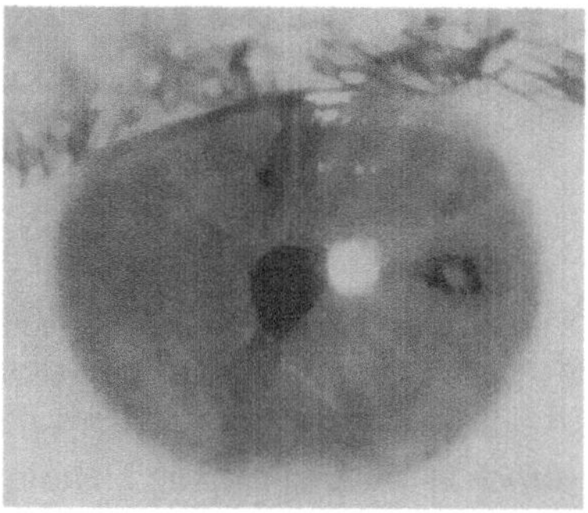

Fig. I-3. — Localized iris atrophy caused by friction. (Courtesy E. Epstein.)

Sterilization of the implant was initially a matter of great concern. Since polymethylmethacrylate could not be sterilized with heat, alcohol, or formaldehyde, the first choice was sterilization by immersion in a 1% solution of quaternary ammonium base, tetradecyl-trimethylammonium bromide (cetrimide). This method, however, often gave rise to postoperative iridocyclitis, sometimes with hypopion. Frederick Ridley introduced a new sterilisating method in the mid-fifties. It solved the problem and has remained in use to the present.

Immediate postoperative problems were generally related to the occurrence of marked inflammatory reactions that were difficult to treat with the methods then available. Occasionally, secondary glaucoma and pupil occlusion by dense membranes resulted. With the advent of better sterilization techniques and more effective medication, such as the corticosteroids, the severity of inflammatory reactions was reduced.

Opacification of the posterior capsule always constituted a serious problem because the bulky lens precluded ready access to the posterior capsule. Secondary capsulotomies had to be performed either through the iridectomy or through the pars plana. Ridley suggested performing a posterior capsulotomy at the time of the implantation but he himself never did it.

The late complications were mainly anterior or posterior lens dislocation, secondary glaucoma, and iris atrophy from the pressure of the rim of a badly centered lens. Anterior dislocation was reported to be rare but serious when it did occur, since contact between the implant and the posterior surface of the cornea generally resulted in corneal dystrophy. Posterior dislocation, which only occurred when the posterior capsule was ruptured, was reported to be less serious—though still very distressing—than a dislocated human lens and did not generally result in chronic uveitis or glaucoma. Ridley did not attempt lens extraction out of the vitreous.

Although Ridley and others initially obtained some good and lasting results, the posterior chamber lens was superseded some 10 years later by the anterior chamber lenses.

The immediate drawbacks of the posterior chamber lens thus were the technical difficulty of extracapsular cataract extraction and the rather severe postoperative reactions. The late drawbacks were the high incidence of dislocation, iris atrophy, and glaucoma (Ridley, 1960). Ridley (1964) cited an incidence of 13% dislocations and 10% glaucoma. The implant had to be extracted in some 15% of the cases (Jaffe et al., 1978).

E. Epstein (1957) from Johannesburg designed two posterior chamber lenses and implanted a small number of them. In contrast to Ridley's lenses, they were very thin and light (Fig. I-4).

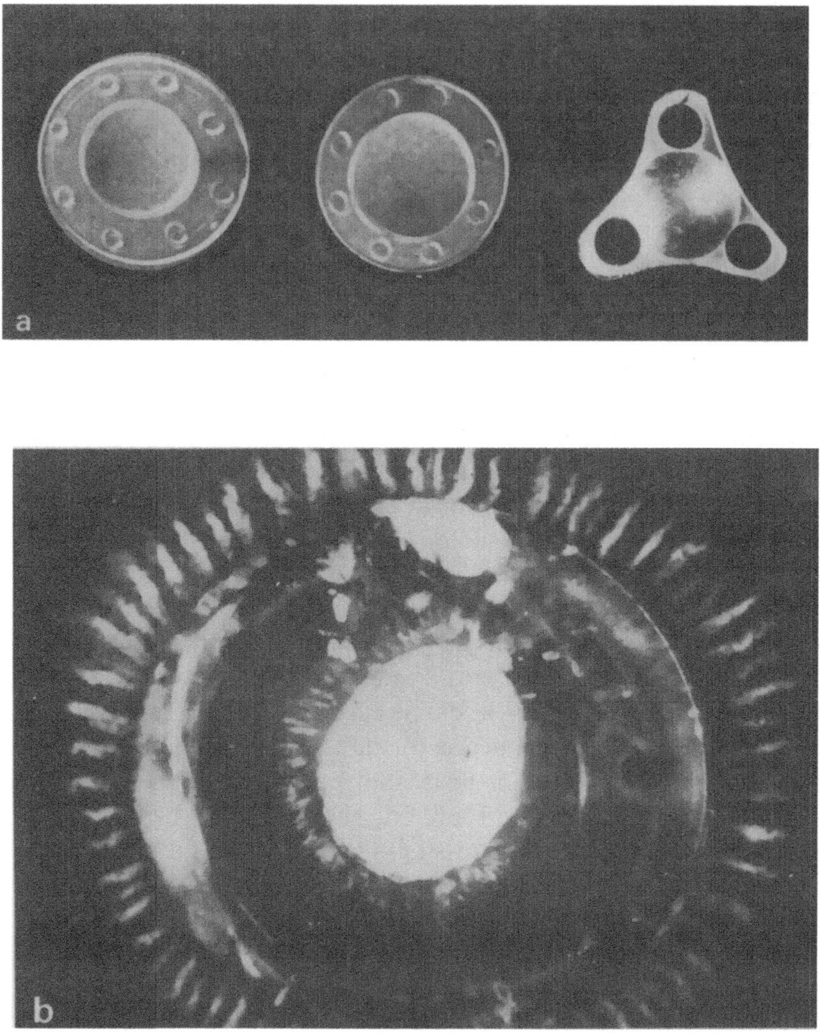

Fig. I-4a. — Various posterior chamber lenses as designed by E. Epstein in 1954. b. — Postmortem specimen which became available in 1978 of an Epstein posterior chamber lens successfully implanted in 1954. (Courtesy E. Epstein.)

T.G. Parry (1954) suggested fixating the original Ridley lens with a tantalum wire in situ. The wire was anchored above the lens in the sclera (Fig. I-5).

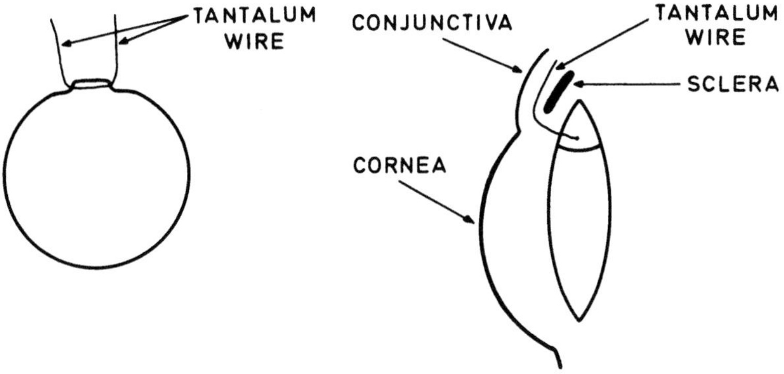

Fig. I-5. — Posterior chamber lens designed by T.G. Parry (1954).

Conclusion

In many ways the concept of using the fixation possibilities of the natural eye lens for the suspension of an artificial lens was ahead of its time. Fifteen years later, C.D. Binkhorst was the first to return to the idea of capsular fixation. Undoubtedly, as was observed by J. Pearce, who was the first to reapply the concept of posterior chamber implantation, a less bulky lens, routine use of the operating microscope, precise handling of the posterior capsule, and watertight wound closure with modern suturing techniques would have given far better results than those achieved with the Ridley lens.

II. Anterior Chamber Lenses

Beginning in the early fifties, lens models with haptic supports extending towards the anterior chamber angle were designed. Rigid and flexible supports entered clinical practice.

The prototype of the rigid lens was the original Strampelli lens, and the Dannheim lens is representative of the flexible models. Anterior chamber lenses were also tried with external fixation by B. Strampelli, W. Lieb, and Dupont-Guerry.

There were many variations in the design of the rigid lens types. The lens designed by A. Baron (1953) of France resembled a round contact lens that covered the posterior surface of the cornea almost completely. His later two lenses were square. One of them had a meniscoid profile and the other plano-convex with the convex side posteriorly (Fig. I-6).

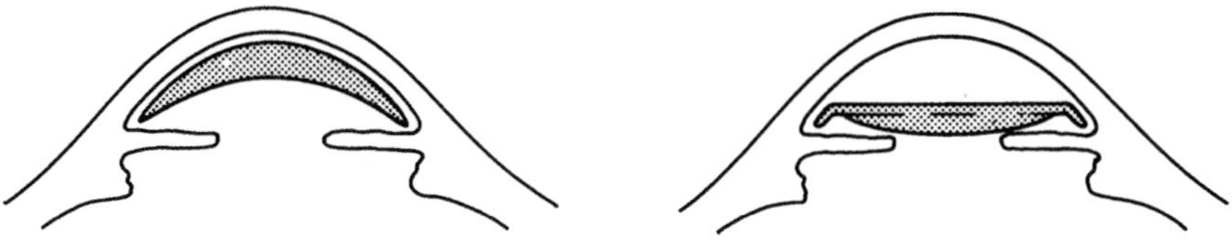

Fig. I-6. — Two types of anterior chamber lenses designed by A. Baron.

The first rigid lens devised by B. Strampelli of Italy was roughly rectangular, 5 mm by 13 mm. It had three tips resting in the chamber angle with the optic in front of the haptic support (Fig. I-7).

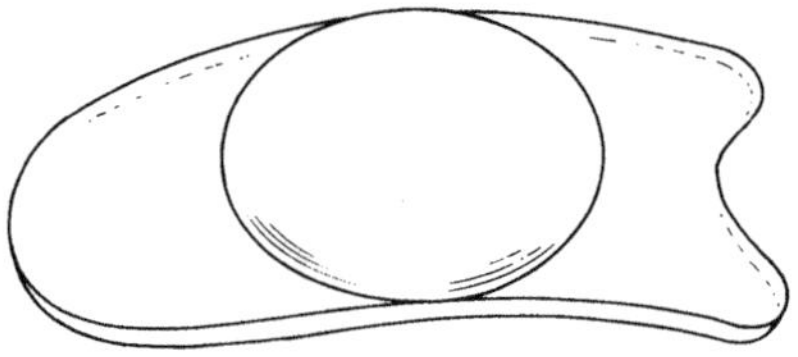

Fig. I-7. — Early model of an anterior chamber lens designed by B. Strampelli.

G.B. Bietti, also of Italy, first designed a lens with 4 thin legs resting in the chamber angle, but ultimately settled on a rectangular model. The lens designed by J. Scharf of Germany also had four legs. The lenses designed by E. Schreck of Germany and A. Apollonio of Italy, as well as Ridley's model, had 3 legs (Fig. I-8). One of the lenses designed by G.B. Bietti and one by E. Shreck had only 2 opposing supports.

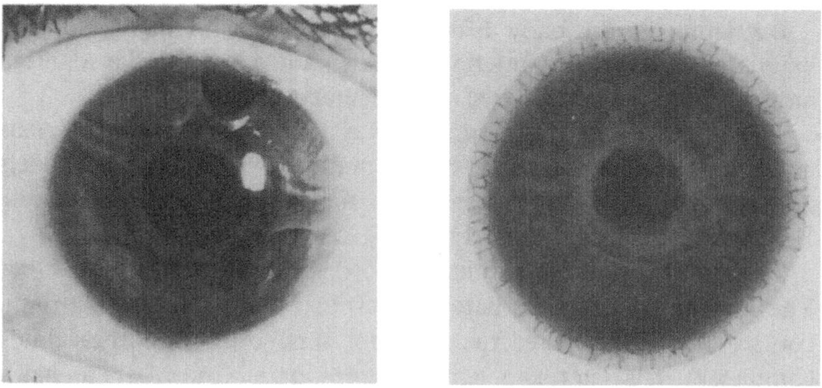

Fig. I-8. — Anterior chamber lenses in situ with three and four haptic legs respectively. (Courtesy C.D. Binkhorst.)

The shape of the Ridley Mark II anterior chamber lens (Fig. I-9) is historically important for its design innovation: it had "flattened feet" and so the tips would be directed more toward the sclera than towards the root of the iris, thus keeping the lens in front but just clear of the iris (Ridley, 1960).

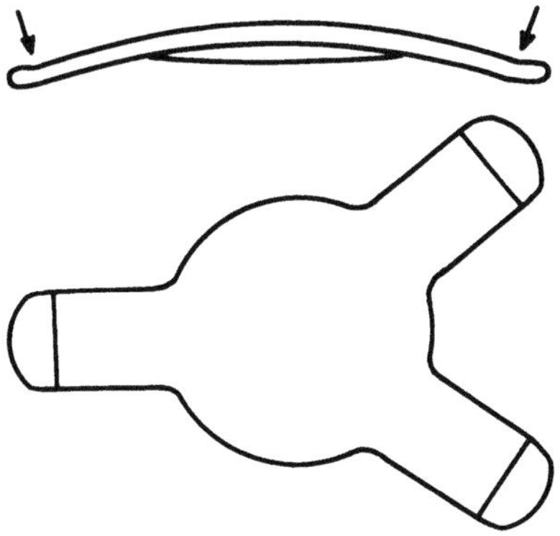

Fig. I-9. — The Ridley Mark II anterior chamber lens with flattened feet.

The first non-rigid or flexible lens was the Dannheim (Fig. I-9), a small lenticulus 5 mm in diameter with 2 wire loops of 1 mm nylon (Supramid). To fit well into the chamber angle, the overall length of this lens had to be somewhat longer than the middle line of the anterior chamber so that it could remain halfway between the iris and the cornea.

J. Barraquer (Fig. I-10) modified this lens by opening out the loops. Very few of these lenses were ever used. In the late seventies this design reappeared (Shearing lens), but, unlike the Barraquer lens, it is used as a posterior chamber lens.

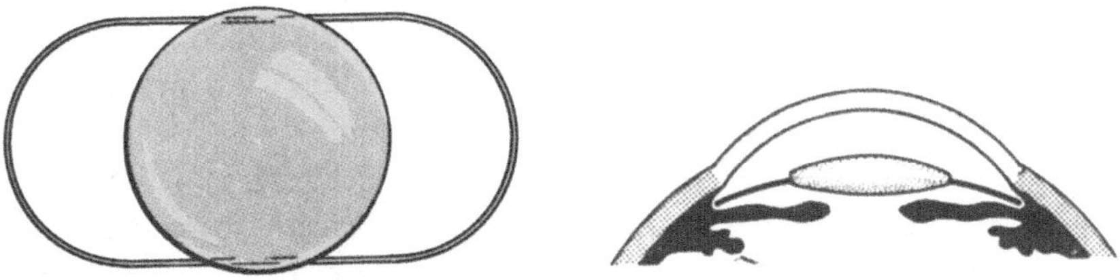

Fig. I-10. — A lens with flexible supports designed by H. Dannheim.

The Boberg-Ans model is another interesting lens. Its inferior leg was flexible, which allowed a certain tolerance in the length.

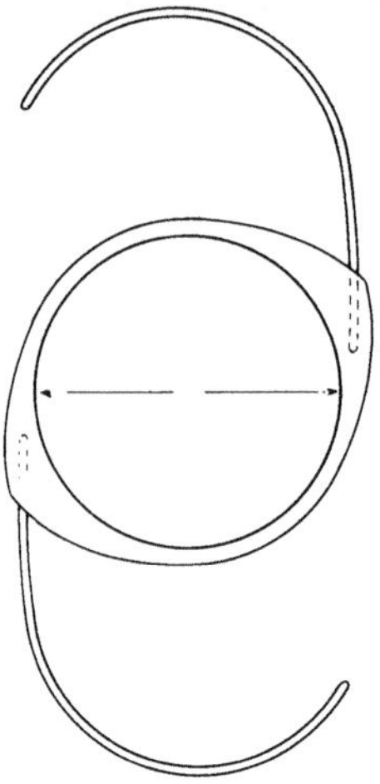

Fig. I-11. — J. Barraquer's lens with flexible supports.

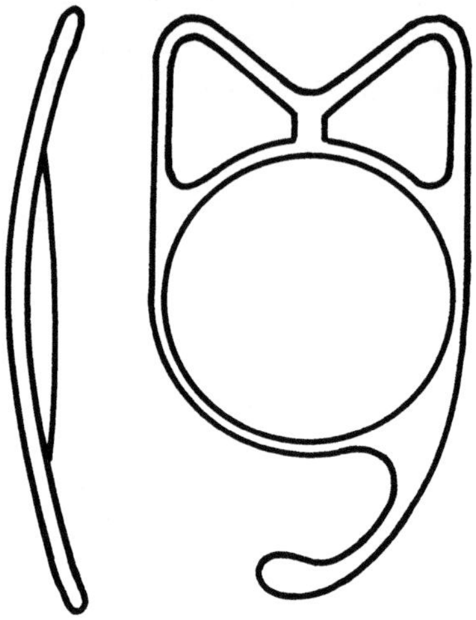

Fig. I-12. — The Boberg-Ans lens.

Polymethylmethacrylate was always the preferred raw material. Zeiss Jena did make a few models out of silicate glass under the direction of K. Emmrich (1958). We have not been able to discover the design of these lenses.

H.R. Ridley (1960) summarized what he considered to be the advantages of the anterior chamber lenses over the posterior chamber lenses:

1. The anterior chamber lenses could be inserted after modern intracapsular cataract extraction.
2. Their exact positioning was felt to be easier.
3. They could be implanted in aphakic eyes in a secondary procedure, so the implantation could be delayed until the eye had completely recovered from the extraction. This made it also possible to calculate the power of the artificial lens very precisely on the basis of the aphakic spectacle correction.
4. After previous extracapsular extraction, the incision of the posterior capsule membrane was not a major problem since there was enough clearance between the optical portion of the pseudophakos and the posterior capsule.

5. Posterior luxation of the lens into the vitreous was virtually impossible.
6. If the lens had to be removed for one reason or another, taking it out of the anterior chamber was relatively simple.

The most important disadvantage with rigid anterior chamber lenses, as Ridley also observed, was the danger it constituted for the corneal endothelium and the other delicate structures of the eye, which are very sensitive to pressure or contact. Thus the major task for this lens was to achieve maximal stability with minimal pressure on the surrounding ocular structures, so one of the common peroperative problems was estimating the exact overall lens diameter required. A lens that was too short would move around inside the eye, twisting and turning on its axis and creating problems that were often complicated by endothelial corneal dystrophy. And a lens that was too long would distort the globe and damage the angle structures (Ashton and Choyce 1959, Ashton and Boberg Ans 1961).

To resolve these problems, haptics with varying degrees of flexibility were proposed. However, as Ridley remarked, "if truly flexible they cannot be as stable as a well-fitted rigid implant and to achieve adequate fixation, the flexible haptic must press into the anterior chamber angle" (H. Ridley, 1960, p. 709).

For some 10 years, the anterior chamber lenses were popular in Europe, but none of them succeeded in giving good long-term results. The major complication was the late development of endothelial corneal dystrophy, which led to almost complete abandonment of this fixating principle in the early sixties.

Of the 9 eyes in which A. Baron implanted his own original models in 1952 and 1953, 4 corneas decompensated definitively (Baron, 1957). These experiments, fortunately, were conducted in eyes that were already functionally lost.

B. Strampelli (1958) of Italy began to implant his rigid anterior chamber lens in 1953. After a period of quiescence, 2/3 of the eyes developed bullous keratopathy within 5 years. This was due to late necrosis of the endothelium starting in the periphery because of compression of the haptic support of the lens. To eliminate this type of contact dystrophy, Strampelli tried several modification, the best known of which is the anterior chamber implant with external fixation (Fig. I-13). It has a 5 mm optic portion with tiny threads (0.12 mm nylon) at the top and bottom that were buried in the sclera under a conjunctival flap.

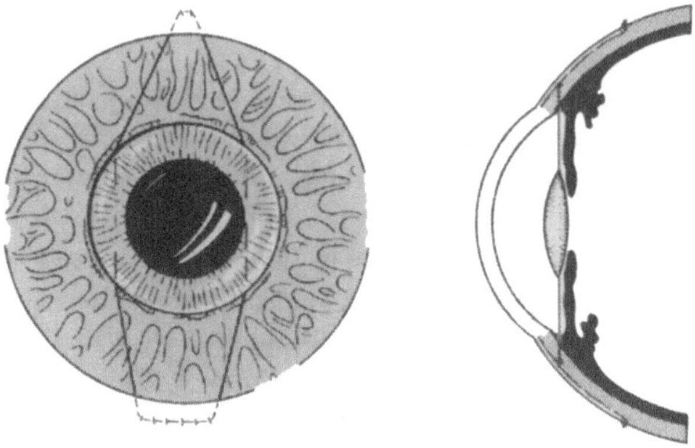

Fig. I-13. — B. Strampelli's anterior chamber lens with external fixation.

In Stuttgart, Germany, H. Dannheim failed to achieve good long-term results with his flexible lens. Between 1955 to 1958 he had implanted 29 such lenses and the results were initially promising. The results of the first cases were published in 1955. In addition to those inserted by Dannheim himself, other surgeons implanted 604 of the Dannheim lenses. Unfortunately, some of the nylon loops dissolved in the angle, which often resulted in glaucoma and corneal dystrophy (see Fig. I-14).

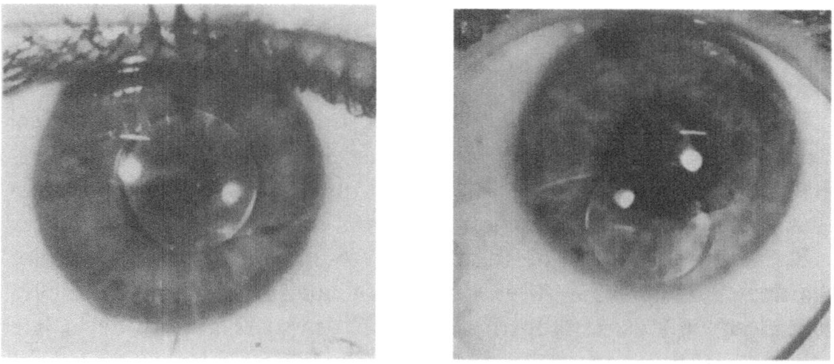

Fig. I-14. — Dannheim lens in situ (left) and dislocated Dannheim lens due to failure of the nylon loops (right). (Courtesy C.D. Binkhorst.)

In 1962, Dannheim mentioned that 5% of 650 of his lenses were "incompatible", with endothelial corneal dystrophy being the most common cause (Nordlohne, 1975). H. Dannheim, Jr. (1979) confirmed these clinical observations.

J. Barraquer also failed to achieve good long-term results with various anterior chamber lenses. In 1959, he reported on 411 cases: 342 Strampelli, 60 Dannheim, and 9 of his own design. This series contained more phakic myopic eyes (239) than aphakic eyes, which means that Barraquer used lens implantation to correct myopia in more than half of his cases. The complication rate with these phakic cases was higher, and, as time went on, the incidence of endothelial corneal dystrophy increased and more and more of the lenses had to be removed.

Barraquer gave the following results (Nordlohne, 1975):

1956	100 cases	No E.C.D.	No implants removed
1959	411 cases	9 E.C.D.	19 implants removed
1961	493 cases	30 E.C.D.	55 implants removed
1970	493 cases	?	±250 implants removed

Though it seems that endothelial corneal dystrophy was the principal complication with all these lenses, its exact incidence will never be known. Only a few surgeons published their results and many of these failed to report on the long-term behavior of the eyes. Thus not only can we not even estimate how many anterior chamber lenses were implanted in Europe between 1953 and 1963, but also we do not know how many eyes were lost because of bullous keratopathy and how many lenses had to be removed in the attempt to cure this complication.

Other eye structures in addition to the cornea were also reported to have been damaged. Iritis was observed when the iris rubbed against the posterior surface of a rigid lens, and this could lead to adhesions between the iris and the lens and even to membrane formation in the pupillary aperture (Barraquer, 1960). Hyphemas occurred during the postoperative course, sometimes attributable to traumatic insertion and sometime for no apparent reason. Finally, late changes of the angle due to pressure resulted in localized atrophy (Ashton and Choyce, 1959; Bresnick, 1969). The exact incidence of these complications is unknown.

Several investigators noted that not only the design but also the finish of the rigid angle supported lenses contributed to the complications. J. Barraquer (1959) for example warned against sharp edges, which could damage the iris.

B. Strampelli (1958) drew attention to irregularities on the extremities of haptics of lenses that had to be removed, and considered that tolerance would be better with refined lenses. E. Schreck (1958) also stressed that only lenses with smooth edges should be used. C. D. Binkhorst suggested in 1958 and again in 1977 that the irregularities on the haptics of these lenses could be due to the very active dissolving power of the angle where the feet of the anterior chamber lenses are lodged. R. Drews examined several dozens of the lenses that J. Barraquer had had to remove and found that many of them had poorly finished tips and edges (Drews, personnal communication, 1979).

Although there are relatively few reports on the long-term behavior of eyes containing anterior chamber lenses, we may conclude the following:

1. Over a period of 10 years, at least 2 dozen different lens models were proposed, each type being advocated by the inventor as an improvement that resolved the problems of previous models. Eventually, they all disappeared from the implant scene.
2. Because determination of the exact length was one of the crucial factors in the success of a rigid implant, the lenses with flexible supports of the Dannheim type were considered to be slightly superior. Unfortunately, the loop material (Supramid) did not hold up.
3. Apart from some problems with the iris and the angle structures, the most serious problem was endothelial corneal dystrophy. It was a particular insidious problem since it most often appeared only after a few years, the eye apparently doing well initially.

III. Toward the Modern Implant Lenses

Frustrated by the catastrophically high rates of complications, most eye surgeons abandonned lens implantation in the late fifties. D.P. Choyce, however, continued to pursue the idea of anterior chamber lenses with angle support, while E. Epstein and C.D. Binkhorst turned to the iris diaphragm for the support for an artificial lens.

Already in 1953, E. Epstein from South Africa had inserted a pupil-supported lens after intracapsular extraction. This lens was a modification of the original Ridley lens and resembled a collar stud. The main portion of the optic was situated behind the iris in the posterior chamber with the iris itself fitting into a deep equatorial groove (Fig. I-15).

He tried various modifications of his lens, but finally had to abandon it because of its instability, which led to frequent dislocation. Epstein introduced a new lens, the Maltese Cross lens, in 1959.

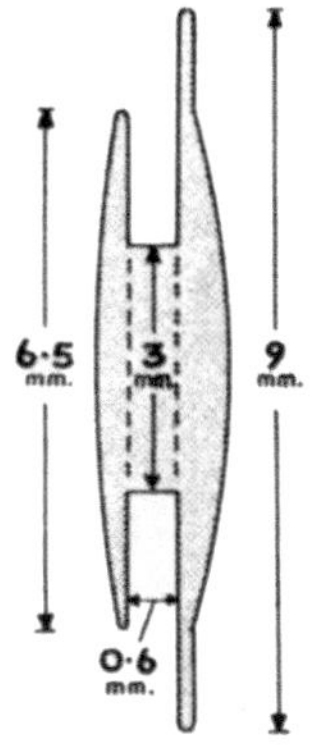

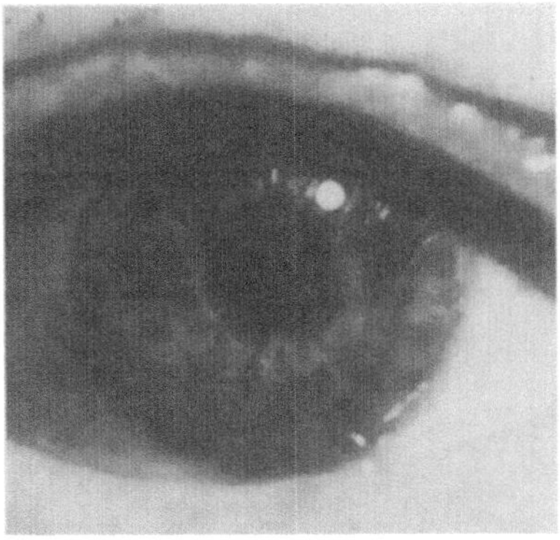

Fig. I-15. — The collar stud lens designed by E. Epstein. The photograph shows such a lens 24 years after implantation (1956-1980). (Courtesy E. Epstein.)

All the supports were at first solid, but he later modified them: 2 solid supports were designed to be placed behind the iris and 2 fenestrated supports in front (Fig. I-16).

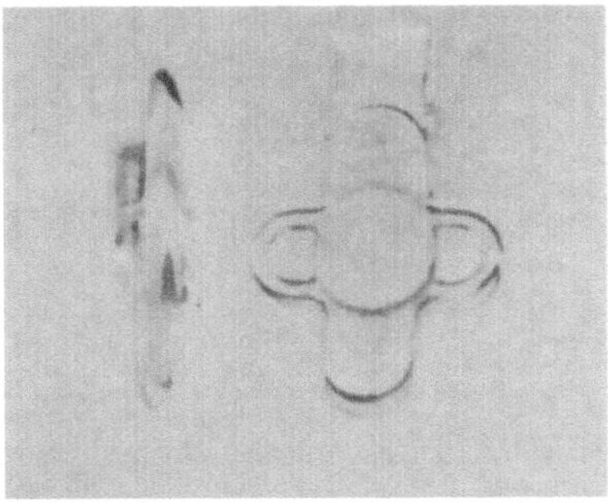

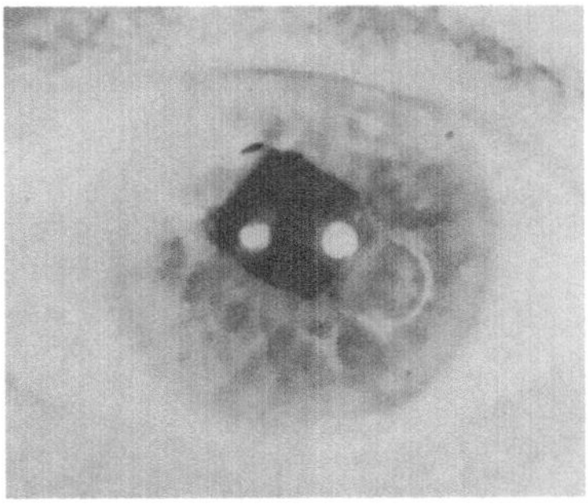

Fig. I-16. — Original Epstein Maltese Cross lens and lens in situ 16 years after implantation (1963-1979). (Courtesy E. Epstein.)

This lens was modified in the U.S.A. by R. Binkhorst and has been manufactured since 1968 by M. Copeland. It is still essentially the Epstein Maltese Cross lens, but the haptics are solid and the entire lens is much thinner and lighter.

Independently of Epstein, C.D. Binkhorst turned to the iris as a lens support in 1958. His intention was to develop a lens that did not have the strong propensity to dislocation as did the Ridley lens or the high risk of late endothelial corneal distrophy that was the case with the angle supported lenses.

The evolution of these lenses will be described in detail in the following chapters.

CHAPTER II

THE CLASSIC MODERN LENSES

I. Design and Fixating Principles of the Classic Lens Models

Intraocular lenses may be categorized in three groups on the basis of their fixating principles:

A. Iris supported lenses.

The Iris clip lens
The Copeland lens
The Medallion lens
The Sputnik lens
The Platinum clip lens

B. Iridocapsular and capsular supported lenses.

The Iridocapsular lens
The Platinum clip lens

C. Angle supported lenses.

The Choyce Mark VIII lens

A. Iris Supported Lenses

In this category, the support is provided by the iris so that such lenses can be implanted in conjunction with both intracapsular and extracapsular cataract extraction.

Iris supported lenses are lightweight devices, their weight in aqueous being of the order of a few milligrams. Fixation is accomplished by means of haptic parts that have various degrees of contact with the iris diaphragm and the iris sphincter.

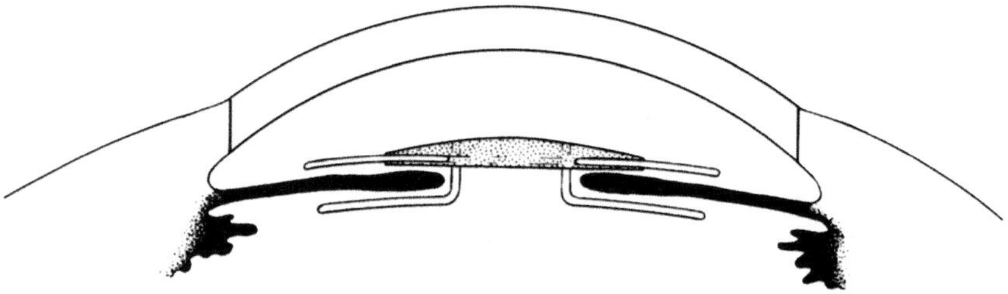

To improve stability and prevent dislocation, some lenses are secured by additional safety devices (sutures or clips).

In view of the anatomy of the iris and its physiological behavior, the iris is not the most suitable structure to provide longstanding fixation. Furthermore, because of pupil motility and iridodonesis, all iris supported lenses are subject to a certain degree of instability. As will be shown, however, satisfactory results can be obtained with such lenses in the short term.

The Iris Clip Lens

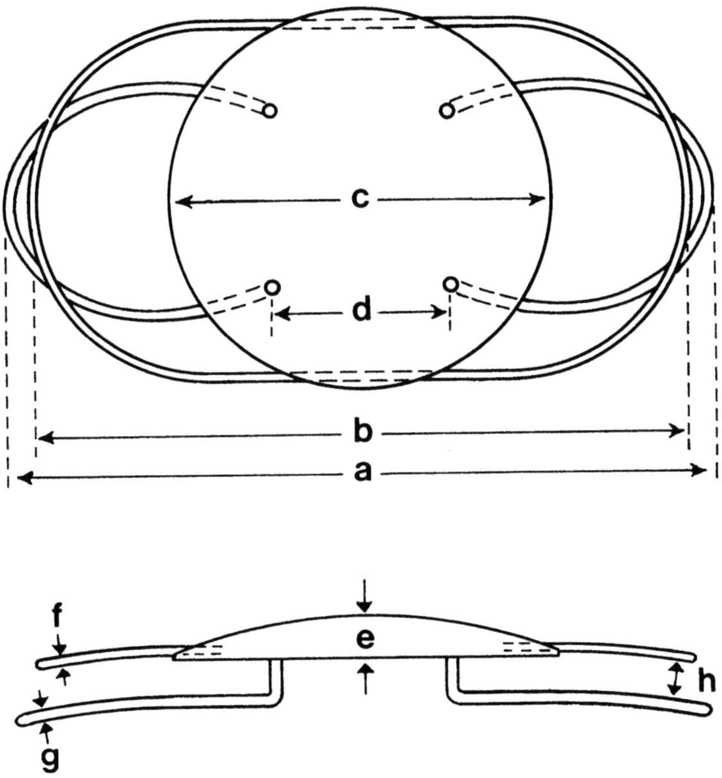

a = 8.5 mm
b = 8 mm
c = 5 mm
d = 2 mm

e = 0.65 mm (standard power)
f = 0.16 mm
g = 0.19 mm
h = 0.50-0.75 mm

Designer: C.D. Binkhorst, The Netherlands.
Manufacturer: K. Morcher, Federal Republic of Germany.
Composition of the optic: Polymethylmethacrylate, Rohm and Haas, Federal Republic of Germany.
Composition of the loops: Polypropylene VIF W.-Germany.
Weight in air: 9.5 mg.
Weight in aqueous: 1.0 mg.
Antiluxating device: Transiridectomy suture.

The Copeland Lens

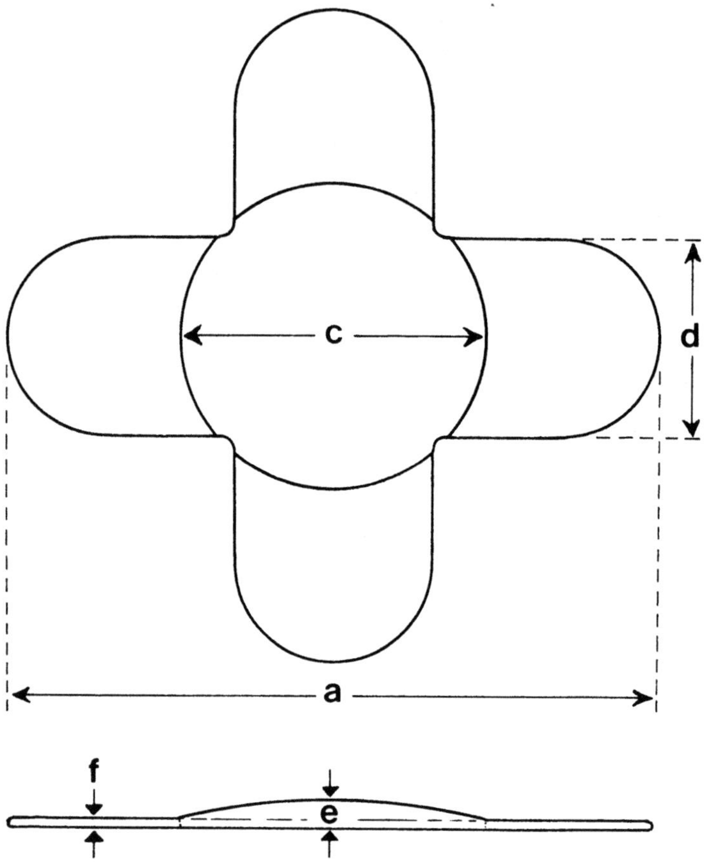

a = 8.9 mm
c = 4 mm
d = 2.3 mm
e = 0.4 mm (standard power)
f = 0.14 mm

Design: Modification of the Epstein lens by R.D. Binkhorst, U.S.A.
Manufacturer: M. Copeland, U.S.A.
Composition: Polymethylmethacrylate, Glassflex®, Dupont, U.S.A.
Weight in air: 8.0 mg.
Weight in aqueous: 1.25 mg.
Antiluxating device: None.

The Medallion Lens

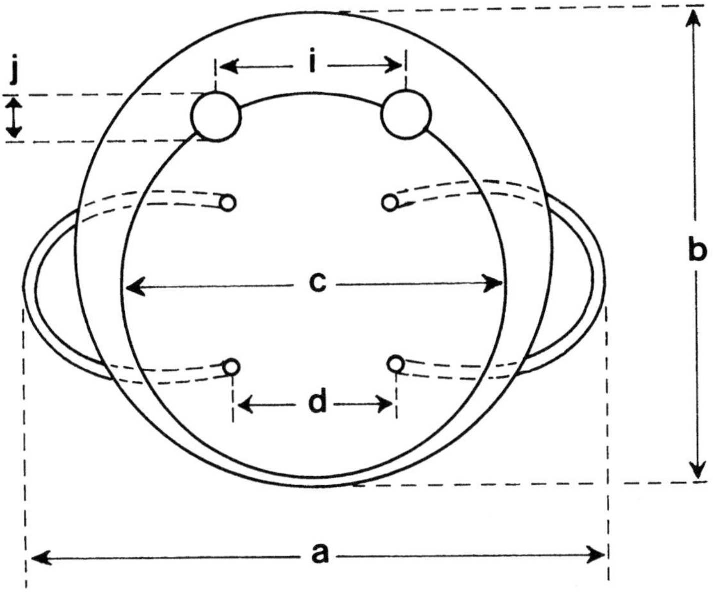

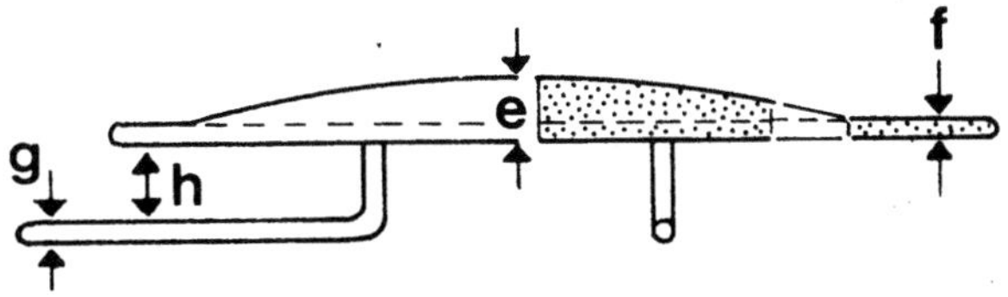

a = 8.0 mm	f = 0.15 mm
b = 6.2 mm	g = 0.2 mm
c = 5.0 mm	h = 0.6 mm
d = 2.0 mm	i = 2.4 mm
e = 0.65 mm (standard power)	j = 0.6 mm

Designer: J. Worst, The Netherlands.
Manufacturer: Medical Workshop, The Netherlands.
Composition of the optic and the haptic rim: Polymethylmethacrylate Perspex, C.Q., Imperial Chemical Industries, Great Britain.
Composition of the loops: Prolene®, Ethicon, Federal Republic of Germany
Weight in air: 10,3 mm
Weight in aqueous: 1,6 mm
Antiluxating device: Suture through the iris stroma.

The Sputnik Lens

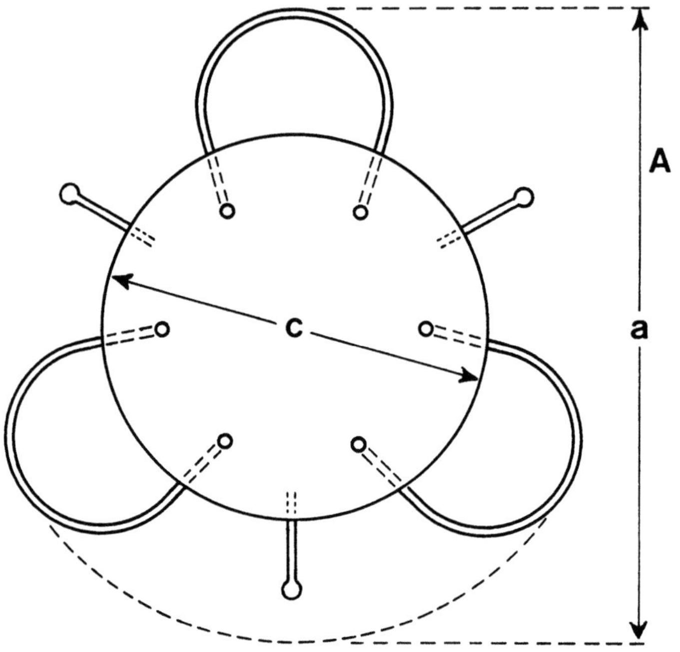

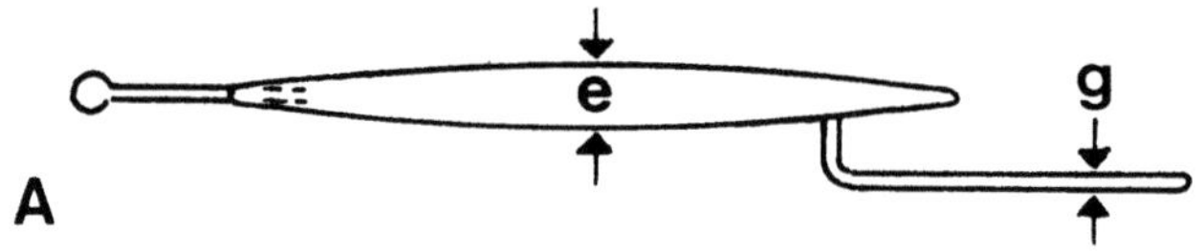

a = 8 mm
b = 5 mm
e = 0.32 mm (standard power)
g = 0.12 mm

Designer: S. Fyodorov, U.S.S.R.
Manufacturer: Medexport, U.S.S.R.
Composition of the optic: Polymethylmethacrylate made in U.S.S.R.
Composition of the loops and struts: Nylon made in U.S.S.R.
Weight in air: 7.5 mg.
Weight in aqueous: 0.5 mg.
Antiluxating device: None.

The Platinum Clip Lens

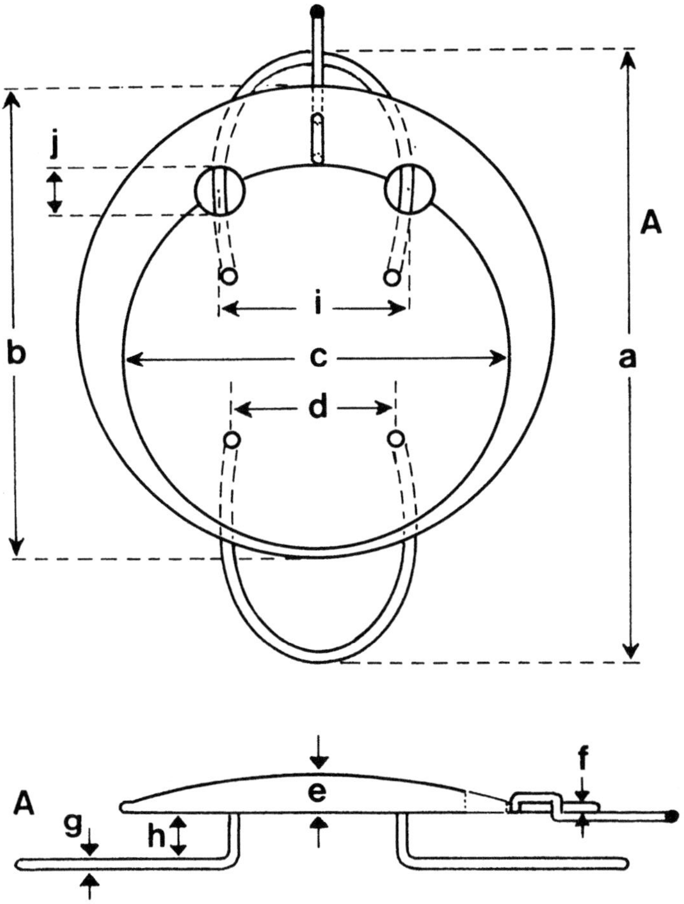

a = 8.9 mm
b = 6.2 mm
c = 5.0 mm
d = 2.0 mm
e = 0.65 mm

f = 0.15 mm
g = 0.2 mm
h = 0.6 mm
i = 2.4 mm
j = 0.6 mm

Designer: J. Worst, The Netherlands.
Manufacturer: Medical Workshop, The Netherlands.
Composition of the optic and the haptic rim: Same as the Medallion lens.
Composition of the loops: Same as the Medallion lens.
Composition of the stave or clip: platinum wire.
Weight in air: 11,1 mg.
Weight in aqueous: 2,0 mg.
Antiluxating device: Platinum clip through a coloboma.

B. Iridocapsular and Capsular Supported Lenses

These lenses rely on capsular support and sometimes on additional iris fixation. Extracapsular cataract extraction is mandatory. In situ, one or more haptics are located between the anterior capsule and the posterior capsule.

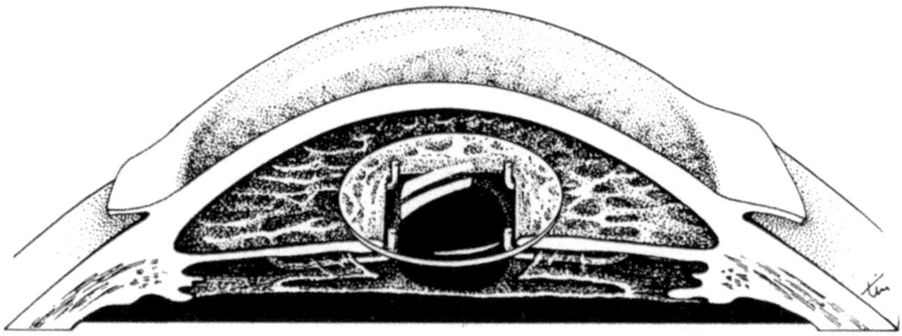

Firm stability is achieved by the development of adhesions between the haptic(s) and the lens capsule. Since the lens capsule is an avascular and insensitive membrane, it constitutes a particularly suitable lens carrier. Typical of the lenses employing this mode of fixation are the Iridocapsular lens and the Platinum Clip lens.

The Iridocapsular Lens

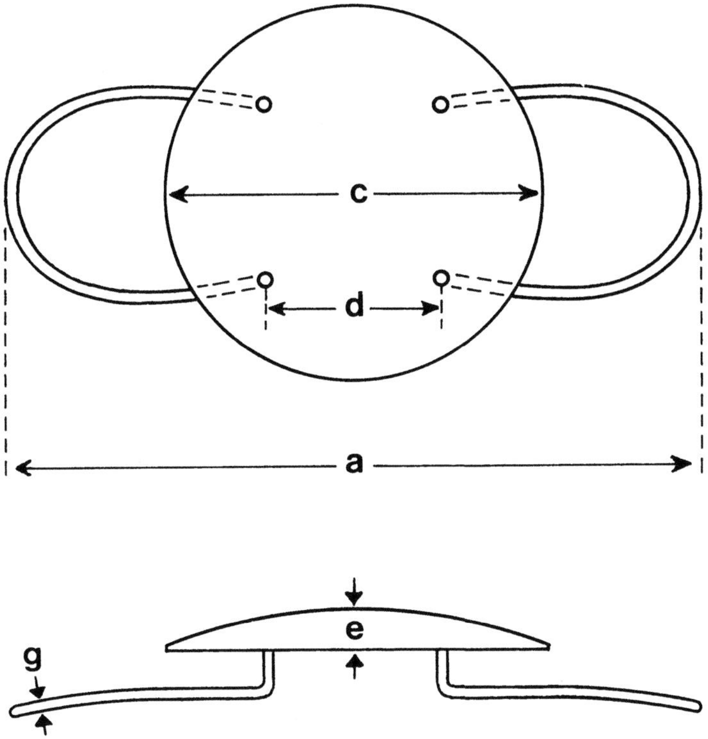

a = 8,5 mm
c = 5 mm
d = 2 mm
e = 0,65 mm (standard power)
g = 0.19 mm

Designer: C.D. Binkhorst, The Netherlands.
Manufacturer: K. Morcher, Federal Republic of Germany.
Composition of the optic portion: Polymethylmethacrylate, Rohm and Haas, Federal Republic of Germany.
Composition of the loops: Polypropylene VIF W -Germany.
Weight in air: 8.0 mg.
Weight in aqueous: 1.5 mg.

The Platinum Clip Lens

Designer: J. Worst, The Netherlands (for full description see p. 23).

C. Angle Supported Lenses

These lenses have tips or footplates that extend into the anterior chamber angle. They can be implanted after intracapsular or extracapsular cataract extraction.

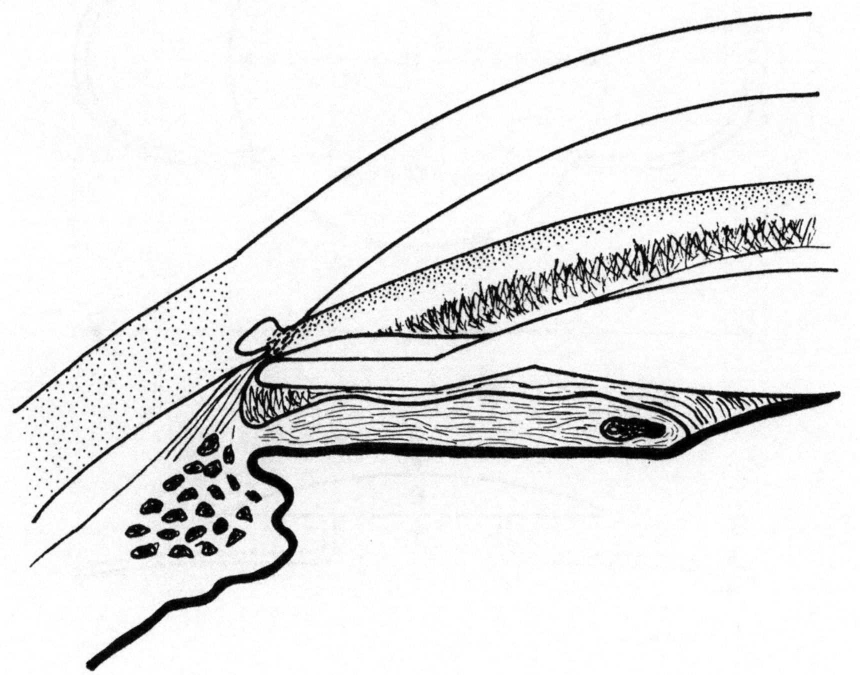

In situ, the tips of the haptic portion are located behind the scleral spur. The stability of these lenses is good: anterior displacement is prevented by the scleral spur, posterior displacement by the iris root, and longitudinal displacement by the scleral wall. An inherent disadvantage of this fixation principle is that the tips of the haptics come in close contact with the delicate tissues of the angle.

The Choyce Mark VIII Lens

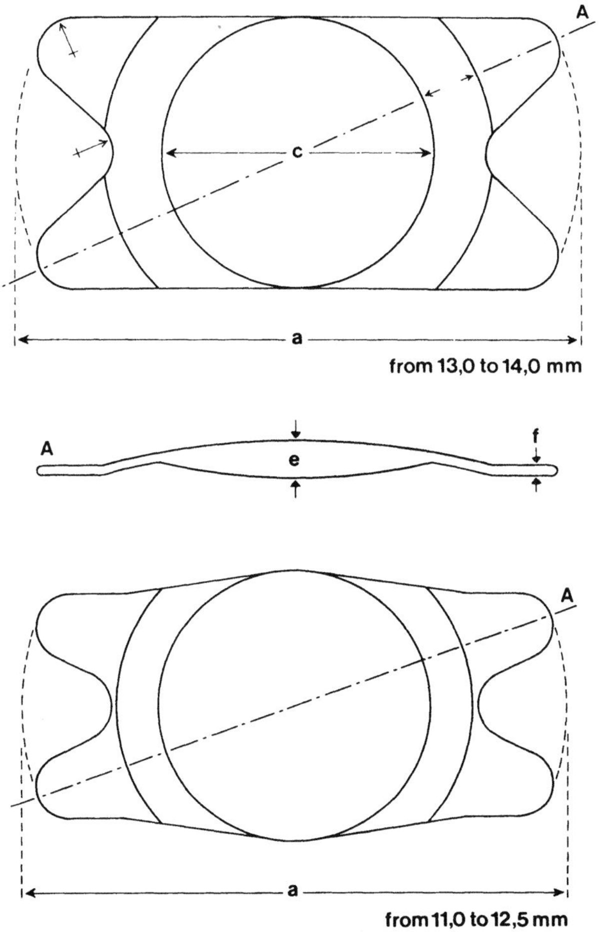

a = 11 mm-14 mm
c = 6 mm
e = 0.63 mm (standard)
f = 0.25 mm

Designer: D.P. Choyce, Great Britain.
Manufacturer: Rayner, Great Britain.
Composition of the optic and the haptic: Polymethylmethacrylate = Perspex C.Q., Imperial Chemical Industries, Great Britain.

II. General Nomenclature

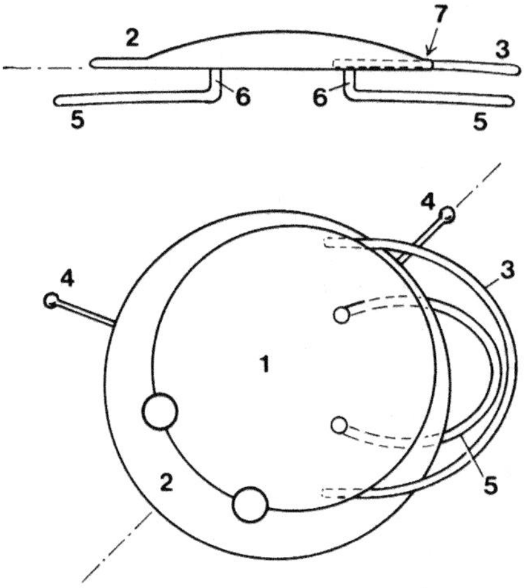

1 = Optic portion
2 = Haptic rim
3 = Loop, anterior loop
4 = Stave, strut, pintle, peg.
5 = Posterior loop
6 = Posterior loop attachment
7 = Lens edge

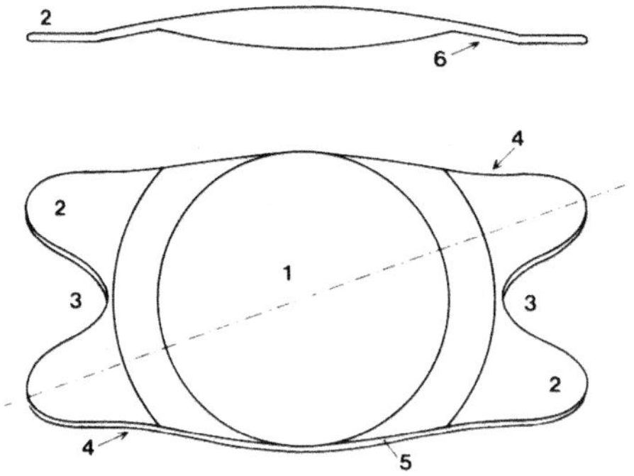

1 = Optic portion
2 = Footplate tip
3 = Recessus, crotch, dovetail
4 = Scallop
5 = Lens edge
6 = Vaulting of the haptic

CHAPTER III

MATERIALS, MANUFACTURE, AND STERILIZATION

§1 BASIC MATERIALS *

The optical component of all currently used modern intraocular implant lenses is made of polymethylmethacrylate (PMMA), the same material that H. Ridley used for his first lens implant in 1948. It is a highly transparent, synthetic material that was already used in sheet form before World War II to replace glass because of its "unbreakability" and because it could be shaped when warm. In Germany it was called "plexiglas" and in England, "perspex". The original Ridley lens remains the prototype for lenses made entirely of PMMA, since it was machined from a solid piece of PMMA. In addition to the optic component, all implants now have a haptic device that is made either of PMMA or another material such as nylon, polypropylene, or even metal. For example:

— Single material lenses with the haptic and optical portions made of PMMA: the Copeland lens, the Choyce lens, and the Pearce lens.
— Two-material lenses: the Iris Clip Lens, the Sputnik Lens, the Medallion Lens and so on. The loops are made of Nylon 6 (Supramid®) Nylon 6.6 and, more recently, from polypropylene (Prolene®).
— Three-material lenses: Among these is the Platinum Clip Lens, which has the optic made from PMMA, the loops from Supramid® or Prolene®, and the stave from platinum.

---

* This section is based on the following:
H.F. Mark, *Encyclopedia of Polymer Science and Technology*, Interscience Publ. Div., J. Wiley and Sons, Inc;
P. Pascal, *Nouveau traité de chimie minérale*, Masson et Co., 1963;
Chemie und Technologie der Kunststoffe, Vol. II, Ac. Verl. Gesell. Geest & Portig K.G., Leipzig, 1963, new edition, R. Houwink and A.J. Staberman;
M.B. Horn, *Acrylic Resins*, New York: Reinhold, Chapman & Hall: London, 1962;
P.G. Stechner et al., *The Merck Index: An Encyclopedia of Chemicals and Drugs*, eigth edition, Rahway, New York: Merck & Co., 1968.

In 1968, J. Worst suggested an intraocular nylon suture as an anti-luxating principle. The materials now used by most surgeons for this are polypropylene and stainless steel thread (30μ).

What may be concluded about the use of all these materials in many thousands of eyes over all these years? The results of the "in vivo clinical experiments" by independent investigators using similar basic materials are concordant, and conclusions may be drawn from these clinical observations.

Polymethylmethacrylate: For 3 decades now, polymethylmethacrylate has proven to be a stable material under certain conditions, that is to say; PMMA used in its clinical quality (CQ) form has not produced any adverse reactions that can be detected by today's investigative methods (slit-lamp biomicroscopy, endothelial cell counts, and anatomopathological examinations). The long-term observations (>20 years), however, are restricted to the lenses made by Rayner (London) and Morcher (Stuttgart). There are no long term in vivo observations exceeding 15 years for lenses made by other manufacturers. The first lenses made by Copeland have now had a 10 year follow-up period, and it may be concluded that the behavior of this material (Lucite, Dupont) is excellent. The first lenses from Medical Workshop are also doing well, the follow-up period now being about 10 years. The polymethylmethacrylate from other sources, mainly in the United States, seems to be behaving similarly, though the follow-up periods are shorter.

Nylon Loops: By the late 1950's, enough clinical evidence had accumulated Supramid® that used as loopmaterial could degrade under certain conditions. For example, the tips of the original Dannheim lenses dissolved after a few years. This problem will be discussed further.

Polypropylene loops: Up till now, the Prolene® material advocated by J. Draeger and R.C. Troutman has not shown any degradation in situ, but there are no long-term ophthalmological observations to guarantee the safety of this material. Indeed, Prolene® loops were used first only in 1976. The stability of this material in vivo, however, has been demonstrated by its widespread use in cardiovascular surgery.

Metal Loops: Metal materials have proven to be stable. However, many eyes with metal loop implants developed chronic uveitis or late iris atrophy, though these complications have been attributed to mechanical properties.

Intraocular Suture Materials: Like the nylon loops of the Dannheim lens, nylon sutures also manifested biodegradibility. The reasons for this are analyzed in the following section. At the present, Prolene® and stainless steel thread seem to be acceptable materials for supplementary fixation of intraocular lenses. The short-term experience with these materials justifies some optimism in their regard.

I. Plastics for Intraocular Use

All the plastic compounds used in lens implantation belong to the same family, which is commonly called the high polymers. This name indicates that these materials are built up of many (*poly*) individual parts (*-mers*) and have a very high molecular weight. Polymethylmethacrylate in sheet form, for example, can have a molecular weight as high as 3 million.

The individual parts are called monomers and are small molecules that make up the structural units that are repeated to form the large molecules. Thus, these polymers are compounds consisting of many individual molecules linked together in a repetitive pattern. For example, polyethylene is a sequence of the monomer CH_2: $CH_2—CH_2—CH_2—CH_2—CH_2—$.

The reaction by which the identical individual molecular units are linked together chemically to form a polymer is called polymerization.

The monomer units need not be the same. Some polymers consist of two or more different monomers. The chemical reaction is then called copolymerization and the end product is called a copolymer.

Figure III-1 shows a single chain of a polymer and a copolymer (linear structure).

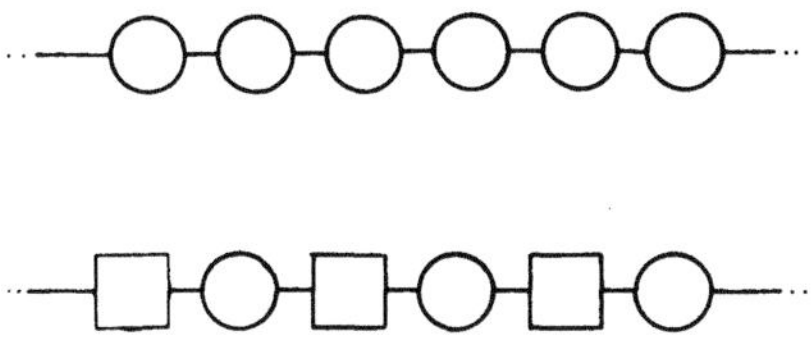

Fig. III-1. — Polymer and copolymer linear chain.

Intermolecular bonds can also be formed between two or more such linear chains, the linkage between the chains being referred to as cross-linkage. The connecting molecule may be of the same kind as in the linear chains or different (Fig. III-2).

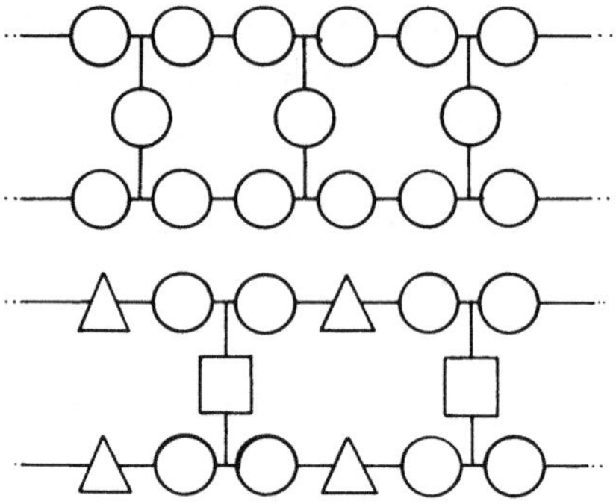

Fig. III-2. — Cross-linked polymer and copolymer.

Linear and cross-linked polymers differ in such qualities as hardness, thermal plasticity, melting point, water absorption, etc. For the manufactoring of most implants linear polymethylmethacrylate is used. The use of cross-linked polymethylmethacrylate is infrequent (Yamanaka 1977).

A. **Polymethylmethacrylate**

Polymethylmethacrylate has a rather simply polymeric structure. Since it is the most commonly used material for the manufacture of implant lenses, we shall present some of the elements of the synthesis process used in producing it.

1. *Synthesis of the Monomer (Methyl Methacrylate)*

The acetone-cyanohydrin process is widely used to synthesize the pure monomer (Horn, 1962). Aceton is caused to react with hydrogen cyanide or sodium cyanide in the presence of potassium hydroxide to yield acetone-cyanohydrin.

$$CH_3{-}CO{-}CH_3 + HCN \rightarrow CH_3{-}\underset{\displaystyle CN}{\overset{\displaystyle OH}{\underset{|}{\overset{|}{C}}}}{-}CH_3$$

The acetone-cyanohydrin is caused to react further with sulphuric acid. With heat, crude methacrylamide sulphate is produced:

$$CH_3{-}\underset{\displaystyle CN}{\overset{\displaystyle OH}{\underset{|}{\overset{|}{C}}}}{-}CH_3 + H_2SO_4 \xrightarrow{125°C} CH_2{=}\underset{\displaystyle CH_3}{\underset{|}{C}}{-}\underset{\displaystyle NH_2 \cdot H_2SO_4}{\underset{|}{C}}{=}O$$

This is caused to react with methanol and water to yield methylmethacrylate and ammonium bisulphate.

$$CH_2{=}\underset{\displaystyle CH_3}{\underset{|}{C}}{-}\underset{\displaystyle NH_2\cdot H_2SO_4}{\underset{|}{C}}{=}O \quad + CH_3OH + H_2O \xrightarrow[90^\circ C]{H_2SO_4}$$

$$CH_2{=}\underset{\displaystyle CH_3}{\underset{|}{C}}{-}COOH + NH_4\ HSO_4$$

The purification of the liquid monomer requires a number of steps:

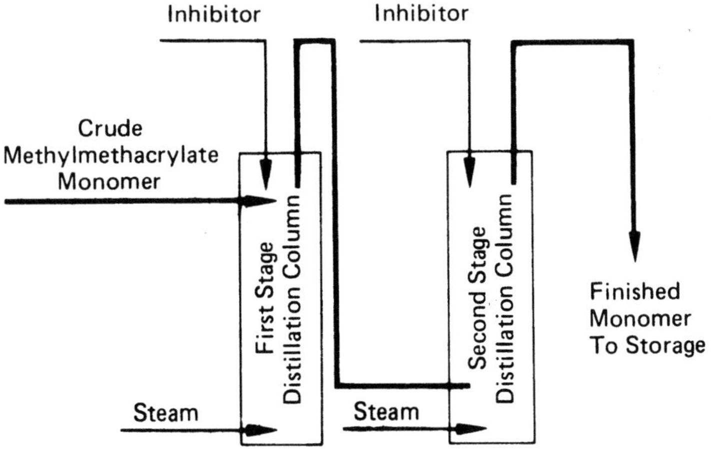

Fig. III-3. — Steps in obtaining a purified monomer. (From E.H. Bekstein, *Am. Intraocular Implant Soc. J.*, *3*: 126, 1977.)

This is a significant stage in the production of the final product since impurities can easily be removed from the monomer by distillation that would be difficult to remove from the finished polymer. This process is sometimes repeated several times in order to "clear the product" as much as possible (Beckstein, 1977).

Because the monomer has a tendency to start uncontrolled polymerization at any time, an inhibitor such as 0.1% hydroquinone is added to allow storage. This substance is washed out at the time of polymerization.

2. *Polymerization*

By the addition of benzoyl peroxide as a catalyst, the double central carbon bond is broken and the separated molecules of methylmethacrylate unite to form the polymethylmethacrylate polymer.

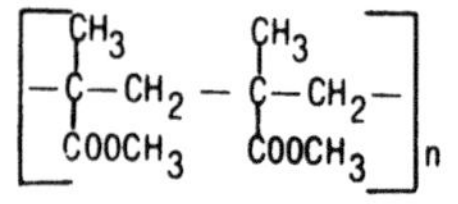

Fig. III-4. — Structural formula of polymethylmethacrylate.

Another popular catalist is a—a′ azo diisobutyronitrile. Unlike benzoyl-peroxide, it has no bleaching action, which makes it more suitable for the production of colored PMMA.

Once polymerization has been started, it tends to continue at an increasing rate because heat in generated. Indeed, the heat of polymerization of methylmethacrylate is around 12 kilocalories per mole, so special measures have to be taken to disperse it.

Depending on the polymerization method used, the end product will be a solid (sheets, rods, pearls, or pellets) or a solution from which sheets or fibers can be made. Also depending on the synthesis method, various residual substances may remain in the polymethylmethacrylate that can eventually migrate from the finished product

TABLE III-1. — *Polymethylmethacrylate Purity*

Polymer Purity		*Rohm & Haas Plexiglas Molded Lenses*	*I.C.I. Perspex CQ Sheet*
Polymer purity		99.6048%	94.27%
Refractive index		1.495	1.492
Peroxide catalyst		0.0013	0.0076
Alcohols		0.0023	4.86 (T-Butyl)
Inhibitor		0.0019	0.0019
U.V. Stabilizer		0.0050	0.0001
Monomer		0.00001	0.0001
Methacrylic acid		0.0047	0.0005
Carboxylic acid		0.38	0.83
Inorganic residue		0.001	0.001
Metals	Fe	0.001	0.001
	Mg	0.0001	0.001
	Al	0.0001	Not detected
	Cu	Not detected	0.001
Others		Not detected	Not detected

such as residual monomers, low molecular weight polymeric molecules, initiators, plasticizers, stabilizers, and other processing agents.

Because of the special quality demanded in the polymeric materials intended for implant lenses, manufacturers maintain rigorous quality controls.

Typical results of quantitative and qualitative tests on polymethylmethacrylate manufactured by two companies are given on Table III-1.

The question then arises about the extent to which the fashioning of the intraocular lens can cause the polymethylmethacrylate to deteriorate. Indeed, molding, heating, lathing, drilling, and other manipulations may be suspected of generating toxic agents. According, to Galin et al. (1977), the most important effect would be an increase in the content of monomers, which are believed to have a deleterious effect on the anterior segment. These authors report the monomer levels in the range of 2% are not toxic to rabbit kidney cell cultures on a short-term basis, and that all the commercially available lenses they examined had monomer levels well below this level. Table III-2 is illustrative in this regard.

TABLE III-2. — *Percentages of Free Monomers in 4 Different Intraocular Lenses from Various Origins as Determined by Gas Chromatography Using Flame Ionization Detectors.*
The lenses were dissolved in chromatographic grade acetone, and standardization was with pure methylmethacrylate monomer. (The analysis was carried out by Analytical Research Laboratories, California, 1974.)

	% of Free Monomers by Weight
Sample A	0.072 ± 0.003
B	0.106 ± 0.003
C	0.081 = 0.002
D	0.044 ± 0.002

The basic properties of polymethylmethacrylate are given on Table III-3. The physical and mechanical properties of Perspex CQ are substantially the same as those of standard polymethylmethacrylate. In optical performance, however, there is a significant difference between Perspex CQ and the standard product: Perspex CQ does not contain any ultraviolet absorbers. The spectral transmission curve for Perspex compared with that of standard Perspex is shown on Figure III-5.

TABLE III-3. — *The Basic Properties of Polymethylmethacrylate*

Specific gravity	1.18-1.19
Refractive index	1.49-1.50
Tensile strength	7000-9000
Hardness	M80 to M100
Heat distribution temperature	160 °C-191 °C
Polymerization shrinkage volume	6%
Water absorption (3 mm spec)	0.2%-0.5% in 24 hours
Effects of acids	Slowly attacked by oxidizing acids Attacked by organic acids
Effects of alkalies	None
Effects of organic solvents	Soluble in ketones, esters, aromatic hydrocarbons, halogenated hydrocarbons
Processing	Excellent machining properties, a rigid, hard material
Clarity	92% light transmission

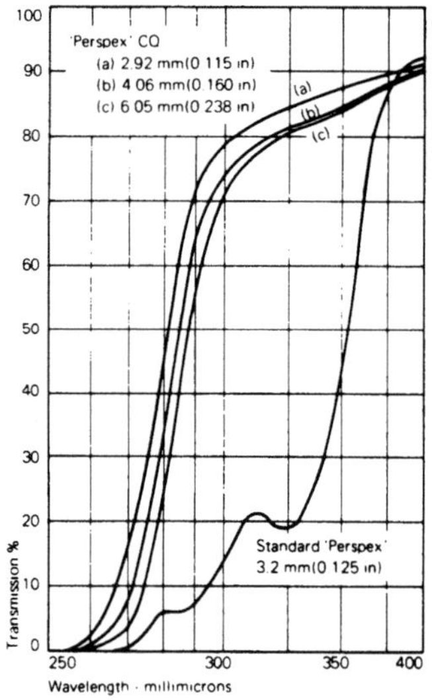

Fig. III-5. — Spectral transmission curves for Perspex CQ and standard quality Perspex (From ICI, Technical Data Sheet PX, TD 232.)

B. Polyamides or Nylons

Polyamides are condensation products that contain recurring amide groups as integral parts of the main polymer chains. Numerous combinations of diacids, diamines, and animo acids have been produced, and copolymers containing various proportions of two or more diacids, diamines, and amino acids have been prepared. Theoretically, it is possible to synthesize any number of varieties of these polyamides. In addition to the linear polymers, cross-linked and network polymers can be obtained. In practice, however, only a few—primarily linear polyamides—have the physical and chemical properties and are able to be produced cheaply enough to make them suitable for commercial exploitation.

Nylon (a generic name for polyamides) is used chiefly in the production of synthetic fibers, the market for which has been growing vigorously since the appearance of Nylon 6/6 in the United States in 1938 and of Nylon 6 in Germany in 1941-1942. These two substances still account for about 50% of the market for fully synthetic fibers. In implant surgery, polyamide is used for lens loops and sutures. The advantages of nylon over natural and other synthetic fibers are its relatively low specific gravity, high tensile strength, and great durability. Like polymethylmethacrylate, nylon was used extensively in the conduct of World War II.

The nomenclature of the nylons is based on the number of carbon atoms in the repeating units of the polyamide. For us, only Nylon 6 and Nylon 6/6 are of interest.

TABLE III-4. — *Trade Names and Basic Products Used in Ophthalmology (Kronenthal 1977 — Am. Intraocular Implant Soc. J. 1977, p.223)*

Suture	*Manufacturer*	*Composition*	*Construction*
Ethilon®	Ethicon	6.0 ↑ Nylon 6 7.0 ↓ Nylon 6/6	A
Supramid®	Kunststofwerk Alfred Huber	6.0 ↓ Nylon 6	A
		5.0 ↑ Nylon 6	B
Perlon®	Perlon trademark Assoc.	Nylon 6	A
Dermalon®	Davis and Geck	Nylon 6/6	A

A = monofilament.
B = Sheet-covered multifilament.

1. *Nylon 6* — (Supramid®)

This polymer contains 6 carbon atoms of ε-caprolactane in its repeating unit and an amide linkage formed by the ring opening (—C—NH—) during polymerization

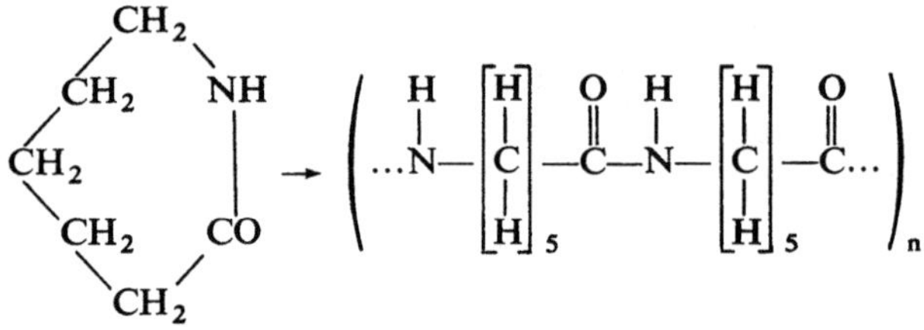

ε-caprolactane Nylon 6 (Supramid)

2. *Nylon 6/6*

Nylon 6/6 is manufactured by causing equal amounts of hexamethylene-diamine and adipic acid to react and produce a high molecular weight polymer.

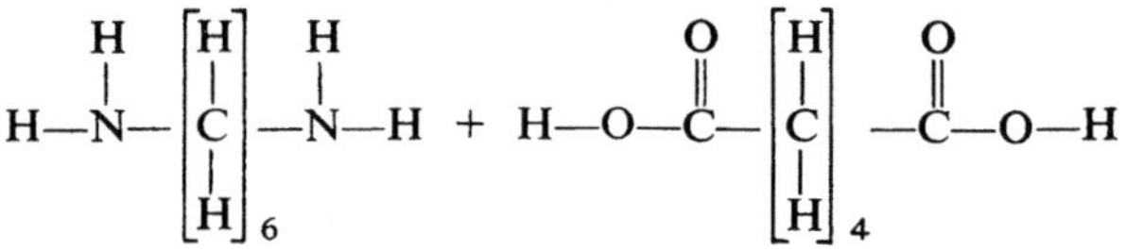

Hexamethylenediamine Adipic acid

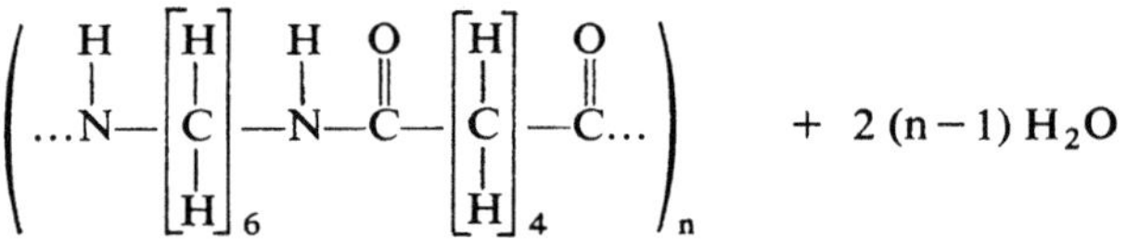

Nylon 66

As shown, in the reaction water is eliminated between the carboxyl and the amino functions in the monomers, which results in the formation of long molecular chains held together by amide linkages (—C—NH—).

Note: In both types of nylon, hydrolysis of the amide linkages (C—NH) results in degradation of the material. In the case of Nylon 6/6, hydrolysis yields adipic acid and hexamethylene diamine. When Nylon 6 degrades by hydrolysis, aminocaproic acid or its metabolic products are formed. It must be noted that the amide linkage encountered in these nylons is similar to that which binds the amino acids together in protein chains.

A detailed treatment of the synthesis of these two nylons is beyond the scope of our study, as is the manufacture of the suture material, a rather complex procedure that is of little interest to the average ophthalmologist. Polyamide fibers were initially made by forcing molten polymers through a hypodermic needle, but more sophisticated technologies soon developed. As the filaments cool after passing through the spinnerette, they are repeatedly stretched, which tends to align the chain-like nylon molecules within the filament. The degree and nature of this alignment along with the length and composition of the polymer chains determine the physical properties.

3. *Properties of Polyamides*

Polyamides are generally resistant to chemicals and solvents, and they are not normally affected by exposure to pure water at low temperatures. The plasticizing action of water at high temperatures for extended periods of time causes the nylon to degrade because of hydrolysis of the amide groups. Hot water also contains dissolved oxygen, which causes degradation in time. Polyamides are inert to most inorganic chemicals including sulfur dioxide and liquid ammonia, but are attacked by oxidizing agents such as chlorine and hydrogen peroxide. Inert solutions of inorganic salts are not harmful, although the water will have some plasticizing effect. Concentrated mineral acids attack polyamide at room temperature, but the effect of dilute acids is minimal.

Resistance to alkalies is good, even at elevated temperatures. Alkyl halides, mercaptans, esters, glycols, organic solvents, oils, fuels, and aldehydes (except formaldehyde) have little or no effect on polyamides.

Phenols, cresols, and similar chemicals dissolve all the nylons. Although none of these substances are present in the eye, delayed degradation of loops and suture material may be caused by improper manufacturing or sterilization. Deterioration in vivo may also occur because of "biological digestion processes".

4. *Nylon Degradation in vivo*

It is well-known that nylon sutures deteriorate in vivo. This phenomenon is commonly observed in ophthalmic practice. All corneoscleral sutures and even pure corneal sutures show a marked thinning after some years or even months. Similar observations in other fields of medicine were made in human beings, dogs, rabbits, etc.

(Dettinger, 1957; Harrison and Adler, 1956; Moloney, 1958; Catchpole, 1958; Postlethwait, 1970, and so on).

In implant surgery, the clinical findings on this subject are controversial. Some nylon implant loops were digested while others were not; some nylon sutures used intraocularly were broken off, others remained intact.

Digestion of the *Supramid loops* (Nylon 6) in Dannheim lenses has been noted at the loop tips. This was seen particularly in those cases where some reactive tissue formation was overlying or embedding the tips (Binkhorst, personal communication).

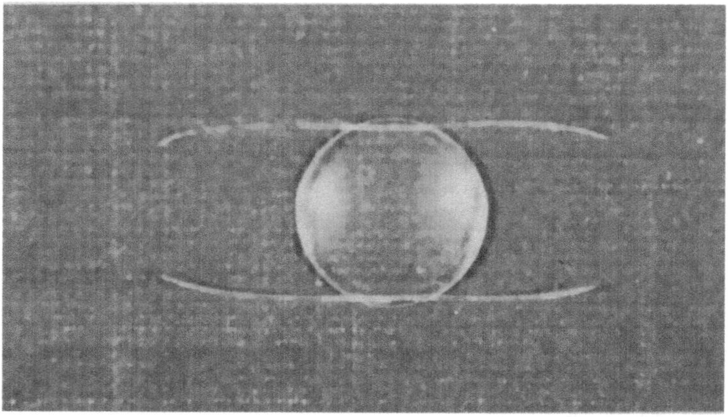

Fig. III-6. — Supramid loops of a Dannheim lens showing dissolved tips. (Courtesy C.D. Binkhorst.)

Marked thinning of this material was observed once by P. Leonard in 1968 with an Iris Clip lens that was embedded for 2 years in vacularized scar tissue and that had to be removed because it was touching the cornea.

But none of the anterior Supramid loops of the Iris Clip lenses used by C.D. Binkhorst and others show changes in reflex, thickness, or transparency when examined in situ with the slit lamp, even after 20 years.

Using electron microscopy, B. Drews et al. (1978) noted surface changes of supramid loop material that was not limited to any one brand of lens, but was frequently seen whenever this material was examined after removal from inflammed eyes.

In 1972, J. Worst (1977) noted that some *iris sutures* that were used to steady certain lens models had failed. Others have reported

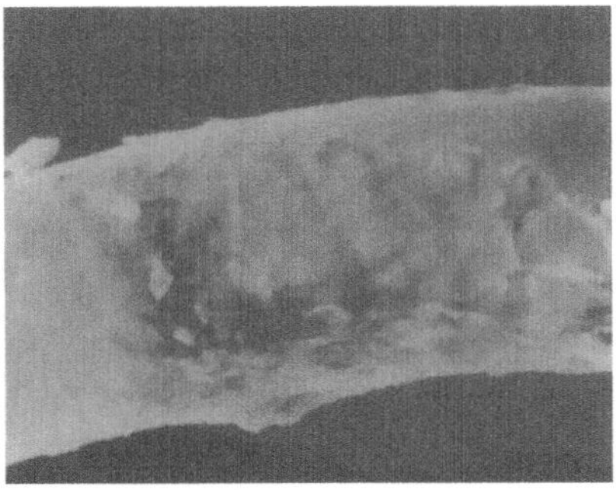

Fig. III-7. — Scanning electron micrograph of a Supramid loop of a medallion lens showing surface biodegradation of the Supramid. This lens had been in place for 2 years and had been associated with chronic inflammation. Note that these changes, although dramatic, do not threaten the integrity of the loops. (Courtesy R. Drews.)

similar observations (Blanksma and Siertsema, 1977; Fechner, 1977; Drews, 1978, and Mawas; personal communication, 1977).

By contrast, Binkhorst, who began using nylon for the transcoloboma suture of his iris clip lens in 1969, has not observed any failure. No iris tissue was involved in this procedure, however.

According to Dettinger (1957), nylon loses about 15% of its original tensile strength when it is wet. This results from hydration or infusion of water between the polymer chains, which weakens the interchain molecular bonds and thus decreases the strength. Doden and Schmitt (1974) found superficial oblique and horizontal tears in 9.0 Nylon kept in distilled water or a normal saline solution for 125 days. Harnisch and Löschau (1975), using a scanning electron microscope, found that fissures occurred in polyamide 6/6 after continuous flexion. They went on to suggest the possibility that water is absorbed through the fissures in the outer mantel.

B. Drews (1977) commented that in some cases the nylon suture holding the Medallion lens in place may also have been eroded by the lens edge; the cutting effect of the lens edge is aggravated when the nylon thread is under tension. Worst also noted the possibility of degradation being caused by sterilization, for example, by γ-irradiation. This hypothesis was later confirmed by Doden and Schmitt (1975) who found that 9.0 Nylon developed irregularities in thickness when it was beamed. The same unbeamed material was uniform in thickness.

Kronenthal (1977) suggested that the improper use of electron beam sterilization may have a thermal effect on the orientation and crystallinity of the fibers that could lead to increased liability to hydrolysis. He also pointed out, however, that ethylene oxide sterilization (standard cycle) reduces suture strength more than does sterilization by γ-irradiation (2.5 megarads from a cobalt 60 source). Kronenthal stressed that resistance of nylon to degradation is primarily related to the manufacturing process. Indeed, insufficient stretching of the fibers produces sutures that are less resistant to hydrolysis.

The degradation of nylon seems also to be aggravated by the presence of surrounding living tissue. As noted above, the amide linkage in Nylon 6 and Nylon 6/6 is similar to that which binds the amino acids in protein chains. Already in the late fifties, Emmrich (1968) cited Hornhauer to the effect that he could demonstrate the release of ε-aminocaproic acid from Nylon 6 as a result of enzymatic attack. In Emmrich's opinion, this was to be considered significant for the behavior of the Dannheim lenses. Schwertaseck and Dvorak (1970: cited by Kronenthal, 1977, and Blanksma and Siertsema, 1977) pointed out the liability of nylon to enzymatic attack by pepsin and suggested that natural body enzymes, possibly lysozymes, may

a b c d

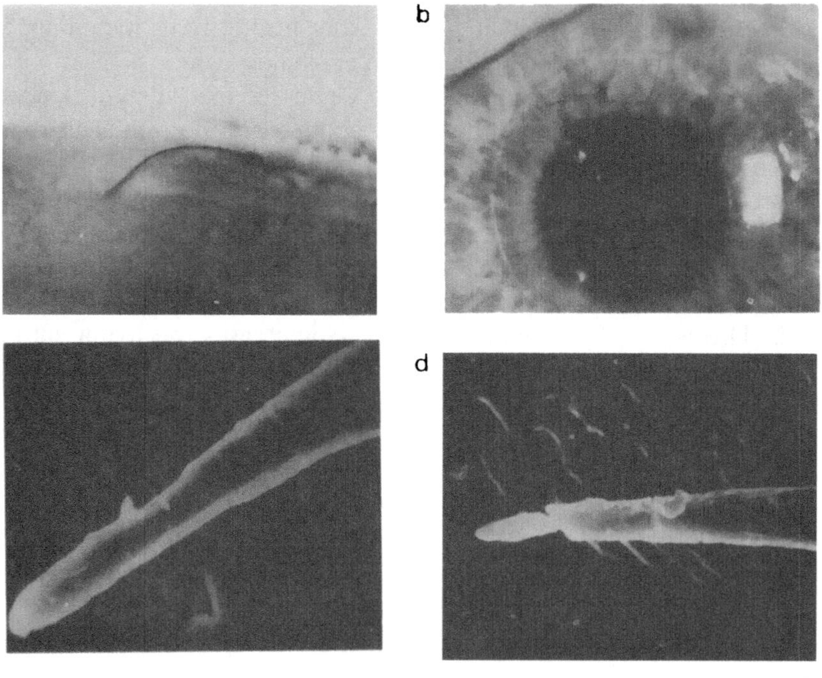

Fig. III-8a. — Broken iris suture in the angle as seen with a gonioscope.

Fig. III-8b. — Broken nylon suture that had supported a medallion lens. This suture broke after $2\frac{1}{2}$ years and no unusual inflammation was present.

Fig. III-8c, d. — The scanning electron micrographs clearly suggest digestion. (Courtesy R. Drews.)

contribute to in vivo degradation of the amide linkages. Harmisch and Löschau (1975) suggested the possibility of enzymatic degradation following mechanical damage such as fissure formation. Dvorak (1975: cited by Kronenthal, 1977) studied the strength and extensibility of nylon, polyester, and acrylic fibers implanted in dogs for periods up to 220 days and concluded that nylon fibers suffered from enzymatic degradation by the second week.

In summary, Nylon 6 and Nylon 6/6 may degrade because of improper sterilization, stress or mechanical aggression, and because of hydrolysis of the amide linkages in vivo. Hydrolysis probably occurs more readily in tissue where the concentration of proteolytic enzymes is significant as is the case for reactive tissue. In normal anterior chamber fluid without inflammatory components, hydrolysis may be minimal.

Nevertheless, there seems to be good reason to avoid the use of nylon in implant surgery, especially when long-term results are desired.

C. **Polypropylene**

Polypropylene suture material became available in the late sixties. It was first used in cardio-vascular surgery because of its long-term stability, a vital factor for cardio-vascular devices such as valves and bypasses.

The chemical structure of polypropylene is:

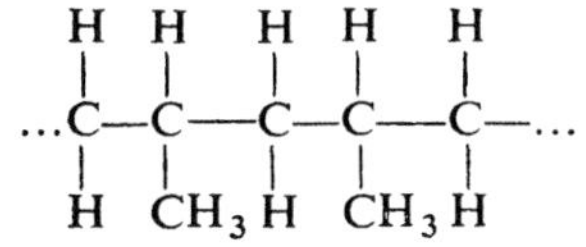

Polypropylene

In "isotactic" polypropylene, all the side-chain methyl groups are sterically similary, i.e., they are located on the same side of the plane of the carbon atom chain. This leads to molecular symmetry and high crystallinity.

There are also two other types of polypropylene that can be synthesized, the syndiotactic and atactic forms. They are of less importance than the "isotactic" polypropylene.

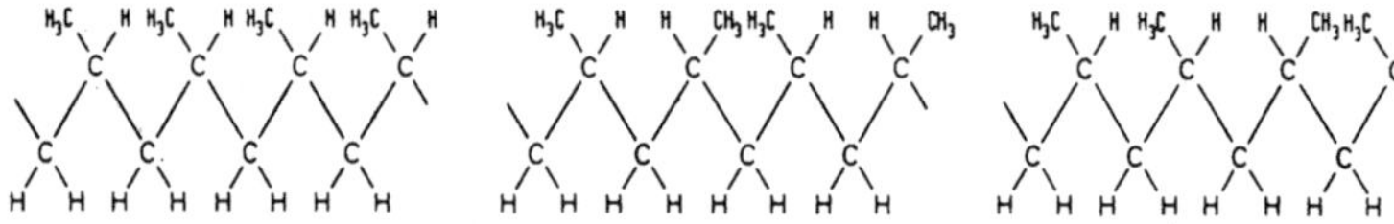

Fig. III-9. — Structural formula of isotactic, syndiotactic, and atactic polypropylene.

The monomer, propylene, is a normal by-product of catalytic or thermal cracking of petroleum in the production of gasoline. It is a liquefiable hydrocarbon gas that boils at $-47\,°C$ at 760 mm Hg. Polymerization grade propylene must be virtually free of impurities that may deactivate the catalyst. Impurities include water, carbon dioxide, carbon monoxide, oxygen, hydrogen, acetylenes, diolefines, and some non-hydrocarbons.

Although the monomer may be polymerized with a wide variety of catalysts, the "Ziegler type" catalyst made it possible to prepare solid, crystalline polypropylene. After the polymerization process, different steps are necessary for purification. In this process, suspended and soluble polymers, residual monomers, active catalyst, and traces of other substances are removed.

Polypropylene has a number of desirable properties that make it a versatile material among the modern thermoplastic polymers. It has high yield strength and rigidity, a high heat distortion temperature, and good surface hardness. It is virtually unaffected by most chemicals at or near the ambiant temperature. Translucent to transparent, it is a hard, rigid material with excellent machining properties. Its specific gravity is less than that of water, 0.90 to 0.92. Its water absorption capacity is very low (0.01 versus 0.4 to 1.50 for Nylon 6/6 and 0.3 to 0.4 for polymethylmethacrylate). It softens at 150 °C and can be steam sterilized.

Advantages of polypropylene over nylon are the absence of hydrolyzable linkages and the long-term exhibition of undiminished tensile strength.

In implant surgery, polypropylene therefore seems to be superior to nylon, although its long-term behavior is still under investigation. So far, the clinical observations are encouraging.

One of the significant negative qualities that must be taken into account is that polypropylene is subject to oxidative degradation. Although it is a saturated hydrocarbon, it responds readily to free-radical oxidation. This process can be initiated by a peroxide or hydroperoxide, by irradiation, or by an ultraviolet source. Normally, this process in inhibited by the incorporation of additives. According to Yamanaka et al. (1979), it is unlikely that ultraviolet rays normally present in the environment would be capable of inducing such an oxidative degradation. E. Svendson et al. (1975) stated that sterilization by γ-irradiation from a cobalt 60 source should not be done with this material, but that β-irradiation from an electron accelerator is innocuous. According to R.L. Kronenthal, Director of Research Ethicon, Inc. (1979), Ethicon has not approved the use of Prolene® suture material for the manufacturing of lens loops because handling and processing polypropylene, particularly by heating, could change, damage, or otherwise affect the quality.

II. The Metals

When C.D. Binkhorst started to use the lens capsule to support his implants, he concluded that the quality of the loops could be improved by making them from an inert metal. Although the specific gravity of metals relative to water exceeds that of nylon many times, the weight of the lens was not the primary concern, since the lens capsule and its suspension system "tolerates" the human lens, which weighs more than 200 mg.

The material used initially for the loops of these iridocapsular lenses by K. Morcher was a platinum-iridium alloy. Later on, other manufacturers used materials such as titanium.

Stainless steel intraocular sutures were introduced by J. Worst in the mid-seventies. He now uses 30μ stainless steel thread for both wound closure and fixation of his Medallion lens to the iris. M.M. Krasnov (1977) reported on the use of a gold alloy for the loops of his "extrapupillary" lenses.

A. **Platinum**

Platinum occurs in its native state alloyed with one or more members of its group (iridium, osmium, palladium, rhodium, and ruthenium). It is a silver-grey, lustrous, malleable, and ductile metal that has a face-centered cubic structure and a density of about 21.45.

Platinum does not react with water or with single mineral acids, but it is attacked by halogens, caustic alkalies, alkali nitrates, and alkali peroxides as well as by arsenates and phosphates in the presence of reducing agents.

Since it is very malleable, it is often alloyed with iridium to give it rigidity.

It is used in thermocouples, resistance thermometers, acid proof containers, electrodes, jewelery, electroplating, and so on. It is also used as a catalyst for oxidation in the manufacture of acetic acid, nitric acid, and sulphuric acid.

B. **Titanium**

Titanium is a dark grey, lustrous metal with an hexagonal structure (below 800 °C). It is brittle when cold, malleable when hot, and ductile when free of oxygen. Its density is about 4.50. It reacts to acid only when heated, and alloys with aluminum, chromium, cobalt, copper, iron, lead, nickel, and tin. It is very resistant to corrosion as it readily forms a protective oxide film on its surface, which is promptly reformed if disrupted. Titanium has a number of industrial applications and was first used in medicine for the fixation of fractures. In implant surgery, titanium wire is used because of its malleability and its lightness.

C. **Stainless Steel**

Stainless steel is an alloy of iron and chromium (20%), nickel (10%), molybdenum, and carbon (0.5 to 0.8%). Contrary to what is generally assumed, stainless steel is subject to corrosion, and, because it contains nickel, it is apt to cause contact dermatitis, though we have yet to see any reports of local reactions to stainless steel used in eye surgery.

Yamanaka (1977) investigated the behavior of platinum-iridium wire and stainless steel wire from the point of view of electrochemistry to evaluate corrosive properties. Polarization curves of the platinum-iridium alloy (75%-25%) did not reveal any corrosion in an N_2-saturated physiologic saline solution and in an air-saturated solution. The polarization curves under the same conditions revealed only limited current density in anodic or cathodic polarization. The cathodic polarization curve for stainless steel was similar to that for platinum-iridium, but the corresponding anodic polarization curve showed small peaks at the limiting current point (flade potentials). According to Yamanaka et al. (1979), the occurrence of flade potentials indicates adsorption of hydroxide ions onto the stainless steel, which means that the ions coat the metal's surface and prevent corrosion (passivation film).

In addition, metal corrosion experimental models in the living body were designed. No significant weight loss was observed after 17 months as long as a single metal was involved. However, as Yamanaka and his colleagues stressed, when metals such as platinum-iridium and stainless steel are used together, the different natural electrode potentials can lead to cell or battery formation. In the experiments, stainless steel combined with platinum-iridium or titanium incurred a fair amount of corrosion that could be measured by weight loss. Therefore, it is well to avoid using stainless steel sutures to fixate a platinum-iridium or titanium loop in the eye.

§ 2 MANUFACTURE

The manufacture of good quality lens implants is a tedious process that requires several steps. Depending on the lens model, the whole lens is made of one piece of material or the parts are made separately and then assembled. Three manufacturing processes are used to shape the lens body out of polymethylmethacrylate: lathe cutting or milling, compression molding, and injection molding. Since the last procedure has yet to be proven safe in the long term, we shall only describe the techniques used by Rayner of Great Britain (milling) and by Morcher of Germany (compression molding).

A. **Rayner's Technique for Manufactoring the Choyce Lens**

The following information provided by Rayner of London gives us an example of how a lens is manufactured from one single material.

The solid portion of all Rayner lenses is made only from polymethylmethacrylate supplied in as pure a form as possible by Imperial Chemical Industries, Ltd., of England and known as Perspex CQ (clinical quality).

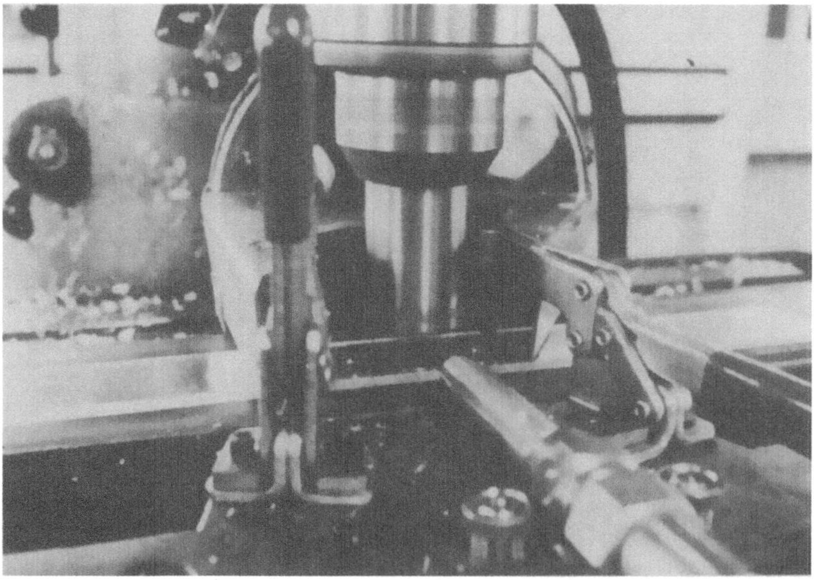

Fig. III-10. — Milling of a perspex sheet. (Courtesy Rayner, London.)

The Perspex is supplied in sheets and is cut into strips about 50 cm long and 2.5 cm wide. From these strips are milled a series of round disks 20 mm in diameter with a central optic of the correct size and curvature and a curved haptic with a flat peripheral band. The disks are removed from the strip, and then polished to remove all cutting marks. A scratch and blemish free blank is produced. After cleaning, these blanks are pressed between polished steel dies to ensure that the lenses are all identical as regards power and to remove any slight polishing irregularities such as the wave formation often found on spectacle lenses. The presses work at controlled low temperatures to avoid chemical changes in the Perspex. The blanks are then cleaned and inspected.

The blanks are mounted on a holder and placed on a modified engraving machine the cutter of which follows a template and cuts the shape and size of implant required. Considerable attention is given to smoothing and hand polishing the edge to ensure it is well rounded, smoothly polished, and entirely free of any roughness or other defect. After ultrasonic cleaning and drying using a filtered air blast in a clean air room the implants are inspected critically and sterilized.

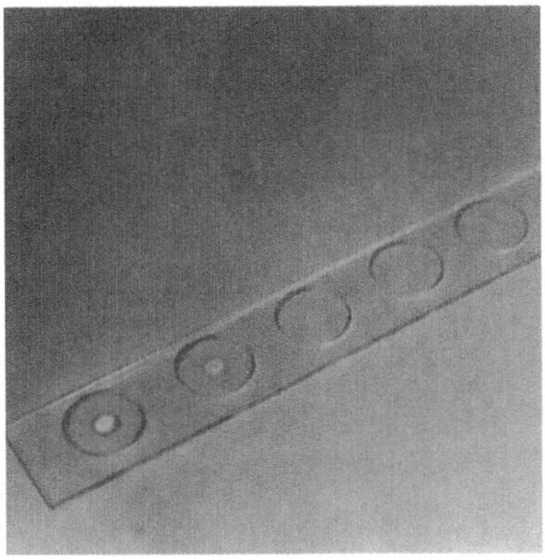

Fig. III-11.

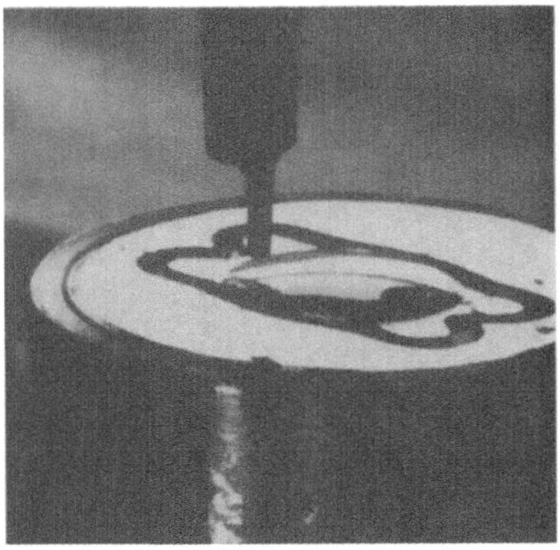

Fig. III-12.

Fig. III-11. — Strip of perpsex with the milled disks. (Courtesy Rayner, London.)

Fig. III-12. — Machine cutting the haptic. (Courtesy Rayner, London.)

B. Morcher's Technique for Manufacturing the Iridocapsular Lens

Morcher uses plexiglass provided by Rohm of Darmstadt, West Germany. Before processing, the polymethylmethacrylate pellets (formmasse 7 N) are dried as much as possible by keeping it at a constant temperature (45 °C) for at least a year.

The optical component of the iridocapsular lens is made by compression molding. The procedure is as follows:

The steel mold is filled with pellets and 500 kg pressure is applied.

The mold is heated to 200 °C and the pressure is increased to 2600 kg. After a period of time, the pressure is released and the mold cooled by ventilation. The optic is taken out of the mold and tested for quality. Any irregularities on the edge are removed on a lathe.

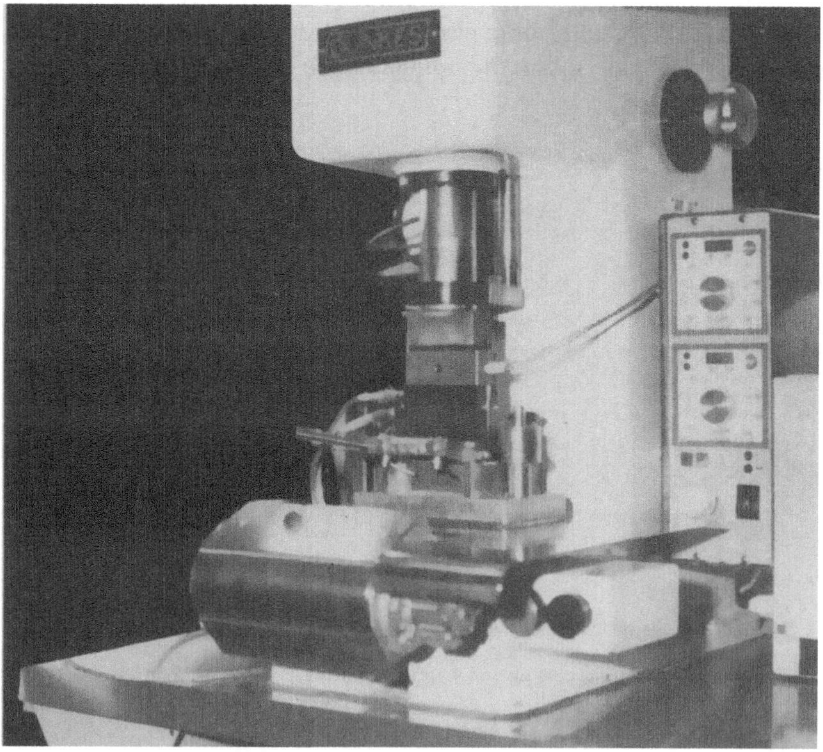

Fig. III-13. — Molding machine for manufacturing the optic portion of the Morcher lens. (Courtesy K. Morcher, Stuttgart.)

Four holes are drilled in the lens to hold the pair of loops. The diameter of these holes is 0.01 mm less than the diameter of the thread from which the loops are made. The edge of the optic is then polished.

The loops are made of polypropylene. The required shaping of the thread is done by clamping it in a steel device and heating it for an hour in an oven at 160 °C.

To fix the loops in the optic, the ends are thinned and threaded through the holes. The excess length is cut off and, if necessary, the position is adjusted.

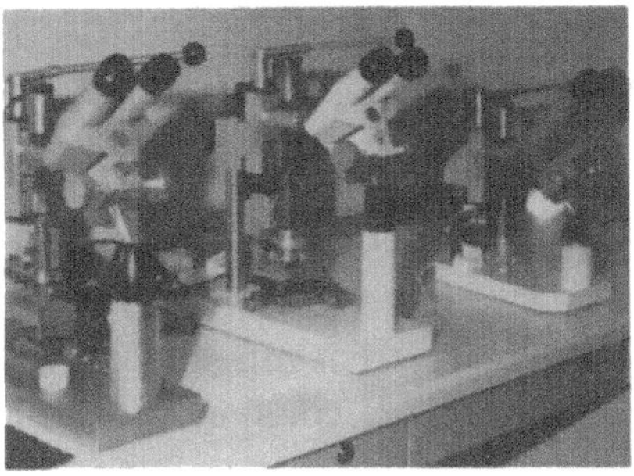

Fig. III-14.

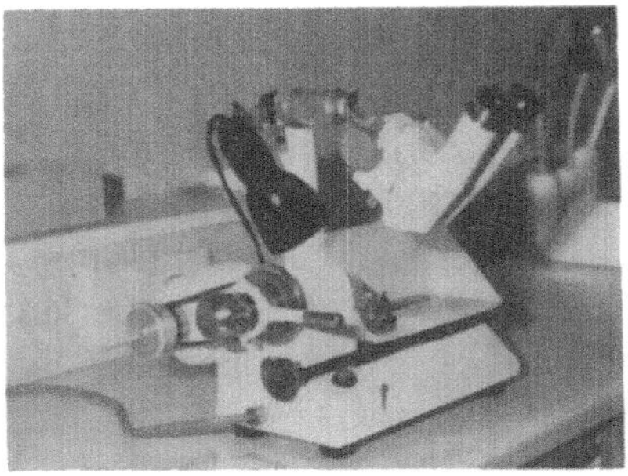

Fig. III-15.

Fig. III-14. — Micro drills for making the holes. (Courtesy K. Morcher, Stuttgart.)

Fig. III-15. — Lathe for the edge finishing. (Courtesy K. Morcher, Stuttgart.)

The lens is then submerged in distilled water for 24 hours at 20 °C. The position of the loops is again checked and corrected if necessary.

Finally, the lens is tested for optical quality and power before it is sterilized.

The iris clip lens is manufactured in almost the same way. The holes for the anterior loops are not drilled, however, but made during the molding phase. This method was first used to make the Dannheim lenses.

§ 3. STERILIZATION

Sterilization means the complete destruction or removal of all forms of life. As implant lenses evolved, so did the methods for sterilizing them.

Harold Ridley's practice was to immerse the lens for at least an hour in a solution of 1 % cetrimide (tetradecyl-trimethylammonium bromide), which is a quaternary ammonium compound and then rinsing it repeatedly in saline.

This method of immersion in an antiseptic solution was followed by several surgeons. Strampelli (1951) mentions using a 1% quaternary ammonium solution, and Schreck, Lieb, and Guerry (1957) mention the use of 0.1% Zephiran (benzalkoniumchloride). Dannheim (1956) mentioned that his lenses were delivered in a solution of bencylcethylammonium.

Since quaternary ammonium compounds are highly surface active and therefore adhere to the lens to be released from the Perspex as time passes, severe postoperative reactions were not infrequent. Furthermore, it was not certain that these antiseptics could assure sufficient sterility of the implant.

To resolve these problems, various other methods were developed. Strampelli (1961) proposed that quartz be used instead of acrylic in

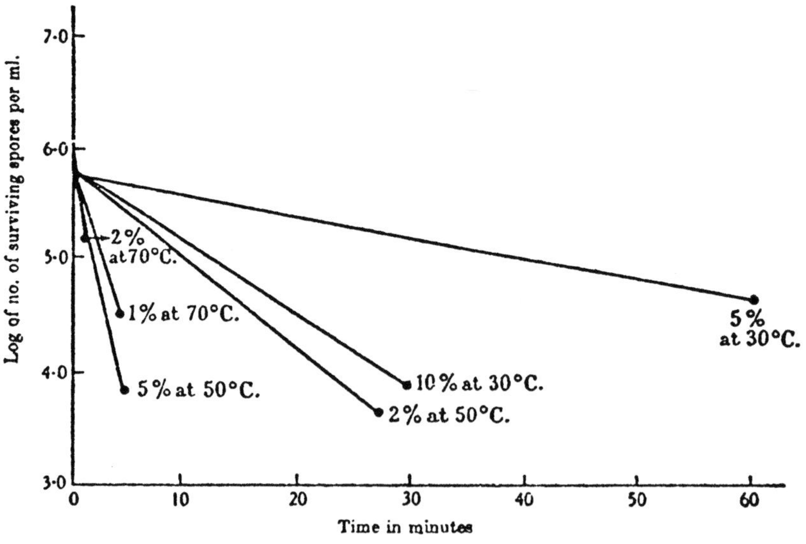

Fig. III-16. — Death rate of *Bacillus subtilis* spores submitted to different concentrations of sodium hydroxide at different temperatures (Hobbs and Wilson, 1942).

the manufacture of the lenses so they could be boiled. And to avoid intraocular toxic reactions resulting from sterilization of acrylic lenses, he proposed that they be implanted for a few months in the patient's subcutaneous tissue, a method he called "humanization".

Binkhorst and Flu (1956) irradiated the lens for 30 minutes with ultraviolet rays with a wavelength of 253.7 nm.

In the opinion of F. Ridley, who proposed in 1957 a method that is still in use, ultraviolet sterilization had some shortcomings. Since ultraviolet rays of the proper wavelength are strongly absorbed by Perspex, it could be a cause of degradation of the acrylic material by producing monomers. In his opinion, too, it was not certain that all spores would be destroyed.

The method proposed by F. Ridley (1957) was based on the studies done by Hobbs and Wilson (1942) and Tilley (1946) that showed that caustic soda (NaOH) 10% at 30°C for 1 hour destroyed even the spores of Bacillus subtilis.

He applied this method to the sterilization of implant lenses. After sterilization, the lens is removed from the caustic soda bath and stored in a 0.1% NaOH solution. Immediately before implantation, the NaOH is neutralized by immersion in a sterile 0.5% solution of $NaHCO_3$ after which the lens is rinsed in saline. Since the application of such a strongly etching material as sodium hydroxide would naturally give rise to objections, Ridley anticipated them by the following:

A. "The caustic soda, 0.1 per cent, used for storage is instantly destroyed by 0.5 per cent sodium bicarbonate introduced in great excess. The resulting ions, sodium and carbonate, are in less than their normal physiological concentration in the tissues, while the bicarbonate in solution is harmless."

B. "The possibility exists that during storage some of the caustic soda solutions may have been absorbed by the acrylic. The material can absorp up to 0.5% by weight in water. For the heavy lens according to Harold Ridley weighing about one-tenth of a gramme, this would represent one two-millionth part of a gramme of caustic soda that might be left in the lens after washing it with sodium bicarbonate. This minute trace of caustic soda would diffuse out very slowly; the sodium ion is harmless, and the hydroxyl ion will be trapped instantly by the 0.18 per cent of sodium bicarbonate normally present in the tissue fluids and rendered harmless as carbonate."

After this method was proven safe in clinical practice for lenses made from polymethylmethacrylate alone, it was soon adopted for all implant lenses. Frederick Ridley's method has withstood the test of time and turned out to be safe and efficient for more than two decades, the only exceptions being the contamination of two lots of sodium bicarbonate solution of different origins (U.S.) of which one was fungal (Paecilomyces lilacenes) and the other bacterial (Pseudomonas aerogenes) (see p. 477) that led to 21 cases of endophthalmitis. In the opinion of Drews (1978) and Worst (1977) all of these cases could probably have been prevented if the neutralizing solution had been passed through a millipore filter at the time of use.

In the late seventies, Galin (1977) and Galin and Turkish (1979) proposed modifications in the original Ridley method. Indeed, according to the investigation they conducted, it was found that a 1 hour passage in 10% NaOH could not guarantee that all microorganisms such as spores of Bacillus subtilis would be destroyed after massive inoculation, especially when the lens had a complex configuration. This applies in particular to lenses with holes in them for the attachment of loops. They therefore proposed to increase the sterilization period to 3 hours at 33 °C, which proved to be sufficient in the experiments they conducted. With this improved method there is a probability of finding a single surviving organism only if 10^6 lenses were cultured—an acceptable level of sterility.

Another modification suggested is to keep the lenses until use in the 10% NaOH solution, which would eliminate the possibility of contamination during the transfer of the lens to the dilute carrier solution (terminal sterilizing method). This solution is a self-sterilizing, highly batericidal medium, whereas the 0.1% solution is only bacteriostatic and vulnerable to protein contamination and to pH changes, which cannot guarantee persistent sterility of the ampule.

Another method of sterilizing plastic materials employs gaseous agents. Of these gases, ethylene oxide has been found to be the most suitable for sterilizing lens implants. Ethylene oxide is a simple cyclic ether of low molecular weight that diffuses very regularly into polymethylmethacrylate. At room temperature it is a colorless gas, and it liquifies readily at 10.9 °C and freezes at −111 °C.

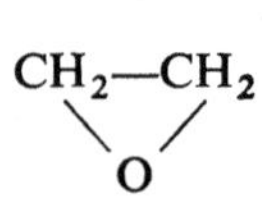

Ethylene oxide

The mechanism by which ethylene oxide kills microorganisms has been linked to its chemical activity as an alkylating agent. According to this hypothesis, ethylene oxide replaces labile hydrogen atoms with hydroxy-ethyl groups ($—CH_2—CH_2—OH$), thus blocking many reactive groups needed in essential metabolic reactions. Along with protein keratin, $-COOH$, $-NH_2$, $-SH$ and $-OH$ groups can all be attacked in this manner (Phillips, 1977).

J. Harry (1977) reported that ethylene oxide was found to destroy all known microorganisms without damaging the materials used in lens implantation. D. Link (1978) stated that the probability of microbial contamination with this method is one in a million (10^{-6}) or less. In other words, the standard of sterility would be that one viable organism would survive out of 10^6 lenses.

Unfortunately, ethylene oxide is a toxic substance that reacts to form additional tissue toxicants such as ethylene glycol and ethylene chlorhydrin. Therefore, all ethylene oxide sterilized materials have to be aerated. This is done by using subatmospheric pressure or by leaving the packaged lens stand in air. Additionally, since the lens material must always be suspected of harboring traces of ethylene oxide, ethylene glycol, and ethylene chlorhydrin, they must be regularly checked. In the United States, where this sterilization method has been required by the Food and Drug Administration since 1978, the manufacturer must determine if the residual concentration of toxic agents is well below the imposed limit by means of regular sampling.

The performance of ethylene oxide has yet to be such as to render the caustic soda method obsolete. Indeed, all the problems with it have not been resolved. Several cases of adverse reactions after implantation of "dry sterilized" lenses have been reported (see chapter XIII). Therefore, the American Intra-Ocular Implant Society (1979) has strongly recommended that all ethylene oxide sterilized lenses be thoroughly rinsed in saline before insertion. This procedure seems to reduce the incidence of irritative reactions. The precise irritant mechanism is unknown.

Another method suggested by the United States Food and Drug Administration as a substitute for the caustic soda method is γ-irradiation sterilization. As many suture materials and other implant devices such as pacemakers are sterilized in this way, the application to pseudophakoi seemed obvious. This method had to be discontinued, however, because of occasional aseptic inflammatory reactions with sterile hypopion (see p. 476). Fortunately, these cases responded well to steroid therapy and good vision was ultimately achieved. The precise reasons for these reactions still remain obscure. As is well known, polymethylmethacrylate may be degraded by γ-radiation (Chapiro, 1962) but it is not impossible that the polypropylene loops also were degraded by γ-radiation. After all, this substance is a prominent example of a material that has no problems with β-radiation, but cannot tolerate γ-radiation very well (E. Svendson et al., 1975).

According to Meltzer (1981), probably neither the PMMA nor the polypropylene were involved, but rather the balanced salt solution (BSS®, Alcon). In his analysis, Meltzer demonstrated the presence of chemical substances resulting from the BSS irradiation that could be irritative in themselves or constitute a trigger for an immune reaction of some sort.

Comment on Sterilization Methods

After an initial period of trial and error, the sterilization method devised by F. Ridley has been generally accepted. In spite of a few failures, it has stood the test of time. Two other methods were proposed by the United States Food and Drug administration: γ-radiation, which has proven unsuitable, and the ethylene oxide method, which sometimes gives rise to excessive postoperative reactions, a matter of serious concern in implant surgery. Even if this problem with ethylene oxide sterilization can be resolved, other disadvantages remain. Distribution of these lenses is more complicated than that of those sterilized with the caustic soda method. Indeed, ethylene oxide sterility can only be guaranteed for a specific period of time, and resterilization can only be done in a specially equipped laboratory. There is also the potential hazard of contamination should the package be accidentally punctured in transit. The wet method has a great advantage in that no complicated apparatus is necessary to perform it and then to test for residual toxicity. Further, the presence of NaOH in the package can be easily confirmed with a pH indicator tape. Resterilization of a suspect lens can also be done anywhere.

CHAPTER IV

THE OPTICS OF INTRAOCULAR LENSES

The basic configuration of the optical portion of the currrent models of implant lenses is either biconvex or planoconvex. The optic of the Choyce Mark VIII lens is biconvex, the anterior surface having a constant radius of 14 mm and the posterior surface varying according to the dioptic power. The optical portion of nearly all of the other lenses are planoconvex, with the radius varying according to their power. Almost all lenses are made of polymethylmethacrylate, which has a refractive index of around 1.49. The thickness at the optic center varies from some 0.4 mm to 0.9 mm.

Since the lens material is permeable for a wide range of wave lengths, including the ultraviolet spectrum, color perception with a pseudophakos is extended toward the shorter wave lengths, as is also the case with plain aphakia.

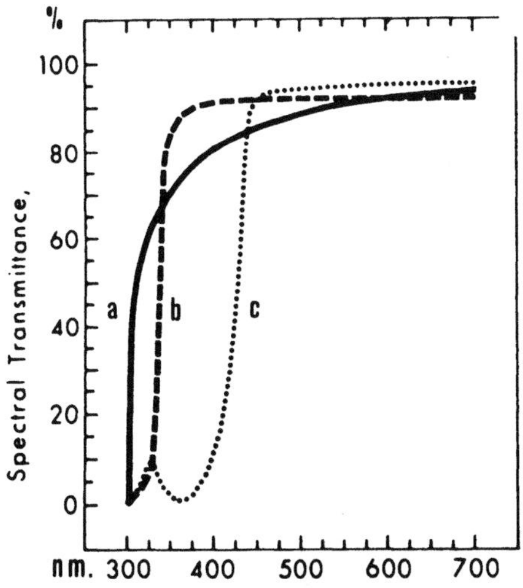

Fig. IV-1. — Near-ultraviolet and visible transmittance measured for clear PMMA intraocular lenses (Curve b), and spectral transmittance of the cornea (Curve a) and the crystalline lens (Curve C) (Mainster, 1978).

So colors appear lighter and more saturated to implant patients. In daylight, sometimes the world also appears more blue (cyanopsia), and complaints of erythropsia after exposure to bright light are not uncommon. However, according to Lui and Krolman (1981) on the basis of the F-M 100 Hue Test and AO-HRR pseudoisochromatic plates, color discrimination is not affected in pseudophakia. Addition of dyes to the polymethylmethacrylate to normalize light perception has been considered, but this has not been implemented in practice. Further studies are necessary to determine how these additives behave in the eye over the long term.

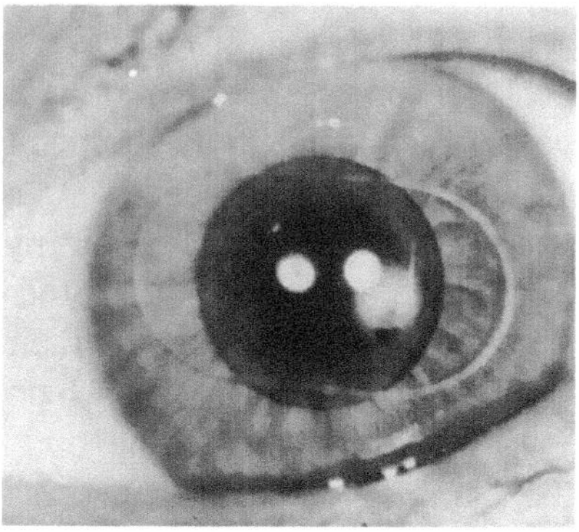

Fig. IV-2. — Iris clip lens with colored optic for the normalization of pseudophakic color perception. (Courtesy C.D. Binkhorst.)

Other materials have also been used for intraocular lenses. Ridley considered the possibility of using glass already in 1952, and Emmerich reported on the behavior of some 30 anterior chamber lenses made of glass in 1958. Strampelli (1961) also implanted a series of anterior chamber lenses made of quartz. Glass has recently reappeared on the implant scene. Barash and Poler (1979) maintain that the optical performance of a glass lens is superior to that of a polymethylmethacrylate lens since its resolving power is higher. Another advantage is glass's greater refractive index (1.62), which permits the optic to be 2/5 the thickness of polymethylmethacrylate implants. For example, a 19 diopter glass lens has a central thickness of 0.3 mm.

I. The Optical Quality of Polymethylmethacrylate Lenses

Like the natural lens, the pseudophakos does not account for the largest part of the refracting power of the eye. The total dioptric power of an emmetropic eye is some 60 diopters, of which the lens provides only a third, acting as an adjunct to the cornea.

The influence of chromatic aberrations on the quality of vision by implant lenses is not significant. According to Blaker (1977), these defects are largely neutralized by other components of the ocular system.

Monochromatic aberrations— spherical aberration, coma, astigmatism, field curvature, and distortion—are of more concern since they directly interfere with the quality of the retinal image.

One of the classic ways of checking the quality of lenses is to determine their resolving power, which gives the limit of efficiency of a lens or an optical system. Resolving power can be expressed in line pairs/mm and determined theoretically for a diffractive limited lens by means of the following formula (Richard, 1977).

$$\text{Resolving power (line pairs/mm)} = \frac{N \times 10^3}{\lambda(f')}$$

where N = the refractive index

λ = wave length in microns

$$f' = \text{relative aperture} = \frac{\text{posterior focal length}}{\text{pupil diameter}}$$

For a perfect lens in air with a relative aperture of $f' = 5.4$, the predicted resolving power for light of 555 microns is

$$\frac{1.0 \times 10^3}{0.55 \times 5.4} = 330 \text{ lp/mm}$$

According to the literature (Richard, 1977; Dunn, 1978), the theoretical resolving power of the eye calculated for a 3 mm pupil and for light with a wavelength of 555 nm—photopic peak sensitivity—is around 320 lp/mm, which is close to the spatial frequency of a perfect lens. But since the cornea is aspheric and thus introduces optical aberrations, the resolution efficiency of the eye is reduced by 15% to 35%. The resultant resolutive power is therefore some 210 to 270 lp/mm. At the fovea, the smallest resolvable receptor element is the 5 μ retinal cone, which is equivalent to a spatial frequency of some 200 lp/mm. Translated into terms of visual acuity, 200 lp/mm corresponds to an angular resolution of 1 minute of arc or a visual acuity of 20/20. From these theoretical considerations, it appears that the optical and the receptor systems of the eye match each other properly.

There have been a few studies of the resolutive power of intraocular lenses. While no lens can ever attain the theoretical upper limit of resolutive power, proper design and manufacturing methods can achieve a substantial percentage of it. Dunn (1978) considers a 75% resolution efficiency desirable, which compares favorably with the resolving power of the retina (±200 lp/mm). The greater the resolution efficiency, the less likely will the intraocular lens constitute the limiting factor for visual performance.

An interesting study of this matter was performed by Olson et al. (1979), who examined 95 lenses from 10 different manufacturers.

TABLE IV-1. — *Intraocular Lens Optical Resolution in Air Using an Air Force Resolution Target with an Automatic Collimator (corrected for lens power and magnification) (Olson et al., 1979, p. 550).*

Lens Manufacturer	*Mean Resolution ±S.D. (Line Pairs/mm)*	*Maximum Resolution (Line Pairs/mm)*	*Minimum Resolution (Line Pairs/mm)*
Cilco	124 ± 63	217	40
Copeland	191 ± 31	239	143
Heyer-Schulte	173 ± 33	219	122
Intermedics	220 ± 35	288	177
Iolab	255 ± 35	313	220
McGhan	110 ± 50	191	43
Medical Workshop	240 ± 28	297	211
Precision-Cosmet	221 ± 37	295	186
Rayner	157 ± 34	214	108
Surgidev	158 ± 13	179	137

TABLE IV-2. — *Intraocular Lens Resolution as a Percentage of the Theoretical Maximum Resolution. Light Wave-Length Used: 546 nm; Collimator Aperture: 3.02 nm (Olson et al., 1979, p. 553).*

Lens Manufacturer	*Mean Resolution, %*	*Maximum Resolution, %*	*Minimum Resolution, %*
Cilco	37 ± 16	63	12
Copeland	58 ± 9	70	45
Heyer-Schulte	49 ± 9	63	40
Intermedics	73 ± 10	88	55
Iolab	73 ± 10	88	63
McGhan	36 ± 16	63	13
Medical Workshop	78 ± 6	88	70
Precision-Cosmet	66 ± 10	88	55
Rayner	49 ± 12	70	31
Surgidev	46 ± 2	55	45

They observed an extreme amount of variation in resolution from a high of 313 lp/mm to a low of 40 lp/mm. As shown on the tables, only 4 manufacturers obtained a resolution efficiency of around 75% of the theoretical maximum of 330 lp/mm for a perfect lens in air.

And 2 manufacturers delivered lenses with a mean resolving power of 36% and 37% respectively, and a minimum of 13% and 12% respectively.

In practice, Dunn states, a level of 50% resolving ability seems to be adequate for ophthalmic purposes. Indeed, many patients have 20/20 vision with such lenses. As we noted above, the pseudophakos is responsible for only a third of the total refractive power of the eye. In Dunn's view, a resolving efficiency lower than 50% is problematical. Olson et al. (1980), after having examined a series of updated lenses, concluded that optical quality has improved significantly since the time of their first study. The following data they provide are illustrative: no lens had less than 52% resolution efficiency nor caused a double image. Ninety (75%) of the 120 lenses examined had better than 74% resolution efficiency (Fig. IV-3).

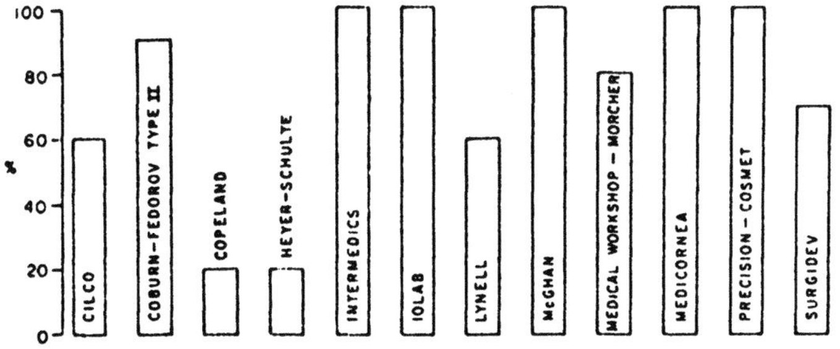

Fig. IV-3. — Percent of lenses for each manufacturer with resolution efficiencies greater than 74% of the theoretical maximum. None of the lenses examined had less than 52% resolution efficiency (Olson, 1980, p. 17).

II. Dioptric Power of Human Crystallin

The total refractive power of the schematic emmetropic eye is +58.38 diopters, according to Tscherning and +58.64 diopters according to Gullstrand. Gullstrand also places the refractive power of the lens in situ for the emmetropic eye at 19.11 diopters (Duke-Elder 1970). Pascal (1952), using Tscherning's data for the radii, indices, and thickness of the crystalline, found that the power of the crystalline lens, treated as a *thin lens,* is greater by 2.29 diopters than the value calculated by Gullstrand, i.e., 21.72 diopters. These values are reduced powers, i.e., air equivalent powers in situ. The same "thin" lens could have an absolute power of 109.25 diopters in air and still an absolute power of over 100 diopters even after a correction factor for the effect of thickness is introduced.

TABLE IV-3. — *The Mean Value, Standard Deviation and Extreme Values of Corneal Radii, Total Refractive Power of the Eye and Refractive Power of The Crystallin in Emmetropia (Delmarcelle et al., 1976, p. 322 – slightly modified).*

Authors	*Refraction*	*N*	*R. Cornea in mm*	*P. Cornea in diopters*	*P. crystalline in diopters*	*P. Total Eye in diopters*
Stenström, 1946	Emm.	1,000			17.35	58.13
Gernet, 1964	−0.5 +1.5	66	7.8	43.3	21.7 (2.95)	64.4 (2.63)
		54	7.68	44	22.9 (2.62)	66.3 (4.3)
		12	all 7.8	43.3	21.6 (15.7-25.8)	64.1 (58.3-68.4)
Gernet, 1964	Emm.	28	all 7.7	43.8	15-26.5	
Gernet, 1964	−0.5 +1.5	73	7.81 (0.2)	43.3	20.3 (9.4%)	62.8 (3.5%)
Fridman and Savitskaya, 1966	Emm.	58			(18.4-43.2)	(60.9-75.8)
Franceschetti and Luyckx, 1967	−1 +1	68	7.8 (0.2)	43.3	22.0 (2.1)	64.5 (2.1)
		38	7.7 (0.2)	43.8	22.0 (3.3)	64.5 (3.9)
François and Goes, 1968	−1.5 +1.5	127	7.67 (0.29)	44	17.74 (2.61)	61.83 (2.71)
Fridman, 1968	Emm.	±100				66.6
Grignolo and Rivara, 1968	+1.31	39			20.81	62.82
François and Goes, 1970	Emm.	222	7.66 (0.30)	44	18.37 (2.82) (10.55-25.22)	

According to various investigators, the power of the crystalline lens is constant neither in emmetropia nor in ametropia. Table IV-3 and Table IV-5 illustrate this.

In the large group of nearly emmetropic eyes, the mean values for the refractive power of the crystallin range from 17.35 to 22.9 diopters.

The results of the study of A. Sorsby (1971) of 107 emmetropes provided the following values for the dioptric power of the cornea, the lens power, the anterior chamber depth, and the axial length.

TABLE IV-4

	Corneal Power (Di)	*Lens Power (Di)*	*Ant. Chamber Depth (mm)*	*Axial Length (mm)*
Range	39.0-47.6	25.5-23.9	2.5-4.2	22.3-26
Mean	43.1	19.7	3.5	24.2
Standard dev.	1.62	1.62	0.34	0.85

As shown on Table IV-4, the mean refractive power of the emmetropic lens tends to be around 20 diopters with a standard deviation of 1.62. Extreme values ranging from 15.5 to 24 diopters were noted, however, which means that there is a 9 diopter difference in emmetropics.

Also illustrative is the study by Gernet and Olbrich (1968), which demonstrated how the power of the crystallin in 60 emmetropic eyes having the same corneal refractive value varies and compensates for the individual differences in axial length (Fig. IV-4).

Similar variations in the dioptric power of the crystalline have been observed by various authors in ametropia. According to the data given on Table IV-5, the mean dioptric power in high myopia rarely exceeds 18 diopters. But with high hypermetropia, the mean dioptric crystallin power exceeds 22.5 diopters with peak values reaching 39.5 diopters.

Several investigators have concluded that the variations in dioptric power of the crystalline lens both in emmetropia and in ametropia are one of the major components of the attempt nature makes to attain emmetropia, a phenomenon that has been actively studied since the beginning of this century in order to explain the predominance of emmetropia in the general population (Fig. IV-5).

TABLE IV-5. — *Mean Value, Standard Deviation, and Extreme Values of Radii of the Corneal Refractive Power and the Crystallin and Total Refractive Power of the Eye in Myopia and Hypermetropia (Delmarcelle et al. 1976 p. 323 – slightly modified).*

Authors	*Refraction*	*N*	*Corneal radius in mm*	*Corneal power in diopters*	*Cristallin power in diopters*	*Total eye power in diopters*
Myopia						
Franceschetti and Gernet, 1965	< −7	18	7.8 (0.29)	43.3	18.8 (1.4)	60.8 (2.5)
	> −7	21	7.9 (0.24)	42.75	17.5 (2.8)	59.8 (2.6)
		12	7.6 (0.08)	44.40	16.0 (3.0)	59.7 (3.9)
		43	7.7 (0.29)	43.80	14.9 (2.4)	58.0 (2.1)
Fridman and Savitskaya, 1966	−0.5 −11	87			(13.1-36.5)	(51.9-74.8)
Franceschetti and Luycks, 1967	−9 (5.3)	38	7.7 (0.2)	43.80	17.9 (2.8)	60.7 (3.2)
François and Goes, 1968	−1.5 −6	30	7.65 (0.29)	44.15	15.28 (1.75)	59.43 (2.1)
	−6 −15	63	7.57 (0.37)	45	14.34 (3.06)	59.1 (2.76)
	>15	28	7.66 (0.26)	44	12.6 (2.05)	56.69 (1.92)
Hypermetropia						
Franceschetti and Gernet, 1965	+11.6 (+7 +14)	8	6.86 (6.8-7.0)	49	33.25 (26.9-39.5)	81.7 (75.0-88.3)
François and Goes, 1970	> +6	38	7.41 (6.67-8.60)	45.6	22.54 (16.6-32.25)	

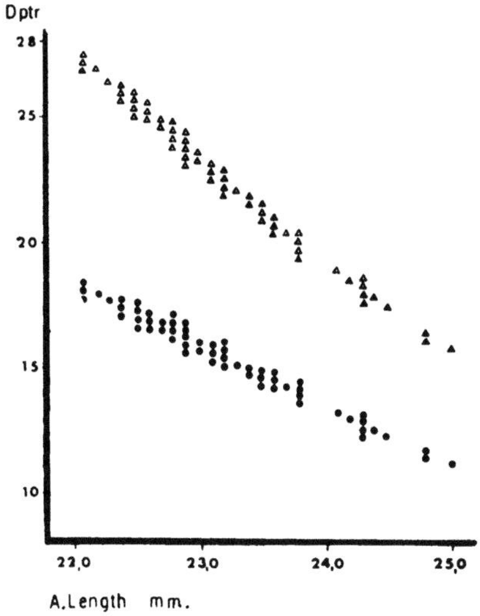

Fig. IV-4.

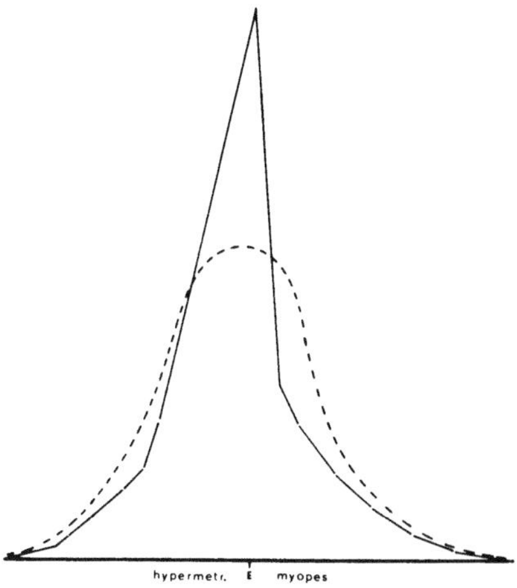

Fig. IV-5.

Fig. IV-4. — Distribution of upper and lower values of refractive powers of the crystalline for 60 emmetropic eyes having the same corneal refractive power. (Gernet and Olbrich, 1968).

Fig. IV-5. — Curves representing the recorded refraction (solid line) and the theoretical binomial values (dotted line) of 2920 adult eyes (F. Wibaut, 1926, cited in Delmarcelle et al. 1976, 316).

The interaction of the parameters—dioptric power of the cornea and the lens, total axial length, and location of the crystalline—have been analyzed by Stenström (1946) and found to have the following relationships. There is:

— a strong correlation between axial length and refraction, $r = -0.76$;
— a correlation between corneal radius and axial length, $r = +0.31$;
— a weak correlation between corneal power and refraction, $r = -0.18$;
— a weak correlation between the eye's total dioptric power and refraction, $r = -0.10$;
— a correlation between anterior chamber depth and refraction, $r = -0.34$;
— a correlation between the eye's total dioptric power and axial length, $r = +0.44$;
— no correlation between refraction and crystalline dioptric power.

Furthermore, according to Stenström (1946; 1948), there seems to be a normal distribution for all the optical factors determining the refraction exception made for the axial length. As Y. Delmarcelle et al. (1976) concluded, this confirms the important role of axial length in the final refraction.

Thus, although the power of the human crystalline in the majority of the emmetropic eyes is about 20 diopters and generally higher in hypermetropia and lower in myopia, striking variations exist.

III. The Pseudophakos as a Substitute for the Crystalline Lens

When the human crystalline lens is replaced by an artificial lens the retinal image is not affected if the implant is located at precisely the same place as the natural lens and if it yields the same dioptric power. In this situation, all six cardinal points of the optical system remain at their same geometric location.

Only the posterior chamber lenses can approximate these conditions, however, since all the other pseudophakoi are located in a more forward position. Table IV-6 gives the mean values of distances from the posterior surface of the cornea to the anterior surface of the different implant lenses taken at the center of the lens.

TABLE IV-6. — *Mean Values of Distances from the Posterior Surface of the Cornea to the Anterior Surface of Different Implant Lenses (Values Measured at The Center)*

	Distances in mm
Angle supported lenses:	
Tennant Lens	2.45
Choyce Mark VIII	2.74
Iris supported lenses:	
Iris Clip Lens	3.20
Copeland Lens	3.80
Capsular supported lenses:	
Iridocapsular 2-Loop Lens	3.45
Posterior Chamber Lens	$\geqslant$4.00

The change in location of the pseudophakos relative to the original lens has two basic consequences:

First, because of the increase in distance between the image plane (retina) and the artificial lens, any implant lens that is intended to restore the phakic situation must be of weaker power than the original crystallin. Thus it was found from experience (with a theoretical basis) that a prepupillary pseudophakos of 18 diopters satisfactorily replaces the original lens in an emmetropic eye having a corneal power of 42 diopters and an axial length of 24 mm. Obviously, any implant placed in a still more forward position would need less refractive power to correct the same eye (Fig. IV-6).

Second, since the weaker lens located in a more forward position has an increased posterior focal length, the resulting retinal image will be enlarged with respect to the original phakic situation.

Using Gullstrand's data for the shematic aphakic eye, Troutman (1962, 1963) calculated the theoretical magnification for an infinitely thin intraocular lens producing emmetropia at different distances behind the anterior vertex of the cornea.

As shown on Figure IV-7, the theoretical magnification of a retropupillary infinitely thin implant lens producing emmetropia in the schematic eye results in insignificant magnification. However, a weaker lens with a longer focal distance situated 3 mm behind the anterior vertex of the corneal give 4% magnification while making the eye emmetropic.

M.C. Colenbrander (1973), also using the data of Gullstrand's schematic eye, calculated for a planoconvex lens of 0.5 mm thickness and a dioptric power of 18 *D* that an anterior shift of 1 mm increases the total refractive power of the eye by 0.60 diopters and produces an enlargement of the retinal image of 2% since the second principal point of the eye is displaced 0.5 mm towards the cornea and the second nodal point 0.34 mm.

Troutman also calculated the theoretical refractive value in the anterior focal plane that would compensate for an intentionally overpowered thin implant in order to maintain the same image size as in the previous phakic state. He did this on the basis of Gullstrand's schematic eye.

As illustrated on Figure IV-8, the theoretical infinitely thin lens in the schematic eye at different distances from the cornea shows different focal lengths resulting in different degrees of myopia. The basis idea behind this intentional myopization is telescopic mimification. This optical effect is obtained by neutralizing the excessive positive power of the implant with negative spectacles. Indeed, the power of the lenses plotted on the iseikonic line increase relative to their value on the emmetropic line.

Also using the data for Gullstrand's schematic emmetropic eye, C.D. Binkhorst (1972) calculated that the implant power of a 0.5 mm

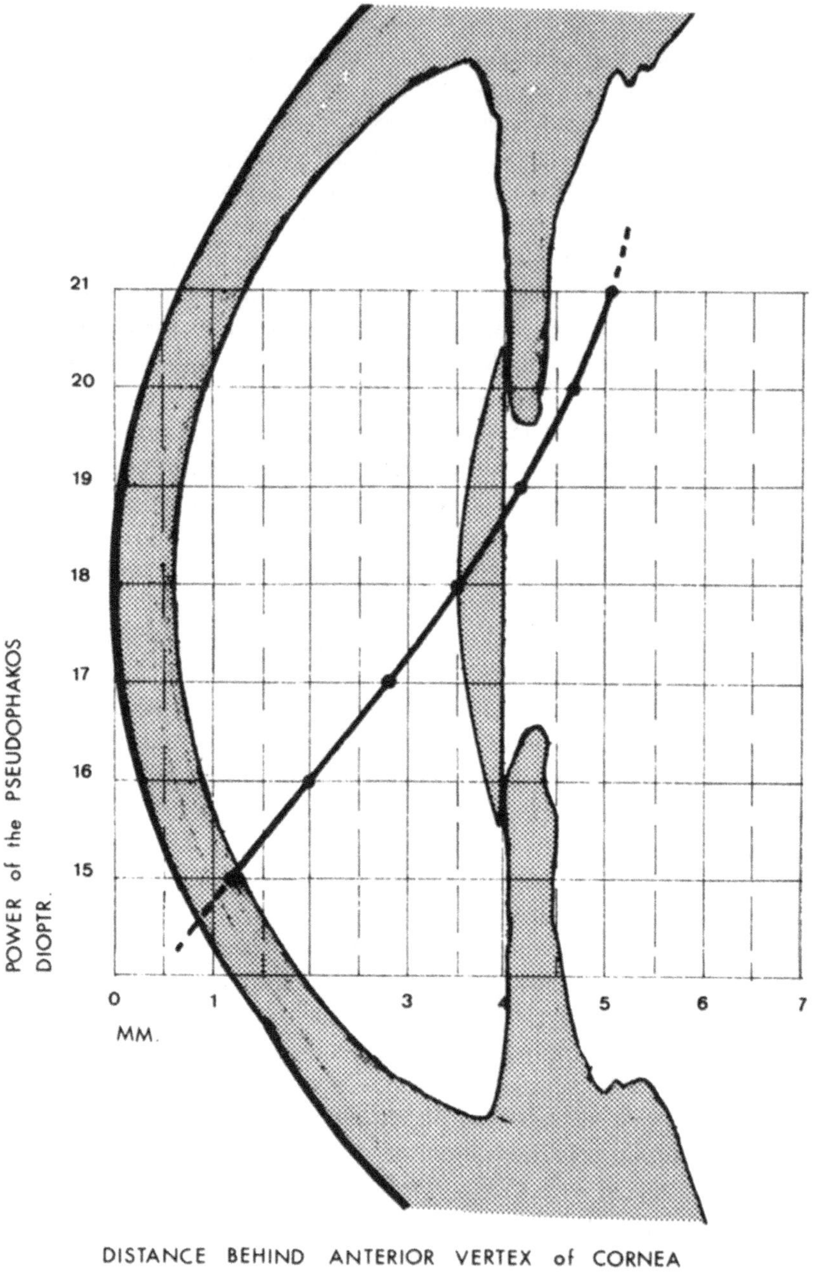

Fig. IV-6. — Diagram giving the corresponding dioptrical power of an emmetropizing pseudophakos placed at any distance behind the anterior vertex of the cornea as calculated by M.C. Colenbrander (1973).

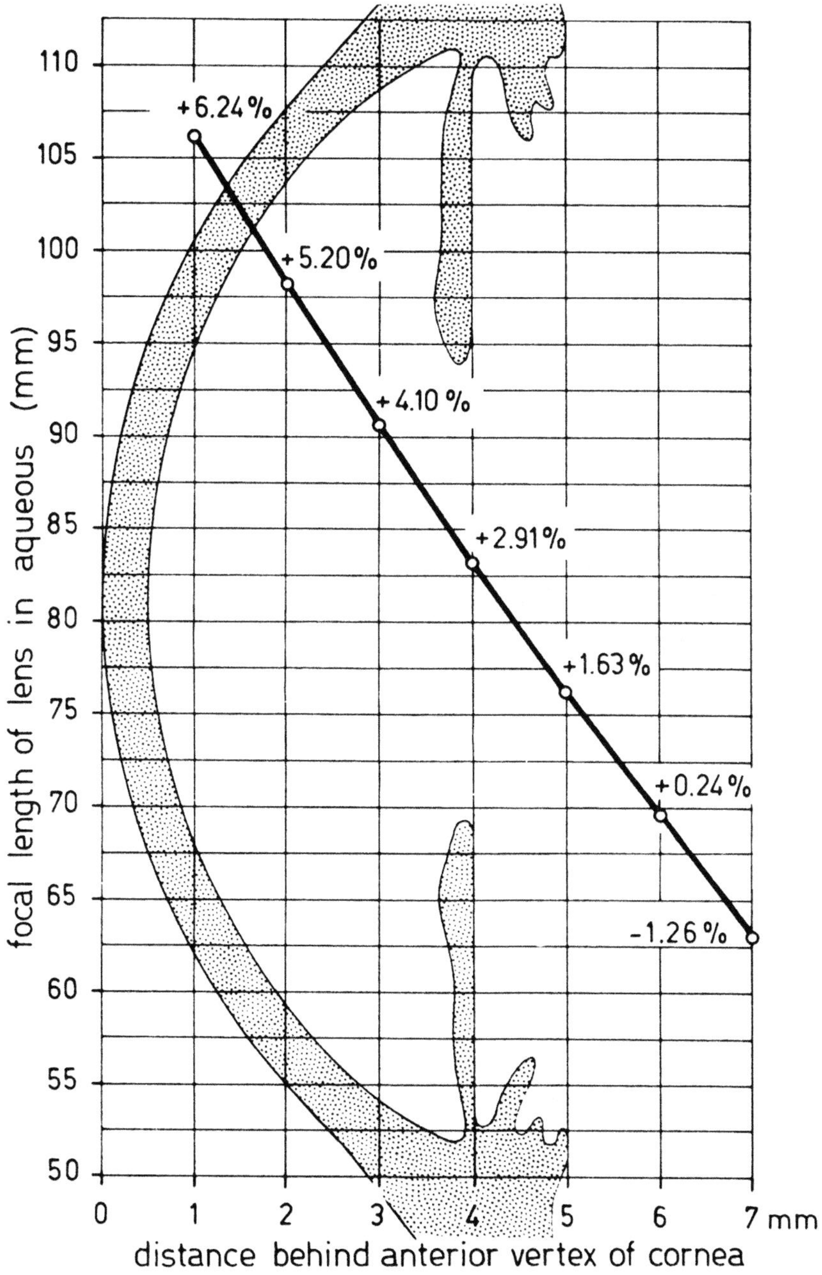

Fig. IV-7. — Theoretical magnification for an infinitely thin intraocular lens producing emmetropia at different distances behind the anterior vertex of the cornea (Troutman, 1962).

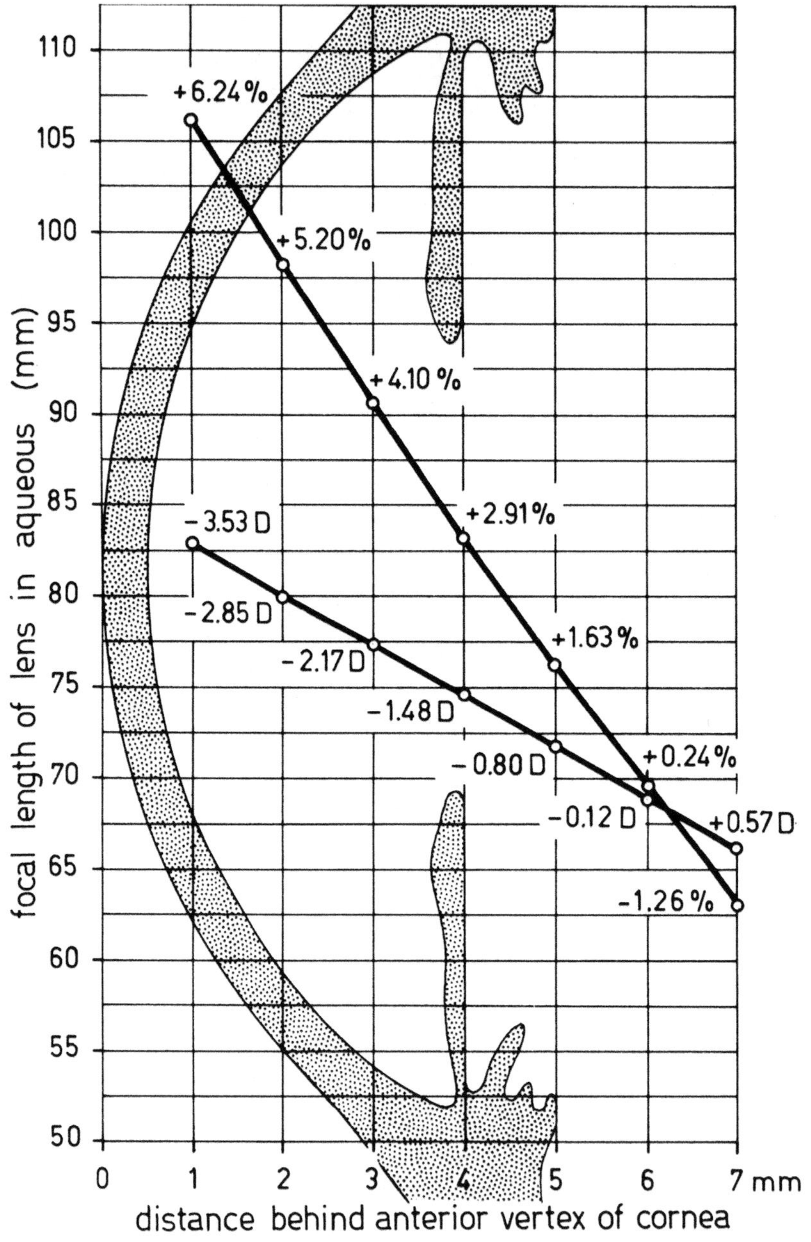

Fig. IV-8. — Theoretical values for an infinitely thin, overpowered iseikonic implant lens at different distances from the anterior vertex of the cornea and the corresponding theoretical values of refraction in the anterior focal plane (Troutman, 1962).

thick planoconvex implant 3.5 mm from the anterior vertex of the cornea, which gives a 1.69 *D* myopia at the anterior focal point, would restore the original image size.

As a rule of thumb, R.D. Binkhorst (1975) suggests that each diopter of spectacle correction represents a variation of image size of approximately 2%.

IV. Determination of Implant Lens Power

As we noted in the historical review, many of the early lens implantations were performed in already aphakic eyes, which had the advantage of the aphakic spectacle correction already being known. On the basis of this data, which was recorded as precisely as possible at a given (back vertex) distance with respect to the cornea, one could look up the required implant lens power on a table. D.P. Choyce, who is still a fervent proponent of secondary implantation, uses the following table for his own lenses, which was calculated for a 10 mm back vertex distance. The recorded aphakic refraction is first converted to its spherical equivalent (Table IV-7).

TABLE IV-7

Refraction	*Lens Required*
+6.50 to +8.00	+14.00
+8.25 to +10.00	+17.00
+10.25 to +12.00	+19.00
+12.25 to +14.00	+21.00
>14.00	+25.00

In primary implantation, the proper selection of the implant power is more complex. For his iris clip lens, C.D. Binkhorst first used a standard power equivalent to a spectacle correction of +13 *D* (at 12 mm back vertex distance). Four years later, this was changed to the equivalent of a spectacle correction of +12 *D* (Nordlohne, 1975). Finally, Binkhorst (1972) adopted a 19.50 dioptic power as the value for the standard pseudophakos in elderly patients. In practice, this power made the emmetropic eye some 2 diopters myopic, which favors iseikonia. For the different age groups, "iseikonic standard pseudophakic powers" were proposed in the early seventies (see Table IV-8).

TABLE IV-8. — *C.D. Binkhorst's Table of Suggested Lens Powers for Different Ages*

Age (years)	1-3	3-10	10-20	20-35	35-50	>50
Diopters	22.5	20.5	19	18	19	19.5

Between certain limits, the values suggested on table IV-8 for prepupillary pseudophakoi are still useful and may serve as guidelines as long as one does not determine the strength of the lens in individual cases by measuring the axial length.

A. The 1.25 Diopter Rule

Some practical guidelines were drawn up by R. Binkhorst (1975). Since there seems to be a normal distribution for all components determining the refraction except for the axial length, it may be assumed that an implant of standard power based on the mean value of the power of the crystalline lens will restore the original or basic refraction of the eye within the limits determined by the variation of the crystalline lens. In general, an 18 diopter prepupillary lens will restore the basic refraction, i.e., the refraction prior to the development of the cataract. In order to determine the basic refraction, a careful anamnesis and an examination of old spectacles and past refraction records are necessary. When it can be determined that the eye was emmetropic before the development of the cataract, there is a good chance that an 18 diopter lens in the prepupillary position will restore it. If the intention is to render a hyperopic or myopic eye emmetropic after the lens implantation, then one applies the 1.25 diopter rule: for each diopter of previous ametropia, 1.25 diopters is added or subtracted from 18. The relationship is not one-to-one because a 1 *D* change in the implant lens power provides a 1.25

TABLE IV-9. — *Theoretical Values for an "Emmetropizing" Pseudophakos (Prepulliary Position) in relation to the Basic Refraction (R.D. Binkhorst, 1975)*

Basic Refraction	*IOL Power*	*Basic Refraction*	*IOL Power*
+5.00	+24.25	−5.00	+11.75
+4.00	+23.00	−4.00	+13.00
+3.00	+21.75	−3.00	+14.25
+2.00	+20.50	−2.00	+15.50
+1.00	+19.25	−1.00	+16.75
0.00	+18.00	0.00	+18.00

dioptric refractive difference when corrected with a spectacle lens worn at a vertex distance of 12 mm.

The main reasons for error in this method even when the basic refraction is known are:

1. The power of the crystalline lens may rather exceptionally reach values of 15 to 25 diopters in the emmetropic eye and from 10 to over 35 diopters in the ametropic eye.
2. The actual value that must be added or subtracted for each diopter of modification of the basic refraction lies between 1.1 to 1.4 diopters. The exact amount depends on K-readings, anterior chamber depth, vertex distance, and the amount and direction of the basic refraction (R. D. Binkhorst 1975).

Of course, when other lens types that occupy a more anterior or posterior position in the eye are implanted, the power has to be adjusted accordingly.

B. **Calculating the Lens Power from Biometric Data**

With the clinical application of ultrasonography, it became possible to measure the axial length easily, which had been the most uncer-

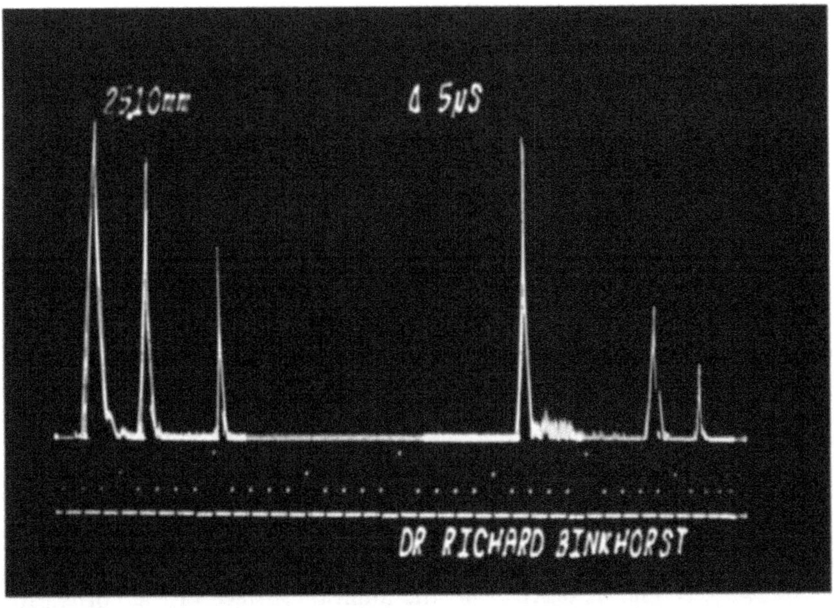

Fig. IV-9. — Axial length measurement with an ultrasonic device. From left to right, the peaks correspond to the echos of the cornea (anterior surface only), the crystalline lens (anterior and posterior surface), and the posterior pole.

tain factor in determining the power of the implant lens. A number of formules have been devised to find the dioptric power from biometric data, which are:

— the exact K reading either in mm or in diopters;
— the estimated postoperative anterior chamber depth, usually the distance from the anterior surface of the cornea to the anterior surface of the pseudophakos;
— the refractive index of the different media;
— the exact axial length.

S.M. Fyodorov was the first to use ultrasonic measurements to calculate implant lens power (Fyodorov pers. comm., 1967). The basic formula he used has since been modified (Fyodorov et al., 1975) and is now as follows:

$$D_p = \frac{h - aD_c}{(a-k)\left(1 - \frac{kD_c}{n}\right)}$$

where:

D_p = the emmetropizing power of the lens in diopters for a thin lens
D_c = the refracting power of the cornea in diopters
k = the estimated postoperative anterior chamber depth in meters
a = the axial length in meters
n = the refractive index of aqueous and vitreous (1.336).

For practical reasons, a nomogram has been constructed based on this formula (Fig. IV-10).

M.C. Colenbrander (personal communication, 1969) suggested the following formula for a planoconvex intraocular lens:

$$F_L = \frac{N_L}{L - v - 0.00005} - \frac{N_L}{\frac{N_L}{F_c} - v - 0.00005}$$

where:

F_L = the emmetropizing power of the lens in diopters
F_c = the power of the cornea in diopters
v = the distance from the anterior surface of the cornea to the anterior surface of the implant lens
L = the axial length

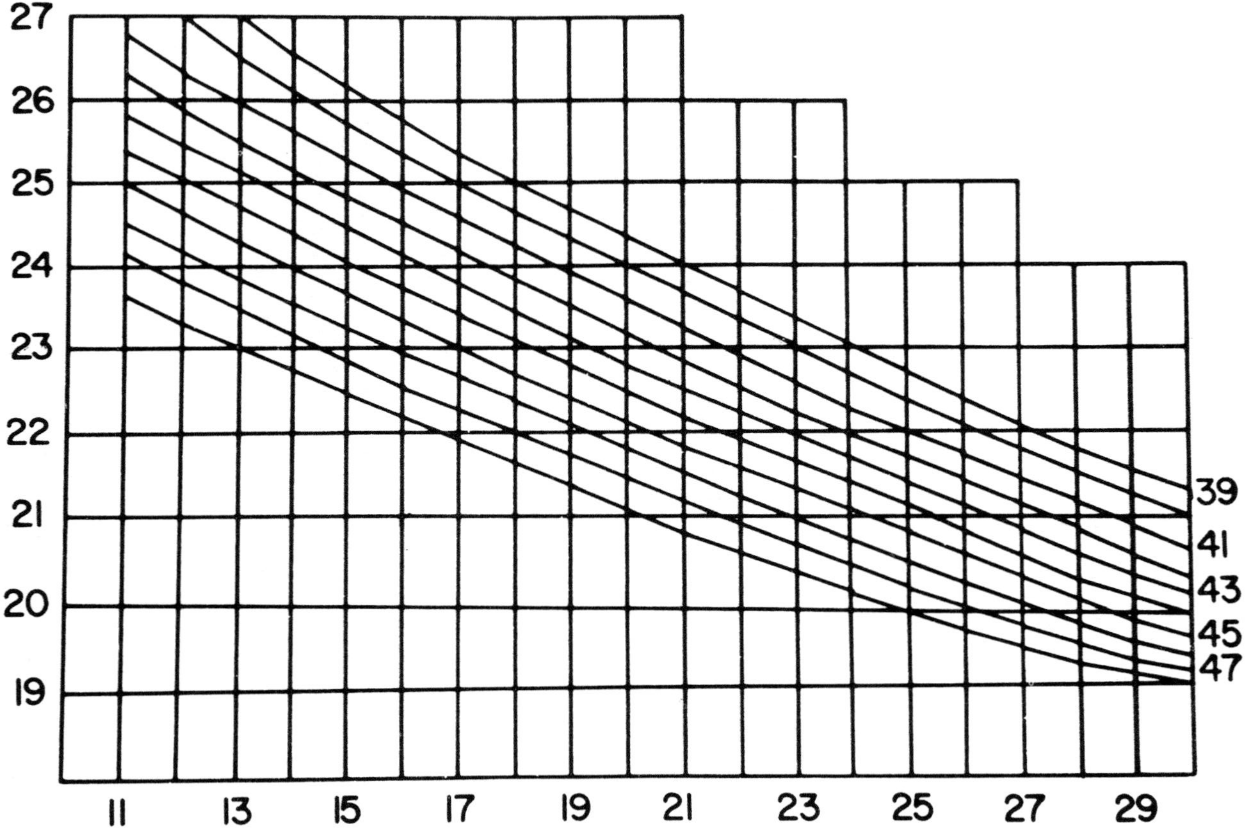

Fig. IV-10. — Nomogram for calculation of implant power based on Fyodorov's formula. Lens power in aqueous (abscis); axial length and corneal power (ordinates).

N_L = the refractive index of aqueous and vitreous (1.336)
0.05 mm = the distance of the second principal point of the lens from its anterior surface.

On the basis of this formula, a graph (Fig. IV-11) was drawn from which the influence of variations in axial length, depth of the anterior chamber, and corneal refractive power on the standard 18 diopter figure can be derived. If indicated, the refractive power of the patient's spectacles can be added to, or subtracted from, the refractive power of the cornea after being converted to the equivalent power at the cornea.

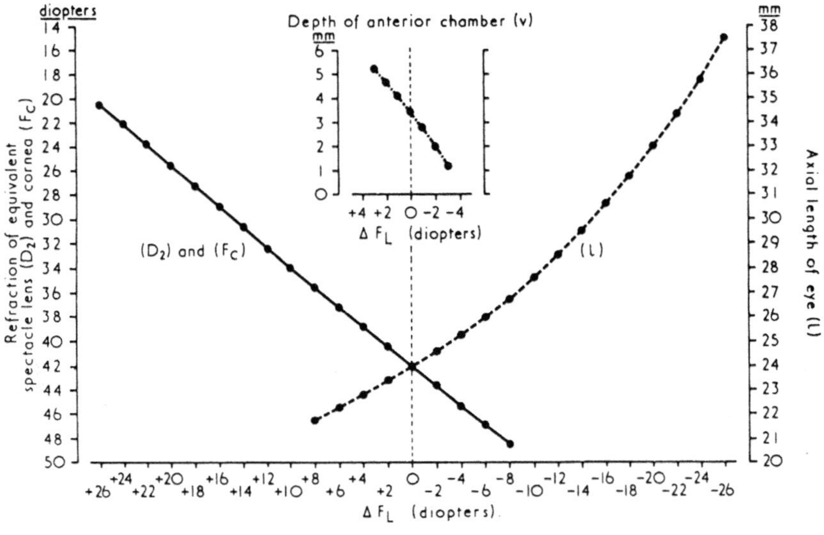

Fig. IV-11. — Deflection (ΔF_L) from normal (18 diopters) of the refractive power of the clip lens as a result of the refractive power of the spectable lens (D) + cornea (F_c), depth of anterior chamber (v), and axial length of the eye (L) (Colenbrander, 1973).

H. Gernet et al. (1971) derived another formula:

$$D_L = \frac{n - LD_c}{(L-d)\left(1 - \frac{dD_c}{n}\right)}$$

where:

D_L = the emmetropizing power of the implant in diopters
D_c = the power of the cornea in diopters
L = axial length
n = the refractive index of aqueous and vitreous (1.336)

d = the distance between the anterior surface of the cornea and the anterior surface of the implant lens.

Gernet has worked out tables with a computer for all the possible combinations and variations of the data.

In 1972, C.D. Binkhorst constructed a diagram based on Colenbrander's formula. In Figure IV-12, the values are given for a plano-convex pseudophakos with a 3.5 mm corneal apex distance. If the corneal apex distance is expected to vary, 0.5 diopter should be added or subtracted for every 0.3 mm deviation.

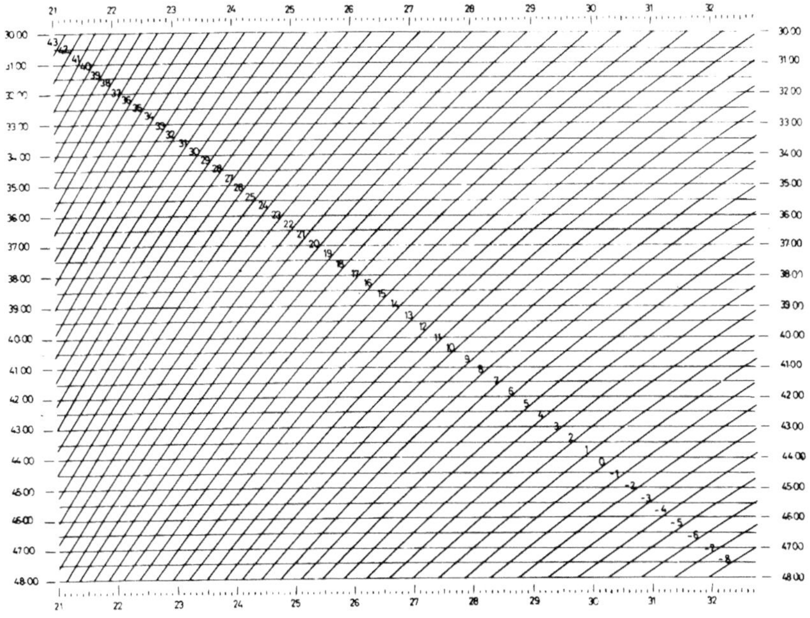

Fig. IV-12. — Diagram giving the relation between the corneal apex distance of the posterior focal point (axial length), the dioptric value of the corneal surface, and the lens power, the lens being placed at 3.5 mm corneal apex distance (C.D. Binkhorst, 1973).

Oguchi and Van Balen (1974) suggested the following formula:

$$D_L = n \frac{1}{L - d - \left(1 - \dfrac{1}{n''}\right) t} - \frac{1}{\dfrac{n}{n' - 1} r - d}$$

where:

D_L = the emmetropizing power of the implant lens

r = the radius of curvature of the cornea in meters

L = the axial length in meters
n = the refractive index of aqueous (1.336)
n' = the refractive index of the cornea (1.332)
n'' = the refractive index of the implant (1.493)
d = the expected depth of the anterior chamber in meters
t = the thickness of the implant lens in meters.

For practical purposes, a nomogram was constructed (Fig. IV-13), in which the expected postoperative anterior chamber depth is assumed to be 3.2 mm.

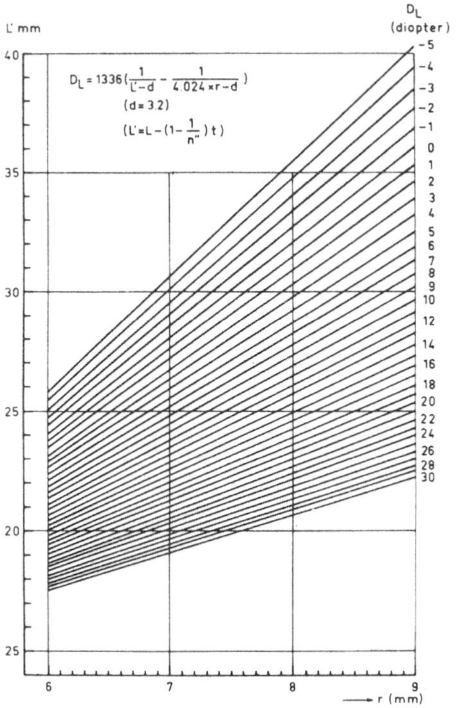

Fig. IV-13. — Diagram for calculating the emmetropizing power of an implant lens. The depth of the anterior chamber is taken to be 3.2 mm; r = the radius of corneal curvature; L = the optical axial length; n'' = refractive index of the implant lens; t = the thickness of the implant lens (Oguchi and van Balen, 1974).

Richard Binkhorst (1975) derived the following formula:

$$D = \frac{1336(4r-a)}{(a-d)(4r-d)}$$

where:

D = the dioptric power in aqueous or vitreous (refractive index = 1.336) of an emmetropizing implant lens

r = the radius of curvature of the anterior surface of the cornea in millimeters

a = the axial length in millimeters

d = the distance in millimeters between the anterior vertex of the cornea and the implant lens.

Unlike most of the other formulas, those of R. Binkhorst and Oguchi and Van Balen use the radius of curvature of the anterior corneal surface instead of its dioptric power. For the refractive index of the cornea, 1.333 (4/3) is used, which is within the range of values used for various keratometers (1.3375 for Haag, Streit, and Bausch and Lomb, 1.336 for American Optical, and 1.332 for Gambs). Since the value of 4/3 is near the lower end of the scale, the formula yields slightly higher implant power values.

R. Binkhorst also worked out other formulas:

— To compute the implant lens power required to create any refractive error at any vertex distance:

$$D = \frac{1336\,\{4r-a-[v(4r-a)+0.003ar]\,Rs\}}{a-d\,\{4r-d-[v(4r-d)+0.003dr]\,Rs\}}$$

R_s = spectacle refraction in diopters

v = vertex distance in millemeters.

— To compute the refractive error at any vertex distance that can be expected from an implant lens of known power:

$$Rs = \frac{1336(4r-a)-D(a-d)(4r-d)}{1336[v(4r-a)+0.003ar]-D(a-d)[v(4r-d)+0.003dr}$$

D = dioptive power in aqueous of the intraocular lens.

Magnetic strips are available to program pocket calculators for these formulas (Texas Instruments and Hewlett Packard).

G.L. Van der Heyde (1975) proposed the following formula for calculating the emmetropizing power of an implant lens:

$$F_L = \frac{n}{b-d_1-d_2-d_3\left(1-\frac{n}{n_2}\right)} - \frac{1}{\left(\frac{1}{F_c}\right)\left(\frac{d_2}{n}\right)}$$

where:

F_L	=	the emmetropizing power of the implant lens
b	=	the axial length in meters
F_c	=	the power of the cornea
d_1	=	the corneal thickness
d_2	=	the postoperative anterior chamber depth
d_3	=	the thickness of the implant lens
n_2	=	the index of refraction of the implant lens

Van der Heyde also published a nomogram (Fig. IV-14) for this formula from which one can read the emmetropizing power of the implant lens for a given depth of the anterior chamber (3.5 mm) by connecting the values of the cornea and the axial length with a

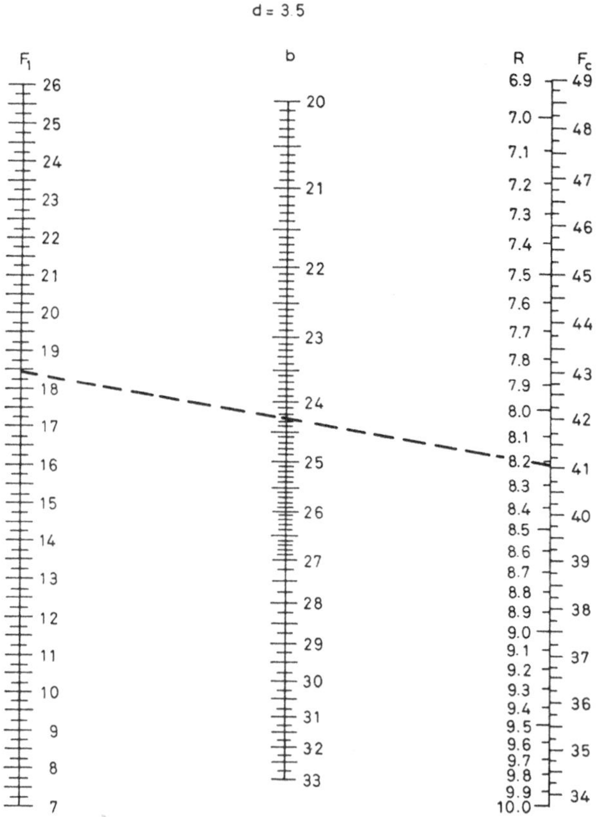

Fig. IV-14. — Nomogram for the determination of the *emmetropizing power* of the implant lens at 3.5 mm behind the anterior corneal surface; F_1 = the power of the implant lens; b = the axial length of the eye; F_c = the power of the cornea; R = the radius of the cornea (Van der Heyde, 1975).

straight edge. The (reduced) refractive index of the cornea used is 1.3375.

This nomogram was also converted to a very convenient circular slide rule (Fig. IV-15).

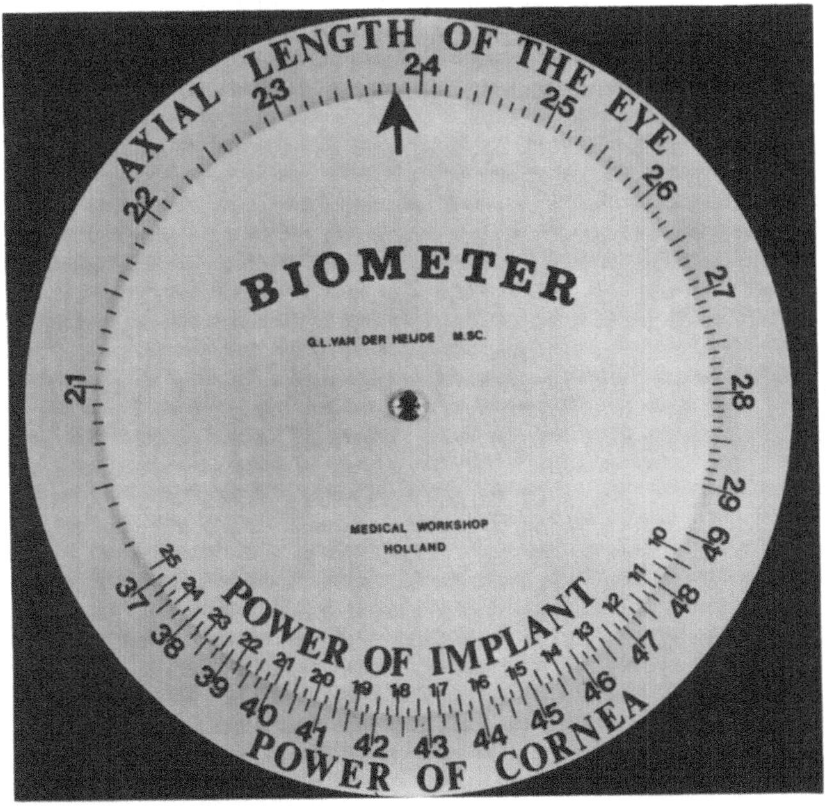

Fig. IV-15. — Circular slide rule for calculating the power of a prepullary lens (Van der Heyde).

J.M. Thyssen (1975) proposed the following formula:

$$P_{LE} = \frac{n_v}{1 - d_2 + \dfrac{d_3 \cdot n_v}{n_L}} - \frac{n_A}{\dfrac{n_A}{P_c} - d_2 + d_3}$$

where:

P_{LE} = the emmetropizing power of the implant lens
P_c = the power of the cornea minus 1 diopter
L = the axial length in meters

d_2 = the corneal thickness plus the postoperative anterior chamber depth in meters
n_V = the index of refraction of vitreous
n_A = the index of refraction of aqueous
n_L = the index of refraction of the implant lens
d_3 = the thickness of the implant lens.

Thyssen also constructed a nomogram (Fig. IV-16).

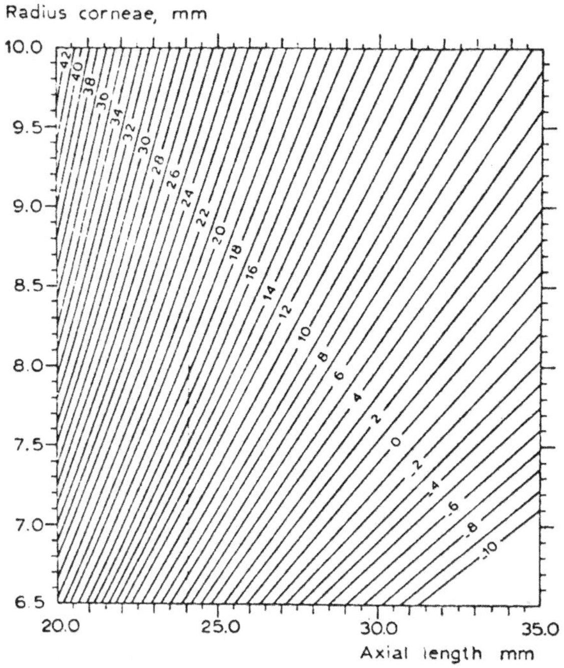

Fig. IV-16. — Nomogram for the calculation of the power of an implant giving emmetropia (Thyssen, 1975).

Discussion

Although the formulas and nomograms given above all have the same purpose, they are not identical nor do they use the same parameters. Fyodorov's formula applies only for a thin lens, for example, while those of Van der Heyde and Thyssen take the thickness of the implant into account.

Thyssen's formula also used three different refractive indices. R. Binkhorst's formula contains a refractive index for the cornea that is established from biometric values and the postoperative refractive status. As R. Drews (1977) pointed out, each formula gives a different answer for the same biometric data, as do the various nomograms. Table IV-10 gives an example of this.

TABLE IV-10. — *Variation in the Results Obtained from Different Nomograms Given: Corneal Power = 42 D, Axial Length = 24 mm, Distance from the Apex of the Cornea to the Implant = 3.5 mm (R. Drews 1977)*

	Results for emmetropizing implant	
	Formulas	*Nomogram*
Fyodorov et al.	17.98	17.40
Colenbrander	18.05	18*
R.D. Binkhorst	18.53	—
Van der Heyde	—	17.8
Thyssen	17.40	18.30

* Taken from C.D. Binkhorst's nomogram, which is based on Colenbrander's formula.

In clinical practice even more variation may be expected than the table indicates for a number of reasons:

1. The K-readings for a patient with an advanced cataract may be inexact because of faulty fixation. Postoperative changes in the corneal radius may also account for some error in this respect. According to R. Binkhorst (1975), a postoperative increase in the corneal radius of 0.1 mm would account for a shortening of the axial length of 0.06 to 0.11 mm, depending on the radius of curvature and the diameter of the cornea. Both the flattening of the cornea and the concomitant shortening of the axial length may be reasons for undercorrection in pseudophakic eyes.
2. The postoperative anterior chamber depth may also interfere with the calculated implant power value: an error of 0.1 mm in the final position of the implant will result in a refractive error of approximately 0.1 diopters.
3. Errors can also occur in the measurement of the axial length. A 1% error in the measured axial length—about 0.25 mm—results in an error of about 1 diopter. This certainly makes large qualitative demands on measurement apparatus. According to R. Binkhorst, modern echographic instruments using frequencies of 20 MHz or more can be accurate to within 0.1 mm (0.1 mm = ±0.25 diopters refractive error).

4. A rather unexpected source of error is mislabeling of the dioptric power by the manufacturer. Already in the mid-sixties S. Fyodorov, aware of this problem, constructed his lenses with the power engraved near the lensedge. In a series of 300 lenses from 8 different companies, McReynolds and Snider (1978) found only 35% of them to have the power indicated by the manufacturer. In 52%, the measured lens power did not exceed 2 diopters of the indicated value, but the remaining 13% varied from 2 to 9 diopters from the manufacturer's label. Loyd et al. (1979) measured 400 lenses from 5 different manufacturers: 58.3% of

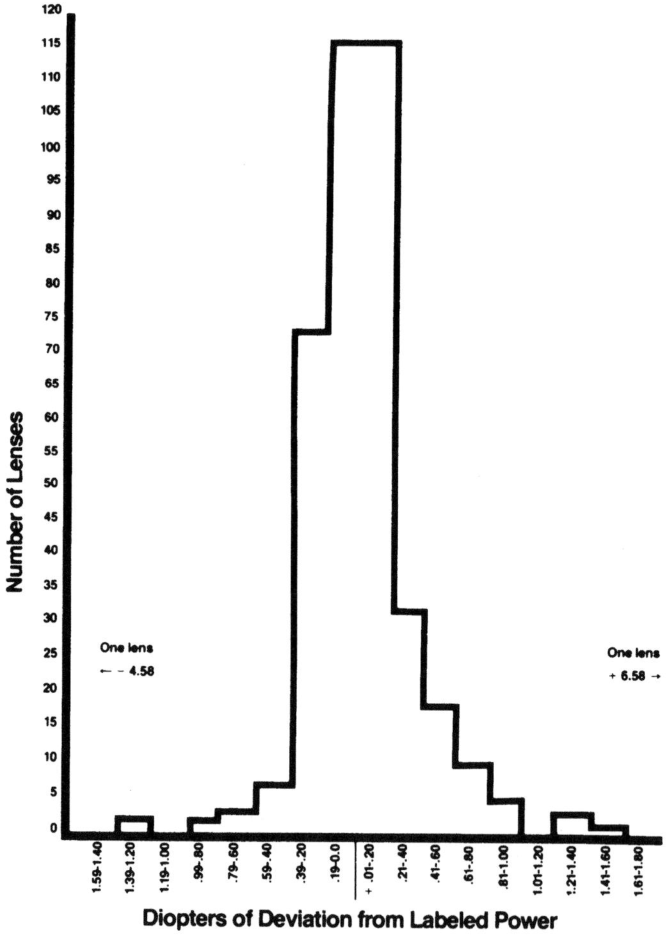

Fig. IV-17. — Histogram of lens labeling errors in 400 lenses (Loyd, Montgomery, and Gills, 1979, p. 229).

them were within ±0.2 diopters of the indicated value; 97.74% were within ±1.0 diopters, but 2.26% were mislabeled by more than one diopter.

The method of measuring the power of an implant lens under sterile conditions was developed by McReynolds and Snider (1978). The lens is placed, convex surface down, in the concave central portion of a glass disc, which is filled with saline and sealed off with a planoparallel second disc. To ensure sterility, the "chamber" is placed in a plexiglas petri dish. The measurement of the dioptric power is then done with a lensometer held vertically. The saline of the chamber reduces the refractive power of an average implant lens from 60 to 20 diopters. The concavity of the chamber further reduces the power another 10 diopters. Thus, 10 diopters has to be added to the recorded dioptric power measured with the lensometer.

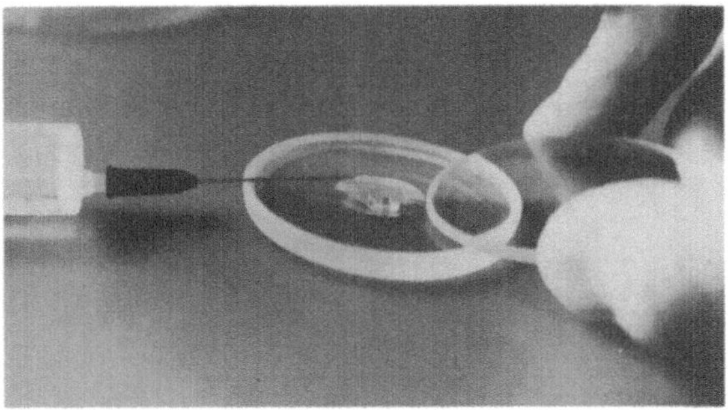

Fig. IV-18. — McReynolds' device for control of the dioptric power under sterile conditions.

V. Determination of the Iseikonic Lens Power

As illustrated above, there are many ways of determining the power of an implant lens and also many sources of error. The surgeon is also faced with various options: he can restore the basic refraction, make the eye emmetropic, or try to achieve a desired degree of ametropia. These options are sharply limited, however, when the binocular needs of the patient are taken into account. For as we have already noted, the replacement of the natural lens by an artificial lens nearly always changed the original retinal image size, thus causing various degrees of aniseikonia that may interfere with comfortable binocular vision. Ridley's posterior chamber lenses had the advantage of being located nearly in the same plane as the original lens. Similarly, the modern posterior chamber lens significantly reduces the problem of residual aniseikonia.

Dudragne (1955) calculated the radius and thickness of a pupillary lens with a concavo-convex optic (meniscus form) that would bring the cardinal points and the principle focal planes into their original position (see Fig. IV-19). Such a lens would be capable of achieving both emmetropia and iseikonia. A few of these lenses have been implanted, but further implantation was discontinued for one reason or another.

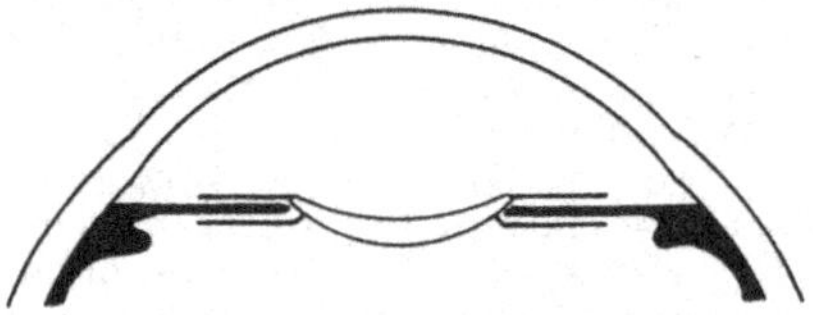

Fig. IV-19. — Modified iris clip lens according to Dudragnes's calculations (Binkhorst, 1961).

In 1964, R.D. Binkhorst, Weinstein, and Troutman proposed a two-element pupillary intraocular lens with an enclosed air space. Theoretically, this doublet composed of a negative and a positive lens acting as an inverted Gallilean system would eliminate aniseikonia (see Fig. IV-20). This design has never been implemented.

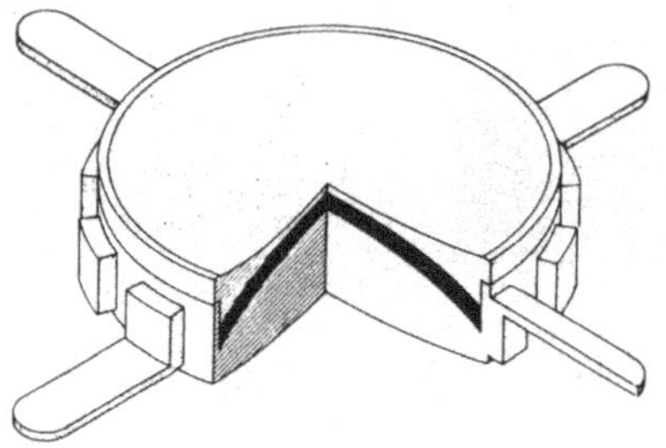

Fig. IV-20. — Perspective diagram of the air space doublet. (Courtesy R.C. Troutman.)

In 1972, C.D. Binkhorst described his method for determining the iseikonic prepupillary pseudophakos based on the data for Gullstrand's schematic eye.

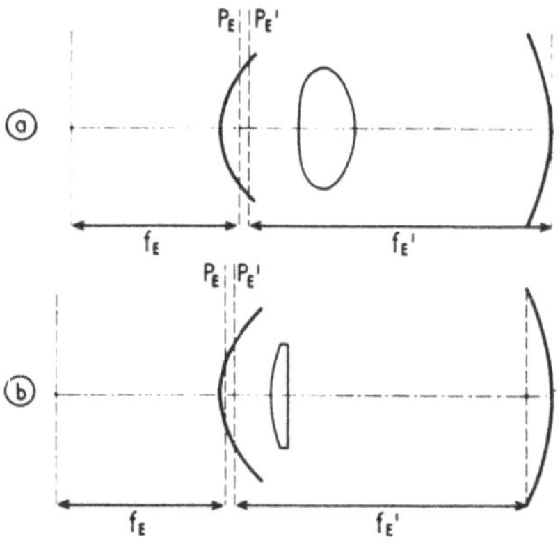

Fig. IV-21. — Schematic phakic eye (a) and schematic iseikonic pseudophakic eye (b) (Binkhorst, 1972).
P_E first equivalent plane
$P_E{}^1$ second equivalent plane
f_E anterior focal length
$f_E{}^1$ posterior focal length

The following relationship for the focal length was used.

$$f_E = \frac{f_c \cdot f_L}{f_L + f_c 1 - d}$$

where:

f_E = the anterior focal length of the complete eye (−17.055 mm)
f_c = the anterior focal length of the cornea (−23.227 mm)
f_c^1 = the posterior focal length of the cornea (31.031 mm)
d = the distance of the first equivalent plane of the pseudophakos from the second equivalent plane of the cornea (3.5506 mm)
f_L = the focal length of the pseudophakos.

The value of d was calculated by assuming a corneal vertex distance of $v = 3.5$ mm.

The focal length of the schematic iseikonic pseudophakos (f_L) turned out to be 75.921 mm, which gives a radius of the anterior surface (r_1) of 8.751 mm and an equivalent power of the pseudophakos (F_L) of 17.6 *D*. Hence,

$$r_1 = \frac{1.49 - 1.336}{1.336} \cdot f_L \qquad F_L = \frac{1.49 - 1.336}{r_1}$$

Since the pseudophakos is in a more forward position than the crystalline lens, the equivalent planes of the pseudophakic eye are further forward than those of the phakic eye. If the focal lengths are the same, this results in a more forward position of the posterior focal point and plus ametropia. For the schematic pseudophakic eye, the anterior displacement of the second equivalent plane and the correlated myopia was calculated as follows:

The distance of the second equivalent plane of the pseudophakos (P_L^1) from its posterior surface is

$$-n_1 \cdot \frac{t}{n_2} \cdot \frac{F_L^1}{F_L} = 0.448 \text{ mm},$$

in which t is the centre thickness of the pseudophakos (0.5 mm), n_1 is the refractive index of the aqueous (1.336), n_2 is the refractive index of the pseudophakos (1.490), and $F_L^1 = F_L$. The corneal vertex distance of the second equivalent plane of the pseudophakos is thus $3.5 + 0.5 - 0.448 = 3.552$ mm.

The distance of the second equivalent plane of the schematic pseudophakic eye (P_E^1) from the second equivalent plane of the pseudophakos (P_L^1) equals

$$\frac{d \cdot f_L}{d - f_L - f_c^1} = -2.607 \text{ mm},$$

in which d = distance of first equivalent plane of pseudophakos (P_L^1) from the second equivalent plane of the cornea P_c^1 (3.5506 mm), f_L focal length of pseudophakos (75.921 mm), and f_c^1 posterior focal length of cornea (31.031 mm). The corneal vertex distance of the second equivalent plane of the pseudophakic eye is therefore $3.552 - 2.607 = 0.945$ mm.

Compared with the corneal vertex distance of the second equivalent plane in Gullstrand's schematic phakic eye of 1.602 mm, the second equivalent plane of the schematic iseikonic eye is in a 0.657 mm more forward position. Calculation with Newton's object image relation $x.x' = f.f'$ shows that this corresponds with a 1.69 *D* myopia at the anterior focal point.

Thus, for the ideal emmetropic eye having a corneal power of 42 *D* and an axial length of 24 mm, a 19.5 D prepupillary lens at 3.5 mm from the apex of the cornea will result in iseikonia if the residual myopia of 1.7 D is corrected with spectacles. So, in emmetropia, there cannot be iseikonia without residual anisometropia when using prepupillary lenses.

Similarly, when using these prepupillary lenses, the axially ametropic schematic eye would theoretically have to be made 1.7 *D* more myopic or less hypermetropic to restore the original retinal image size.

Various practical methods have been proposed to calculate the iseikonic implant power in emmetropia or in ametropia of whatever origin. Formulas, nomograms, and computer programs were developed in which the refractive and biometric data of both eyes can be introduced. The basic principle of all these methods primarily involves equalization of the posterior focal lengths.

Gernet et al. (1971) developed formulas for determining the posterior focal length that are used with a computed table.

For clinical practice, C.D. Binkhorst (1973) recommended using Colenbrander's nomogram. In the case of a unilateral cataract, the corneal power of the eye to be operated on is first corrected with the spectacle power of the fellow phakic eye. Second, the axial length of the fellow eye must be decreased by 0.657 mm because of the forward displacement of the second principal plane in the pseudophakic eye relative to its position in the phakic eye. Hence, this displacement of 0.657 mm corresponds to a −1.69 *D* anisometropia. In the same simple way, the iseikonic lens power can be found when the fellow eye is pseudophakic. In this case, the axial length of the fellow eye need not be corrected by −0.657 mm. If the spectacle correction exceeds 5 *D*, the conversion tables compiled for contact lens power should be used.

Another method employs the nomograms devised by G.L. Van der Heyde. The principle of Van der Heyde's method is as follows: with a unilateral cataract the posterior focal length (f_E) of the fellow phakic eye is calculated by using the spectacle correction (F_s), the corneal power (F_c), the anterior segment depth (d) and the axial length (L) of that eye. These values are introduced into

Nomogram B, which is derived from the following formula (Van der Heyde, 1976):

$$\frac{n_6}{f_E} = \frac{1 - d_2 F_s}{n_3}\left(1 - \frac{d_1}{n_2} F_1\right)\left(\frac{n_6}{L - d_3}\right)\left(1 - \frac{d_3}{n_4} F'_c\right)$$

where:

n_2 = refractive index of spectacles
n_3 = refractive index of air (1.000)
n_4 = refractive index of aqueous (1.336)
n_6 = refractive index of vitreous (1.336)
d_1 = thickness of the spectacles
d_2 = vertex distance from the spectacles to the cornea
d_3 = depths of the anterior chamber plus the corneal thickness (d_3 should be corrected by +62.5% of the lens thickness as measured by echography).

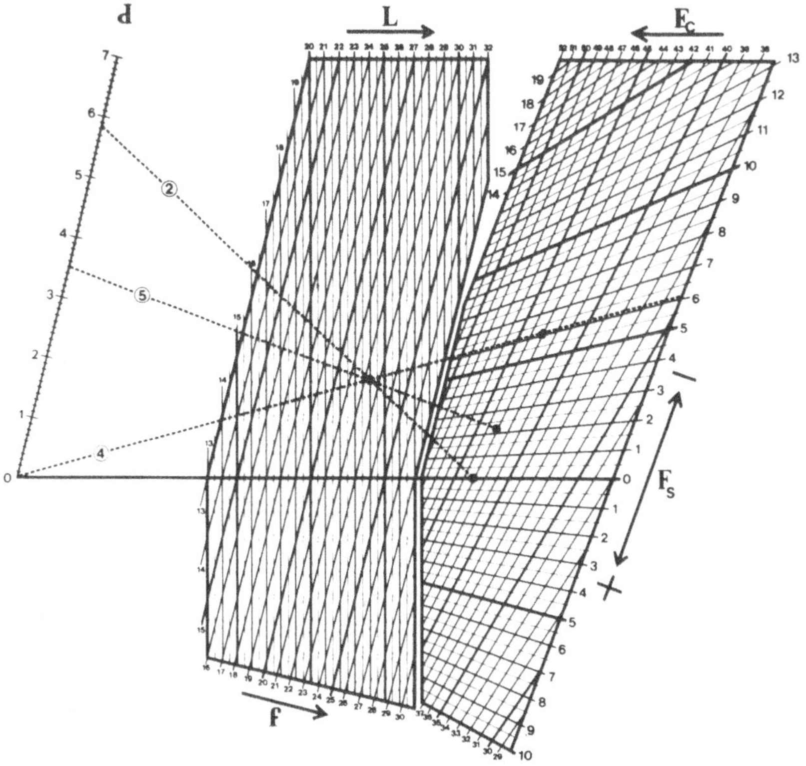

Fig. IV-22. — Nomogram B of Van der Heyde (1976) for the determination of the post-operative refraction of the pseudophakic eye when rendered iseikonic.

Using the thus determined posterior focal length (f_E) along with the corneal power (F_c), the axial length (L), and the expected anterior segment depth (d_E), the postoperative refraction of the pseudophakic eye is also obtained with Nomogram *B*.

Finally, the power of the iseikonic implant lens (F_L) is obtained by means of Nomogram *A*, which is based on the following formula (Van der Heyde, 1976, p. 85):

$$F_1 = \frac{n_6}{L-d_s} - \frac{1}{\dfrac{1-d_3}{F'_c n_4}}$$

where:

d_3 = depth of the anterior chamber plus corneal thickness
n_4 = refractive index of aqueous (1.336)
n_6 = refractive index of vitreous (1.336)

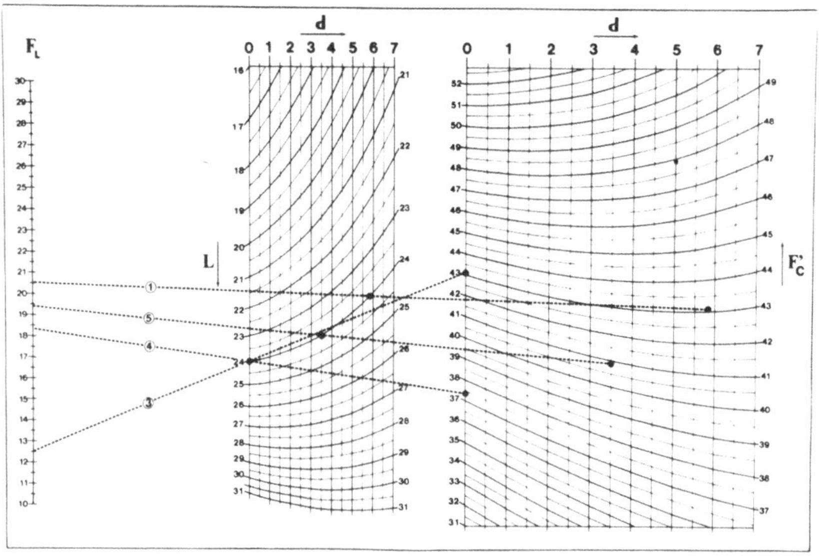

Fig. IV-23. — Nomogram A according to Van der Heyde (1976) for the determination of the power of the iseikonic implant lens (F_L).

In this nomogram, $F'c$ represents the corneal power of the cataractous eye corrected by the spectacle correction as found above, d is the assumed postoperative anterior chamber depth, and L the axial length of the cataractous eye.

The same method can be used to determine the iseikonic pseudophakic power when the fellow eye is already pseudophakic or aphakic. However, it is not necessary to correct the depth of the anterior chamber (d_3) of the already pseudophakic fellow eye with 62.5% to find its posterior focal length. It should also be noted that d_3 for an aphakic eye corrected with a contact lens is zero.

R.D. Binkhorst (1975) used a different method to calculate the iseikonic implant power with a unilateral cataract. In his method, the determination of the axial length of the eye to be operated on is not used to find the iseikonic lens power, which eliminates ultrasonic measurement errors due to either fixation problems or variations in the velocity transmission of the crystallin. The method involves 3 steps:

Step one: Calculation of the posterior focal length of the crystalline lens in the fellow eye with the following formula:

$$F = \frac{(a-ACD-2.21)\left(\dfrac{1336}{D_c+R_c} - ACD-2.08\right)}{\dfrac{1336}{D_c+R_c} - a+2.21-2.08}$$

where:
F = the focal length of the crystalline lens in mm
a = the axial length in mm
ACD = the anterior chamber depth in mm
D_c = the dioptric power of the cornea
R_c = the refraction at the cornea in diopters
and 2.08 and 2.21 are the respective schematic values for the distances of the anterior and posterior principal planes for the crystalline lens from its anterior vertex in mm.

Step two: Determination of the anterior focal length of the phakic fellow eye:

$$F_1 = \frac{1000F}{D_c[F-(ACD+2.08)]+1336}$$

where F_1 = the anterior focal length in mm

Step three: Calculation of the iseikonic power of the implant lens using the anterior focal length (F_1) of the fellow eye:

$$D = \frac{1336\left(\frac{3r}{F_1} - 1\right)}{4r-d}$$

where:

D = the dioptric power in aqueous of the intraocular lens
F_1 = the anterior focal length of the fellow eye in mm
r = the radius of curvature of the anterior surface of the cornea of the cataractous eye in mm

As R.D. Binkhorst notes, if the spectacle corrections of both eyes were placed at their respective anterior focal points, the two eyes would theoretically have the same image size since their anterior focal lengths would be equal. However, since the spectacle correction is usually worn closer to the eye and the refraction of the pseudophakic eye is less hyperopic or more myopic, there will still be a difference in image size, i.e., the image of the pseudophakic eye will be slightly larger. This error can be anticipated by selecting an implant that usually would have to be 0.25 to 0.50 diopters stronger

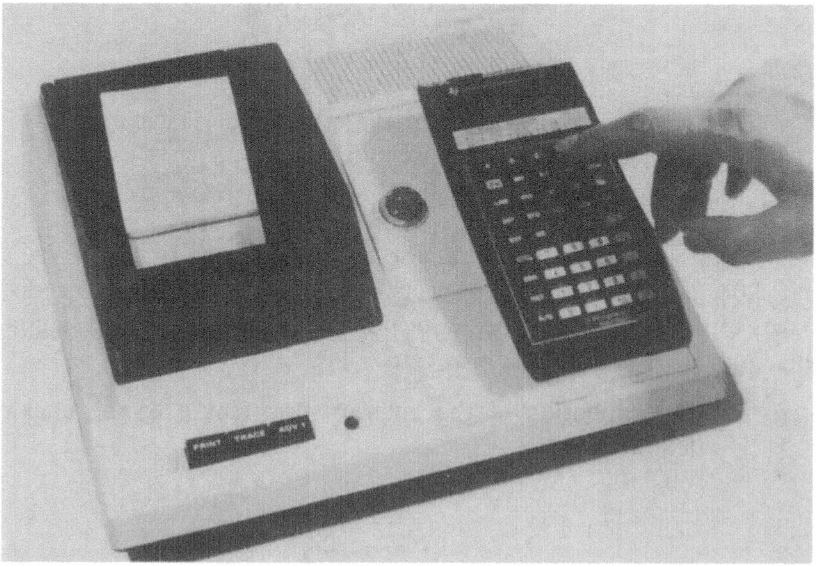

Fig. IV-24. — Pocket calculator programmed for IOL power calculation and printer. (Courtesy R.D. Binkhorst.)

than the value calculated by means of the above formula. R.D. Binkhorst also noted that if one wants to know the final spectacle refraction of the pseudophakic eye, the axial length of the cataractous eye has to be measured and introduced into the following formula:

$$R_s = \frac{1336(4r-a) - D(a-d)(4r-d)}{1336\,[v(4r-a) + 0.003\,ar] - D(a-d)\,[v(4r-d) + 0.003\,dr]}$$

where:
D = the dioptric power of the iseikonic implant
V = the vertex distance in meters.

For practical purposes, the calculation of iseikonic implant power for different situations can be performed with the programs designed by R.D. Binkhorst for pocket calculators. Calculator programs have also been designed by other authors (Drews, Hoffer, Thyssen).

VI. Practical Considerations on the Proper Selection of the Implant Power

As we have explained, specifications of the lens power that rest on clinical, non-biometric data are subject to various degrees of error. The systematic use of standard power lenses is, therefore, limited. Even if the data of the basic refraction can be accurately traced, the application of the 1.25 diopter rule is only valid for those cases in which the power of the original crystalline lens does not deviate very much from the average crystalline lens power. With the advent of ultrasonography, nearly all the parameters can be evaluated preoperatively, so that the lens power can be determined in function of what one wants to achieve. A number of options are open:

— For patients with advanced bilateral cataracts whose needs, for example, are met sufficiently with cataract extraction and lens implantation in one eye, one may aim to restore either the previous ametropic condition or to render the eye emmetropic or slightly myopic. The last condition is preferable for the elderly patient whose life is largely conducted indoors.

— When bilateral implantation is considered for elderly patients, the same options for the first eye are open. The power of the implant lens for the second eye should be selected to restore binocular comfort.

— In contrast to these cases are those of strict unilateral cataract where the restoration of binocular vision is essential. In children, for whom one must take account of the great power of accommodation of the fellow eye, binocular vision in general is best served by choosing the power of the implant in such a way that the uncorrected pseudophakic eye is equiped for near vision. This eliminates the magnification inherent in additional spectacle corrections for the pseudophakic eye.

— For adults, the restoration of binocular vision should be considered in function of occupational demands. A number of situations can arise. For example, if emmetropia and binocular vision for distance are both required, it can be that emmetropization of the pseudophakic eye is not always synonymous with iseikonia, as has been substantially demonstrated. On the basis of biometric data, one then has to determine whether a lens in the prepupillary position or one in the posterior chamber will best resolve the problem. When the use of spectacles is not contraindicated iseikonia can be obtained with various implant lenses.

— Another category of patients are those with bilateral evolutive lens opacifications for whom the selection of the lens power for the worst eye may be significantly influenced by the status of the fellow eye. Indeed, when the fellow eye shows pronounced lenticular myopia but still with good visual acuity, a great deal will depend on when the cataract surgery must be performed. When there is a slow evolution, the first eye has to be made iseikonic with the fellow eye if serious complaints about binocular discomfort are to be avoided. As we have demonstrated, the spectacle correction of the pseudophakic eye will be about 1.5 diopters greater than the myopic correction of the phakic fellow eye when a prepupillary pseudophakos is implanted. Although this postoperative condition is iseikonic, it can be very frustrating for the patient. Indeed, a patient who was nearly emmetropic for several decades will be rarely pleased with strong myopia in the operated eye and with the prospect that the other eye will be about as myopic after the second intervention. One possible solution is, therefore, to neglect temporary binocular vision and to aim at any desired postoperative refractive status. This must, of course, be discussed with the patient. Another option is to provide the lenticular myopic fellow phakic eye with a contact lens temporarily. This would allow the selection of a weaker implant lens power while still providing binocular comfort.

— Another situation is that of bilateral developmental cataract in patients with longstanding precataractous aniseikonia. Indeed, as Huber and C.D. Binkhorst (1979) have observed, some of these patients may well have adapted to this longstanding aniseikonia, so that making the two eyes iseikonic will create subjective aniseikonia of the opposite sign. It might therefore be preferable to make the pseudophakic eye iseikonic with its pre-cataract refraction rather than with the other, assymetric eye. This will preserve the difference in posterior focal lengths and the degree of pre-cataract optical aniseikonia.

— Yet another situation occurs in the patient who is already aphakic in one eye that is corrected with a contact lens and who strongly prefers an implant lens for the fellow cataractous eye. Here, too, various possibilities are available depending on the biometric status of both eyes. If the eye pair is emmetropic, the phakic eye wearing the contact lens would present a magnification of some 6%. To achieve iseikonia, a prepupillary lens could be used (e.g., an angle supported lens), which offers the greatest possible magnification because of its location. But still, this choice could be inadequate. Another possibility would be to select any lens type that could render the pseudophakic eye some 3 diopters hyperopic, which, in turn, would require an additional spectacle correction of 3 diopters to enlarge the image by some 6%. Again the exact calculation of the iseikonic dioptric power of any given lens type can be done with the available formulas, nomograms, or computer programs.

CHAPTER V

PRE-, PER-, AND POSTOPERATIVE MANAGEMENT OF LENS IMPLANTATION

In this chapter, we shall consider some special aspects of lens implantation. We presume that the selection of both the lens model and the eye takes place according to criteria representative of the current state of the art and that the patient has been fully informed of the advantages and risks involved in the new techniques. Because the implant procedure may have to be aborted due to factors that arise during surgery, the patient should be told that a lens cannot always be implanted. And, in some countries, the medico-legal situation requires that "informed consent" be obtained from the patient in writing.

I. Preoperative Management

A. Clean and Aseptic Surgery

Since the introduction of germs and foreign material into the eye may cause inflammatory reactions and infection, clean and asceptic surgery is one of the first conditions for successful implant surgery.

1. *Clean Eye Surgery*

Clean eye surgery involves taking reasonable, though the maximum possible, measures to keep unwanted foreign material out of the eye. C.D. Binkhorst routinely inspects all instruments for lint and dust and places them on a lint-free sheet of synthetic material. When gloves are used, special attention must be paid to keep glove powder away from the operation field because its toxicity (Drews, 1976).

To reduce the amount of atmospheric particles, lint-free drapping should be used. In addition, Worst (1975) recommends directing a laminar flow of filtered air across the operating field.

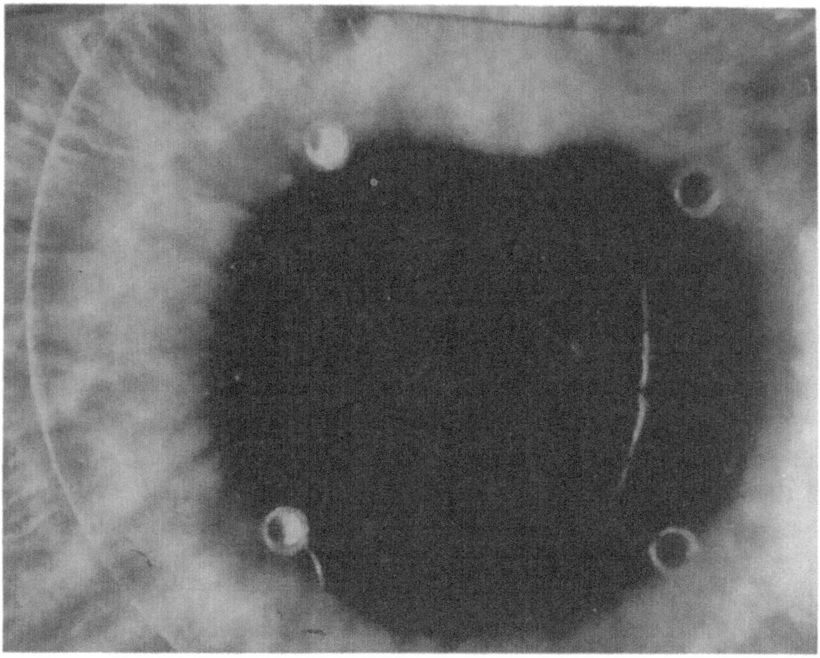

Fig. V-1. — The curved silvery foreign body in the pupillary aperture was unadvertently introduced into the eye during surgery and caused a vitreous abscess and endophthalmitis (which fortunately responded to antibiotics). (Courtesy R. Drews.)

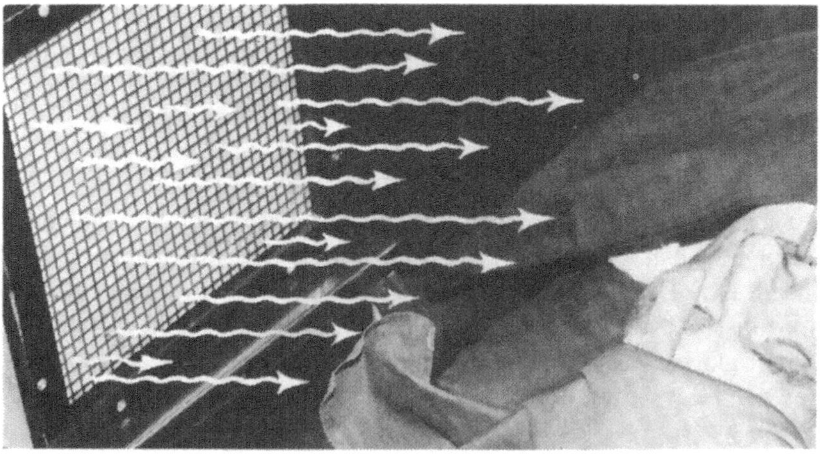

Fig. V-2. — J. Worst's technique of directing a laminar flow of filtered air across the operating field to eliminate lint and dust.

Due to the electrostatic properties of plastic, dry implant lenses have the unfortunate property of attracting foreign material. Therefore, as soon as the lens is removed form its container, it should be immersed in fluid. It should never be touched with the fingers, not even when gloved, but only with the appropriate instruments. If the implant has foreign material adhering to it or spots, it is better to discard it instead of attempting to clean it. The implant should never be laid on the cornea or the conjunctiva.

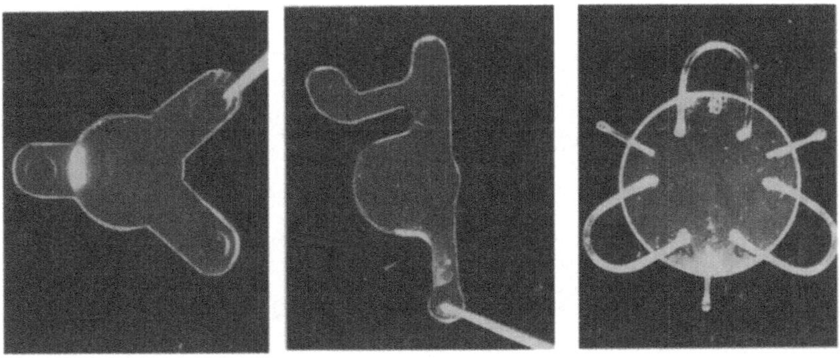

Fig. V-3. — Dust and deposits on lenses.

During implant surgery, more fluid is required than is necessary for simple cataract extraction. But this can cause unwanted foreign material to enter the eye. R. Drews and J. Worst (1975) recommend that all intraocular solutions be passed through millipore filters (see also the discussion on irrigating solutions below, pp. 453). However, according to W. Meltzer, R. Drews, and S. Hajek (Meltzer et al., 1981), not all types of millipore filters are innocuous. Indeed, membrane filters need to be treated with wetting agents or detergents to facilitate the passage of fluids. Unfortunately, as these authors point out, some manufacturers use highly toxic agents such as Triton X-100.

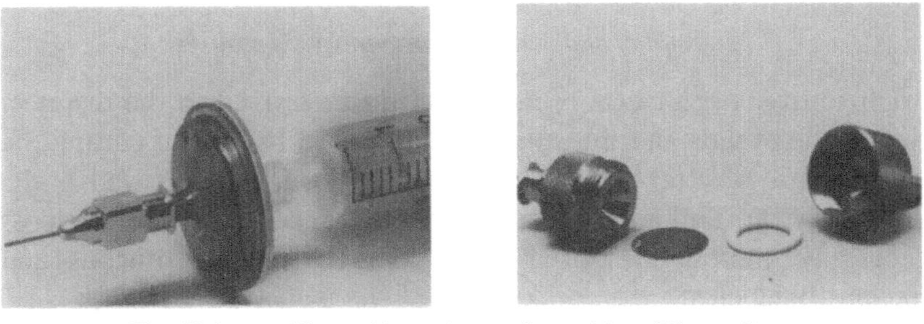

Fig. V-4a. — Disposable and non-disposable millipore filters.

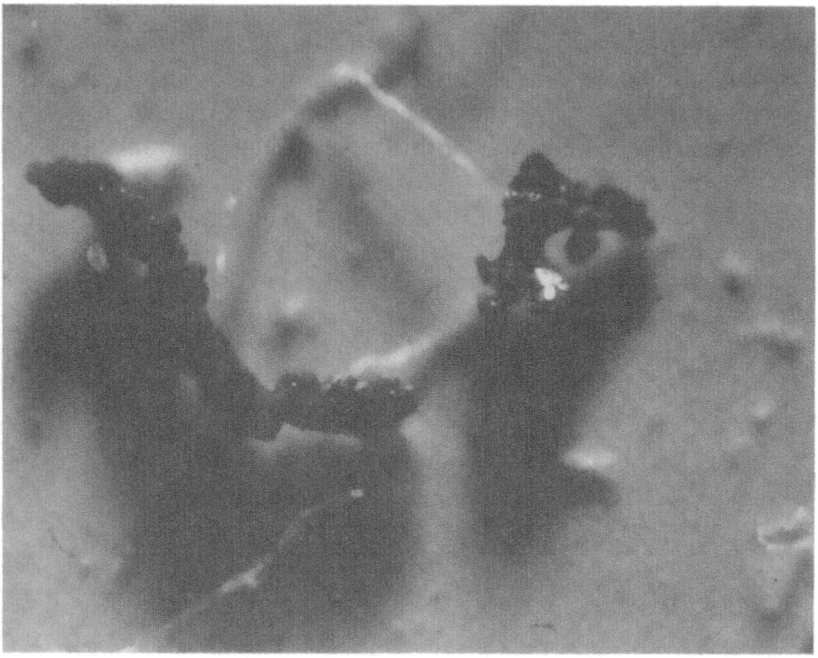

Fig. V-4b. — This is debris trapped on part of the surface of a millipore filter after filtering 1 cc of irrigating solution taken from a medicine glass on an operating room table at the end of a case. One sees lint, rubber, metal, and many small amorphous pieces of debris. Counts after such experiments have shown up to 900 particles per cc. All solutions that are not known to be particle free should be filtered before use. (Courtesy R. Drews.)

When intraocular suturing is necessary—when the lens must be fixed or a coloboma must be closed, for example—care should be taken to handle the needle only with clean instruments. Drews suggests passing the suture through subjunctival tissue before introducing it into the eye in order to remove possible contaminants.

2. *Aseptic and Anti-Inflammatory Measures*

Obviously, a great deal of attention must be given to the disinfection of the eyelids and the surrounding tissues. Instead of cutting the eyelashes, it is better to use Steridrape® to cover them as well as the skin. As C.D. Binkhorst recommends, the upper and lower fornices should be thoroughly rinsed with saline to remove mucous and foreign material.

Although the wisdom of routine preoperative administration of topical antibiotics and corticosteroids may be questioned, there are several surgeons who do so. The advantages of systemic use of antibiotics in routine lens implant surgery is also controverted.

The preoperative use of non-steroidal anti-inflammatory agents such as indomethacin eyedrops may possibly be indicated, though the benefits of these agents have yet to be confirmed.

NB: It is advisable to perform a tap of anterior chamber fluid at the end of the surgical procedure. The fluid should be inoculated in two different media, one for aerobic and one for anaerobic culture. Should postoperative infection occur, one then has information about the type of microorganism involved.

B. **The Pupil**

Whether or not the pupil is to be dilatated depends on the technique used to extract the cataract and on the type of lens to be inserted. Most lenses that are designed to be inserted after intracapsular cataract extraction do not require a large pupil; indeed, a rather small pupil is advantageous since it prevents vitreous interference in positioning the lens. But with extracapsular cataract extraction, adequate pupil dilatation is mandatory to facilitate removal of cortical remnants and to allow the proper insertion of some of the lens types that are designed to be fixated between the capsular flaps.

In general, one should aim at a mydriasis that can be reversed at the end of the procedure. Routine intracameral use of commercially available mydriatic and myotic agents should not be considered lightly, since serious complications such as corneal dystrophy may result.

C. **General or Local Anesthesia**

Whether local or general anesthesia is better for lens implantation has not yet been demonstrated. The arguments in favor of general anesthesia are:

— The surgeon may give all his attention to the surgical procedure.
— There is no risk of any sudden movements by the patient.
— The duration of the intervention is not limited.

In favor of local anesthesia:

— Patients with a borderline cardiovascular condition need not be subjected to the risks of general narcosis.

— The patient can be mobilized sooner.

Ultimately, it seems to come down to the personal preferences of the surgeon and the patient.

There are indications in the literature that many implant surgeons favor local anesthesia with pre- and peroperative administration of sedativa by an anesthesiologist, who also monitors the cardiovascular condition. With the advent of long-lasting local anesthetic agents with low toxicity (Marcaine), the time factor is no longer a problem. A mixture of equal doses of Xylocaine® and Marcaine® is gaining popularity.

D. **Visibility**

Good visibility is of paramount importance for the correct positioning of an intraocular lens, and so operating magnifiers or surgical microscopes are used. Lateral illumination significantly enhances the effectiveness of operating magnifiers.

As most intraocular maneuvers have to be observed through the cornea, it must be kept as transparent as possible. And as this transparency is largely dependent on the status of both the epithelium and the endothelium, regular irrigation of the cornea and avoidance of endothelial trauma are necessary. B. Drews and J. Worst advocate using a continual dripper to keep the cornea moist.

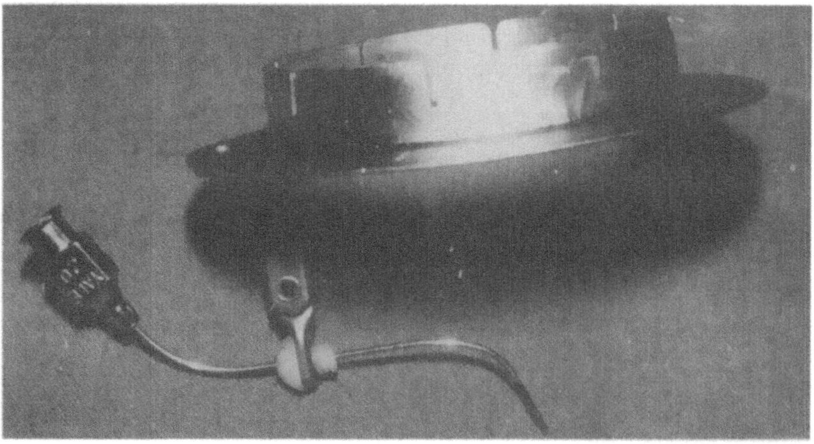

Fig. V-5. — The "Drews Dripper". This device is simply attached to the objective lens of the operating microscope. I.V. tubing supplying a balanced salt solution is connected to the lower lock and the rate of flow is adjusted so that a gentle continuous drip is maintained on the operating field (Drews, 1977).

Loose pigment and blood in the anterior chamber must be removed by means of gentle irrigation lest they interfere with visibility. Air in the anterior chamber can sometimes limit visibility, so the surgeon must decide if replacing it with fluid would improve the situation.

E. **Preparation of the Lens**

Depending on the sterilization technique, lenses come in wet or dry packets. Wet sterilized lenses have to be neutralized according to the manufacturer's directions. All lenses have to be thoroughly rinsed in saline before insertion. It is prudent to have spare lenses available should the lens at hand be inadvertantly dropped or become unsterile.

Obviously, too, each lens must be carefully inspected for design or manufacturing defects. Unfortunately, defects in manufacture can be manifold and their recognition requires a great deal of familiarity with the configuration of the particular lens type.

F. **Obtaining a Soft Eye**

More than does routine cataract surgery, lens implantation requires the presence of a deep anterior chamber after the lens extraction. Ideally, the iris will show a fair tendency to fall back, which indicates negative vitreous pressure. This allows insertion and positioning of the implant without damage to the anterior hyaloid or the corneal endothelium.

In view of the factors that may influence the position of the iris diaphragm and the anterior hyaloid face, the elements of the problem are as follows:

— Once the eye is opened, intraocular pressure equals atmospheric pressure, and it is unlikely that vitreous bulge will occur unless force is applied to it.

— Since the vitreous body shares the posterior eye cavity with the retina and the choroid, an increase in volume of either will influence the relative position of the vitreous. The volume of the choroid, a highly vascularized membrane, is known to be particularly influenced by changes in arterial and especially in venous circulation.

— Deformation of the outer scleral wall is also known to create positive vitreous pressure. This phenomenon may be a result of lack of rigidity of the sclera or of outside forces on the globe. External pressure on the globe can occur if the ocular muscles are not completely anesthetized or if the orbital content or eyelids are swollen by an excess of local anesthesia or by hemorrhaging. Deformation can also occur from traction by bridal sutures and from pressure exerted by eyelid specula, steridrapes, etc. Bearing this in mind, we shall analyze some of the measures available to obtain a so-called "spontaneous deep anterior chamber" or "soft eye" or "negative vitreous pressure".

1. *Diuretics and Osmotic Agents*

a. *Acetazolamide*

First, there are the so-called secretory inhibitors, of which acetazolamide is the best known. After I.V administration to adults, intraocular pressure begins to fall within a few minutes with the minimum being reached between a half hour and 4 hours. After oral administration, intraocular pressure begins to fall in 1 to 2 hours, reaching the minimum in 3 to 5 hours and recovering in 6 to 12 hours (Becker and Shaffer, 1976). Duke Elder (1969) emphasizes that precisely how acetazolamide acts is unknown. Although preoperative administration of acetazolamide is advocated by a number of implant surgeons, it is unlikely that it reduces vitreous pressure in an open eye. It may be of value in that it certainly does lower the intraocular pressure and thus diminishes the decompressive effect of opening the anterior chamber. D.D. Shepard (1978) has observed that acetazolamide seems to augment the effect of osmotic agents, which can have a very clear influence on the vitreous. In the presence of acetazolamide osmotic agents work quicker, drop the intraocular pressure lower, and keep it down longer.

b. *Osmotic Agents*

Osmotic agents were first used in ophthalmology to lower intraocular pressure in the case of an acute glaucoma. Although various agents are applied in various ways, the mechanism is similar in that they all produce an increase in blood osmolality that causes water to go from the eye to the hyperosmotic plasma. Effective lowering of intraocular pressure is obtained when blood osmolality increases by some 20 to 30 m osmol/l (Becker & Shaffer, 1976). In cataract surgery, osmotherapy is especially advantageous since it has a direct effect on the volume of the vitreous (Jaffe and Light, 1965). Kornblueth and Gombos (1963) have observed that the vitreous in aphakic eyes significantly reduces in volume within 2 hours after I.V. administration of ureum. R. Robbins and M.A. Galin (1969), in animal experiments, substantiated the clinical observation that the vitreous volume can be reduced by osmotic therapy. Since there are too many side effects associated with ureum, however, only manitol and glycerol are used in modern ophthalmic surgery.

1) *Manitol* has to be administered intravenously and is the osmotic agent of choice when oral administration of glycerol is undersirable. The usual dose varies between 2.5 and 10 ml of a 20% solution per kilogram of body weight. The osmotic effect depends not only on the amount given but also on the time allotted for administration, usually from 20 to 45 minutes. Theoretically, a large volume is to be given in a relatively short period of time (for example, max. ±700 ml to a patient weighing 70 kg), which involves some risk for cardiac patients. In practice, smaller doses seem to be effective. Jaffe (1976) suggested that the dose be halved. Havener (1974) has reported a sudden, marked softening of the eye upon I.V. administration of 40 ml of a 20% manitol solution in about 2 minutes, and several implant surgeons have claimed favorable results with intravenous administration of small doses (50 cc of 20% manitol solution for 3 minutes just prior to surgery; the "Manitol Push").

Since manitol is not metabolized to a significant degree, it may be given to diabetic patients. Nor are renal disorders a contraindication. Unlike ureum, extravasation of manitol does not result in local tissue necrosis, and thrombophlebitis is less likely. In general, the undesirable side effects are not especially dangerous, but they do bear watching. A rise in diuresis may require catheterization. Headaches, chills, agina-like chest pains and acute allergic reactions have also been reported (Havener, 1974).

2) *Glycerol.* In combination with local anesthesia, preoperative administration of oral agents can be used to reduce the intraocular pressure. Although they act more slowly than those given intravenously, the greater safety of these drugs largely compensates for this disadvantage. The possibility of overloading the circulatory system is minimal, which is an advantage with borderline cardiac patients. Generally, a 50% glycerol solution is given with a dosage of

1 to 1.5 grams per kilogram of body weight. A drop in intraocular pressure is usually perceptible within 10 minutes and quite clear in 30 minutes, so it is usually administered 90 minutes before surgery. The pressure rises again in a few hours. The patient may not drink anything during the period of osmotic dehydration as the therapeutic effect will be lost.

Glycerol preparations are now available in a number of different flavors.

Antiemetics are recommended if headache or nausea ensues. According to Jaffe (1976), gastrointestinal distress and significant degrees of diuresis are uncommon. Hyperglycemia and glucosuria may be complicating factors.

2. *Ocular Massage*

Another method of enhancing peroperative softness of the eye is mechanical removal of fluid from the vitreous by massage. Duke Elder (1962) notes that Maklakoff had already stressed the importance of massage in lowering intraocular pressure in 1893 and that it was thoroughly studied by Knapp (1912), who found that massaging the globe for several minutes resulted in a perceptable decrease in intraocular pressure lasting from 30 to 45 minutes.

According to Kirsch and Steinmann (1955), P.H. Chandler was the first to apply digital massage after retrobulbar injection for cataract surgery. Investigations by Kirsch and Steinmann (1955) and by Hildreth (1961) have demonstrated that reduction in vitreous volume and weight could be attained by massage. In addition, Quin and Porter (1963), Robbins et al. (1970), and François et al. (1973) concluded from their studies of animal and human eyes that the reduction of vitreous volume resulted from a loss of liquid. Several authors stress that ocular massage is fully effective only with adult patients, whose vitreous is somewhat liquified (François et al. 1973). Since a child's vitreous contains less fluid, massage is probably of less importance.

In practice, the eye is massaged from 3 to 5 minutes, and the drop in intraocular pressure can be measured with a Schiøtz tonometer. In Jaffe's opinion, if the intraocular pressure can be massaged to a Schiøtz scale reading of 12 or more within 2 minutes (which means <5 mm Hg with a 5.5 gr weight), the eye has a markedly dehydrated vitreous (Jaffe, 1972).

Obviously, digital massage and ocular compression do not just influence intraocular fluid alone. Pressure on the globe is also transmitted to adjacent structures, thereby expelling fluid from the orbital cavity as well (J. Copper, 1948).

Another method of exerting external compression on the eyeball is to place an elastic band around the head. A mild but constant pressure can thus be exerted over an extended period of time. J. Gills (1979) uses a soft rubber ball with an elastic band passing through it. He applies it for an hour. J. Worst has designed a similar device made of silicone. P.R. Honan (s.d.) designed a "pneumatic eye softener". Very soft eyes are obtained by using 20 or 30 mm Hg of monitored pressure for 30 to 60 minutes. Releasing the pressure every few minutes has not been found necessary.

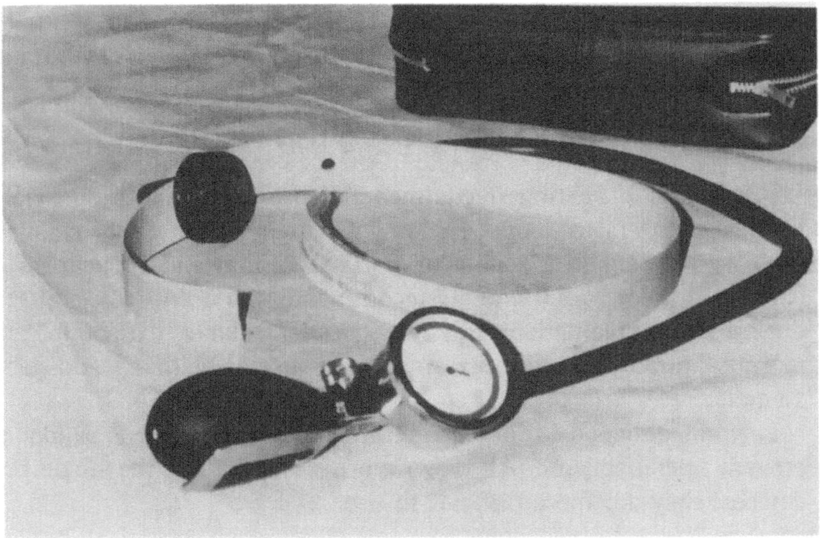

Fig. V-6. — Pneumatic eye softener designed by P.R. Honan.

3. *Separation of the Eyelids*

Effective devices to prevent the eyelids from exerting pressure on the eyeball are more important in intraocular implant surgery than in ordinary cataract surgery. This is one of the first things that should be checked when there is peroperative forward bulging of the iris diaphragm. Regardless of the procedure being used, the eyeball has to be free of all external pressure from eyelids, eyelid holders, or traction sutures.

W.J. Rich (1977) has used pneumatonography to measure the influence of different types of lid retractors on intraocular pressure. In his opinion, adjustable retractors are to be preferred. He also recorded the variations in intraocular pressure caused by traction on bridle sutures for the superior rectus. Since traction on the superior suture has been shown to lead to considerable rise in intraocular pressure, he recommended that it be avoided unless absolutely necessary.

A large variety of devices are available for eyelid separation, and personal preferences diverge widely. But the advice profferred by D. Shepard applies to all of them: "Using a muscle hook or similar instrument one should run around between the globe and the eyelids looking for pressure points, if found, they should be released."

Finally, to provide better separation of the eyelids or to neutralize pressure on the temporal side of the globe, a lateral canthotomy should be considered.

4. *The Scleral Ring*

In 1953, H.J. Flieringa recommended suturing a ring to the scleral to prevent scleral collapse. The ring he used was made of stainless steel with a diameter ranging from 20 to 22 mm and a thickness of 0.3 mm. J. Worst also strongly recommends the use of a scleral ring during lens implantation with intracapsular cataract extraction, and recently introduced a model of his own design with an adjustable diameter.

Legrand designed a double ring and Girard a scleral expander to prevent scleral collapse. Although more effective than the single ring devices, they are more difficult to use.

5. *The Pars Plana Vitreous Tap Vitrectomy*

In 1966, C.E. Iliff suggested posterior sclerotomy to drain fluid vitreous before opening the anterior chamber. The procedure was restricted to those cases in which conservative means could not achieve a Schiotz scale reading of at least 10 units with the 5.5 gr weight. According to Iliff, fluid vitreous can be extracted from the superior, temporal region of the globe by making a scleral incision with a small Graefe's knife 6 mm behind the limbus in the superior temporal quadrant.

The technique has since been slightly modified and its application extended to cases of vitreous prolapse and vitreous presention after the eye has been opened. Instead of making the incision with a Graefe's knife, disposable 25 or 27 guage needles are now used to make a tap of the vitreous fluid (Jaffe, 1972). Vitrectomy devices are now also used for this purpose. It would be premature to recommend any of these procedures as only a few reports dealing with small numbers of cases are available.

6. *Anesthesia: Local and General*

With the advent of modern local anesthetics with long-lasting effects and minimal toxicity, one can achieve satisfactory relaxation of both the ocular and the periocular muscles. Combination with

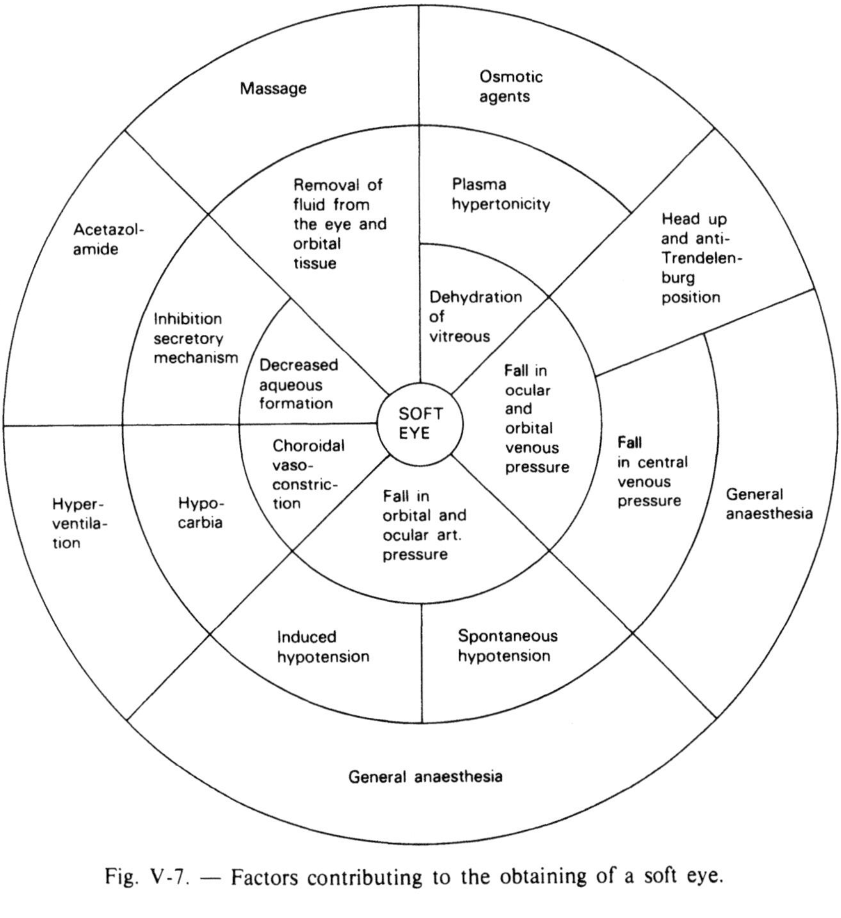

Fig. V-7. — Factors contributing to the obtaining of a soft eye.

Hyaluronidase is advisable. Apart from an occasional retrobulbar hemorrhage (which is an indication that the surgery should be postponed), some problems may occur with patients with shallow orbits, tight eyelids, or proptotic globes. In such cases, the volume of anesthetic injected into the orbital cavity may seriously interfere with the desired behavior of the iris diaphragm. More than in routine cataract surgery, special attention should be paid to effective akinesia avoiding an increase in volume of the eyelids. O'Brien's method of achieving akinesia may be of interest here.

With general anesthesia, several mechanisms can help to get a soft eye as is illustrated on Figure V-7.

In the opinion of A.K. Bermingham, the anesthesiologist who assists C.D. Binkhorst, a constant, deep narcosis can bring about a soft eye, and the most reliable method of achieving this is by curarization and maintenance of the narcosis by intermittant positive pressure ventilation and administration of nitrous oxide, oxygen, and small increments of halothane. Occasionally, extra fentanyl or dehydrobenzperidol or both are added. According to Bermingham, this method has the advantage of allowing the monitoring of all the parameters that contribute to the maintenance of a soft eye.

As the schema above shows, general anesthesia, which precludes coughing, straining, vomiting, etc., produces a fall in the central venous pressure, which in turn decreases the orbital and intraocular venous pressure. Slight hyperventilation produces hypocarbia, which in turn causes choroidal and retinal vasoconstriction (the upper limit of exhaled carbon dioxide concentration should not exceed 5%).

As a rule systolic pressure is maintained between 90 and 100 mm Hg. This systemic hypotension reduces the arterial blood flow, which decreases the capillary hemodynamic pressure. Contraindications for induced hypotension are coronary diseases (angina pectoris, recent infarction) and cerebral ischaemic problems.

This type of general anesthesia also provides adequate ocular muscle relaxation since it uses a neuromuscular blocking agent.

Finally, regardless of the type of anesthesia used, the position of the head and the body is important, since engorgement of the intraocular veins results in positive vitreous pressure. Ease of blood flow from the neck vein into the thorax requires a higher positioning of the head. In addition, a slight anti-Trendelenburg position is advantageous since it decreases the venous pressure in the upper region of the body.

II. Peroperative Management

A. The Incision

Implant surgery employs different kinds of incisions—pure corneal, limbal, and scleral—and their orientation can vary from perpendicular to parallel to the iris. The length of the incision is largely dependent on the cataract extraction procedure and the type of implant. Since implant surgery involves more instrument passages through the incision, the preferred incision would be the one that allows the easiest access to the formed anterior chamber without harming the endothelium or stripping the Descemet's layer at the inner edge of the cornea. An incision that roughly parallels the iris in the 12 o'clock area greatly facilitates this.

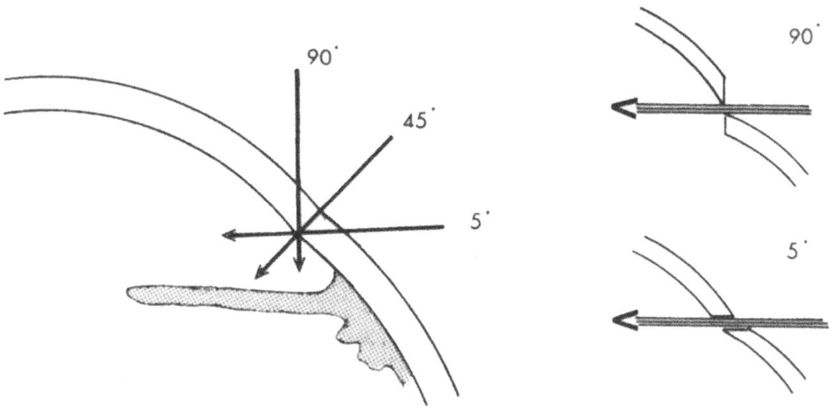

Fig. V-8. — Left: incisions used in implant surgery. Right: effect of incision types on subsequent instrumental access.

NB: Special attention must be given to the location of the incision for angle supported lenses (see chapter VIII).
Stopping the bleeding takes on more importance in implant surgery than in ordinary cataract extraction since blood hampers visibility and, if it coagulates on the iris, interferes with pupil constriction.

Generally, one or more preplaced sutures are used. The surgeon must take special care to lay the suture loops to the side: inadvertent snaring of the suture with the implant lens is not infrequent, and, when intraocular sutures are used, identification of the various threads can be troublesome.

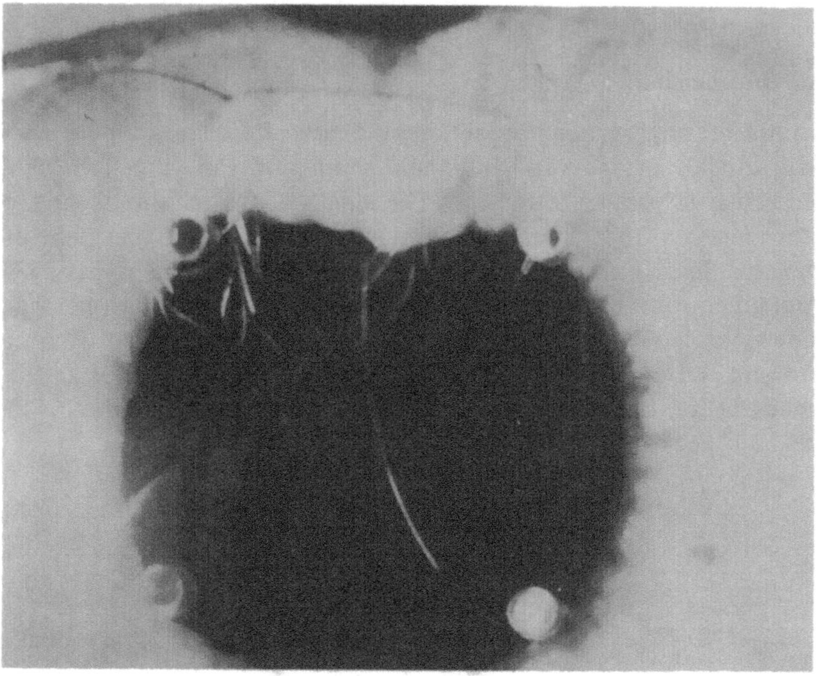

Fig. V-9. — The suture has been accidentally snared around the inferior temporal foot of an implanted medallion lens. (Courtesy R. Drews.)

B. Cataract Extraction

1. *Intracapsular Cataract Extraction (ICCE)*

Most novice implant surgeons prefer intracapsular cataract extraction, a technique they are already familiar with. But whichever technique is employed, the cataract must be removed atraumatically. Subclinical injury may be harmless under normal circumstances but can engender serious consequences when aggravated by the additional trauma of a pseudophakos.

When iris-supported lenses are implanted, the sphincter and pupil margin must be preserved. When the pupil is rigid, a radial iridotomy followed by iris repair is indicated for cataract extraction. And while slight vitreous bulge is very rarely a problem in cataract extraction, the insertion of an artificial lens in such an eye gives rise to serious problems, with most resulting from the rupture of the anter-

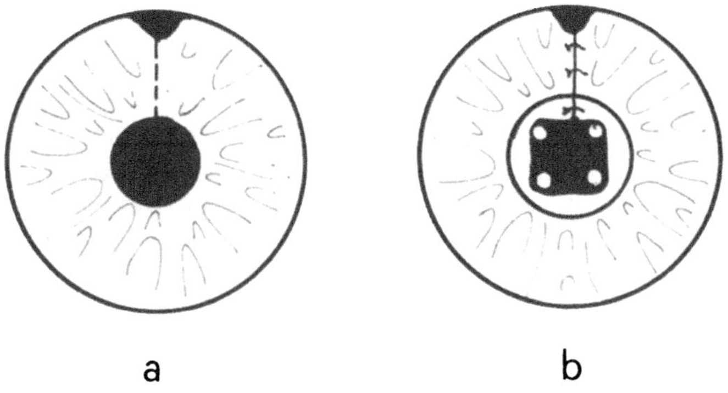

Fig. V-10a. — Radial iridotomy in the case of a rigid pupil and b. — iris repair using 2 or more intraocular sutures.

ior hyaloid by the implant. With an iris supported lens, decentration, caused, for example, by an updrawn pupil, can provoke contact corneal dystrophy. Also a vitreous knuckle sharing the pupillary aperture with the lens may sooner or later dislocate the lens. As a rule, the neophyte should not insert a lens when there is vitreous bulge unless it can be adequately managed. Such management includes detection of the underlying reasons, repressurization of the

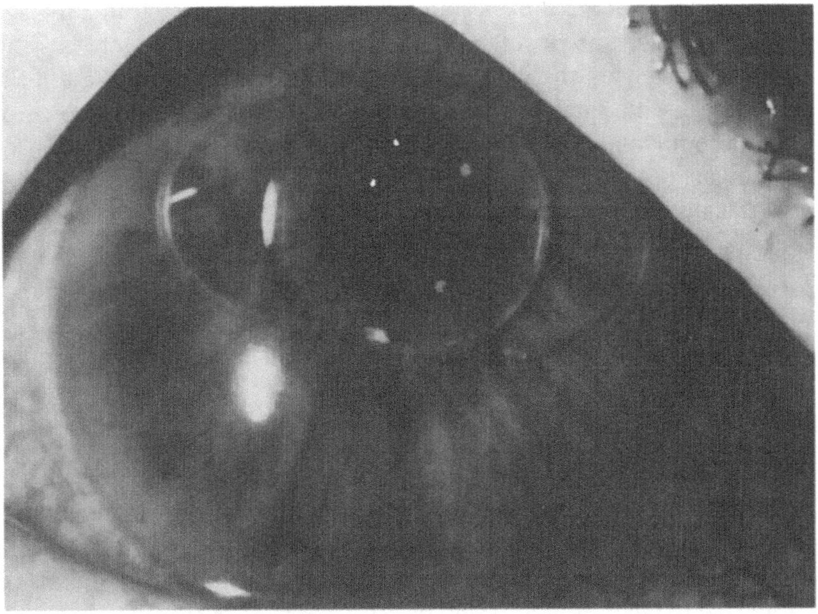

Fig. V-11. — Upward decentration of an implant because of vitreous loss.

anterior chamber with air, the use of viscuous agents and introduction of the implant in close contact with the iris while sliding it into the pupil sideways. Also a lensglide can be used.

According to C.D. Binkhorst, if vitreous loss occurs, aborting the implant procedure should be the rule, even when this complication has been adequately managed (freeing the anterior chamber and the pupillary aperture with a vitrectomy). After a vitrectomy, the stability of iris-supported lenses is compromised since there is a more iridodonesis, which in turn will lead to marked "pseudophakodonesis". Furthermore, as will be discussed later, such eyes have a higher rate of specific complications such as cystoid macular edema and retinal detachment even without lens implantations. The surgeon must decide if the risks are commensurate with the expected benefits.

2. *Extracapsular Cataract Extraction (ECCE)*

In the late sixties, C.D. Binkhorst introduced the practice of routine extracapsular cataract extraction in combination with lens implantation. Since this practice is becoming more widespread, we include some aspects of extracapsular surgery in this section.

In our experience, not all cataracts are equally easy to remove. Total white or "mature" cataracts are easy to extract in any age group. Posterior subcapsular cataracts in adults are relatively easy to remove, but lenses showing only a central nuclear sclerosis are difficult to deal with since the nucleus is often small and the removal of cortical remnants is time consuming and frustrating, especially for the novice.

Extracapsular cataract extraction combined with lens implantation consists of three major steps:

a. Capsulotomy or capsulectomy of the anterior lens capsule;
b. Removal of the nucleus (in adults);
c. Removal of the cortical material.

STEP 1: Capsulotomy—Capsulectomy

Techniques to open the anterior capsule are as old as extracapsular extraction itself. According to Duke Elder (1969), Jacques Daviel used a sharp needle for this purpose in the middle of the 18th century; Georges de la Faye in Paris used a cystitome in this same period; and Gerhard ten Haaf of Rotterdam (1768) and Guillaume Pellier de Quengsy of Montpellier (1789) simplified the procedure by opening the capsule with the point of the knife used for puncture and contrapuncture of the anterior chamber.

Today a variety of instruments are used to perform capsulotomies and capsulectomies, and the patterns followed are as many as there are surgeons.

The aim of the procedure is twofold: to make an opening in the capsule large enough to allow the nucleus to pass, and to leave "enough" of the anterior capsular flap to hold the lens in place. Implants that rely on pure iris fixation or angle fixation do not need anterior capsule flaps, so for these lenses as much of the anterior capsule is removed as possible.

Capsulotomy

Many different incision patterns are used (see Fig. V-12).

In this procedure, the anterior capsule is not excised but only incised. D. Kratz has tried out probably the most variations on this theme.

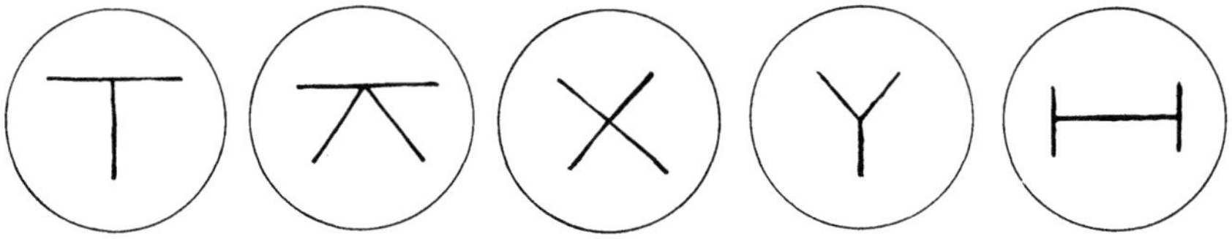

Fig. V-12. — Incision patterns for the anterior capsule.

In addition to the classic cystitome (Fig. V-13), other devices are also used such as the Kelman cystitome and a variety of practical instruments made from injection needles. Adequate protection of the endothelium is generally achieved by making only a small incision of perhaps 3 mm and maintaining a formed anterior chamber by using irrigating fluid or air.

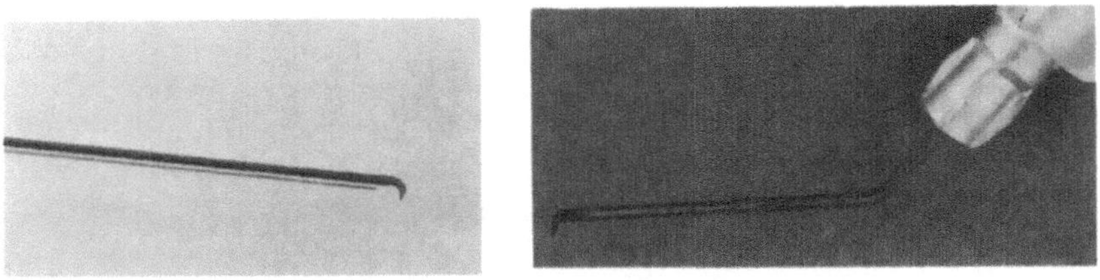

Fig. V-13. — Cystitomes: Left: Cystitome designed by C. Kelman. Right: Self-made needle cystitome for mounting on a syringe or irrigating device.

Capsulectomy

Depending on the lens to be inserted, more or less of the anterior capsule is removed. Here, too, different patterns are possible (see Fig. V-14).

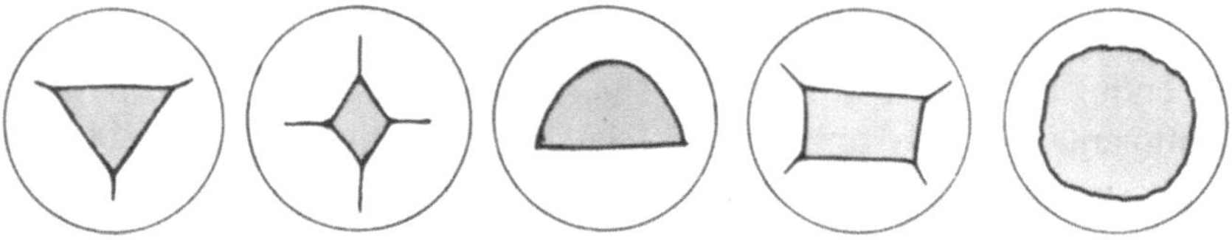

Fig. V-14. — Patterns of anterior capsulectomies.

A cystitome can be used for this, though some surgeons prefer a Vannas scissors (Gills, Charleux). A scissors generally requires a larger opening in the anterior chamber than does a cystitome, which makes the maintenance of the formed anterior chamber difficult. At first, C.D. Binkhorst used the small-toothed capsule forceps designed by Vogt, but he now makes a T-shaped capsulotomy with a Haab's knife.

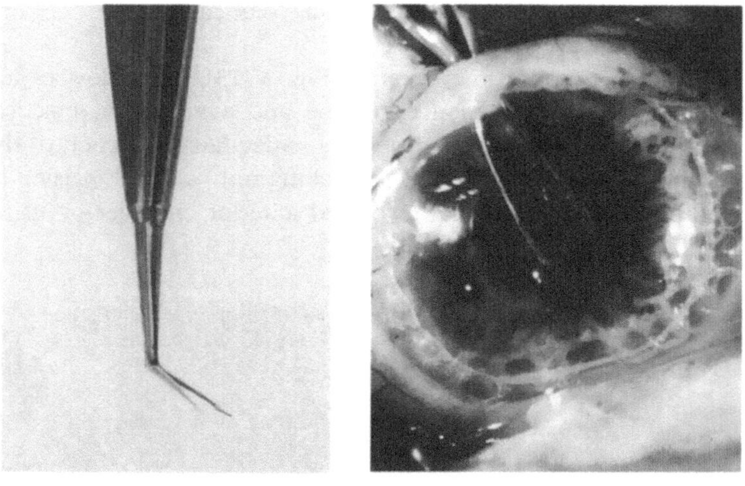

Fig. V-15. — Left: Capsule pincet designed by Vogt. Right: Vogt's pincet in situ for removal of the central portion of the anterior capsule. Note the presence of an air bubble preventing corneal contact. (Courtesy C.D. Binkhorst.)

One interesting method is the so-called "can opener" technique in which small slits are made in the anterior capsule, thus performing a guided capsulectomy.

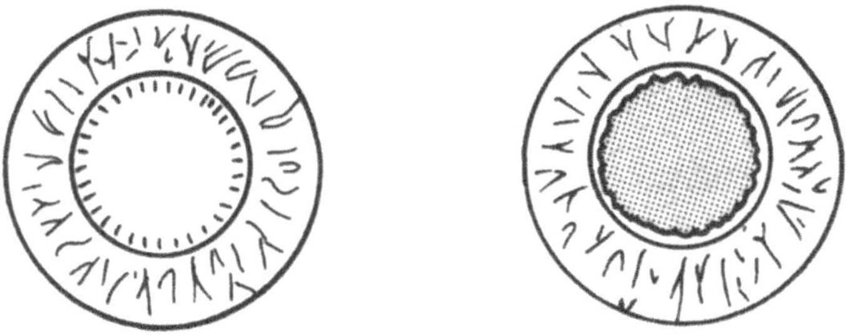

a b

Fig. V-16. — "Can-opener technique": many small slits are made in the capsule (a), permitting the removal of an anterior capsular flap (b).

To facilitate easy separation of the nucleus and the remaining anterior capsule, gentle irrigation between them with a small cannula is recommended (Binkhorst, personal communication, 1979).

STEP II: Removal of the Nucleus

Large Incision Techniques

In the classic extracapsular technique, the nucleus is expressed in one motion out of the capsule and worked out throught the

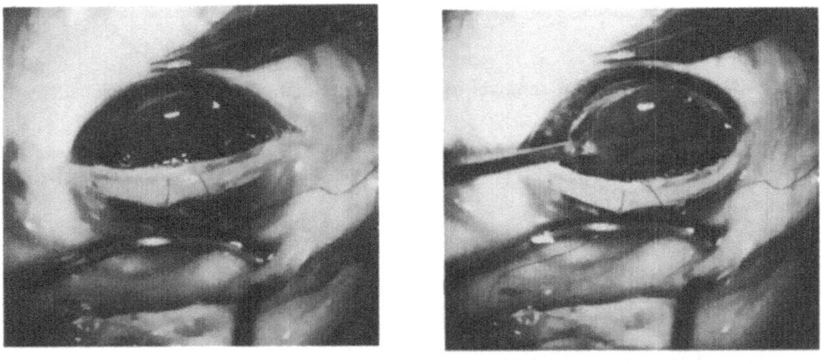

Fig. V-17. — Bimanual maneuver for the expression of the nucleus. Left: the superior lip of the incision is depressed while counter pressure is exerted in the limbal area below with the heal of a squint hook. Right: an assistant may harpoon the nucleus with a sharp instrument such as a Graefe's knife or injection needle to facilitate the expression.

incision (this technique is described in detail in Chapter VII). This method has the advantage of not needing any special instrument, and it can also be applied when the pupil is only moderately wide. The anterior chamber has to be opened over at least 130° to 150° (corneo-scleral section) to allow easy passage of the nucleus. If the nucleus is very large, the incision might have to be extended to 170°.

Other methods that require a large incision as well as a wide pupil are the following:

— Forward luxation of the nucleus followed by expression or extraction: with an olive tip irrigating cannula, the back of the nucleus is separated from the posterior subcapsular layers to bring it into the anterior chamber. From here it can be extracted with a toothed forceps or expressed with the classic bimanual maneuver.

— Another way to remove the nucleus is the method J. Gills has applied to several thousand extractions. A lens loop (Fig. V-18) is inserted carefully between the nucleus and the posterior capsule while the scleral lip of the incision and the superior iris sector are pushed back. Once the lens loop is under the nucleus, it is rocked back and forth very gently and slowly to deliver the lens from the eye—a "rock-me-gentle-rock-me-sweet" movement.

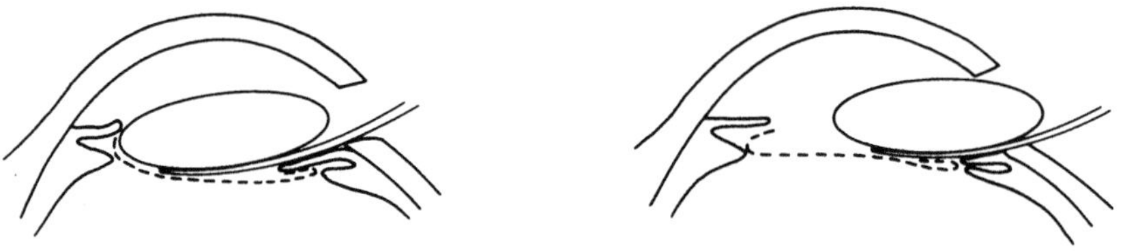

Fig. V-18. — Method for removal of the nucleus using a lens loop designed by J. Gills.

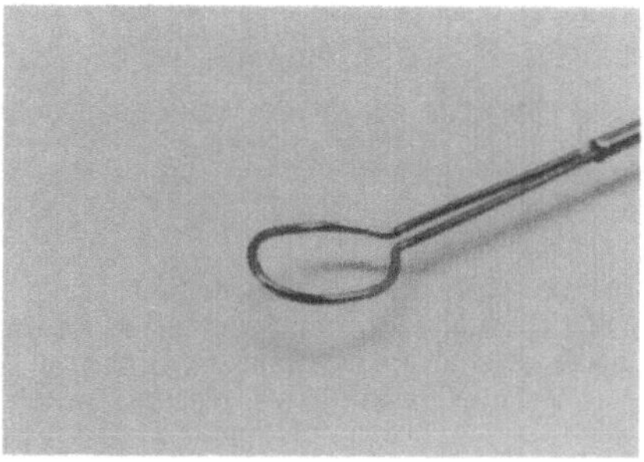

Fig. V-19. — Pearce's irrigating lens oop for removal of the nucleus.

— Another method uses an instrument designed by J. Pearce. An irrigating lens loop, which is called an "irrigating vectis", is inserted between the lens and the posterior capsule as in the preceding method so as to form a slide for the nucleus.
— Finally, the nucleus can be removed by grasping it with a forceps or by "spearing" it.

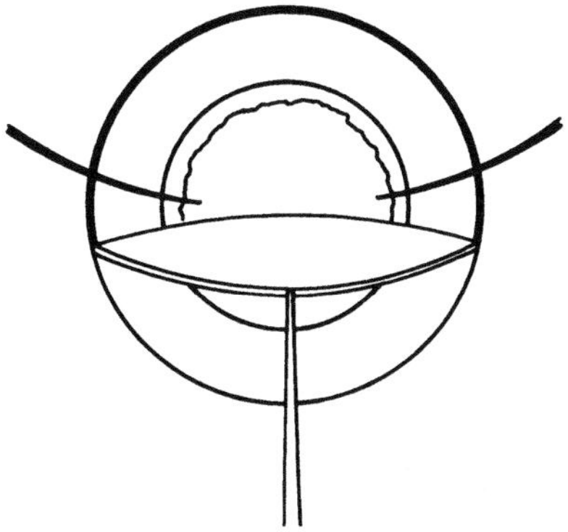

Fig. V-20. — Removal of the nucleus using 2 needles.

Small Incision Techniques

Currently, there are a number of devices available to break up the nucleus and to remove the fragments from the eye through a small incision. In the early seventies, C. Kelman evolved an original method he called "phakoemulsification". Kelman's apparatus has a probe with a 3 mm tip that emits ultrasound at 40 kHz. The tip also has an irrigating and aspirating cannula system. Both the time the ultrasound is emitted and the rate of irrigation and aspiration can be easily controlled. It is also provided with an automatic safety device to release the aspiration vacuum if necessary. Some surgeons emulsify the entire nucleus in the anterior chamber after it has been moved forward by means of a cystotome (see Fig. V-21, original Kelman technique). Others emulsify the top layer of the nucleus in situ (Kratz's sculpture method) and then shift the bottom layer forward.

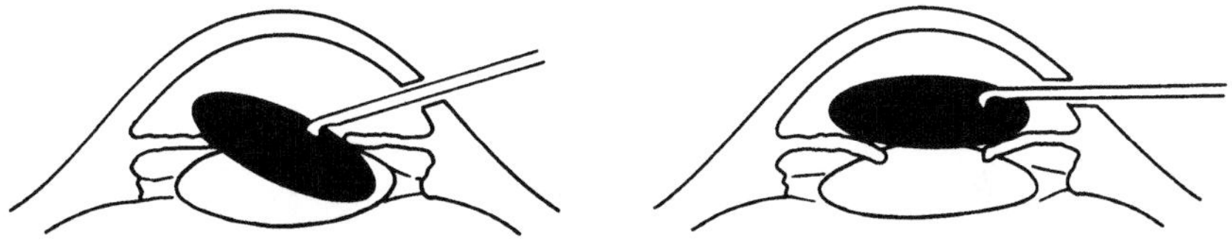

Fig. V-21. — Kelman's technique for luxation of the nucleus in the anterior chamber.

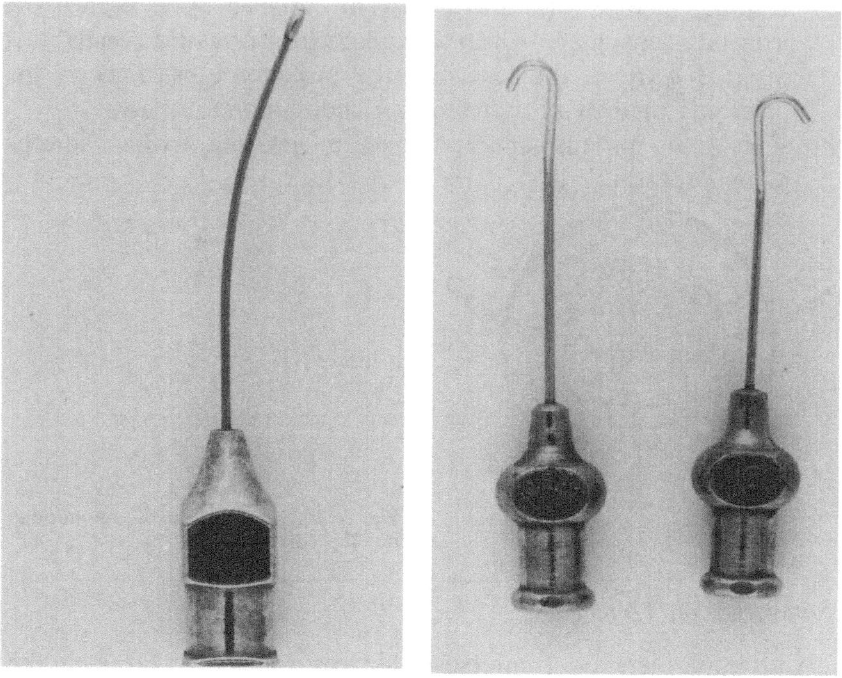

Fig. V-22a. — Cannulas used by C.D. Binkhorst for removing cortical material.

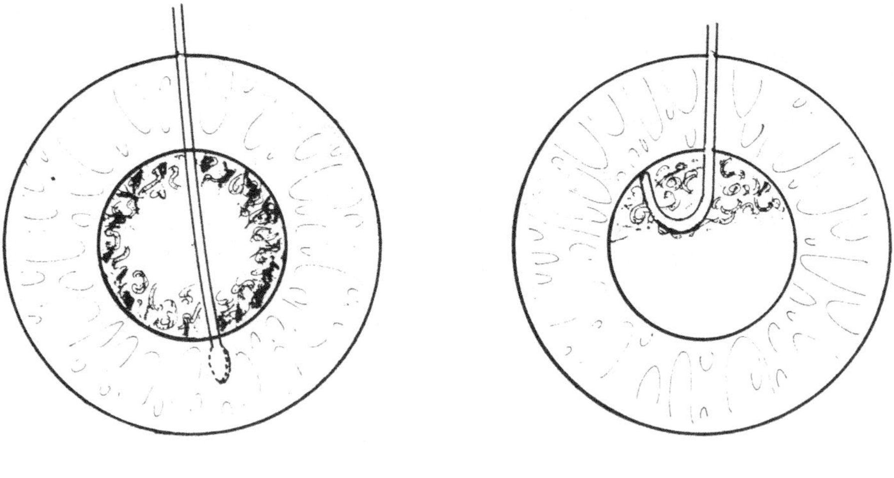

A B

Fig. V-22b. — Evacuation of cortical remnants using a straight olive tip cannula and a bent cannula.

Girard's phakofragmentation is based on Kelman's idea of using ultrasound to fragment the nucleus in senile cataracts, so that the material may be aspirated through a 23 guage cannula (Girard, 1976).

STEP III: Evacuation of Cortical Remnants

Large Incision Technique

Most of the cortical material can be rinsed out with simple irrigation (irrigation solutions are discussed in Chapter XII). The loose material will follow the flow and be brought out of the eye. The front of the iris can be lightly massaged from the periphery to the center to collect material hidden in the periphery. Binkhorst suggests using a slightly curved olive tip cannula to remove the remnants from the lower sector and a cannula that is bent 170° to rinse out the upper sector (Fig. V-22).

In order to evacuate cortical material, J. Worst designed a set of "golf clubs": a set of handpieces fitted with straight and curved cannulas connected to an irrigation source (infusion bottle or syringe) (Fig. V-23).

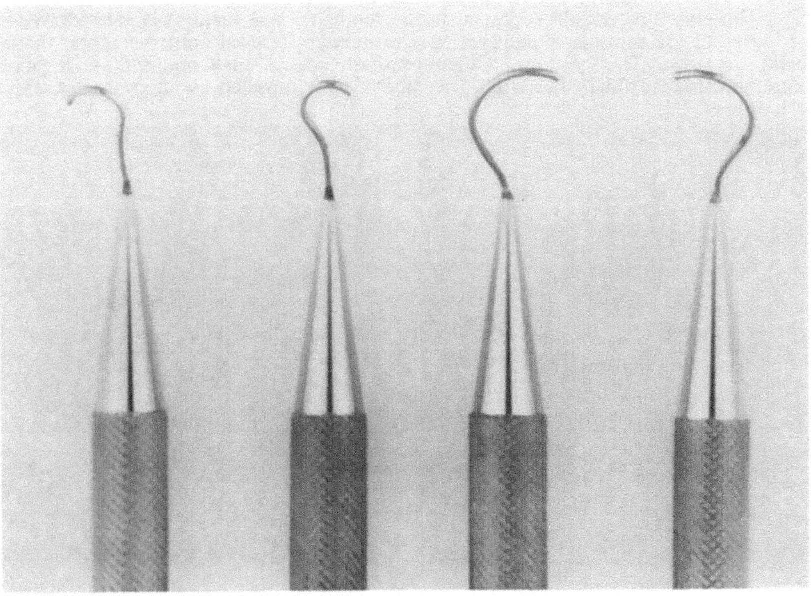

Fig. V-23. — Irrigating devices designed by J. Worst for removal of cortical remnants.

Clinging lens remnants and subcapsular adhering layers have to be removed mechanically. The technique used is variously called the "non-irrigating, non-aspirating method", the "push-pull method".

The principles of this technique are simple. First the tip of a cannula, which is mounted on a syringe, is brought in contact with the lens material, and the lumen is plugged by vacuum application. While maintaining the vacuum, the lens material is pulled gently towards the center, which generally results in the stripping of a

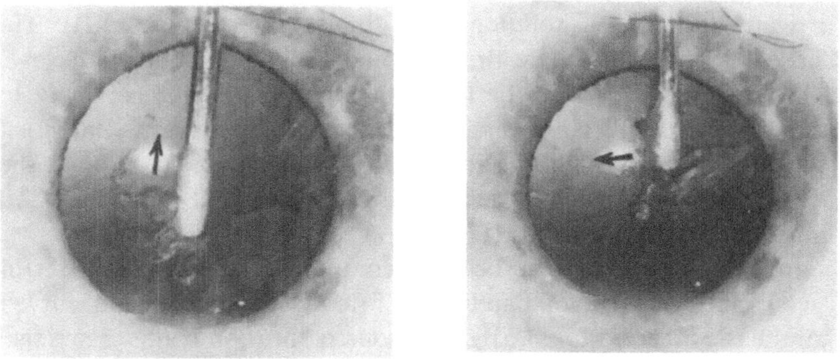

Fig. V-24. — Stripping out of cortical remnants from the *lower capsular bag and the sides:* The olive tip cannula is dipped in the remnants and vacuum is applied. When the lumen of the cannula is plugged, it is withdrawn (arrows) until the center of the pupil is reached. The vacuum is then released, and a small amount of irrigation solution is used to flush the pupil. The maneuver is repeated as often as necessary.

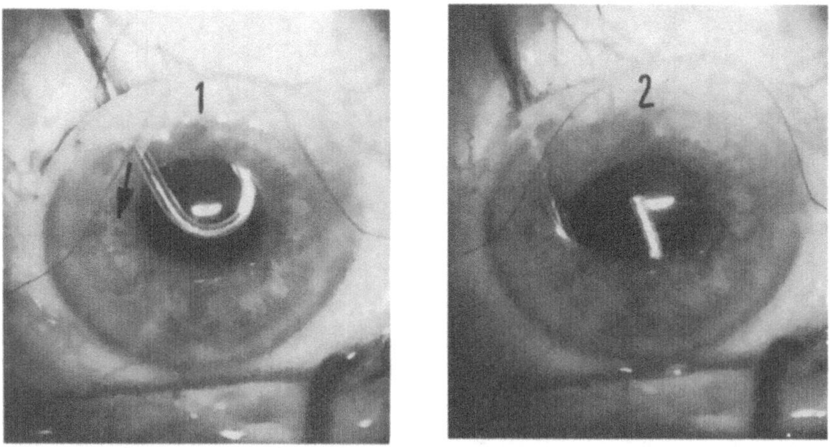

Fig. V-25. — Cleaning the *superior quadrant:* Using the "pull-push" technique, the remnants can be stripped out with a cannula bent 170°. Note that this method as illustrated does not require a well-dilated pupil.

triangular piece of cortex. Once the lens material is in the pupillary area, the vacuum is released and the pupil is cleared by irrigation. The procedure is repeated in the other sectors. Of particular interest is the use of a curved or bent cannula to strip off the cortical remnants in the superior sector. As with the straight cannula, the tip is brought into contact with the cortical material, which is then stripped out by vacuum pull. The whole procedure can be performed in a partially closed eye, which has the advantage of maintaining a deep anterior chamber and facilitating access between the capsular flaps.

C. W. Simcoe (1977) proposed the use of an elastic bulb filled with fluid and fitted with a long blunt 23 guage cannula with a side port opening near the tip. The cortical remnants are stripped off by

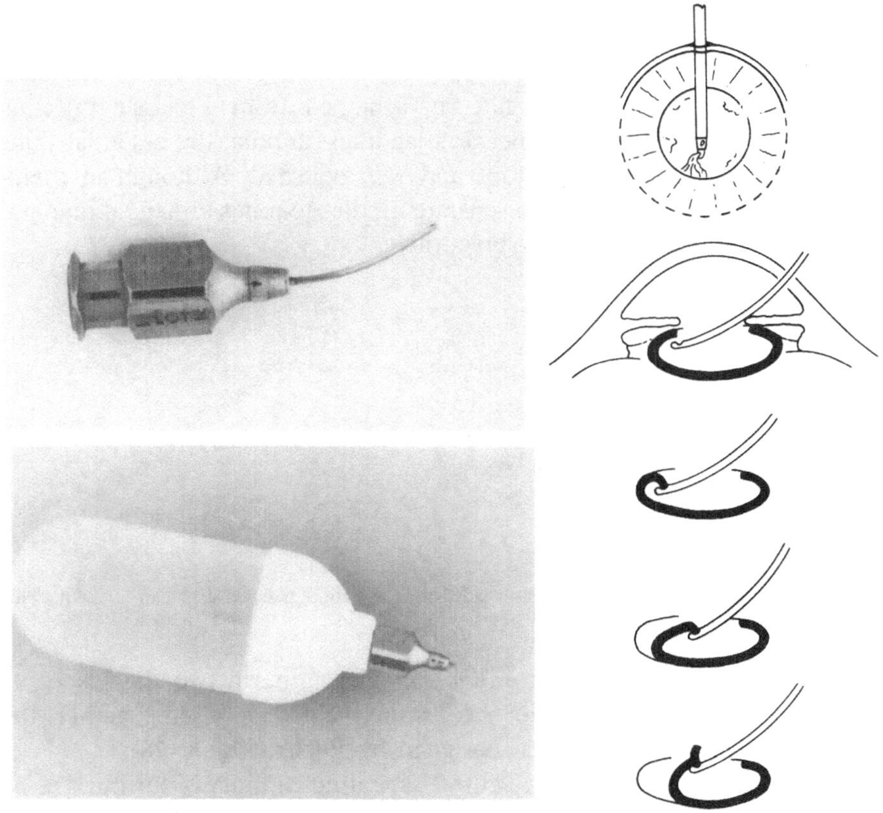

Fig. V-26. — Simcoe's microcrysiphake and his technique for the removal of cortical remnants using a blunt cannula with side port opening, mounted on an elastic bulb.

alternately squeezing and relaxing the bulb (micro-erysiphake technique).

Small Incision Technique

When the incision is very small, evacuation of cortical and soft lens material requires aspiration, so fluid has to be introduced constantly to keep the anterior chamber formed. A variety of devices are available for this purpose. They may be classified into two categories on the basis of the configuration of the tip introduced into the eye:

— separate irrigation-aspiration instruments;
— combined irrigation-aspiration instruments (parallel and coaxial models).

Separate irrigation-aspiration cannulas are useful for the removal of "soft" cataracts from younger patients (Fig. V-27). The tips of the cannulas are blunt and the opening may be at the top or the side. Many of these devices can be fashioned from a classic injection needle, a disposable needle, or a lacrimal cannula, the essential thing being that the tips be blunt and well polished. Although in themselves effective, using two separate needles requires bimanual manipulation, which is not very practicable.

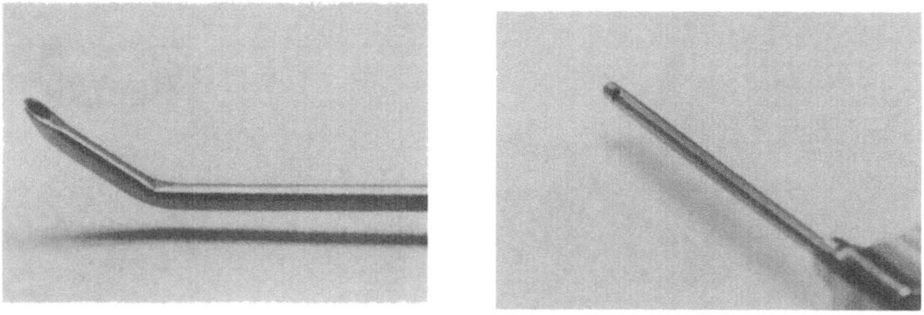

Fig. V-27. — Blunt cannulas made from injection needles and cannula with side port opening.

Combined irrigation-aspiration cannulas come in two models:

— Parallel cannulas: two needles are welded or fused together, the prototype having been designed by Fuchs (Fig. V-28);
— Coaxial cannulas: the central aspirating cannula is surrounded by the larger irrigation cannula. The prototype is the Cavitron irrigation aspiration probe that was designed by C. Kelman. D. McIntire (1976) has proposed a similar combined cannula system.

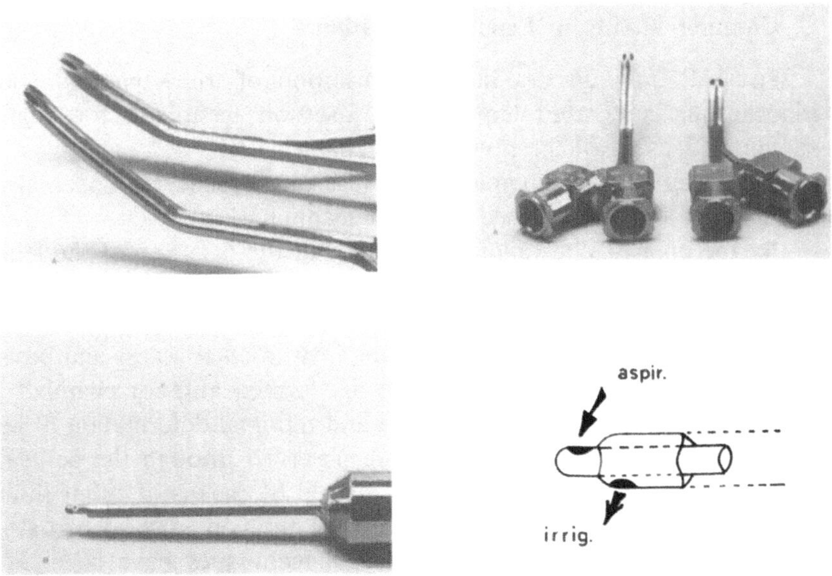

Fig. V-28. — Top: parallel cannula system: 2 cannulas fused together.
Bottom: Schema of coaxial cannula system for simultaneous irrigation and aspiration and disposable coaxial device.

Irrigation-aspiration devices are, of course, to be connected to fluid and vacuum sources. Irrigation fluid is generally supplied from an infusion bottle with the dripper maintained at a level calibrated with respect to the eye. Vacuum can be supplied with a syringe or a vacuum pump. It is essential to be able to stop the aspiration at any moment. For this purpose, different cannula holders have been designed that can be controlled manually. Most of the automated devices (Cavitron, Medical Workshop, etc.) can be controlled by means of a foot switch.

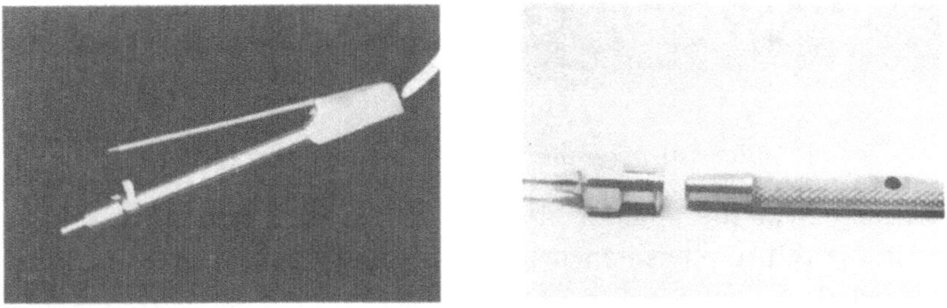

Fig. V-29. — Left: Cannula holder designed by P. Leonard, with handle for interrupting the irrigation or vacuum supply. Right: Cannula holder with shunt opening that can be plugged with the finger tip to achieve suction.

C. **Common Points in Lens Implantation**

We shall only discuss here the insertion of iris supported and iridocapsular supported lenses. The insertion technique for angle supported lenses will be reviewed in chapter VIII.

There are two basic approaches for inserting a lens: the "open sky technique" and the "closed chamber technique".

— By the open sky technique is meant that the insertion of the lens and most of the positioning and fixating maneuvers are done under direct visualization for which the cornea is lifted.

— With the closed chamber technique, instrumental access and positioning of the lens take place in a "formed anterior chamber" with minimal lifting of the cornea and minimal deformation of its architecture. All manipulations are observed through the cornea, and the anterior chamber is kept formed by means of either fluid or air. Depending on the situation, the incision may be partially or almost totally closed. A variety of techniques have been devised to perform the delicate intraocular maneuvers using small instruments that can be introduced between the sutures. Some arguments in favor of this technique are given in the section on lens implantation and the endothelium.

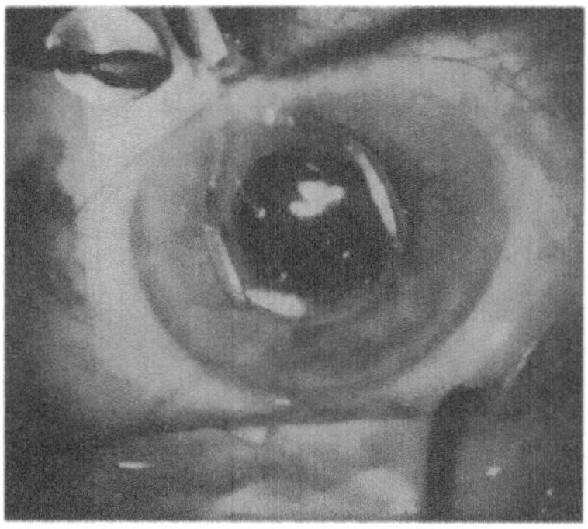

Fig. V-30. — "Formed chamber technique": While the lens is inserted, the corneal architecture is not disturbed, and all maneuvers can be observed through the cornea.

1. *After Intracapsular Cataract Extraction (ICCE)*

After ICCE, the anterior chamber is reformed, and, if necessary, the iris is gently repositioned. If the iris diaphragm is concave, fluid is injected to float it.

Iris supported lenses have at least one pair of haptic parts or loops that must be introduced behind the iris; the optic portion is generally situated in front of the pupil.

A number of different instruments can be used for the proper positioning of the lens:

— The original Binkhorst forceps with cross-action is suitable for lens types that have a 5 mm optical component. This instrument has an inbuilt cannula through which fluid can be injected.
— Slightly different lens forceps have been designed by several surgeons.
— Further a number of small instruments can be used for inserting lenses such as tying forceps and needle holders.

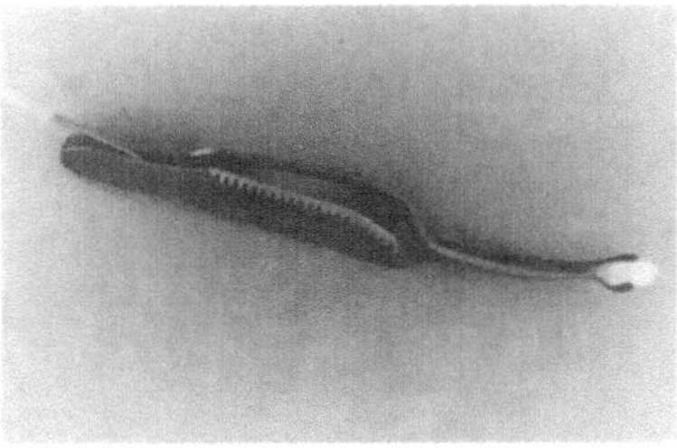

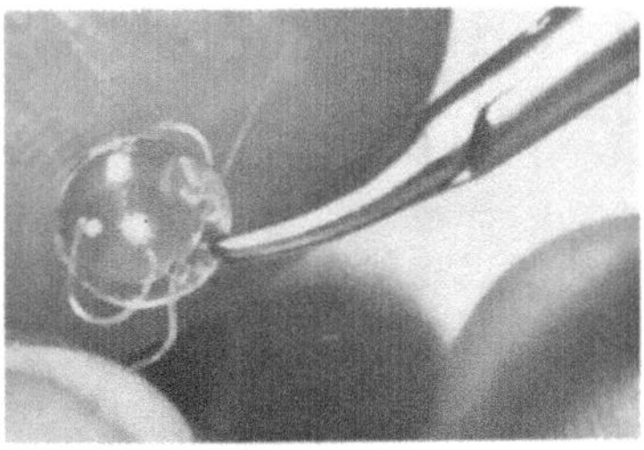

Fig. V-31a. — Original Binkhorst lens forceps. b. — Needle holder used for inserting the medallion lens.

According to the preference of the surgeon, the lens is grasped either at the optic portion or at its haptic (loop, strut, rim, etc.). What is essential is that the lens not be damaged and that the instrument provide a firm grip so that the maneuvers inside the eye can be performed without harming the most delicate of the eye structures, the endothelium and the vitreous.

Common techniques for inserting iris supported lenses:

a. *Single Maneuver*

With a gentle movement, one of the posterior haptics is introduced through the pupillary aperture and slid behind the iris. The movement is continued until the opposite haptic clears the underlying pupil border whereupon that haptic is guided through the pupil with a "zig-zag" or "to-and-fro" movement. It may be necessary to use a fine iris forceps to retract the underlying iris sector (see Fig. V-32). The implant should be kept as parallel as possible to the iris plane in order to avoid tilting or dipping a loop or haptic with the risk of endothelial contact.

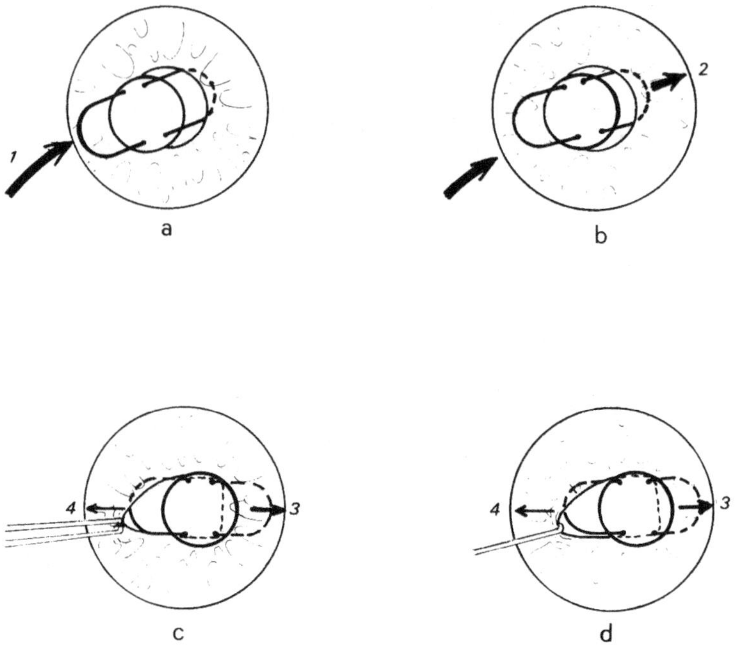

Fig. V-32. — Consecutive steps for inserting a lens with the loops in the horizontal meridian by means of a zig-zag maneuver. If necessary, a fine iris forceps (c) or a blunt iris hook (d) can be used to engage the second loop.

b. *Two-Step Insertion*

Again, the first haptic is put in position behind the iris by means of a gentle movement through the pupillary aperture. The forceps is released and the other haptic or haptics are allowed to rest on the iris surface. The anterior chamber is then reformed and one or more sutures can be tied. A two-handed maneuver is used to bring the iris sector or sectors in front of the corresponding loops or haptics: while the lens body is steadied with a fine spatula held in one hand, the iris is pulled or hooked over the corresponding loop or haptic. For this "tire-hooking maneuver", a fine-toothed forceps or a blunt iris hook can be used. Some micro-hooks are modified injection needles with which the anterior chamber can be kept formed at the same time.

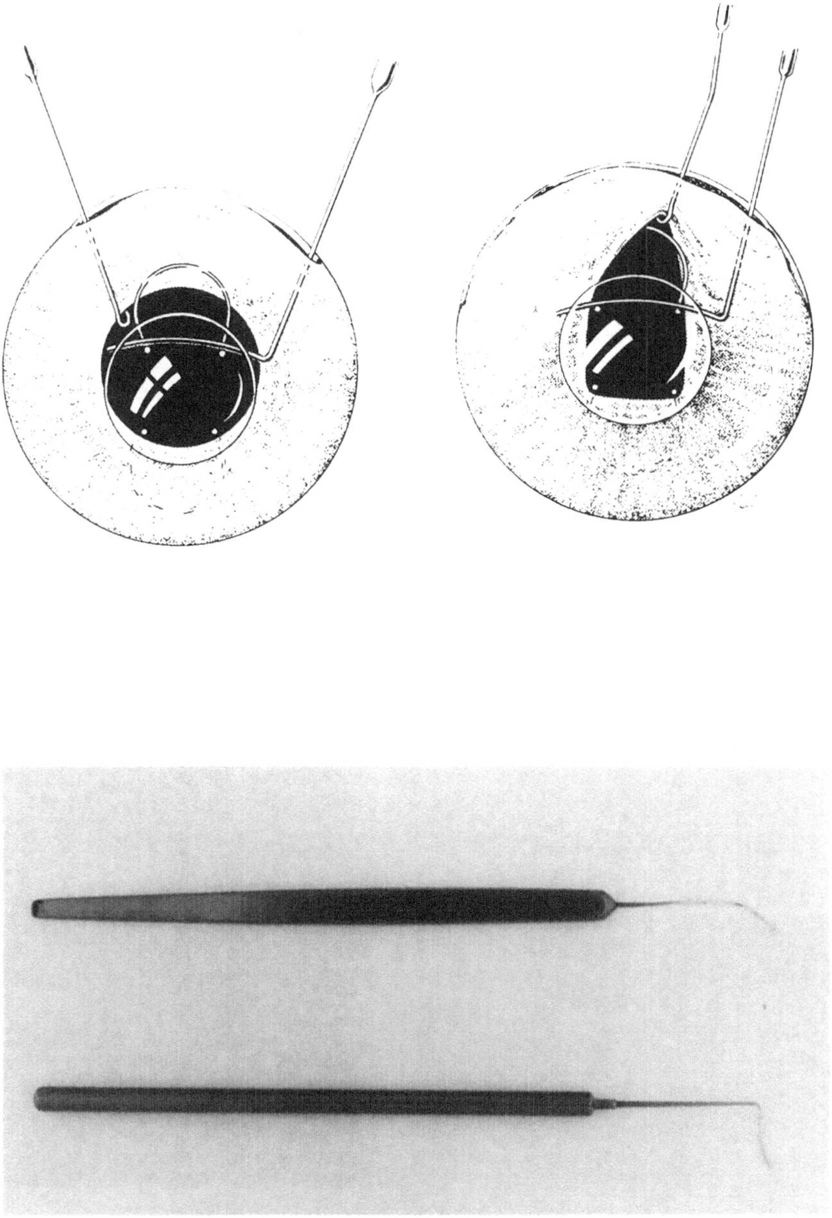

Fig. V-33. — Method and instruments for bringing an iris sector in front of a loop or haptic.

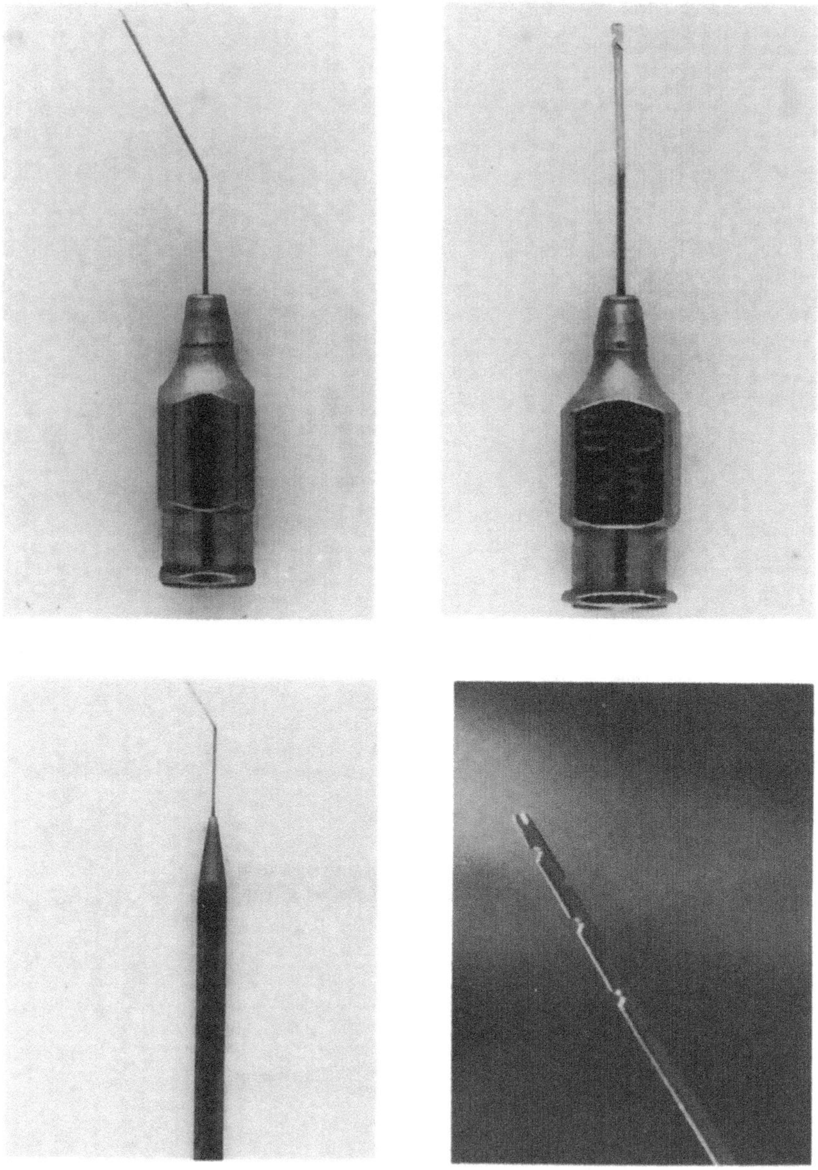

Fig. V-34. — Top: microhook made from an injection needle (left) and notched irrigating spatula (right).
Bottom: notched Hirschmann spatula for steadying the lens in the eye.

2. *After Extracapsular Cataract Extraction (ECCE)*

a. If only iris support is intended, the lens is inserted in the same way as with intracapsular cataract extraction.
b. If capsular support is intended, the lens is inserted in such a way that one or more of the posterior haptics (generally loops) fit between the anterior capsular flaps and the posterior capsule. In essence, the one- or two-step procedures given above are suitable, and, from the technical point of view, the opening in the anterior capsule may be considered an additional pupillary aperture.

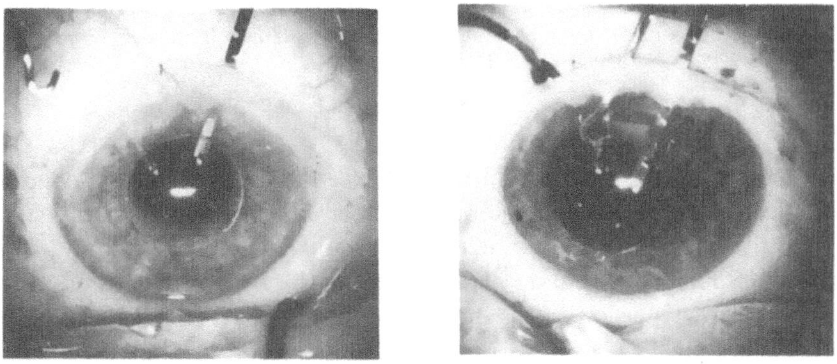

Fig. V-35. — Left: Iridocapsular lens with the inferior loops in position. The preplaced suture is tied while the lens is steadied with a Hirschman spatula. Right: A blunt iris hook is used to pick up the superior capsular flap and position it in front of the superior loop.

Note: The proper identification of the anterior capsule may be difficult: insertion is always easier when the pupil is rather large. When magnifiers are used, intensive lateral illumination, e.g., from a fiber optic source, is extremely useful. When a microscope is used, the anterior flaps can be easily identified with either lateral or coaxial illumination.

3. *Glides and Sleeves*

Already in the fifties, a blunt, flat spatula was used to depress the iris in order to facilitate insertion of the implant (Schreck, 1958): DuPont Guerry mentioned the use of a similar instrument. In the mid-seventies, J. Sheets devised a plastic guide that can be easily fashioned prior to use (the Sheets glide).

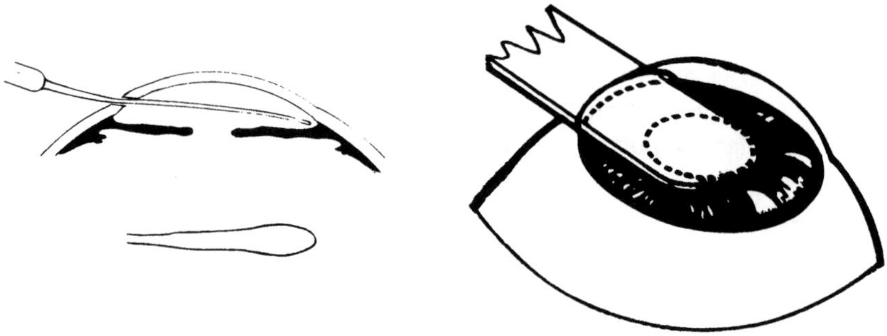

Fig. V-36. — Left: Flat, blunt spatula used as a glide to facilitate the introduction of an angle supported lens over the iris. Du Pont Guerry 1960.
Right: Schema representing how the "modern glide" is held in the eye. In general, only the upper iris sector and the pupil are covered.

There is little advantage in using such lens glides when the conditions are ideal. In a deep anterior chamber, any lens can be easily slid over the iris if the lens is held with a suitable forceps.

But problems may arise if the lens has to be inserted through a very narrow incision as is the case when the cataract is removed through a small incision as in phakoemulsification or phakofragmentation, or when the anterior chamber must be closed because of a forward bulge of the iris diaphragm. A lens glide is then useful in pushing the iris back and keeping the lens from sliding along the endothelium.

In extreme cases of bulging iris diaphragm, we prefer using a sleeve. With it, one can gradually work the lens into position or simply drop it into the anterior chamber and manipulate it into position after further closure of the incision. Such a sleeve can be made from a plastic sheet (see Fig. V-38). For most lenses, a width of 6 mm is suitable and a length of 12 to 15 mm.

Dardenne (personal communitation, 1978) has designed a metal lens glide for the two.loop iridocapsular lens.

The lens retaining suture suggested by C.W. Simcoe (1978) is also helpful for the implantation of a lens under difficult circumstances. This is a preplaced suture crossing the anterior chamber to prevent endothelial contact by the implant (Fig. V-39). A retaining suture combined with the use of a sleeve will generally resolve the most difficult problems, such as those that arise when the anterior chamber collapses as it is apt to do with younger patients.

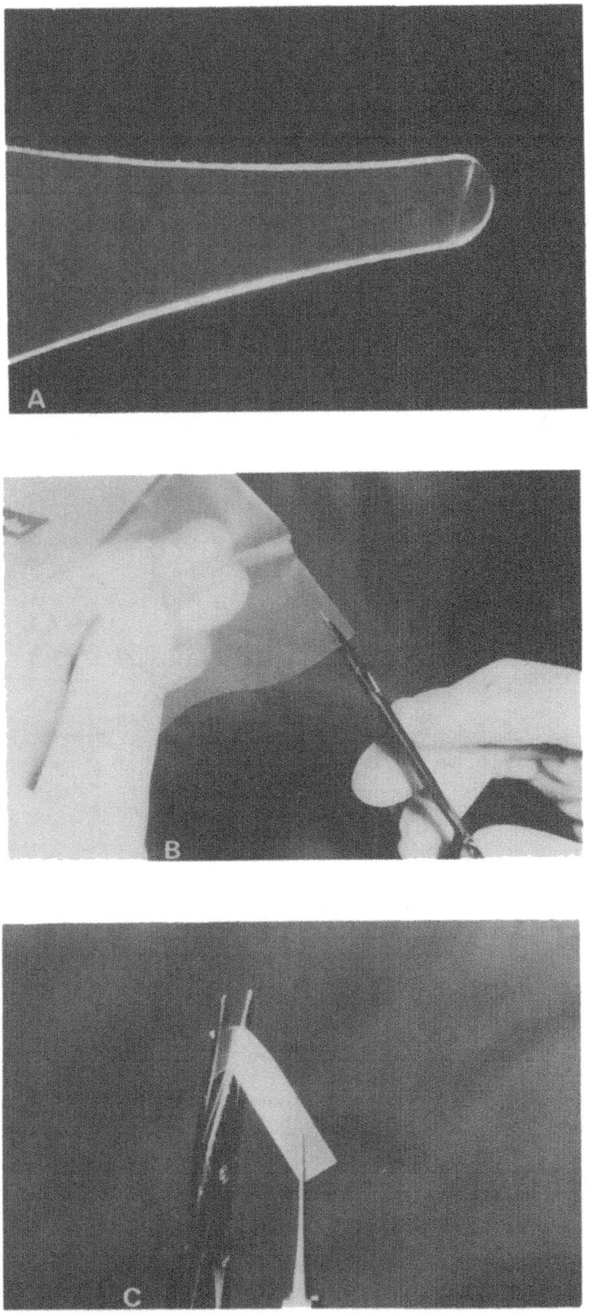

Fig. V-37a. — The commercially available plastic guide designed by J. Sheets.
b, c. — Method of fashioning a lens glide from a plastic sheet.

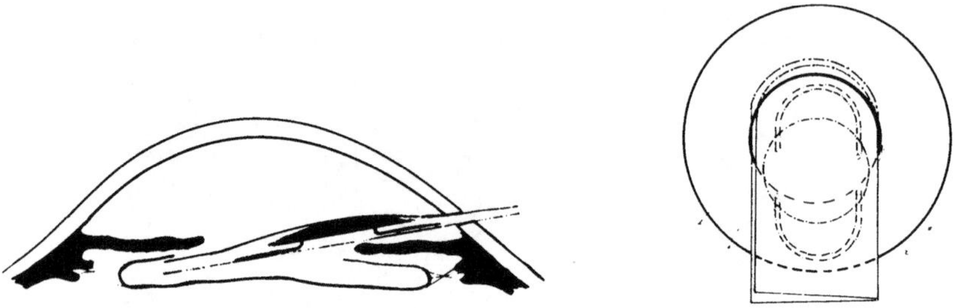

Fig. V-38. — Schematic side and front views illustrating the function of a sleeve. In this case, the distal end of the sleeve is placed in the capsular bag to assure the correct placement of the lens loop.

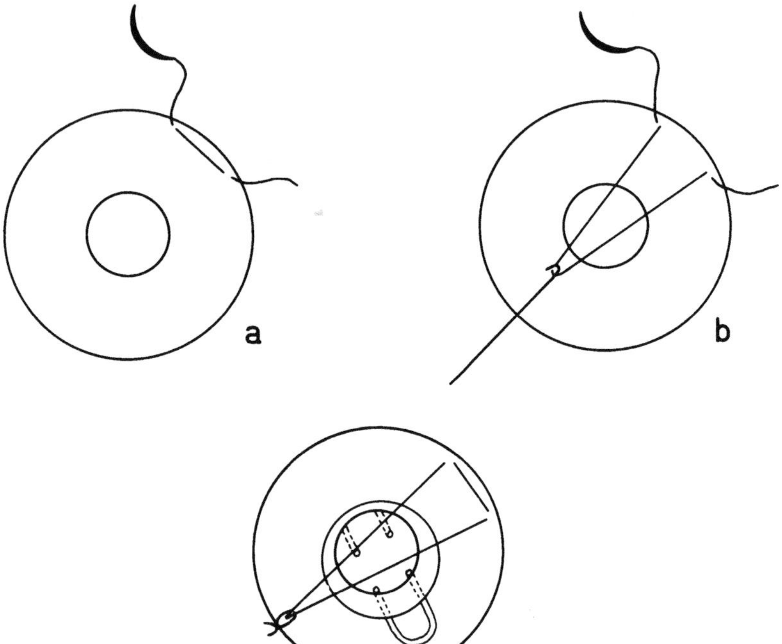

Fig. V-39. — Lens retaining sutures proposed by C.W. Simcoe.

Another way to facilitate atraumatic lens insertion is reformation of the anterior chamber with viscous solutions containing Na-hyaluronic acid (Miller 1979) or methylcellulose (Fechner 1978). Once the anterior eye segment is filled with such a jelly-like substance, the insertion of an implant is simplified and less traumatic. Little is known, however, of the long term effects of these products on the eye.

4. *Pupil Constriction*

Depending on the type of lens implanted, the pupil can be narrowed at this stage. Both intracameral and extraocular miotics are used.

5. *Iridectomies*

One or more iridectomies or iridotomies are performed either before or after implantation. There are some disadvantages of performing iridectomies before implantation:

— If bleeding occurs, visibility is temporarily hampered.

— If the lens is brought into the eye over an iridectomy, it may catch on it, which can lead to an iridodialysis.

As will be discussed below, some lens types require a specific kind of iridectomy because the coloboma is needed for the positioning of an antiluxating device such as the transiridectomy suture for the iris clip lens and the transcoloboma clip for the platinum clip lens.

6. *Finishing Touches*

The anterior chamber should be irrigated to evacuate all the pigment that may have come loose during the introduction of the lens.

At this stage, too, any large blood clots should be evacuated since excessive blood in the angle may lead to goniosynechiae. Blood on the iris prevents pupil constriction, and blood between the iris border and the lens itself may promote synechiae.

Iris colobomas should always be checked for patency and any peripheral iris adhesion should always be released. The presence of a large air bubble at this stage is of great help in the inspection of the iris root and the chamber angle (air gonioscopy). The angle structures and the colobomas can be easily inspected with a magnifier by looking at the superior part of the iris root (Binkhorst's air gonioscopy). With the microscope, air gonioscopy can be done with the aid of a dental mirror (Kelman, 1979). And, of course, gonioprisms can also be used.

It is prudent to center the lens before the incision is completely closed, even though pupil constriction will generally center an iris supported or an iridocapsular lens.

D. **Wound Closure and Astigmatism**

Even though there are many suitable techniques and materials available for closing a cataract incision, lens implantation has some special requirements:

— While the wound is being closed, the anterior chamber must always be kept perfectly formed in order to avoid endothelial contact by the lens. The best way to do this is with an air cushion, which stays in place better than fluid.
— During wound closure, the air is gradually exchanged for fluid, with care being taken to avoid endothelial contact.
— Only a perfectly watertight closure technique should be considered. The patient should leave the operating room with a well-formed anterior chamber, and postoperative collapse must be virtually impossible. In contrast to wound closure after simple cataract extraction, a flat anterior chamber after the operation will nearly always be disastrous. Corneal dystrophy is then almost inevitable.
— Early and prolonged use of topical corticosteroids can interfere with wound healing. Therefore, durable suturing materials are preferrable. The literature reports a trend toward the abandonment of virgin silk for nylon 9.0 and 10.0, polypropylene, or even fine stainless steel thread. Absorbable sutures (Vicryl®, Dexon®) lose a great deal of their tensile strength in a few weeks and are, therefore, not recommended.

Astigmatism after cataract extraction conforms to certain rules, which are no longer a mystery. R. Troutman has often emphasized that astigmatism with the rule occurs with the use of nylon 9.0 or 10.0 when one takes a rather large and deep bite through the wound lips and the suture is well-tightened. Since nylon will hold its tensile strength for months, this induced astigmatism with the rule will not alter spontaneously. Therefore, once the wound has partially healed (6 to 8 weeks after the operation), excessive astigmatism with the rule must be corrected by cutting one or more of the sutures situated in the meridian showing the highest refractive value.

Note: There are devices that can be used to check the degree of astigmatism during surgery. R. Troutman has devised a keratoscope to be used wich the microscope; Van Loenen Martinet, and Vijfwinkel have designed a simple device (see Fig. V-42) that gives useful information about the degree of astigmatism; and Terry developed a

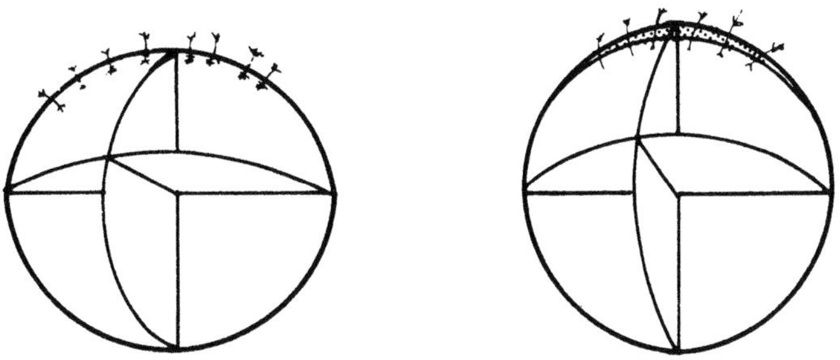

a b

Fig. V-40a. — "With the rule" astigmatism and b. — "against the rule" stigmatism resulting from too much and too little suture tension, respectively.

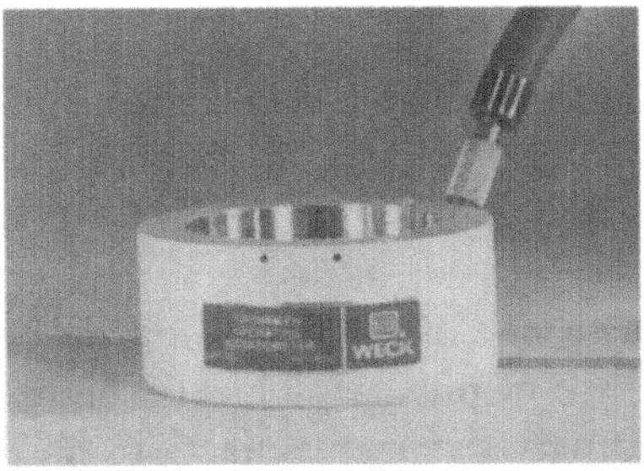

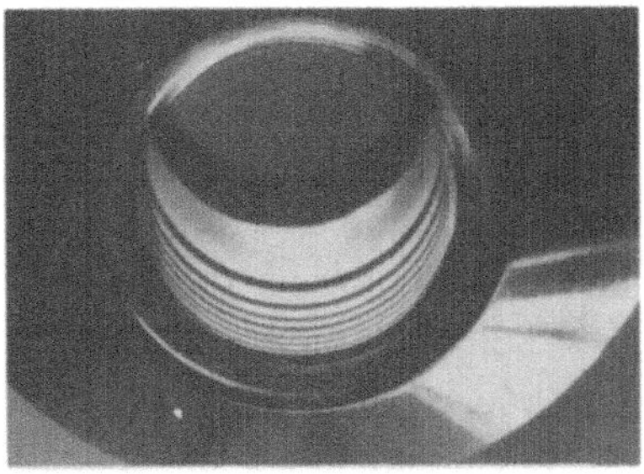

Fig. V-41. Fig. V-42.

Fig. V-41. — Troutman's keratometer for attachment to the surgical microscope, for the per-operative control of astigmatism.

Fig. V-42. — Simplified keratoscope designed by Van Loenen-Martinet and Vijfwinkel (inside view).

keratometer with which one can make a good determination of the degree of astigmatism during wound closure.

III. Postoperative Management

A. Postoperative Care

Depending on the type of lens that is used, miotics or mydriatics are administered in the days following the implantation. All eyes are given local steroids and antibiotics. Some surgeons inject antibiotics and/or corticosteroids subconjunctivally at the end of the surgical procedure. Acetazolamide or timolol are often used.

The patient may be allowed to get up on the same day. An eye patch is not mandatory, but a protective eye shield is highly advisable.

Beginning already on the first day after surgery, the eye should be regularly examined with a slit lamp. A great deal can be learned by observing the eye during the early postoperative period. For example, the status of the cornea is a good parameter for the assessment of surgical aggression. It is also useful to record the ocular tension as well as the degree of cellular reaction and flare in the anterior chamber, since these can provide the surgeon with information on the therapeutic course to be followed.

B. The Management of Some Postoperative Complications

1. *Shallow and Flat Anterior Chamber*

Serious problems may arise if the anterior chamber becomes shallow. In such a situation, a lens with parts protruding in front of the iris may come in contact with the endothelium and cause localized endothelial corneal dystrophy.

When the anterior chamber is shallow, one of the first things to be checked is pupillary block. The incidence of pupillary block is higher with lens implantation than with ordinary cataract extraction since the pseudophakos may hamper aqueous flow through the pupillary aperture. Well functioning iris colobomas can compensate for this. Judicious pupil dilation can release a pupillary block, but care must be taken to avoid lens luxation. Surgical management includes transfiction of the iris or additional iridectomies.

Wound leakage may be another cause for a shallow anterior chamber, and if it occurs, it must be treated without delay.

Should the anterior chamber be flat and contact between the endothelium and the lens occur, surgery is necessary. This may not be postponed lest total corneal decompensation result. The implant is separated from the endothelium by air and the causal factor dealt with.

2. *Subluxation and Luxation*

The subluxation of a part of the lens can sometimes be treated by pharmacological and sometimes by instrumental therapy. Occasionally, if no harmful side effects are expected, some lenses, such as a strut of a Sputnik lens, can be left in the subluxated position. Medical treatment of a subluxation often consists of mild dilation that may allow the subluxated part—a strut, a foot, or a loop—to return to its original place. A bit of imagination is helpful to place the head of the patient in such a position that gravity will induce the subluxated part to fall back into position. If these methods do not work, a discision needle can be used to resolve the problem. Should a vitreous knuckle prevent repositioning, osmotic agents can be considered. Most of these procedures can be carried out on an outpatient basis, unless significant dose of an osmotic agent is administered.

Since most patients are unaware that a part of their lens can be subluxated, J. Worst designed a simple instrument that permits the patient to observe the position of his own implant.

Total lens luxation or dislocation can occur anteriorly or posteriorly.

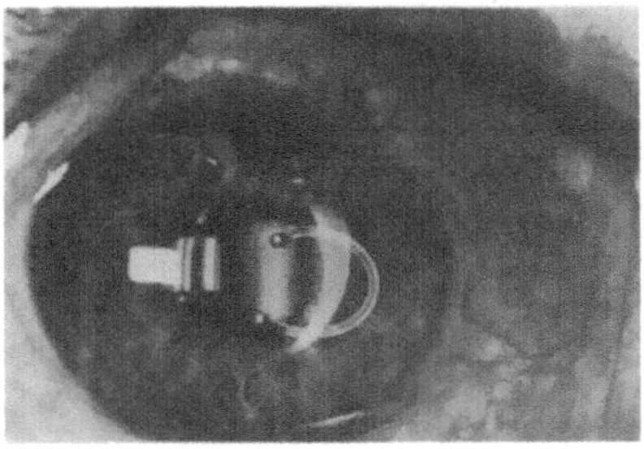

Fig. V-43.

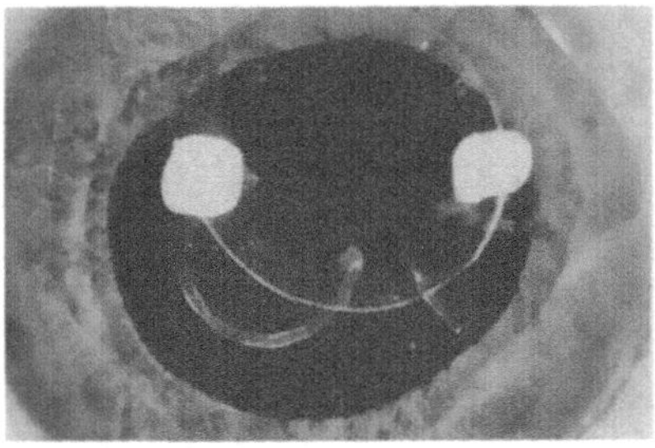

Fig. V-44.

Fig. V-43. — Subluxation of a medallion lens. (Courtesy J. J. Alpar.)

Fig. V-44. — Posterior dislocation of an anterior strut of a Sputnik lens. (Courtesy J. J. Alpar.)

Posterior dislocation must be approached leisurely. Indeed, some lightweight lenses have been left in the vitreous without further sequellae. Fishing a lens out of the vitreous cavity is a troublesome task, though various techniques are available. Lenses with loops may be picked up with a microhook, while other models, such as the Copeland Lens, require forceps removal. Vitrectomy devices are useful because a channel can be made to the luxated lens. With judicious dilation and the patient in the prone position, some lenses will cooperate by gliding into the pupillary aperture. Light taps on the

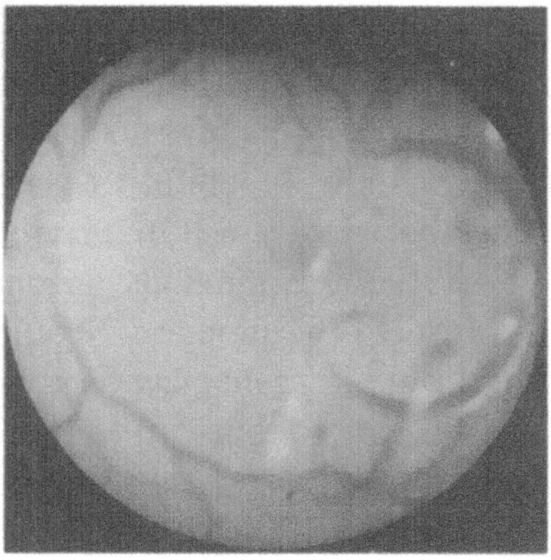

Fig. V-45.

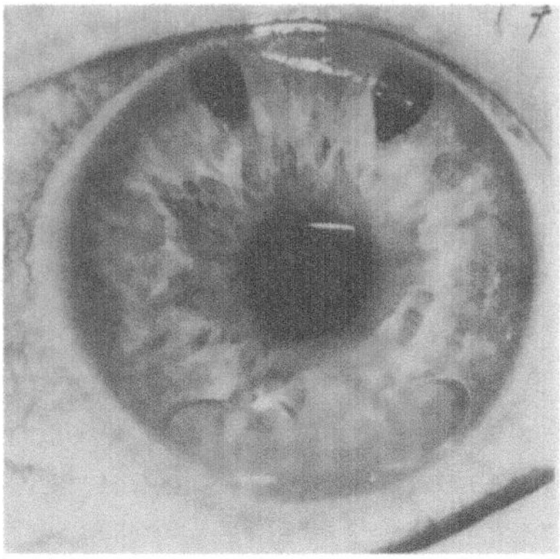

Fig. V-46.

Fig. V-45. — Dislocation of an unsutured iris clip lens into the vitreous. (Courtesy C.D. Binkhorst.)

Fig. V-46. — Anterior dislocation of an iridocapsular lens.

sclera of the eye can help to move the implant towards the desired position.

Total dislocation of the implant into the anterior chamber is a serious complication as the lens usually comes in contact with the endothelium (see chapter XII on lens implantation and the cornea). This kind of luxation is an emergency. Here, too, pharmacological repositioning must be considered first. If this is unsuccessful, the implant must be promptly repositioned by means of a micro-instrumental approach.

3. *Decentration*

The most common reason for lens decentration after ICCE is the extension of vitreous strands into the wound, which will pull up the pupil and the lens. An atonic pupil, a vitreous knuckle in the pupillary aperture, or an iris-to-lens suture located too peripherally can also cause lens decentration. Iris incarceration and peripheral anterior synechiae can also cause pupil deformation and subsequent lens decentration. After ECCE, lens decentration can occur as a result of asymmetric adhesions between loops and the iris, lens cortex, or capsule.

As long as the lens is not dangerously near the endothelium, therapeutic measures are not called for. But should corneal touch be

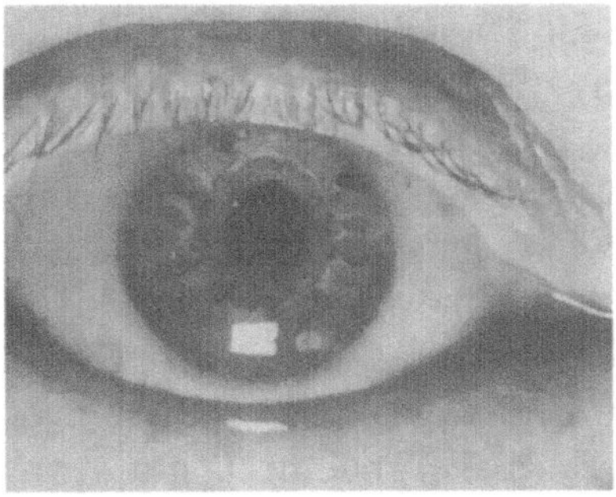

Fig. V-47. — Decentration of an irido-capsular lens.

likely, the offending part must be amputated, with due attention being given to the danger of lens instability. If the body of the lens makes contact with the cornea, more complicated procedures are necessary, i.e., the causal factor must be dealt with, e.g., cutting vitreous strands, releasing peripheral synechiae, or correct resuturing of the lens to the iris. All these procedures, it must be noted, require a high degree of skill on the part of the microsurgeon.

4. *Secondary Procedures for Lens Remnants*

After extracapsular cataract extraction, lens remnants are sometimes left in the pupillary aperture. Such material should not be removed hastily, since the situation may clear up in a few weeks by spontaneous resorption of the soft material.

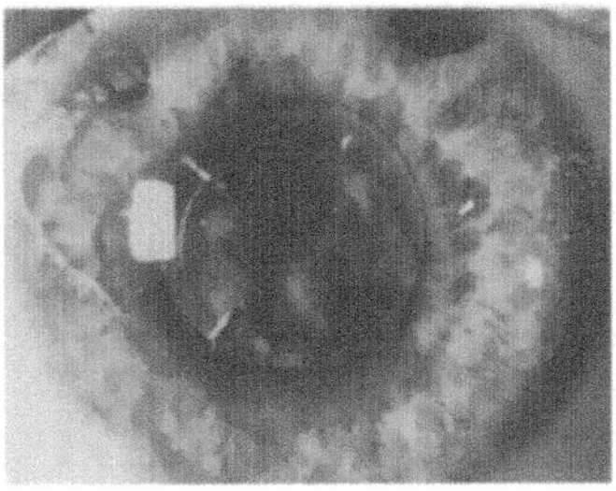

Fig. V-48.

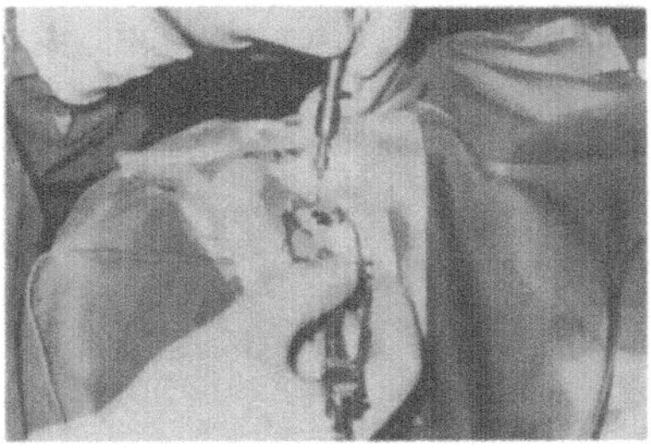

Fig. V-49.

Fig. V-48. — Soft lens material left after surgery. In this case, the pupil cleared spontaneously within 4 weeks.

Fig. V-49. — Irrigation-aspiration of excessive cortical material using 2 separated cannulas.

One intervention that may be effective is to dislodge the soft material and to " place " it between, for example, the iris and the lens capsule outside the pupillary aperture. The technique is simple. The anterior chamber is entered with a small, sharp discission needle such as a Haab knife 0.5 mm wide, and the soft material is swept away either superiorly or inferiorly. The lens remnants can also be brought into the anterior chamber where they will be resorbed.

Another method to remove small amounts of residual cortical material is simple aspiration. The cornea is punctured and the eye is entered with a blunt cannula (e.g., 25 guage) mounted on a syringe half-filled with fluid. The tip of the cannula is brought behind the lens and introduced between the cortical lens material. After careful aspiration, the needle is withdrawn. If the anterior chamber tends to collapse, an air cushion must be maintained between the lens and the endothelium.

When large amounts of cortical material are left over, both irrigation and aspiration are indicated. Two separate blunt cannulae may be introduced at 3 and 9 o'clock respectively. The soft material is then aspirated gently from behind the lens, the anterior chamber being kept formed by means of an infusion bottle with the dripper level some 20 cm about the iris level. Since the aspiration must be controllable by the surgeon himself, there must be a device that can cut of the vacuum (we use a cannula holder of our own design, which is described on p. 000).

5. *Incision of the Posterior Capsule and Secondary Membranes*

The incision of an opaque posterior capsule can be done either immediately after the lens is inserted or at a later stage. There is a great variety of capsulotomy instruments. The simplest is a 30

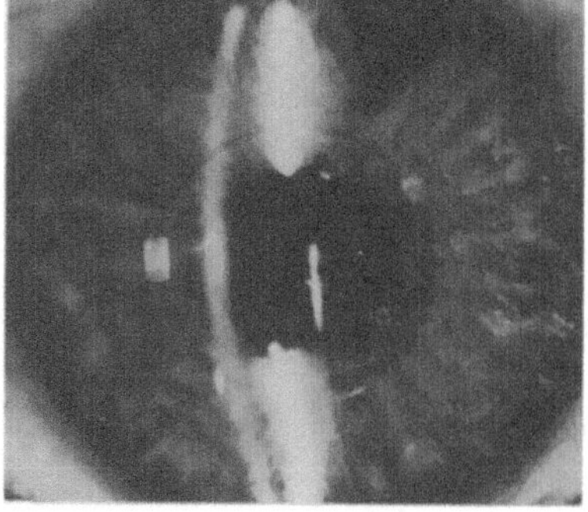

Fig. V-50. — Opacification of the posterior capsula.

guage disposable needle with its point bent 90° or more. Another is the very small discision Haab knife, which C.D. Binkhorst uses.

With the bent disposable needle, the posterior capsule is punctured on the nasal side of the pupillary aperture and the "micro hook" is gently brought toward the temporal side while ripping the capsule open. If necessary, the procedure can be repeated in any direction. For very thin membranes, a 30 guage needle, with or without a bent tip, can be sufficient to make a sufficiently large tear.

C.D. Binkhorst generally tries to make the incision(s) perpendicular to stress lines that can sometimes be seen on the capsule with a slit lamp.

A combination of the hooking and cutting principle is our own modification of the Haab knife (Fig. V-52).

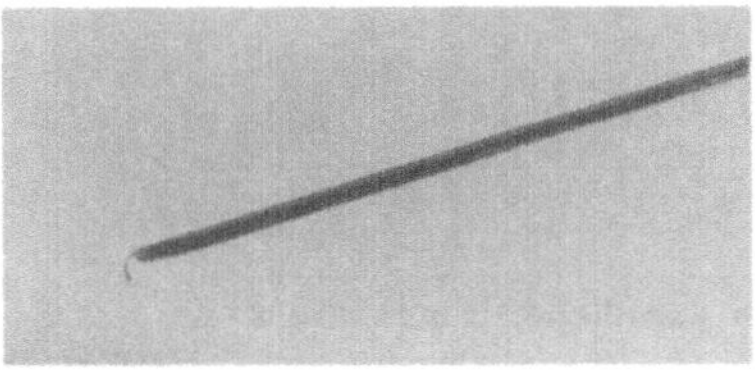

Fig. V-51. — Microhook made from a 30 gauge disposable needle for the opening of a tin membrane behind the pseudophakos.

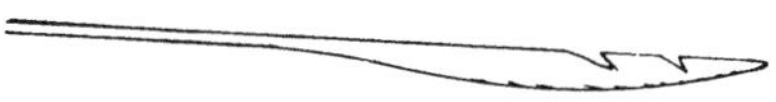

Fig. V-52. — Modified Haab's knife for cutting and hooking a retroimplant membrane.

Note: With a discision knife or a small needle, an adequate opening can be made in the central part of the posterior capsule, often without disturbing the anterior hyaloid face. This is easily achieved in cases when there is a space between the capsule and the anterior hyaloid because of adherences between the posterior loops and the capsule.

For rather thick membranes, two bent disposable needles may be necessary. They are introduced in opposite directions and are worked together (Galin, 1976).

Some surgeons prefer to remove retrolenticular membranes by using the so-called VISC devices (vitreous suction and cutting) (Girard, 1974; Eichenbaum, 1977, Jaffe et al., 1978; Deutman, 1978; Galand et al., 1979). After the membrane is punctured with a rather large capsulotomy knife, the flaps are aspirated and fragmented with

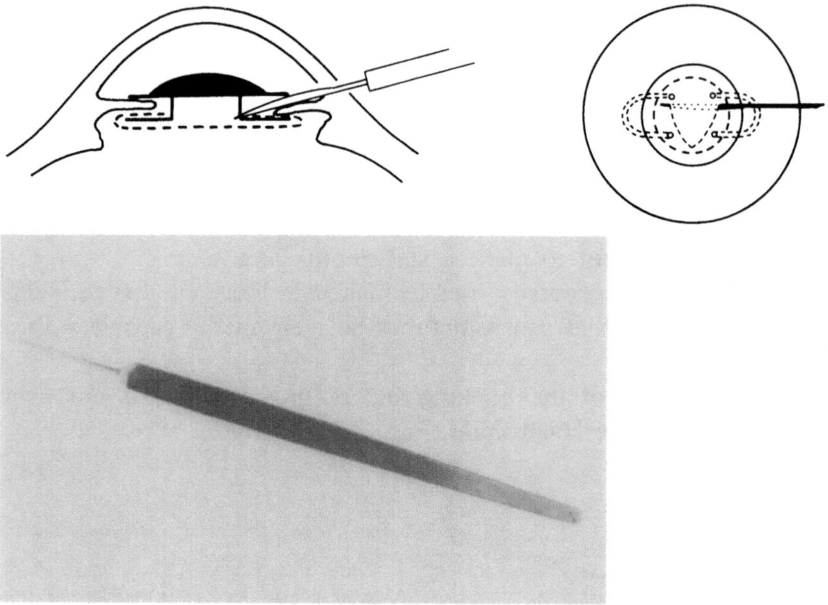

Fig. V-53. — Discision of the posterior capsule with a Haab's knife.

the VISC probe introduced through the pars plana. Although this procedure is certainly effective, in our opinion it should be used only exceptionally. In our own series of 1000 extracapsular cases, we never had to have recourse to it, nor have C.D. Binkhorst and J. Worst, who have performed many thousands of extracapsular procedures.

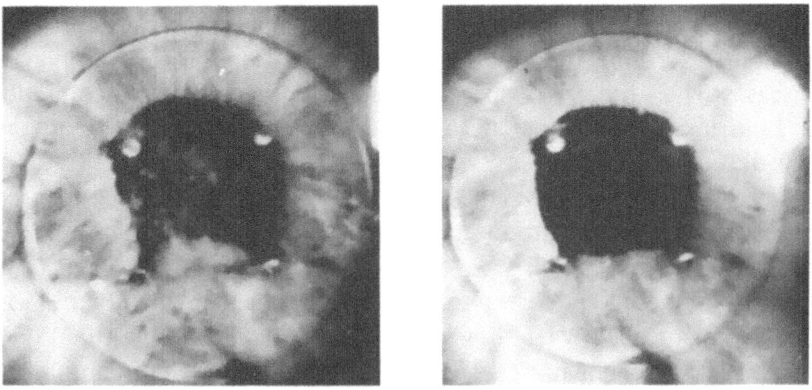

Fig. V-54. — Retroimplant membrane removed by a VISC device using the pars plana approach. (Courtesy A. Galand.)

Another method deserving of our attention is one using a pulsed laser beam that primarily was developed to destroy membrane structures and strands in the vitreous. According to D. Aron Rosa (personal communication, 1980), also the destruction of a secondary membrane behind a polymethylmethacrylate implant is a rather simple procedure.

6. *Lens Removal*

The removal of an implant is a complex procedure that should only be undertaken by an experienced implant surgeon. A distinction must be made between partial and total removal.

a. *Partial Removal*

Most often, only the anterior part—the optic portion or a haptic component—of an implant protruding into the anterior chamber has to be removed (e.g., because of corneal contact). For example, a small incision in the anterior chamber peripherally is made and the optic portion is cut off with fine scissors from the posterior loop attachments while the anterior chamber is kept formed with air, fluid, or coating agents. Retaining devices may also be helpful in preventing contact between the implant and the endothelium. Finally, the inci-

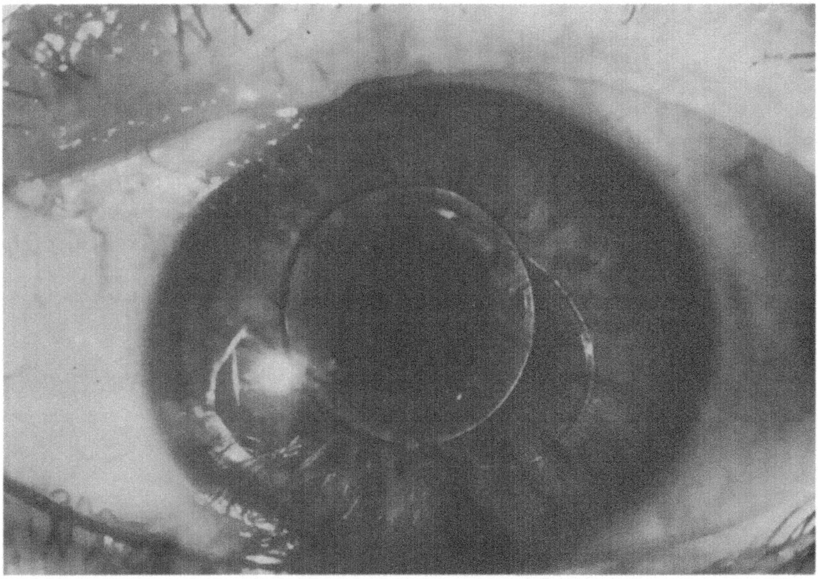

Fig. V-55. — Amputation of an offending anterior loop.

sion is widened just enough to allow the part to be removed with a small forceps. For the removal of an anterior loop or strut, a corneal incision is made in the area overlying the offending part, which is then cut off with a scissors. Usually a stab incision in the periphery of the cornea will suffice for the removal of the loop or strut with a fine forceps.

b. *Total Removal*

When a loose lens is involved, the procedure is relatively simple. Through a small incision, all parts of the lens are brought in front of the iris by means of a spatula a needle, a discission knife, a micro-hook or the like. Here, too, the anterior chamber should be maintained with fluid, air, or coating agents, and the use of retaining devices should be considered. A small forceps is used to take the lens out through the incision, which must be enlarged just enough to allow it to pass.

Total removal of an iris supported or an iridocapsular supported implant that is well-fixed in the eye with multiple synechiae is nearly impossible without excision of a part of the iris, and possibly even a part of the posterior capsule. Since these procedures depend on anatomical conditions that can vary widely from case to case, no general rules can be formulated.

IV. Stabilization of Implants by Sutures

Sutures can be used to stabilize an implant lens during and also after surgery. Techniques specific to particular lenses are described in the respective chapters dealing with the implantation techniques.

Polypropylene (9.0 or 10.0) or 30μ steel wire are used for this purpose. According to J. Worst, the latter is best for fixation of his "slotted Medallion lens".

1) *Alpar's Approach*

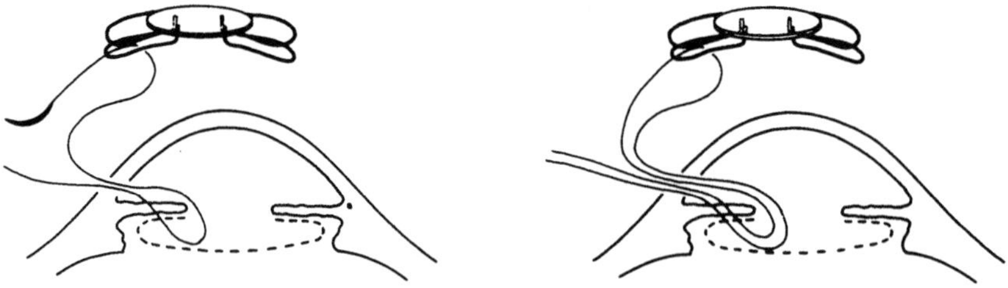

Fig. V-56. — Peroperative stabilization of an implant using sutures as suggested by J. Alpar.

2) *Simcoe's Approach*

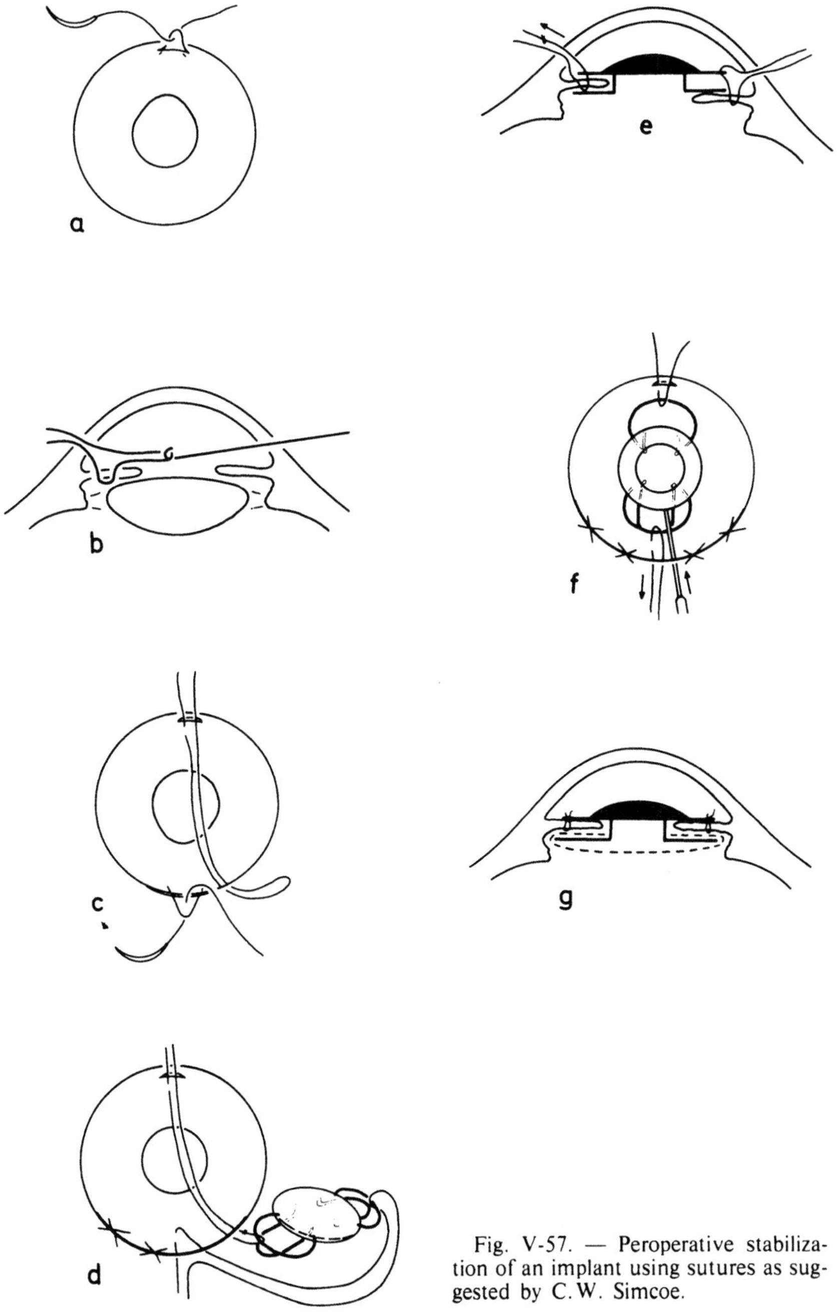

Fig. V-57. — Peroperative stabilization of an implant using sutures as suggested by C.W. Simcoe.

3) *McCannel-Binkhorst Suture*

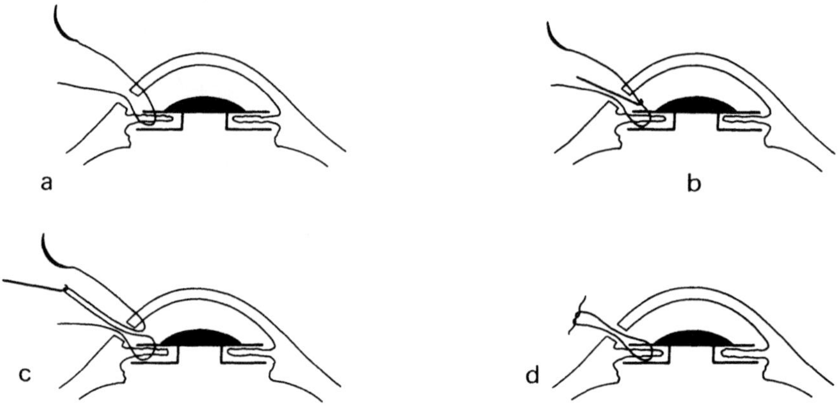

Fig. V-58. — Steps of the Binkhorst-McCannel technique for peroperative and postoperative stabilization of an implant.

The McCannel-Binkhorst suture can be used with lenses that have loops extending in front of or behind the iris and with implants that have holes drilled in their haptic portion. A curved needle swaged with a 10.0 polypropylene thread is passed through a small stab incision in the cornea. A bite of the iris tissue is taken along with the loop. The point of the needle is turned gently upwards and is passed through the overlying cornea by making a counterpuncture. The suture between the iris and the corneal counterpuncture is retrieved by means of a microhook through the stab incision. The suture ends that come out of the stab incision are carefully tied and trimmed off flush, the knot being allowed to enter the anterior chamber.

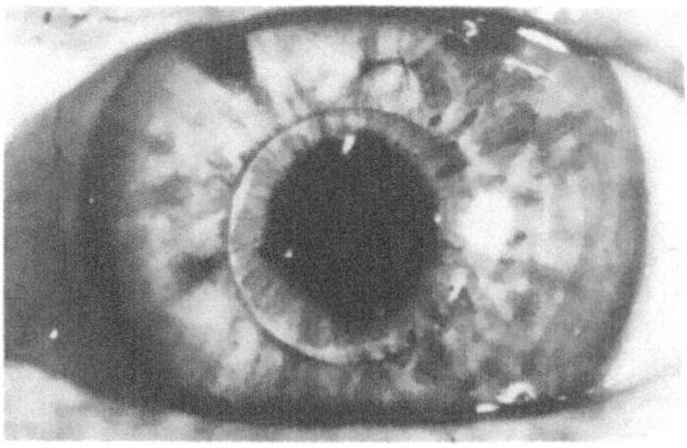

Fig. V-59. — An iridocapsular lens being steadied with a Binkhorst-McCannel suture.

4) *The Strampelli Thread*

Finally, as proposed by J. Worst (1980), permanent retaining sutures crossing the anterior segment can be used to stabilize a loose or decentered lens. He suggests using stainless steel thread with the ends being buried under a scleral flap, and he calls this retaining device the "Strampelli Thread".

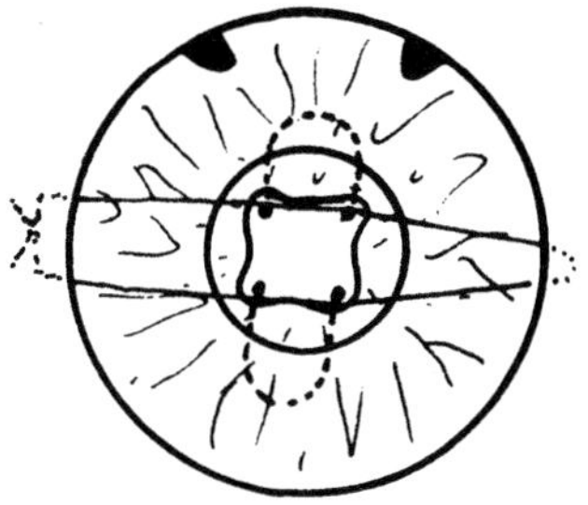

Fig. V-60. — Schematic view of a permanent suture crossing the anterior chamber to steady a lens. The thread lies in front of the iris and behind the optic portion of the implant.

Up until now, the range of needles available has been rather incomplete. For open sky techniques, the curved corneo-scleral needles are used. The ski-shaped needle designed by Drews is very useful in suturing through the iris.

Long needles, which are particularly important for the closed chamber techniques, can be made by oneself. J. Worst has shown how one can use very thin, disposable injection needles (30 guage) for all sorts of thread.

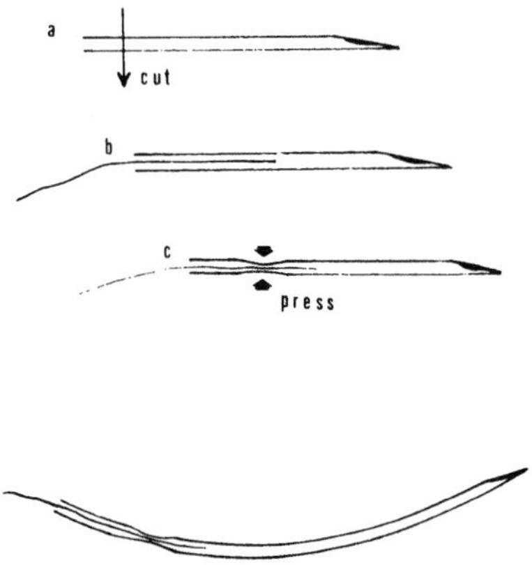

Fig. V-61. — Method for adapting long needles: a) a long, 30 g needle is cut off or broken at the required length; b) a 9-0 of 10-0 polypropylene thread or 30μ stainless steel wire is introduced in the lumen; c) the needle is pressed tight a few mm from the end. The needle can be given a particular curvature by means of 2 forceps or needle holders. Note: Long and very sharp injection needles (30 g) are used in dentistry.

CHAPTER VI

IRIS SUPPORTED LENSES

Introduction

After having used the different lens types that were available in the mid-fifties such as the Ridley lens and a variety of angle supported lenses, C.D. Binkhorst concluded that the iris probably would be a suitable carrier for a lightweight implant. It is important to note that he was not disappointed with the result he obtained from 12 cases of Ridley lens implants (Binkhorst, 1957). But, as he pointed out, "this technique is too much of a strain on the surgeon and especially it is asking too much of the human hand never to fail in completely sparing the delicate suspension system of zonule and posterior capsule" (Binkhorst, 1959). On the other hand, the results he obtained with the first anterior chamber lenses with rigid supports were disappointing, the major complication being early or late endothelial corneal dystrophy (Binkhorst, 1960).

As an alternative solution, Binkhorst designed the iris clip lens in 1957. Actually, this was not the first iris supported lens in use at that time. D.L. Epstein had already inserted a few of his "Collar Stud" and "Maltese Cross" lenses, but his clinical observations were not published until 1959.

During the following years, these iris supported lenses were followed by a variety of other models based on the same principle:
— the Fyodorov I lens in 1968;
— the Copeland one plane lens in 1968;
— the Fyodorov II lens in 1970, nicknamed the "Sputnik" lens;
— the medallion lens in 1970 and later modifications.

All these lenses were initially designed to be inserted after intracapsular cataract extraction, obviously they could also be used in the presence of a posterior capsule. Up till now, most of the iris supported lens insertions have taken place after intracapsular cataract extraction. In the future we may expect an increasing number of these lenses to be implanted after planned extracapsular cataract extraction since this technique seems to provide substantial advantages.

In this chapter, we shall deal with the possibilities and limitations of iris supported lenses after intracapsular cataract extraction (ICCE). Special attention will be given to the underlying why's and how's of the various modifications in lens design and techniques that have been introduced.

§1 THE IRIS CLIP LENS

I. Introduction to the Lens and Its Evolution

The iris clip lens is an iris supported lens having two components: an optical part made of polymethylmethacrylate with a diameter of 5 mm, and a haptic part consisting of two pairs of loops made of nylon or polypropylene. In the model currently used, the anterior loops have an overall diameter of 8 mm, and the clearance between the anterior and posterior loops is 0.50 mm to 0.75 mm. Both pairs of loops are bent backward at an angle of 15°. The weight of the lens in aqueous depends on whether nylon or polypropylene material is used to make the loops. With nylon loops, it is 10.0 mg in air and 2.5 mg in aqueous; with polypropylene, it is 9.5 mg in air and 1.0 mg in aqueous.

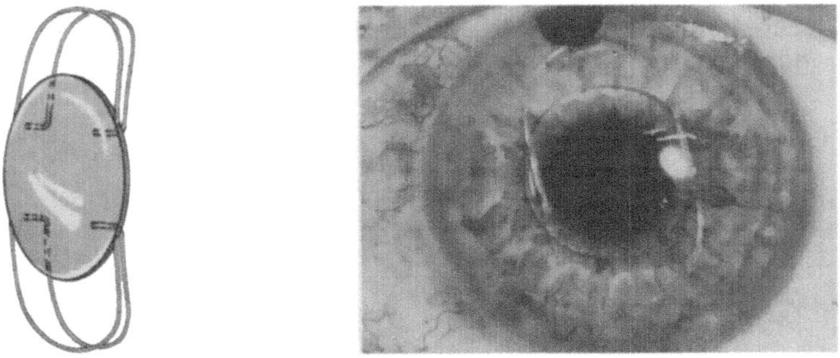

Fig. VI-1. — The iris clip lens of C.D. Binkhorst.

Binkhorst called his lens the "iris clip lens" because of its resemblance to a paper clip. This was somewhat misleading and caused some who were unfamiliar with the lens to conclude that the "loops would pinch the iris".

During the two decades that have since elapsed during which Binkhorst as well as other surgeons used this lens, some apparently small but significant modifications were introduced into the design of the lens itself as well as in the fixation technique.

The reader may profit from the thesis on lensimplantation written by M.E. Nordlohne (1975) in which he fully documents the evolution of the iris clip lens.

A. Binkhorst's Design Changes

1. *Loop Length*

The length of the loops may be defined as the length of the line connecting the extremeties of the diametrically opposed loops (Nordlohne, 1975). In the first hundred models, the anterior loops had a length of ≈7 mm. Between 1962 and 1965, the length was increased to 8 mm, and during the three following years a 9 mm lens was used. From 1969 on, the length has been reduced to 8 mm.

7 mm →	8 mm →	9 mm →	8 mm
1958	1962	1965	1969

2. *Loop Design*

Initially, the anterior loops and the optical component were located in the same geometrical plane. Since the end of 1971, the loops have been bent backward at an angle of about 15° with respect to the plane of the optical component.

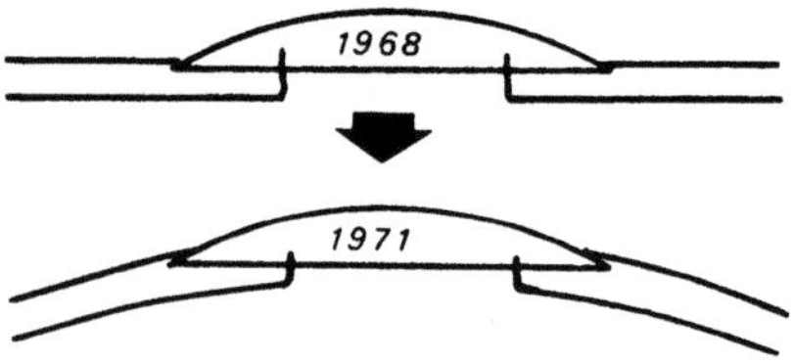

Fig. VI-2. — Change in the profile of the iris clip lens by backward bending of the loops.

3. *Material*

Since 1977, the loops have been made of polypropylene thread. The lens body itself is still being made of polymethylmethacrylate. Changing the material of the loops reduced the weight of the lens from 2.5 mg to 1.0 mg in aqueous.

B. Binkhorst's Changes in Loop Orientation and Additional Fixation Aids

Until 1969, most of the iris clip lenses were inserted with the largest diameter in the horizontal direction. Later on vertical insertions became routine.

In order to provide additional stability for the lens, the use of miotics was introduced in 1965 to keep the pupil constricted.

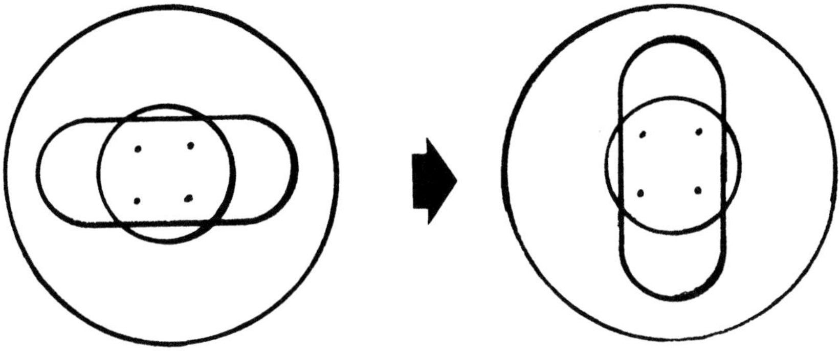

1958 1969

Fig. VI-3. — Horizontal and vertical positioning of the iris is clip lens.

After trying out various kinds of sutures, Binkhorst finally opted for the so-called transiridectomy suture to prevent luxation even when miotics were not used.

C. **Modifications of the Iris Clip Lens by Other Surgeons**

1. *The Fyodorov Mark I Lens (1968)*

After having inserted several iris clip lenses, S. Fyodorov of the USSR modified the iris clip lens as shown in Figure VI-4. In this model, the axes of the anterior and the posterior loops are not parallel but intersect at an angle of 90°. Still in use today on a moderate scale, its insertion is felt to be simpler than that of the

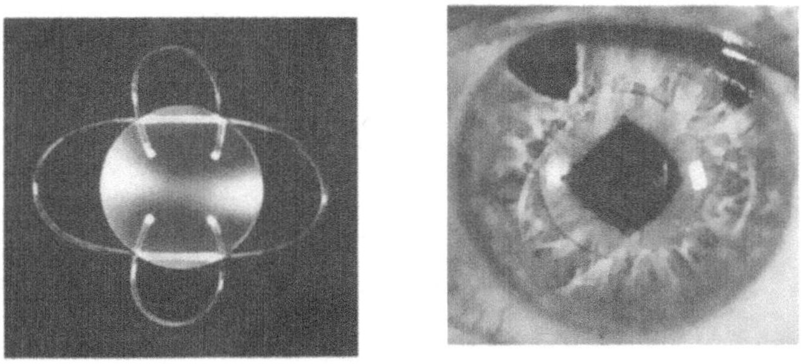

Fig. VI-4. — The Fyodorov Mark I lens.

original iris clip lens because the posterior loops can be easily identified. And like the iris clip lens, the loops of the Fyodorov Mark I are also bent backward at an angle of 15°. This lens was recommended by Hirschmann as being a simple lens for beginners, but he also stressed that long-term stability may become a problem unless there is additional suturing through the iris.

According to K.J. Hoffer (1978), at least 2700 such lenses were inserted by members of the American Intraocular Implant Society before 1977. Fyodorov himself abandoned this lens for his "Sputnik" lens, which will be discussed below.

2. *Modification by L. Lurie (1965)*

In order to facilitate identification of the loops during insertion, L. Lurie of London introduced black posterior loops.

3. *Modification by P. Leonard (1968)*

In 1968, P. Leonard asked K. Morcher, the lens manufacturer, to change the axis between the anterior and posterior loops: an angle of 15° to 20° was shown to facilitate insertion of the lens as it was felt that identification of the anterior and the posterior loops would be easier. Although Leonard soon abandoned it, some surgeons still prefer this modification of the iris clip lens (K. Morcher, personal communication).

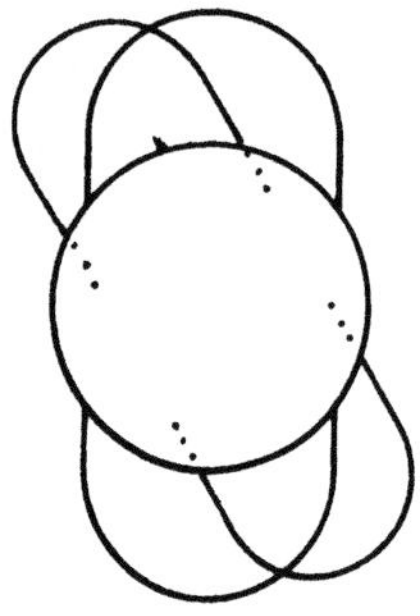

Fig. VI-5.

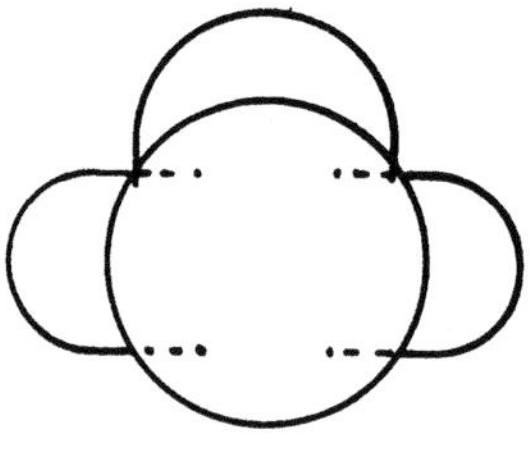

Fig. VI-6.

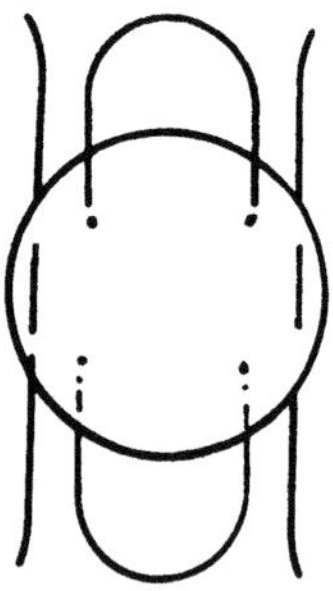

Fig. VI-7.

Fig. VI-5. — Leonard's modification of the iris clip lens.

Fig. VI-6. — Schott's modification of the iris clip lens.

Fig. VI-7. — Kwitko's modification of the iris clip lens.

4. *Modification by J. Worst*

As will be presented in detail below, J. Worst after having introduced various techniques for suturing the iris clip lens to the iris, designed an iris supported lens with only two posterior loops and an additional haptic rim at the upper edge of the optic portion. Fixation and stability of the lens is achieved by a suture passing through the iris and the two holes in the haptic rim.

5. *Modification by K. Schott*

In order to provide the lens with an iris suture, K. Schott of Germany designed an iris supported lens with one anterior loop. It is similar in many respects to the medallion lens, but the suturing is felt to be easier.

6. *Modification by M. Kwitko (1974)*

Since 1974, M. Kwitko (1976) has been using a modified iris clip lens without the distal portion of the anterior loop. Kwitko is of the opinion that the four atennae-like anterior supports reduce the possibility of corneal contact.

II. Implantation Techniques

A. **Binkhorst's Technique**

1. *Vertical Positioning of the Lens*

After the extraction of the cataractous lens if the diameter of the pupil exceeds 6 mm, it is narrowed with a minimal dose of acethylcholine (1/100). The purpose of this step is to make sure that the sphincter will constrict after lens insertion and that no vitreous is present in the pupillary area. All the loose pigment is evacuated with fluid, and the iris diaphragm is floated. The anterior chamber is reformed with air or fluid, according to the judgment of the surgeon. The iris clip lens is prepared and mounted in the special Binkhorst forceps, the irrigating cannula having been tested for obstructions and the air evacuated. While the left hand lifts the cornea just enough to allow the implant and forceps to pass, the lens is slid into the anterior chamber with the posterior loops kept close to the iris in order to avoid endothelial contact. In the meantime, the assistant begins irrigating the anterior chamber by operating the syringe connected to the irrigating cannula of the forceps. The surgeon gently moves the lens towards 6 o'clock until the iris sector slides between the two inferior loops (Fig. VI-8). Sometimes a gentle zigzag movement facilitates this step. When the pupillary margin shows the typical square deformation at 6 o'clock that is produced by the posterior loop attachments, it is a sure sign that the iris is engaged properly between the loops and not in front or behind them.

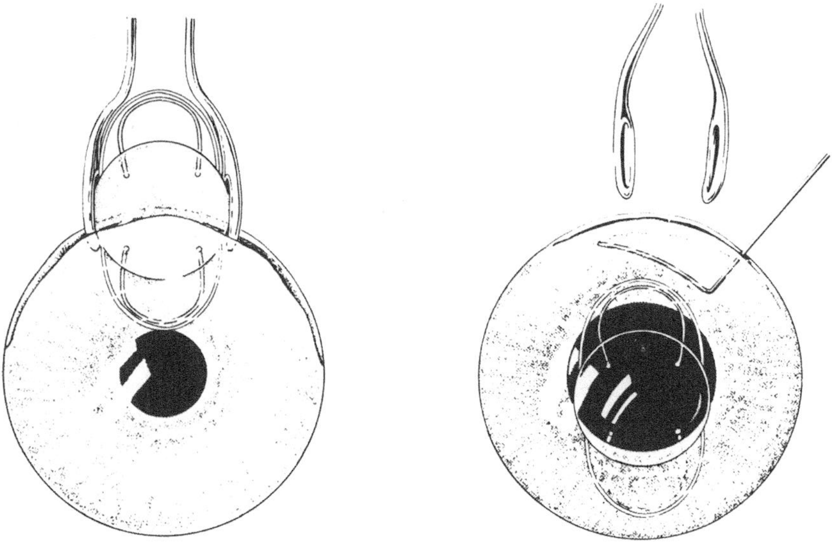

Fig. VI-8. — Vertical insertion of the iris clip lens and positioning of the inferior loops.

There are different ways of engaging the superior loops:

1. When the pupil is *rather large* (but no more than 5-6 mm), the insertion maneuver towards 6 o'clock is continued until the pupil is fairly pear-shaped, thus allowing the superior posterior loop to be brought through the pupillary aperture. When the pressure towards 6 o'clock is released, the pupillary margin at 12 o'clock will spontaneously engage between the two superior loops providing the lens is held in the correct position. Once the lens is in place, the forceps are opened and removed from the eye, always by sliding them over the iris.

2. When the pupil is *rather small,* the lens forceps are removed as soon as the inferior loops are properly placed, leaving both superior loops in front of the iris. A two-handed maneuver is necessary in order to perform the proper insertion of the superior loops: while a

fine wire repositor is held between the superior loops to steady the lens, a blunt iris hook is used to pull the sphincter over the posterior loop with a circular movement (Fig. VI-9). If necessary, the assistant keeps the anterior chamber formed by irrigation. Another way of engaging the superior posterior loop is to steady the lens with a repositor and to grasp the upper iris sector with a fine-toothed forceps in order to pull it over the posterior loop.

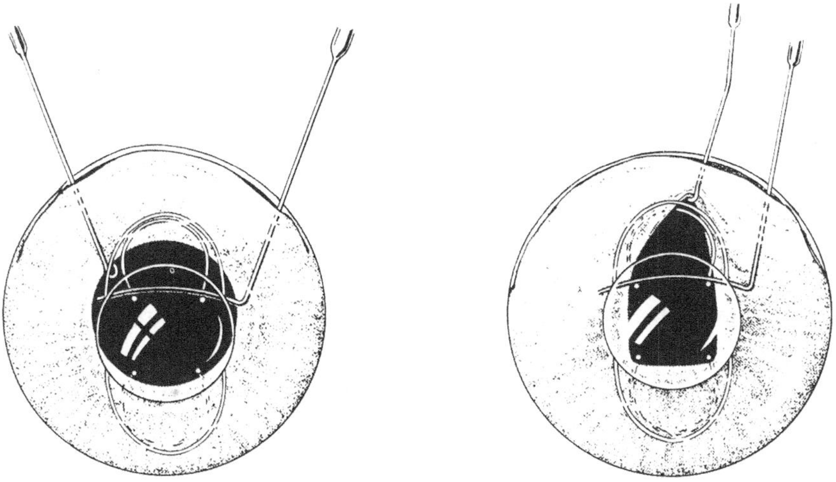

Fig. VI-9. — Bimanual maneuver for the positioning of the posterior superior loop of the iris clip lens.

2. *Transiridectomy Suturing*

An iridectomy of the appropriate size is made in order to expose the tip of the posterior loop. While the assistant gently lifts the cornea, the anterior loop is grasped with fine forceps and lifted to present the tip of the posterior loop through the coloboma. Using a specially prepared blunt needle (BIF 4 Ethicon®), a 10-0 Prolene® suture is passed through both superior loops (Fig. VI-10), starting with the posterior one, and brought out of the eye. A surgical knot is made to connect both loops, with enough clearance being left to allow the iris to move between them. The ends of the knot are cut as short as possible. The anterior chamber is closed watertight; before closure, it is generally filled with air, which is gradually replaced with fluid during the suturing procedure. If required, acetylcholine is used after the lens is put in place. As a rule, pilocarpine eye drops are administered on the outer eye while the wound is being closed.

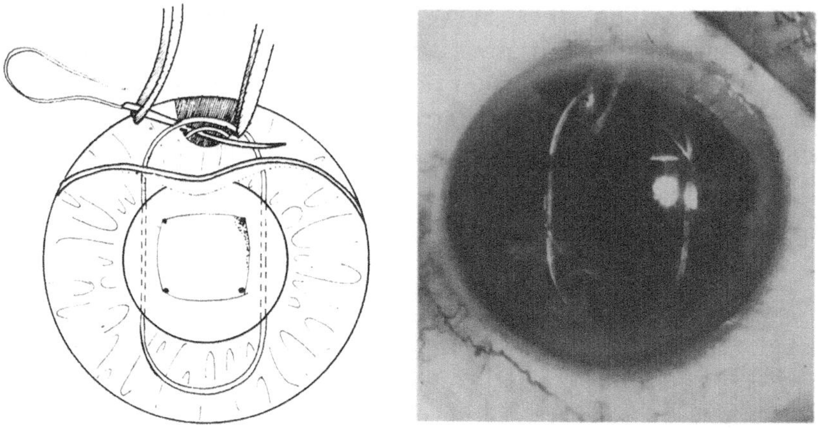

Fig. VI-10. — Technique for the placement of a transiridectomy suture connecting both superior loops of the iris clip lens and iris clip lens with transcoloboma suture in situ.

A modification of the original transiridectomy suturing technique has been proposed by J.O. Beauchamp, M.H. Clayman, and N.S. Jaffe (1976). The specially prepared needle is first passed through both superior loops using fine tissue forceps (non-magnetic) after which the needle is extracted by means of a small magnet (Beauchamp Magnesure).

R.C. Drews (1979) has proposed a pigtail suture guide to introduce the transiridectomy suture into the formed anterior chamber. First, a suture is threaded through the hole in the pigtail guide. The suture is brought under the posterior loop of the iris clip lens in the iridoctomy and forward out through the loop with a rotating motion. The suture is retrieved in front of the anterior loop with a fine iris hook. The guide is rotated back again and brought out of the wound, trailing some suture after it posterior to the loop. The iris hook is also drawn from the wound, bringing out the other end of the suture anterior to the lens loop. The suture is then tied around the loops.

B. Other Techniques

1. *The "Closed Chamber" Technique*

After delivery of the lens, the eye is temporarily closed except for 6-7 mm at the 12 o'clock position. The lens is held with McPherson forceps or a similar instrument at one of the posterior loop attachments and introduced into the anterior chamber, which is kept formed with air or fluid (some forceps have built-in irrigating cannulae). Depending on the surgeon's skill and the particular situation, both the inferior and the superior iris sectors can be engaged between the corresponding loops in one movement. Of course, the upper iris sector can also be engaged by using small iris forceps or a blunt iris hook.

Particularly in the U.S., the "lens glide" is used to facilitate the insertion of the lens through a small incision. (See p. 131).

2. *Horizontal Positioning of the Lens (not recommended)*

A pupil of at least 5-6 mm in diameter is required. The lens is grasped as illustrated (Fig. VI-11) and introduced into the eye close to the iris. Performing a zigzag movement with the lens, the surgeon engages either the temporal or the nasal sector between the two loops. In order to engage the opposite iris sector, the lens is brought into a more eccentric position and recentered after the pupillary margin is trapped between the remaining anterior and posterior loops. Since the pupil has to be rather large for a horizontal insertion, the use of intraocular miotics is indicated after the lens is in position. If necessary, the lens can be rotated 90° by using a blunt iris hook.

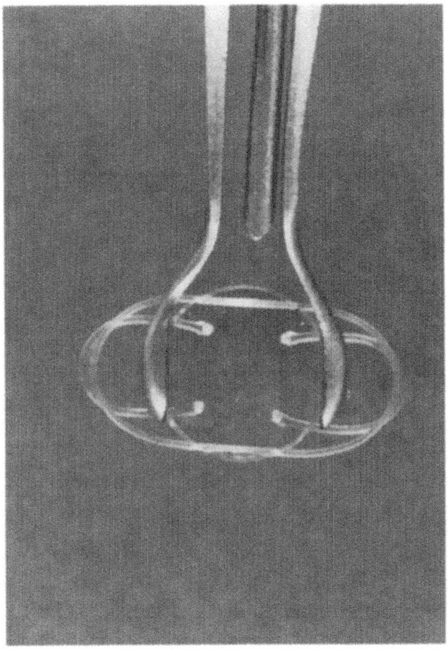

Fig. VI-11. — Iris clip lens held in correct positioning for horizontal insertion.

3. *Modified Suturing Techniques*

In addition to the above-described transiridectomy suturing techniques a variety of other suturing techniques have been developed to provide the iris clip lens with an additional anti-luxating device.

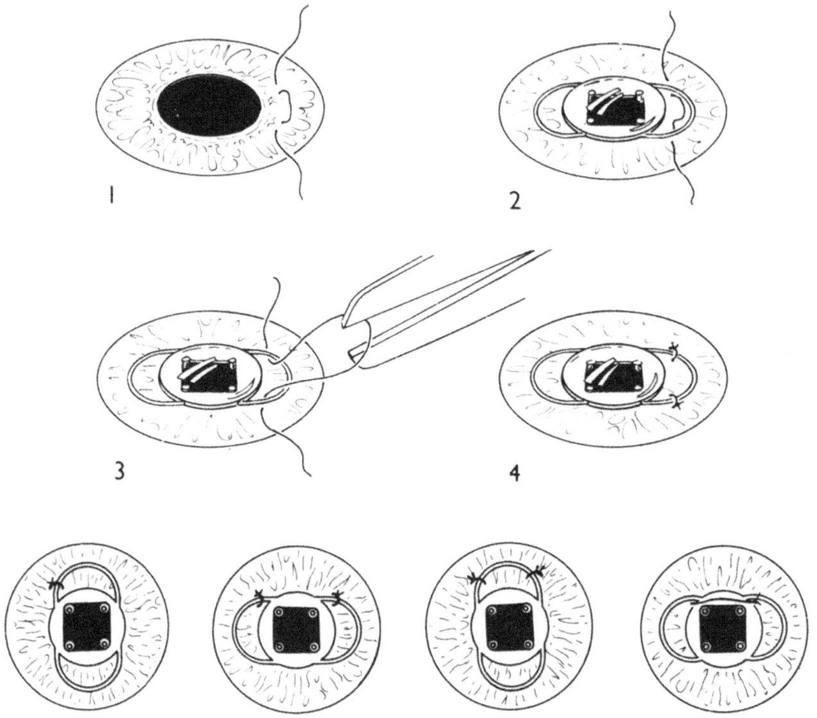

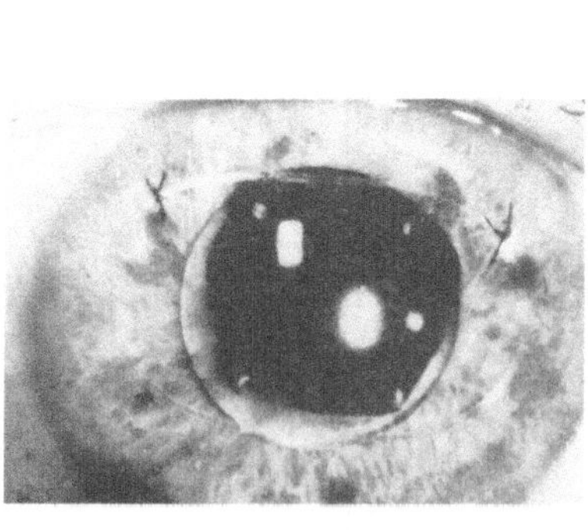

Fig. VI-12. — Top: Various techniques devised by J. Worst for securing the iris clip lens to the iris with sutures. Bottom: iris clip lens sutured to the iris. (Courtesy C.D. Binkhorst.)

According to C.D. Binkhorst (1975), securing the lens with a trans-iridectomy suture has the advantage of allowing pupil dilation without decentering the lens. Furthermore, the iris stroma is not involved, which is a great advantage since the suture cannot cut through the iris later on (Binkhorst, 1975).

J. Worst (1970, 1971) introduced the use of sutures through the iris in order to prevent luxation of the iris clip lens. The sutures may be either pre-placed or post-placed. Some of Worst's techniques are illustrated above.

In 1977, J. Alpar (1977) proposed the following suturing technique to provide the iris clip lens with an additional fixation principle. The main steps are illustrated in the following figure:

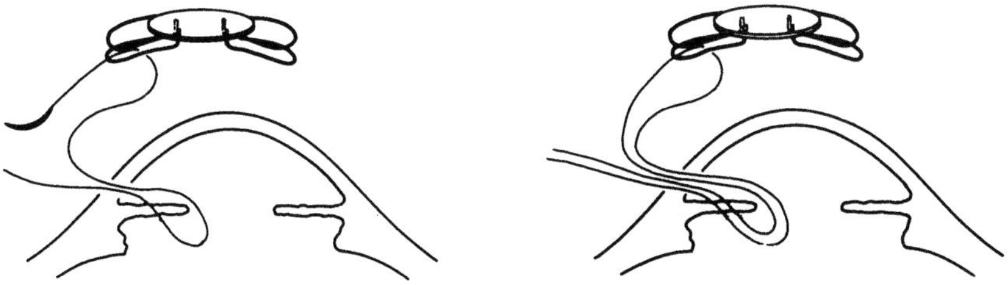

Fig. VI-13. — Alpar's suturing technique for the fixation of the iris clip lens.

C.W. Simcoe (1977) proposed another technique to steady the iris clip lens. Both the anterior loops are sutured to the iris.

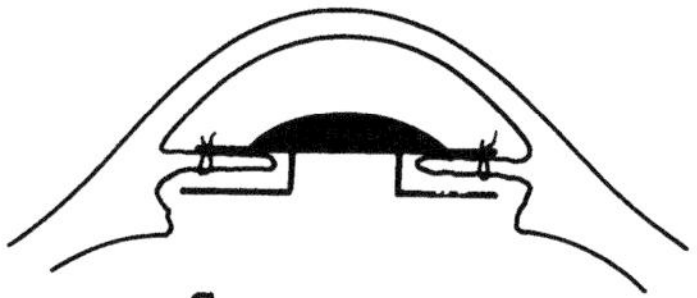

g

Fig. VI-14. — Simcoe's technique for steadying the iris clip lens.

J. Charleux (1978 personnal communication) routinely places an iris suture through the superior anterior loop and uses the Binkhorst-McCannel technique for steadying the inferior loop.

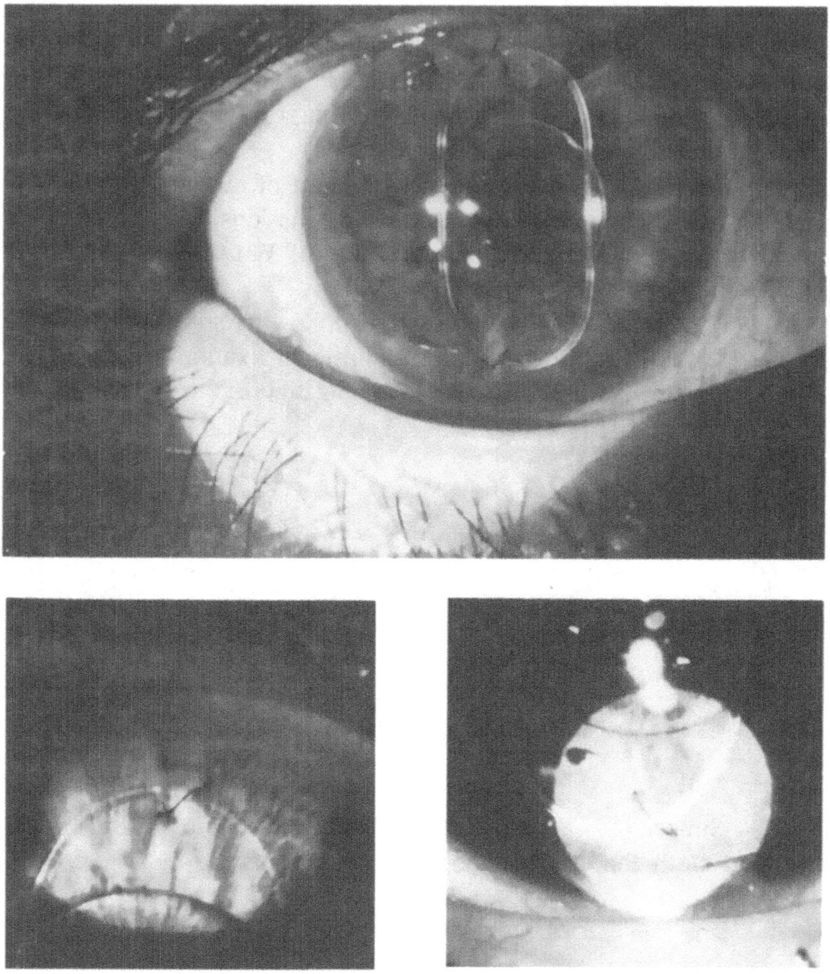

Fig. VI-15. — An iris clip lens with superior and inferior sutures. (Courtesy J. Charleux.)

III. Twenty Years of Experience with the Iris Clip Lens: 1958-1978

We shall treat first the evolutionary period, when the primary changes were introduced in both lens design and techniques. This period falls naturally into two phases: the first when secondary implantation predominated (1958-1961), and the second when the practice of primary implantation was adopted (1961-1971). Then we shall review the current literature on iris clip lenses.

A. The Developmental Period: Binkhorst's Experience, 1958-1971

1. *Secondary Implantations: Binkhorst's First 70 Cases*

For his first cases (1958-1961), Binkhorst selected unilateral aphakics who were unable to wear contact lenses or who could not adapt to contact lenses. From the technical point of view, the proper insertion of an iris clip lens in an already aphakic eye presented many problems. Vitreous presentation or loss was sometimes inevitable, and occasionally anterior or posterior synechiae had to be released in order to obtain an adequate pupil or a deeper anterior chamber. Management of these adverse conditions required extra manipulation in the anterior chamber that was directly responsible for post-operative complications such as keratitis, vitreous strands, and macular changes. In spite of these difficulties, the results were encouraging as regards the restoration of binocular vision and patient rehabilitation, with the "happiness factor" undoubtedly being a primary contributor to psychological rehabilitation.

The lessons provided by these early cases were many and, for Binkhorst, served as guidelines for the further development of the technique. The case selection and the results he obtained are summarized on Table VI-1.

TABLE VI-1. — *Summary of Binkhorst's Cases and Visual Acuity Attained (Binkhorst and Leonard, 1967)*

Type of Cataract	*Age*	*Number of Eyes*	*Corrected ≥20/60*	*Visual 20/60*	*Acuity ≥20/40*
Senile	46-82 yrs	52	6	1	45
Traumatic	17-74 yrs	5	1	–	4
Cyclitic	53-69 yrs	2	1	–	1
Radiation	12-65 yrs	2	–	–	2
Unknown	32-73 yrs	9	–	1	8
		100%	11%	3%	86%
			Uncorrected	Visual	Acuity
		100%	41%	22%	37%

This group of 70 aphakics consisted of 5 extracapsular and 65 intracapsular cases. The follow-up period ranged from a minimum of 5 years to a maximum of 8 years.

There were 5 other secondary insertions but the data relating to them is not included in the survey because:

— 1 lens was erroneously placed behind the iris and was removed the next day;
— 1 lens was removed after four weeks because of the development of a serious bacterial infection in the eye (the condition was cured);
— 3 patients died within a few years (their case histories were uneventful).

Visual Acuity

Unaided visual acuity of better than 20/40 was attained by 37% of the patients; 86% attained visual acuity of 20/40 or better after correction; and 89% regained visual acuity of value for binocular performance ($\leqslant$20/60) according to the Polaroid Fly Stereo Test. But in 11% of the cases, visual acuity dropped to less than 20/60.

Endothelial Corneal Dystrophy (7.1%)

In 2 cases (2.9%), there was total corneal edema, and in 3 cases (4.2%) edema was juxtalimbal and did not interfere with visual acuity. The relation between surgical trauma and subsequent corneal problems was obvious.

Macular Changes (31%)

The figure of 31% reflects the incidence of all macular pathology including senile degeneration, diabetic maculopathy, and a number of macular changes that were recorded as macular holes, pseudo-holes, or edema. Probably, all the cases of the Irvine Gass Syndrome (cystoid macular edema) were not recognized and could not be traced retrospectively. An incidence of at least 10% cystoid macular edema may be accepted (Binkhorst, personal communication, 1968).

Uveitis (1.4%)

Only in one case (1.4%) was an uveal reaction lasting a few weeks noted. Uveal reactions were uncommon after secondary implantation.

Retinal Detachment (1.4%)

The retinal detachment that occurred once was found to be unrelated to the implant.

Vitreous Problems

Vitreo-corneal adhesions were present in 13 eyes (19%) with several showing peaked pupils or slight decentration of the pseudophakos. Less severe vitreous abnormalities were the occurrence of a vitreous knuckle between the iris and the lens and opacities in the anterior part of the vitreous. A relationship between some edematous macular changes and peroperative vitreous problems has been suggested.

Dislocation (12%)

Dislocation occurred, sometimes repeatedly in the same eye. Reasons for dislocation were:

— inadequate loop length (7 mm);
— age, because the population was rather young and thus still had mobile, non-rigid pupils;
— unsuspected variations in pupil size due to physiological and emotional influences (sexual activity).

Conclusions from the First Series of 70 Secondary Implantations

The re-opening of an aphakic eye and the insertion of an iris clip lens resulted in a high incidence of peroperative vitreous problems and post-operative edematous macular changes. There was also a clear relationship between preoperative conditions, surgical trauma, and post-operative corneal pathology. Post-operative uveal reaction was of minor importance. Regarding the problem of dislocation, it was noted on several occasions that the pupil showed unexpected mobility that resulted in partial or total lens luxation (except for those cases in which posterior synechiae between the pupillary margin and the lens had developed). The diameter of the iris clip lens, which was then only 7 mm, was felt to be a contributing factor.

Some 86% of the cases regained corrected visual acuity of 20/40 and 69% were even able to achieve 20/60 without any additional correction. However, about 11% of the patients ended up with a final visual acuity of less than 20/60 because of corneal damage or macular problems or both. This led Binkhorst to conclude that secondary implantation of an iris supported lens in an aphakic eye without a capsular membrane involves serious risks that have to be weighed against the benefits.

2. *Primary Implantations by Binkhorst from 1961 to 1971*

In 1961 C.D. Binkhorst began to use primary implantation, thus the insertion of the pseudophakos being performed immediately after the intracapsular delivery of the cataractous lens.

The pioneering work done by Binkhorst in this field has been thoroughly assessed. The results of the first 133 cases were published by Binkhorst and Leonard (1967) and later data were assembled by M.E. Nordlohne in his doctoral thesis, *The Intraocular Implant Lens* (1975). Binkhorst also published his findings and conclusions in many articles (see bibliography). In addition, J. Pearce (1972) re-examined a random selection of Binkhorst's patients. What follows is an analysis of these often overlapping data. Finally, some reports on the use of the iris clip lens by other surgeons during this evolutionary period will also be discussed (A.T.M. Van Balen, M.E. Nordlohne, N. Dallas, and J. Worst).

We first analyzed visual performance and the influence of the pseudophakos on the cornea, the retina, the uvea, and intraocular pressure. This permitted us to evaluate the possibilities and limitations of this particular lens. Second, we tried to clarify the underlying reasons for the modifications of the lens and techniques.

a. *The First Primary Implantations of Iris Clip Lenses*

Table VI-2 gives the results of the first 133 primary iris clip lens implantations by Binkhorst after intracapsular cataract extraction.

Comment

Eight patients are not included because of illness or death. No abnormalities were reported. The pseudophakos had to be removed from the eye of one patient one week after implantation because the eye turned out to suffer from high degenerative myopia. The history of this patient's unilateral cataract was unknown to the surgeon.

Until 1967, the problem of endothelial corneal dystrophy (ECD) after primary implantation did not arise (this was in contrast to the 7% incidence of ECD reported after secondary iris clip insertion). Four years later in 1971, however, M.E. Nordlohne detected an incidence of 3.7% of total ECD when reviewing the same cases. Lens dislocation and contact between the tips of the lens loops and the endothelium turned out to be the main causes. We shall discuss this problem later on in this chapter.

TABLE VI-2. — *The First 133 Primary Iris Clip Lens Implantations after Intracapsular Cataract Extraction by C.D. Binkhorst*

Source	C.D. Binkhorst and P.A.M. Leonard (1967)
Surgeon	C.D. Binkhorst
Lens Type	Iris Clip Lens
Surgical Procedure	Intracapsular, primary
Number of Cases	124
Follow-up	1 to 5 years
Corrected Visual Acuity	
⩾20/40	80%
Endothelial Corneal Dystrophy	0%
Clinical Cystoid Macular Edema	3% to 5%
Retinal Detachment	2.4%
Dislocation	12.3%
Uveal Reaction	
Iritis (transient)	7.2%
Uveitis (persistent)	0.8%
Secondary membranes	4%
Vitreitis	0%
Endophthalmitis	0%
Glaucoma	
Transient	0.8%
Persistent	0%
Lens Removal	0%
Enucleation	0%

Macular disorders of varying origins were encountered in 17 out of the 124 eyes (12.7%). Eight patients, however, were reported to have either diabetic retinopathy or senile macular degeneration. Cystoid macular edema probably occurred in 3% to 5% of the cases.

The dislocations (12.3%) were ascribed to the inadequate length of the lenses and uncontrolled pupil width.

b. *The Survey of J. Pearce*

In 1972, J. Pearce published the results of his independent investigation of Binkhorst's patients. Out of the nearly 500 lens implantations that had been performed up till then, he selected 72 cases at random, excluding traumatic cases and any with a history of previous intraocular surgery. Table VI-3 gives Pearce's results.

Comment

Pearce placed the cases of endothelial corneal dystrophy into two categories:

Total: 3% or 2 cases. In one case surgical manipulation or intracameral use of epinephrine was the cause. In the other case, no obvious reason was found.

TABLE VI-3. — *Pearce's Survey*

Source	J. Pearce (1972)
Surgeon	C.D. Binkhorst
Lens Type	Iris Clip
Surgical Procedure	Intracapsular, Primary
Number of Cases	72
Follow-up	9 m. to 10 y.
Mean Age	73.9 years
Corrected Visual Acuity	
⩾20/40	72%
Endothelial Corneal Dystrophy	
Total	3%
Partial	10%
Clinical Cystoid Macular Edema	5%
Retinal Detachment	1%
Dislocation	10%
Uveitis	7%
Glaucoma	0%

Partial or minimal: 10% or 7 cases. Visual acuity was not impaired.

The 10% dislocation rate is comparable with the figure given in Table VI-2) and reflects one of the major problems with the iris clip lens at the time.

c. *Nordlohne's Survey of Binkhorst's Patients*

The study conducted by M.E. Nordlohne on lens implantation covers a period of ten years during which the Binkhorst lens and its

TABLE VI-4. — *Data on the Results Obtained by C.D. Binkhorst with 505 Primary Iris Clip Lens Implantations*

Source	M.E. Nordlohne (1975)
Surgeon	C.D. Binkhorst
Lens Type	Iris Clip Lens
Surgical Procedure	Intracapsular, Primary
Number of Cases	505
Mean Age of Patients	68 years
Corrected Visual Acuity	
⩾20/40	64%
Endothelial Corneal Dystrophy	
Total	5%
Partial	2%
Clinical Cystoid Macular Edema	4%
Retinal Detachment	2%
Dislocation	7%
Uveitis	0.2%
Glaucoma	0%
Lens Removal	0.6
Enucleation	0.3%

insertion technique underwent major modifications. It contains a great deal of data of primary importance, and we will often have occasion to refer to it (see Table VI-4).

Comment

Regarding endothelial corneal dystrophy, Nordlohne lists all edematous changes of the cornea, even localized and minimal. He separated the cases showing "total ECD" from those with "partial ECD". The figures given reflect the average percentages of ECD that occurred both before and after adequate preventive measures were taken (see Fig. VI-16).

In this retrospective study, an incidence of ±4% clinical cystoid macular edema was established. (Fluorescein angiography was not available at that time.)

Like the incidence of ECD, the nearly 7% dislocation rate reflects the average incidence of lens luxation both before and after adequate preventive measures had been developed (see Fig. VI-16).

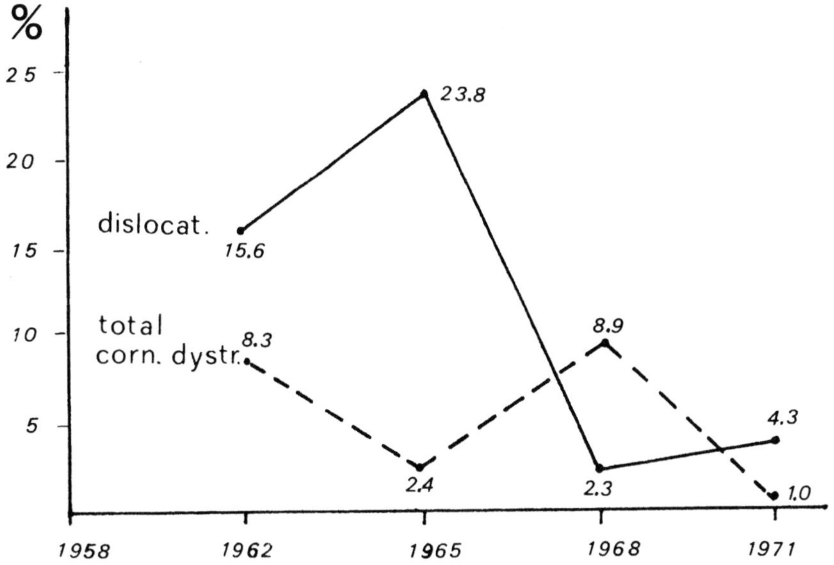

Fig. VI-16. — Incidence of lens dislocation and total endothelial corneal dystrophy in eyes with iris clip lenses in the period when major modifications in technique and lens designs were being introduced: 1958-1971.

3. *Discussion and Conclusions about C.D. Binkhorst's Use of Iris Clip Lenses after Intracapsular Cataract Extraction during the Developmental Period*

a. *The Materials Used*

Polymethylmethacrylate and Supramid proved to be stable over this period; the loops and optical components showed no clinical signs of deterioration; and there were no reports of any adverse reactions.

b. *Tissue Reaction*

Late uveitis was not a problem and there was no "rejection" of the implant.

Transient iritis tended to be slightly more intensive in the early postoperative period but, as a rule, it could be reduced to a minimum by local administration of corticosteroids. In any event, prolonged uveal reactions were more frequently seen after primary implantation than after secondary implantation. M.E. Nordlohne reported that early and late uveitis turned out to be of little or no consequence as far as the final result was concerned. J. Pearce confirmed this.

Pigment deposits: Fine pigment deposits were occasionally noted on the lens, on the hyaloid face, and even on the endothelium. The last case may suggest Krukenberg's Spindle. According to Binkhorst, the amount of pigment seen immediatly after surgery is related to surgical trauma, and therefore irrigation of the anterior chamber before and after insertion of the lens is mandatory. Continuous loss of pigment was seen in various degrees, especially where the posterior loop tips touched the pigment layer of the iris. This can be demonstrated by transillumination. This phenomenon neither disturbed visual acuity nor influenced intraocular pressure.

Greyish white precipitates on the lens, resembling Descemet precipitates, were encountered a few times after intracapsular extraction. The etiology is not clear, though Nordlohne considers infection to have been the underlying cause. These kind of deposits could interfere with visual acuity, but they disappeared after corticosteroids were administered.

c. *Secondary Membrane*

Nordlohne reports a frequence of 1.30% for needling after intracapsular surgery. This figure is significant in that it demonstrates the low-grade inflammatory response of the eye.

d. *Glaucoma*

As stated by Binkhorst and confirmed by the surveys of Pearce and Nordlohne, the iris clip lens did not disturb intraocular pressure. Using gonioscopy, Pearce found no visible modification of the angle, except in 19% of the eyes where some synechiae were detected. It is to be noted that Binkhorst paid utmost attention to the chamber angle and to the patency of the colobomas during surgery. He always injected air after insertion of the pseudophakos, inspected the angle, and released peripheral iris adhesions if necessary.

e. *Cystoid Macular Edema (3.76%)*

Retrospectively, Nordlohne could find no obvious lens-related reason in the majority of cases of cystoid macular edema. He noted that in 1% of the cases, both cystoid macular edema and corneal endothelial dystrophy developed in the same eye, with the cystoid macular edema being observed before the partial or total endothelial corneal dystrophy. He, therefore, considered these conditions to be related somehow, and suggested a common etiological mechanism.

f. *Retinal Detachment*

The figure of 2.3% probably indicates that the incidence of retinal detachment was not influenced by the presence of an iris clip lens.

g. *Hemorrhage*

No significant hemorrhaging was reported.

h. *Dislocation and Endothelial Corneal Dystrophy*

Both problems demand further attention because they are the reasons for all the modifications of the iris clip lens that were introduced between 1958 and 1970.

1) *The Problem of Dislocation*

Dislocation was a common problem in the early years of the history of the iris clip lens. Some occurred the night after surgery, while others after months or even years. Table VI-5 gives the total incidence and Table VI-6 the intervals between insertion and dislocation for 694 primary and secondary iris clip implantations.

TABLE VI-5. — *Incidence of Lens Dislocation for 694 Iris Clip Lens Implantations (Nordlohne, 1975)*

Period	*Number of Implants*	*Eyes with Implant Dislocations*	*Total Incidence of Dislocation*
1958-1971	694	53 (7.64%)	73 (10.52%)

TABLE VI-6. — *Interval between Implantation Date and Dislocation Date for 694 Iris Clip Lens Implantations (Nordlohne 1975)*

Interval	*0-¼ year*	*¼-1 year*	*1-4 years*	*After 4 years*
Number of Dislocations	29	13	20	11

— *Types of Dislocation*

1. Total dislocation may be either anterior or posterior. In the former case, the lens moves into the anterior chamber; in the latter,

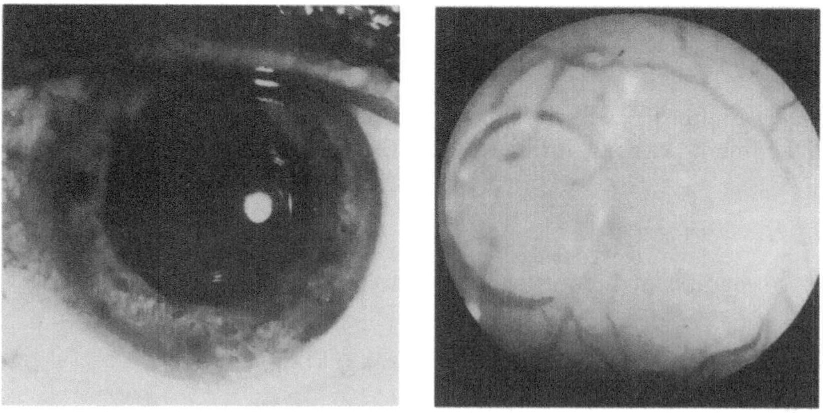

Fig. VI-17. — Total posterior dislocation of an iris clip lens: Left implant lodged between the iris and the anterior hyaloid face; Right implant dislocated into the vitreous.

the lens may shift into the posterior chamber between the iris and the anterior hyaloid face or into the vitreous itself.

2. Partial dislocation may occur in all possible combinations. Initially, the phenomenon of dislocation was not fully understood, but it is now ascribed to two main causes:

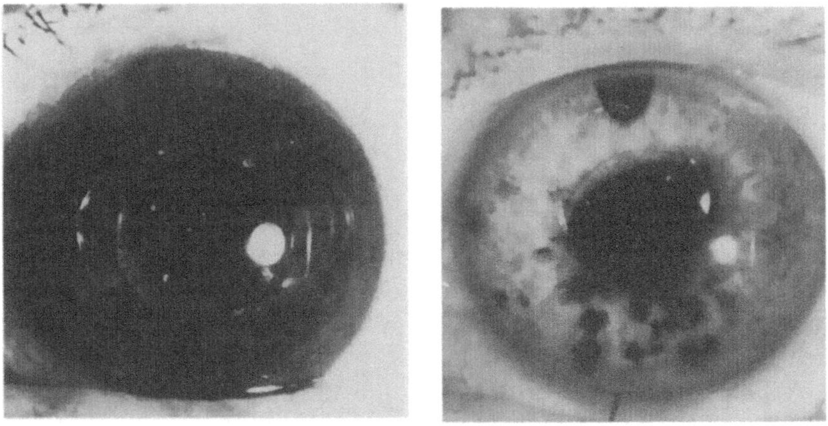

Fig. VI-18. — Left: Partial anterior dislocation of an iris clip lens. Right: Partial posterior dislocation of a sutured (transcoloboma) iris clip lens.

1. *Inadequate Loop Length*

With the 7-8 mm iris clip lens, the incidence of dislocation was nearly 24%, sometimes occurring more than once in the same eye. A.T.M. Van Balen (1973) reported one patient having partial or total anterior luxation 9 times. Binkhorst did not initially favor enlarging the loops for fear of other complications.

2. *Changes in Pupil Width*

Because the iris clip lens is essentially a pupil supported lens, an increase in pupil width may result in partial or total dislocation. Examination of some dislocation cases revealed the following:

a. Pupil behavior is very unpredictable in younger patients.
b. Unexpected changes in pupil width occur at night.
c. Spring-like dilation of the pupil can be caused by sexual activity (H. Hirschman, 1972).
d. In some eyes, control of pupil width was lost when sphincter erosions developed. Indeed, with the passage of time, localized atrophy of the pupillary border occurred at those points where the pupil margin met the posterior loop attachments (cheese wiring).

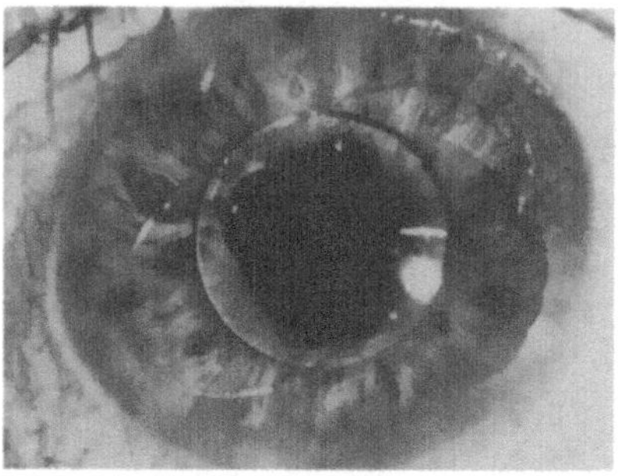

Fig. VI-19. — Localized contact atrophy of the pupillary margin.

Note:

Posterior synechiae formation occasionally provided additional fixation. The possibility of enhancing post-operative synechiae formation has been considered, but as yet no satisfactory results have been achieved.

A blunt injury was occasionally the direct cause of dislocation. Nordlohne (1975) reported three cases of such dislocation out of the 694 iris clip lenses Binkhorst implanted.

On a few occasions, instillation of mydriatics was found to be responsible.

— *Dislocation Prevention*

1. *Modification of the Loop Length*

In 1962, Binkhorst increased the loop length from 7 to 8 mm. Three years later, he tried a 9 mm lens but it turned out to be too large for the average eye. After 1969, the loop length was reduced to the standard 8 mm.

2. *Miotics*

In 1965, the use of pilocarpine 2% twice a day was routinely prescribed. With this, better control of pupillary behavior was expected and, to a certain extent, realized. Initially, this measure was indeed very effective (Binkhorst & Leonard, 1967). As time went by, however, many patients neglected to use their eye drops.

3. *Suturing*

At the suggestion of Worst, who had begun to suture the iris clip lens to the iris in 1969, Binkhorst started to perform transiridectomy suturing in March 1970.

The effectiveness of these measures in eliminating luxation was thoroughly assessed by M.E. Nordlohne (1975). The figures he reported are significant and cover 694 eyes, including the first 70 secondary implantations.

TABLE VI-7. — *Luxation Incidence with 694 Iris Clip Lens Implantations Performed by C.D. Binkhorst (Nordlohne, 1975)*

Period	*Number of eyes*	*Loop Length*	*Miotics*	*Suturing*	*Eyes with Luxations*	*Total Incidence of Luxation*
1958-62	96	±7 mm	No	No	15.6%	26.0%
1962-65	84	±8 mm	No	No	23.8%	28.6%
1965-68	214	±9 mm	Yes	No	2.3%	3.8%
1969-71	300	±8 mm	Yes	Yes after 1970	4.3%	5.3%

As can be seen from Table VI-7, the incidence of luxation dramatically decreased between 1965 and 1968 which was attributed to the use of longer loops and the routine administration of miotics.

The difference in incidence between the 7 mm and the 8 mm groups is difficult to account for. But, as we have noted, there was a different basis used for case selection (secondary versus primary implantation). The rigidity of the pupil in aphakic eyes was suggested by Nordlohne as a possibly contributing to the stability of the lens. Nevertheless, in spite of all these measures, the incidence of partial or total luxation still exceeded 5% at the end of 1971.

2) *The Problem of Endothelial Corneal Dystrophy*

After investigating the factors contributing to endothelial corneal dystrophy, Nordlohne (1975) reported the following useful information: of 694 eyes operated on by Binkhorst up until 1971, 64 eyes (9%) manifested various degrees of endothelial corneal dystrophy. In half of them, the dystrophy was total, and in one-third it was

TABLE VI-8. — *Interval between Implantation and First Detection of Incipient Endothelial Corneal Dystrophy (Nordlohne, 1975)*

Percentage of Endothelial Corneal Dystrophy	*Interval in Years*			
	0-¼	*¼-1*	*1-4*	*4*
100% (=64 eyes)	8%	14%	51.5%	26.5%

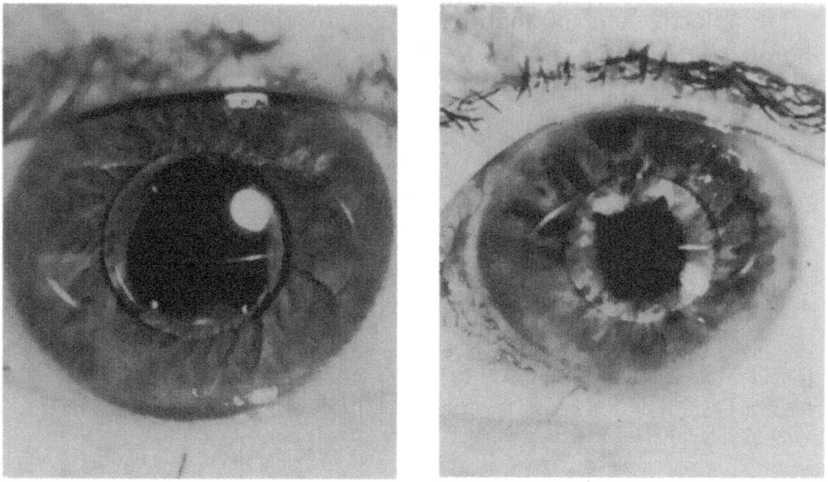

Fig. VI-20. — Left: Marked degree of localized iris atrophy and subsequent localized endothelial corneal dystrophy. (Courtesy C.D. Binkhorst.)
Right: Localized endothelial corneal dystrophy in the area overlying an anterior loop tip. (Courtesy C.D. Binkhorst.)

minimal, being localized mostly in the areas overlying the tips of the loops. As shown on Table VI-8, endothelial corneal dystrophy was a late problem. Indeed, it took several years of follow up before the total incidence of endothelial corneal dystrophy could be established.

— *Analysis of Factors Contributing to Endothelial Corneal Dystrophy*

TABLE VI-9. — *Factors Contributing to Endothelial Corneal Dystrophy in 694 Iris Clip Lens Implantations Performed by C.D. Binkhorst (Nordlohne, 1975)*

Etiological Factors	*Number of Cases*	*Percentage*
Preoperative Fuch's ECD	13	20%
Operative and Postoperative Complications	14	22%
Endothelial Contact by the Lens	32	50%
Unknown	5	8%
Total	64	100%

a. *Pre-Existing Conditions:* Nordlohne could demonstrate pre-existing corneal pathology in 13 eyes.

b. Although *surgical trauma* during implantation was minimal, additional surgery in some cases—particularly for repositioning of luxated lenses—contributed to endothelial corneal decompensation in 14 eyes.

c. *Endothelial damage* by the lens itself was the primary cause in half of the cases. The following mechanisms are to be considered (see also chapter XII on lens implantation and the endothelium below).

1. *Early Post-Operative Corneal Contact by the Lens*

a. Flattened anterior chamber because of wound leakage, wound rupturing, or pupillary block was rare.

b. Early decentration or tilting of the lens, resulting in persistent or intermittant contact between the anterior loop tips and the endothelium, was also of minor importance in this series. The following mechanisms were identified:

— residual air that was introduced during surgery, either in front of or behind the iris diaphragm (rare);
— deformation of the pupil by residual blood, or vitreous knuckles or strands (rare after primary implantation);
— peripheral anterior synechiae (rare);
— sphincter dehiscence due to surgical trauma (sphincter rupture) allowing the lens to ride in any direction.

c. Subluxation or luxation of the lens in the early postoperative period.

2. *Late Post-Operative Corneal Contact by the Lens*

Nordlohne reports that the vast majority of incipient ECD developed not before the end of the first year after implantation. Two mechanisms are involved:

a. Late lens decentration, subluxation, or luxation;
b. Intermittent contact because of the following contributory causes:

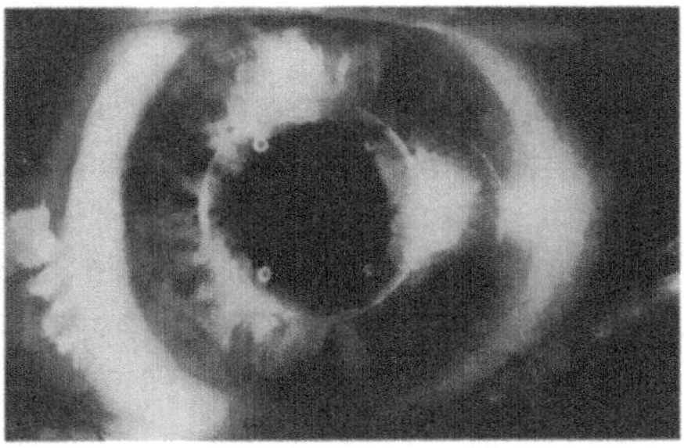

Fig. VI-21. — 9 mm iris clip lens in the horizontal position, which were factors contributing to late endothelial corneal dystrophy.

(1) *Inadequate Lens Design*

- The longer the anterior loops, the more likely there will be endothelial contact sooner or later.
- The more the loops point forward (anteriorly), the closer they are to the endothelium. As already noted, the first few hundred lenses used by Binkhorst had the anterior loops in the same geometrical plane as the optical component. This turned out to be potentially dangerous for the cornea, especially if the loop length exceeded 8 mm.

(2) *Pseudophakodonesis*

Because of the normal occurrence of iridodonesis after intracapsular cataract extraction, all lenses that rely on iris support move to a certain extent. This is called pseudophakodonesis. The amplitude of the "donesis" is dependent on the weight and momentum of the lens and on individual anatomical conditions such as laxicity and mobility of the iris diaphragm and the degree of sphincter atrophy. Clinical observation has established that a vertically oriented iris clip lens has a smaller amplitude of pseudophakodonesis than one that is horizontally oriented.

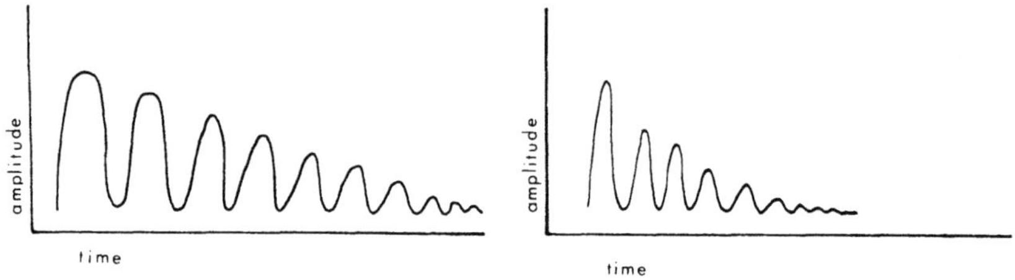

Fig. VI-22. — Graphic representation of the oscillation of an iris clip lens as a result of a single horizontal movement. When the loops are in the horizontal position, a very regular and decreasing pendular movement around the vertical axis is noticeable (left). This movement is damped and also much shorter than when the loops are in the vertical axis (right).

Obviously, the combination of inadequate lens design and significant pseudophakodonesis increases the danger of corneal contact, especially when the anterior chamber is rather shallow. (M.E. Nordlohne (1975) observed that the anterior chamber depth of an eye containing an iris clip lens after intracapsular extraction shows a variation of 0.2 mm between the prone and the supine positions.)

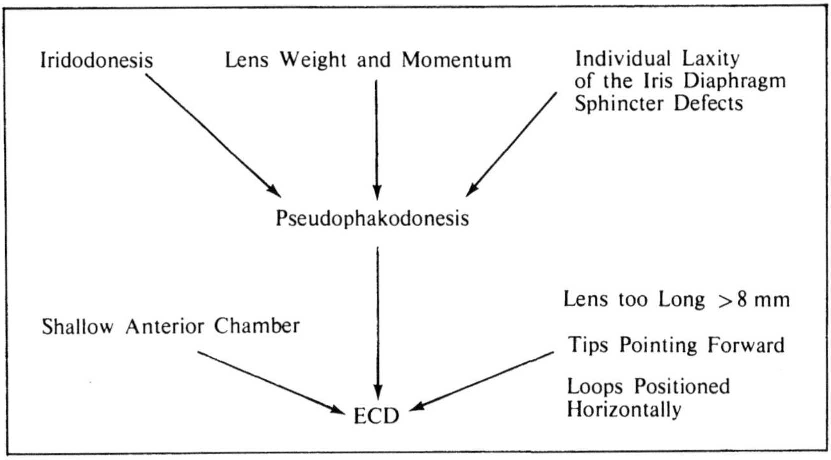

Fig. VI-23. — Factors contributing to endothelial corneal dystrophy.

— *Endothelial Corneal Dystrophy Prevention*

1) *Changes in Lens Design*

a. *Modification of the Loop Length*

In order to decrease the incidence of luxation and its possible consequences for the endothelium, the loop length was gradually increased. While this effectively reduced luxation, (see Table VI-10), it turned out to be the main cause of intermittent corneal contact and late endothelial corneal dystrophy. From an incidence of 8% with the early 7 to 8 mm lenses, the incidence gradually climbed to around 19% with the 9 mm lenses. As mentioned above, the interval between implantation and the first detection of endothelial corneal dystrophy ranged from 1 to 4 years. In January 1970, the loop length was reduced to 8 mm where it has since remained.

b. *Backward Bending*

For an additional margin of security, the loops were bent backward (end 1971), the radius of the bend being 30 mm.

2) *Vertical Positioning of the Lens*

It was noted that the incidence of intermittent corneal contact was dependent on the orientation of the lens.

This phenomenon was virtually absent when the loops were oriented vertically instead of horizontally. Since 1970, therefore, all iris clip lenses have been placed in the vertical position.

TABLE VI-10. — *Incidence of Endothelial Corneal Dystrophy and Lens Luxation in Relation to Lens Design, Lens Orientation, Use of Pilocarpine, and Loop Suturing*

Period	*Number of Eyes*	*Loop Length*	*Loops Bent Backward*	*Lens Horiz.*	*Lens Vert.*	*Pilocarpine*	*Loop Suturing*	*ECD*			*Luxation of Eyes*	*Frequency*
								Tot.	*Part.*	*Min.*		
11 Aug 58 to 3 Aug 62	96	≈7 mm	No	Yes	No	No	No	8.33%	—	—	15.62%	26.4%
9 Aug 62 to 3 Jun 65	84	≈8 mm	No	Yes	No	No	No	2.38%	1.19% =7.14%	3.57%	23.80%	28.60%
10 Jun 65 to 12 Dec 68	214	≈9 mm	No	Yes	No	Yes	No	8.88%	3.74% =18.70%	6.07%	2.35%	3.75%
9 Jan 69 to 31 Dec 71	300	≈8 mm	Yes	No	Yes	Yes (optional)	Yes (optional)	1.00%	0.33% =3.33%	2.00%	4.33%	5.33%

3) *Transiridectomy Suturing*

The reduction of the length of the anterior loops to reduce the incidence of ECD aggravated the problem of luxation. After trying out various methods of suturing the lens to the iris, Binkhorst concluded that transiridectomy suturing was the most effective solution.

4) *Elimination of the Anterior Loops and Capsular Fixation*

Converting the method of fixation from iris to capsular yielded two main advantages: first, the anterior loops became superfluous and could be eliminated, and, second, the lens, supported by the lens lens capsule became very stable. Other advantages also were apparent:

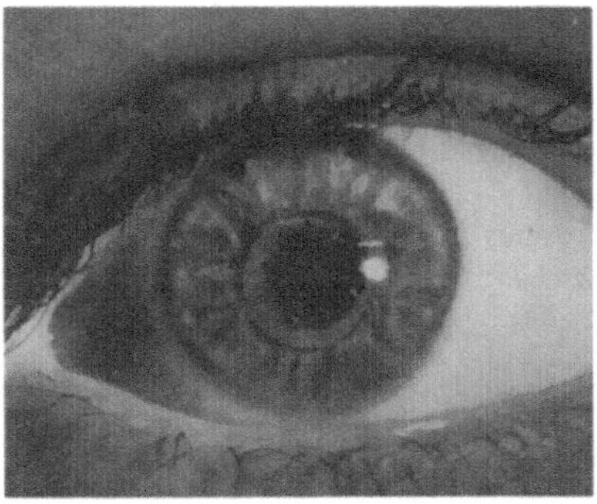

Fig. VI-24. — An iridocapsular lens in situ.

— There were no vitreous problems during insertion.
— Luxation into the vitreous was impossible.
— Iridodonesis and pseudophakodonesis decreased or occurred very rarely.
— There was no reason to expect this type of fixation to fail in the long run.

4. *Other Reports on the Iris Clip Lens after Intracapsular Cataract Extraction during the Development Period*

a. *Results of Different Surgeons in 321 Cases*

N. Dallas (1970) and M.E. Nordlohne (1975) reported on their personal experiences with, respectively, 92 and 72 implantations of the iris clip lens, and A.T.M. van Balen (1973) analyzed the results of 157 iris clip implantations performed by the staff of the Rotterdam Eye Clinic. These results are given on Table VI-11.

TABLE VI-11. — *Results from Early Models of the Iris Clip Lens Reported by Dallas, van Balen, and Nordlohne*

Source	N. Dallas (1970)	A.T.M. van Balen (1973)	M.E. Nordlohne (1975)
Surgeon	N. Dallas	Rotterdam Eye Clinic	M.E. Nordlohne
Surgical Procedure	Intracaps. Primary	Intracaps. Not available	Intracaps Primary
Number of Cases	92	157	72
Follow-Up	max. 5 yrs.	6 mos. to $3\frac{1}{2}$ yrs.	$1\frac{1}{4}$ average
Age of Patients	44-89 yrs	mean: 69 yrs.	mean: 71 yrs.
Corrected Visual Acuity ≥20/40	≥6/24=77%	80%	0.60% avg.
Endothelial Corneal Dystrophy	7.6%	1.9%	6.94%
Cystoid Macular Edema	Not available	6.3%	5.50%
Retinal Detachment	None	1.8%	None
Luxation	7.6%	5.7%	6.94% Early: 5.53% Late: 1.41%
Tissue Reactions			
Iritis	12%		
Uveitis		4.46%	4.17%
Endophtal.	1%	0.6% phthisis	
Secondary Membrane	1%		
Glaucoma, Transient or Persistent	4.3%	4.4%	6.94%
Hemorrhage in Anterior Chamber	None		
Vitreous Problems	2.1%		12.5%
Lens Removal	7.8%	1.2%	None
Enucleation	2.1%	None	None

Comment

The differences and similarities of these reports are striking.

Endothelial Corneal Dystrophy: This varied from 2% to 7%. The 5 cases (7%) of ECD in Nordlohne's series could be attributed to excessive intraocular manipulation during surgery, contact between the lens and the endothelium, or pre-existing corneal pathology. The underlying reasons for the 7 cases (7%) of ECD of N. Dallas were surgical damage, postoperative shallowness of the anterior chamber, or decentration of the lens resulting in contact between the lens loops and the endothelium.

Cystoid Macular Edema: For van Balen, this was the most distressing and disturbing complication (10 cases, 6.3%). Two cases developed after prolonged uveitis, two after acute glaucoma, one after obstruction of the central retinal vein, and five cases developed without any apparent reason two years after implantation.

Luxation: The approximately 7% luxation rate reported by all three authors seems to be the luxation rate for the iris clip lens before suturing techniques were used. Nordlohne reported the same rate for 505 cases operated on by Binkhorst.

Iritis-Uveitis: Nordlohne and van Balen reported an incidence of 4.5% whereas Dallas noted 12%. In Dallas's series, 2 cases were associated with vitreous loss during surgery, 1 case was of uncertain origin, and in 1 case the lens had to be removed because of corneal dystrophy.

Glaucoma: Transient glaucoma (pupil block) was noted by van Balen and Nordlohne. The latter ascribed his 7% incidence to inadequately functioning iridectomies. Van Balen reported that the glaucoma was mostly associated with keratopathy and lens luxation. Dallas had a 4% incidence of persistent glaucoma of varying origins.

Enucleation: Dallas had 2 cases: 1 because of a gross infection resulting from defective wound closure and the other because of lens luxation that required explantation.

The rather high incidence of some complications compared to Binkhorst's results led Nordlohne and van Balen to conclude that the surgical technique could be improved.

b. *Nordlohne's Survey of 485 Iris Clip Lens Implantations by J. Worst*

Nordlohne's report on 485 iris clip lens implantations done by J. Worst after intracapsular lens extraction is particularly interesting

TABLE VI-12. — *Results of 485 Iris Clip Lens Implantations by J. Worst (Nordlohne, 1975)*

Source	M.E. Nordlohne (1975)
Surgeon	J.F.C. Worst
Surgical Procedure	Intracapsular (primary)
Number of Cases	485
Not Sutured	238
Sutured	247
Follow-Up	Up to ±3.7 yrs.
Mean Age of Patients	72 yrs.
Corrected Visual Acuity	
⩾20/40	56.5%
Endothelial Corneal Dystrophy	2.3%
Not Sutured	1.7%
Sutured	2.8%
Cystoid Macular Edema	3.51%
Retinal Detachment	1.86%
Luxation	2.7%
Not Sutured	3.4%
Sutured	2.0%
Uveitis	2.06%
Glaucoma (transient)	0.62%
Lens Removal	0.82%
Enucleation	0.21%

because Nordlohne used the same standards in evaluating the results obtained by this skillful surgeon. In this series, about half of the iris clip lenses were provided with an iris suture.

With regard to ECD and luxation, the use of the various suturing techniques Worst developed, decreased the incidence of luxation (3.4% to 2%), but the extra manipulations involved in this new procedure were responsible for a slight increase in ECD (from 1.7% to 2.8%). Once the lens was secured with a suture through the iris, total lens luxation was prevented. This was a dramatic improvement. Still, partial luxation remained at 2%.

5. *Conclusions for the Development Period*

During the initial period of more than 10 years during which the iris clip lens was used by Binkhorst and others, the main problem was fixation. Another problem was endothelial corneal dystrophy. In addition to the well-documented series discussed above, clinical observation by many other surgeons confirms these findings, although individual differences are occasionally striking. The incidence of lens luxation, which was reported by Binkhorst and others to be about 7%, decreased because of suturing of the lens to the iris. In Worst's series, the dislocation rate was 2% for his sutured cases, which compares favorably with the 2.2% luxation incidence in 360 cases of J. Pearce, of which 95% were sutured iris clip lenses (Pearce, 1974).

The majority of ECD cases in the Binkhorst series occurred either as a consequence of surgical manipulation or of intermittent or persistent corneal contact by the lens. However, at least 4 years elapsed before the total incidence of this pathological condition could be established. This confirms the utmost importance of sustained follow-up before definite conclusions regarding ECD can be drawn.

The incidence of endothelial corneal dystrophy was also found to be significant in most of the series performed by other surgeons. M. Dallas (1970) reported 7.6%, M.E. Nordlohne (1975) 7%, G.M. Stubbs (1967, 1977) 10%, and J. Boberg-Ans (1977) 6.6%. Reported a lower incidence: A.T.M. van Balen (1973) 1.9%, J.J. Worst (Nordlohne, 1975) 2.3%, and J.L. Pearce (1974) 1.9%.

Finally, it must be noted that all the modifications of both lens design and implantation technique were responses to imperfections revealed by clinical experience. The changes in lens design were never spectacular, though the consequences, which only became fully apparent years later, were.

B. The Current Situation: Recent Data on the Use of the Iris Clip Lens after Intracapsular Cataract Extraction

After having refined his lens, which was primarily intended to be used after intracapsular cataract extraction, Binkhorst in the late sixties adopted extracapsular surgery with the same lens or a modification of it. The advantages he expected from this change were not then clear to everyone who belonged to his "school": some followed him, and some did not.

Some implant surgeons are still using the refined iris clip lens after intracapsular extraction and report acceptable results.

At Draeger's suggestion, Morcher started making the loops out of polypropylene in 1971, which was a major advance since the weight of the lens in aqueous was thus reduced to the point where it could be considered virtually weightless. M.E. Nordlohne also found that the refined model yielded very good results after ICCE in comparison with the incidence of complications that occurred previously. In this section, we shall examine the available data on the refined model (with both nylon and polypropylene loops) to determine if better results are indeed being obtained and, if so, what the advantages and disadvantages of the improved lens are.

1. *The Data Published by J. Draeger, K. Schott, and N.S. Jaffe*

Combining the data published by J. Draeger, K. Schott, and N.S. Jaffe, we have a statistical base of 1250 cases.

TABLE VI-13. — *Recent Data on the Iris Clip Lens after Intracapsular Cataract Extraction*

Source	K. Schott (1977)	J. Draeger (1977)	N.S. Jaffe (1978)
Surgeon	K. Schott	J. Draeger	N.S. Jaffe
Lens Type	Iris Clip	Iris Clip	Iris Clip
Surgical Procedure	Intracapsular	Intracapsular	Intracapsular
Number of Cases	202	350	698
Follow-Up	6 years	6 months-6½ yrs.	max. 3½ yrs.
Age of Patients	40-90 yrs. (avg. 75 yrs.)	22-86 yrs. (avg. 58 yrs.)	55-94 yrs. (avg. 74 yrs).
Corrected Visual Acuity ≥20/40	79%	Not available	90%
Endothelial Corneal Dystrophy	2.4%	1.7%	0.6%
Uveitis	rare	rare	rare
Secondary Membrane	1%	N.A.	1.9%
Glaucoma			
Transient (pupil block)	1%	15%	N.A.
Persistent	4.4%	1.7%	N.A.
Clinical Cystoid Macular Edema	4.4%	3.4%	1.5%
Retinal Detachment	2%	2.3%	1.5%
Luxation	2.4%	4.8%	2.8%
Vitreous Problems	Not available	Not available	6%
Lens Removal	N.A.	0.6%	N.A.

N.A. = Not available.

Comment

It must be noted that Draeger did not use any additional suturing, that Jaffe sutured the lens in about 65% of the cases, and that Schott did not generally suture, but, in 25% of his cases, used a lens with only one anterior loop, which he routinely sutured. The follow-up periods are not identical and range from 3½ years in Jaffe's series to 6 years for the patients of Draeger and Schott. All the lenses were made by Morcher and wet sterilized with Ridley's classic method. It was impossible to trace how many of the lenses had nylon loops and how many had polypropylene loops.

In our opinion, these results may be considered representative of what surgeons with a substantial amount of experience can be expected to achieve with the iris clip lens after intracapsular cataract extraction.

Visual Acuity

Senile macular degeneration was the main reason cited for visual acuity of less than 20/40 in Jaffe's patients. Jaffe noted the correlation between increasing age and decreasing visual acuity. Other reason for poorer visual results were cystoid macular edema, endothelial corneal dystrophy, retinal detachment, and some pre-existing conditions such as vascular or optic nerve pathology.

Endothelial Corneal Dystrophy

The incidence of endothelial corneal dystrophy ranged from 0.6% to 2.4%. The reasons for this wide divergence are not entirely clear. It may reflect differences in surgical techniques or in follow-up periods.

Uveitis

Uveal reactions were rare. The highest incidence of secondary membranes was 1.9%.

Glaucoma

Transient rises in intraocular pressure were ascribed to pupillary block. It occurred particularly in Draeger's first cases and was attributed to excessive use of miotics. Improvement was achieved with the judicious administration of mild mydriatics. Schott listed only the 5 cases (1%) of pupil block for which surgical intervention was indicated. The rises in intraocular pressure during the late postoperative period reported by Schott (4.3%) and Draeger (1.7%) could be satisfactorily controlled by conservative therapy except for one of Draeger's cases for which glaucoma surgery was indicated.

Clinical Cystoid Macular Edema

The incidence of clinical cystoid macular edema ranged from 1.5% to 4.4%. Schott found this condition associated with ECD in two cases of the nine he reports. Most of these cases improved after intensive administration of steroids. Jaffe, who reported an incidence of 1.5%, investigated the problem of cystoid macular edema in a separate study comparing a matched series of aphakic patients after ICCE with a series of pseudophakic patients who had undergone either intracapsular or extracapsular surgery. Although fluorograms performed after 4, 8, and 16 to 24 months after surgery showed a comparable incidence of cystoid macular edema in both the implanted and the non-implanted groups, it turned out that vascular leakage was more pronounced in the pseudophakic patients after intracapsular than after extracapsular extraction (cf. chapter XIV on lens implantation and cystoid macular edema).

Retinal Detachment

As stressed by both Jaffe and Draeger, the incidence of retinal detachment was not influenced by the presence of the pseudophakos. Draeger pointed out that this patients were relatively young and that instances of both traumatic and complicated cataracts were included. Jaffe attributed the low incidence of retinal detachment in his series to rigorous preselection that excluded the younger age group and patients predisposed to retinal detachment.

Luxation

Schott reported only the 5 cases (2.4%) in which surgical repositioning of a subluxated lens was necessary. Draeger, who did not provide additional suturing, had 6 cases of *early luxation:* for 3 cases, conservative repositioning sufficed; for 2 cases, surgical intervention was required; for 1 case, the lens had to be removed. *Late luxation* occurred in 11 cases. Except for one case in which a trauma was involved, the underlying reason was omission of miotics by the patient. In half of these case, surgical repositioning was necessary. Two lenses had to be removed because of persistent corneal contact and associated keratopathy. According to Jaffe, luxation usually occurred early in the post-operative period, but because his follow-up time was only 3½ years, no definitive conclusion could be drawn about the long-term stability of the lenses in his series. Luxation or subluxation ranged from 2.3% for the sutured lenses to 3.2% for the non-sutured. Three of the non-sutured lenses luxated into the vitreous, which demonstrates the superiority of the suturing procedure.

Vitreous Problems

Schott and Draeger found that the presence of vitreous in the pupillary aperture is a contraindication for the insertion of a lens after ICCE. According to Schott, vitreous loss, even after anterior vitrectomy procedures, gives rise to additional complications. For Draeger, the main reasons for aborting the implantation procedure in 32% of the planned cases were ballooning vitreous, a broken anterior vitreous face, and too large a pupil. With regard to his 6% incidence of vitreous problems, Jaffe gives the following details: of the 47 cases, there were

7 cases of vitreous bulge (℞ aspiration),
11 cases of spontaneous prolapse (℞ vitrectomy),
19 cases during lens insertion, and
10 cases during lens suturing.

In Jaffe's opinion, peroperative loss of vitreous does not constitute a contraindication for implantation of an iris clip lens provided it is adequately managed. In his experience, when peroperative loss of vitreous had occurred, the presence of this lens did not alter the incidence of post-operative cystoid macular edema or retinal detachment. According to Jaffe, the incidence of both these complications increases after vitreous loss whether or not the lens is implanted. But, as Jaffe's breakdown of vitreous problems shows, 60% of these problems were lens related and occurred during the insertion or the suturing of the lens itself. This again demonstrates that the insertion of an iris supported lens over bare vitreous is a demanding procedure.

2. *Conclusion*

The data we have reported reflect the results obtained by qualified surgeons using the updated iris clip lens. Unfortunately, these 1250 cases do not tell the whole story. According to K.J. Hoffer (1978), at least 9000 iris clip lenses were inserted before 1978, with the vast majority of them after 1971. If all surgeons who used Binkhorst's refined iris clip lens did as well as Schott, Draeger, and Jaffe, there were between 40 and 170 instances of endothelial corneal dystrophy (0.6% to 2.5%) and luxation in 160 to 320 eyes (2.4% to 4.8%).

However, there are strong indications that the reality does not match these optimistic suppositions and that many more complications have occurred. We know personally of many cases in which, notwithstanding vitreous loss, iris clip lenses were inserted without adequate surgical management. Many of these eyes showed subsequent lens decentration and endothelial corneal dystrophy. There is also evidence to indicate that the true incidence of luxation is higher than the 2.4% to 4.8% cited above, since transiridectomy suturing after intracapsular extraction is a difficult procedure and is reported to be often omitted by beginners. Bearing this in mind, the iris clip lens is certainly not to be used after ICCE when adverse conditions arise during surgery. Furthermore, since the incidence of lens luxation may be estimated at 5% when the lens is not sutured, suturing is mandatory. In our opinion, the beginner should start with a pre-placed suture through one of the pillars of the coloboma. This suture is tied loosely around the upper anterior loop. Obviously, suturing techniques call for a high degree of surgical skill.

But even when the lens is secured with an additional suture, there is a subluxation rate of more than 2%. And although repositioning of a subluxated iris clip lens is possible without surgery, repeated subluxation is a matter of serious concern, especially for the younger patient. Therefore, the iris clip lens after intracapsular cataract extraction is certainly not recommended for cataract patients with a long life expectancy. Suturing the lens to the iris can sometimes be safely omitted with elderly patients who manifest a non-atrophic iris pattern and whose pupil dilation after one drop of 1% homatropine does not exceed 5 mm, which indicates a degree of sphincter rigidity.

Finally, during the preoperative examination, it should always be kept in mind that the internal diameter of the anterior segment of some eyes is definitely too small for an iris clip lens. In these eyes, the slightest decentration or tilting of an 8 mm lens will result in intermittent or persistent endothelial contact.

Note: At least 2000 iris clip lenses were made with metal loops by American manufacturers and inserted after intracapsular cataract extraction. Because the weight of these lenses exceeded by far the physiological limits of the iris diaphraghm as a lens carrier, the ensuing problems were enormous. The metal-looped models were responsible for a high incidence of sphincter erosion and iris atrophy leading to lens dislocation. Chronic uveitis and cystoid macular edema were common, often resulting in secondary glaucoma and corneal dystrophy. Many of these lenses had to be removed (see chapter XIII on inflammatory response and glaucoma).

§2 THE COPELAND LENS

I. Introduction

The Copeland lens was designed in the United States in the mid-sixties and is a modification of the Epstein Maltese Cross lens and the original iris clip lens.

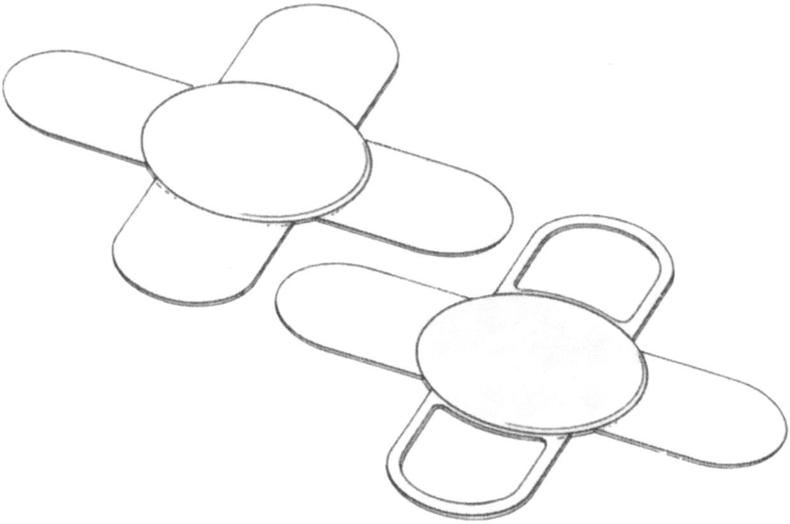

Fig. VI-25. — The Epstein Maltese Cross lens and the Copeland lens.

Intended to be a lightweight, iris supported lens of simplified construction, it is a one-plane lens made of one kind of material without loops or fenestrations. The first models were made in 1968 by its namesake, Michael Copeland. This lens became very popular in the US during the next 10 years with at least 30,000 of them being implanted (Richard Binkhorst, personal communication, 1978).

The Copeland lens is an all polymethylmetacrylate, one-plane lens in the shape of a symmetrical cross. It is sometimes described as a propeller with four blades.

In situ, two opposing haptic feet are in front of the iris and the other two are behind, which gives the iris diaphragm a corrugated configuration.

Technically, it is one of the easiest lenses to insert. This point has been stressed not only by N.S. Jaffe, who performed his first insertion of this lens on 13 May 1968, but also by the later proponents of the Copeland lens.

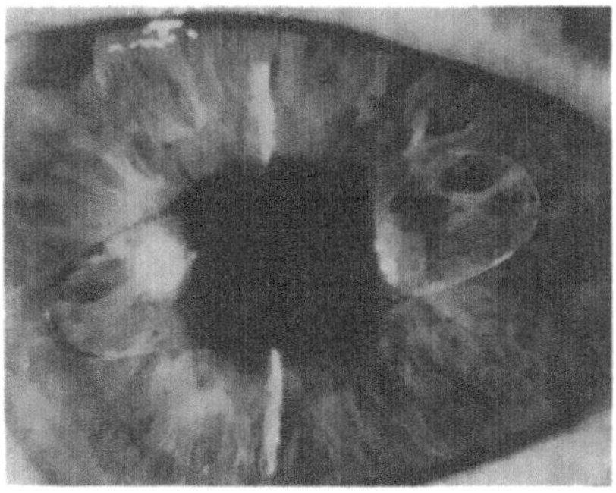

Fig. VI-26. — Copeland lens in situ. (Courtesy R.D. Binkhorst.)

Other advantages are also claimed:

— It is made of a single kind of material whereas other lenses have haptic devices made of nylon, polypropelene, or metal.
— It does not readily luxate.
— As no sutures are required to ensure fixation, intraocular manipulation are kept at a minimum during surgery.
— The haptic components occupy a relatively safe position in the anterior chamber, lying in nearly the same plane as the iris itself (thus it is sometimes called the iris plane lens). Contact with the endothelium is unlikely to occur, therefore, even when the anterior chamber is relatively flat.
— It can be used after both intracapsular and extracapsular lens extraction.

II. Implantation Techniques

A. The Open-Sky Technique

Insertion of the Copeland lens is generally done under direct observation, which technique is called the open-sky method. After delivery of the cataractous lens, the cornea is lifted high by an assistant. A previous incision from 180° to 200° is required. Depending on which pair of opposing haptic supports will be located in front or behind the iris, a slightly different insertion technique is indicated. Figures VI-26a and VI-26b show the final configurations of the lens in situ.

In Configuration A, the horizontal haptics are in front of the iris. This insertion can be done even when the pupil is rather narrow. The iris diaphragm is floated with fluid if required, and then, under direct observation, holding the right lateral haptic with a small smooth forceps, the inferior haptic is slid behind the iris into posi-

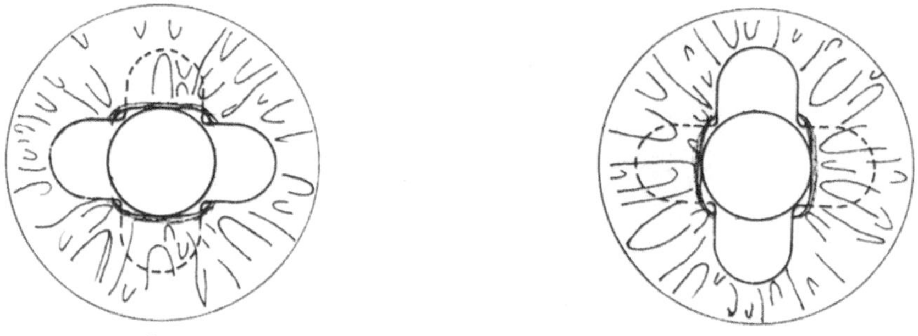

A B

Fig. VI-27. — Copeland lens in situ; a. with horizontal haptics in front of the iris; b. with horizontal haptics behind the iris.

tion. Still holding the right haptic, the surgeon lifts the superior iris sector over the superior haptic with a fine iris forceps.

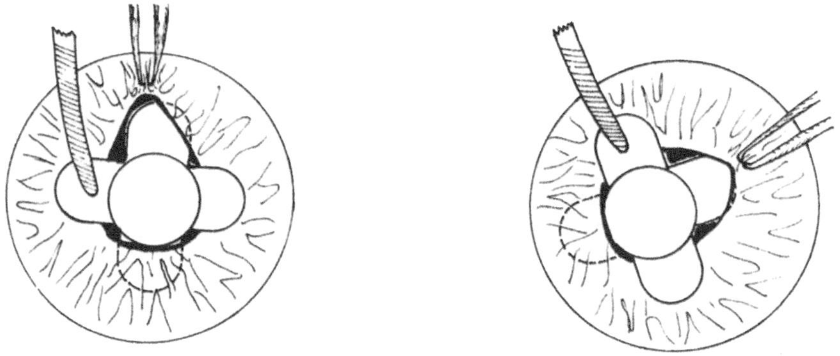

A B

Fig. VI-28. — Insertion of a Copeland lens with:
a) the horizontal haptics in front of the iris and
b) the vertical haptics in front of the iris.

In Configuration B, the horizontal haptics are behind the iris. A miotic pupil makes this insertion difficult, a 4 to 5 mm pupillary diameter being ideal for this maneuver. To position the lens, it is grasped at the superior haptic and one of the horizontal supports is slid under the iris either temporally or nasally. It is then shifted to engage the opposite horizontal support behind the iris. To facilitate this maneuver, the iris may be gently retracted and lifted over the haptic.

If necessary, miotics are injected into the anterior chamber to constrict the pupil. As the tip of the haptic support may obstruct the iridectomy, care should be taken to place them properly.

B. The Formed Chamber Technique

According to C.W. Simcoe (1978), the Copeland lens can be cartwheeled into the eye through a small incision. After delivery of the cataractous lens, the incision is partially closed to 6 mm and the lens is turned into the eye as shown on Figure VI-29.

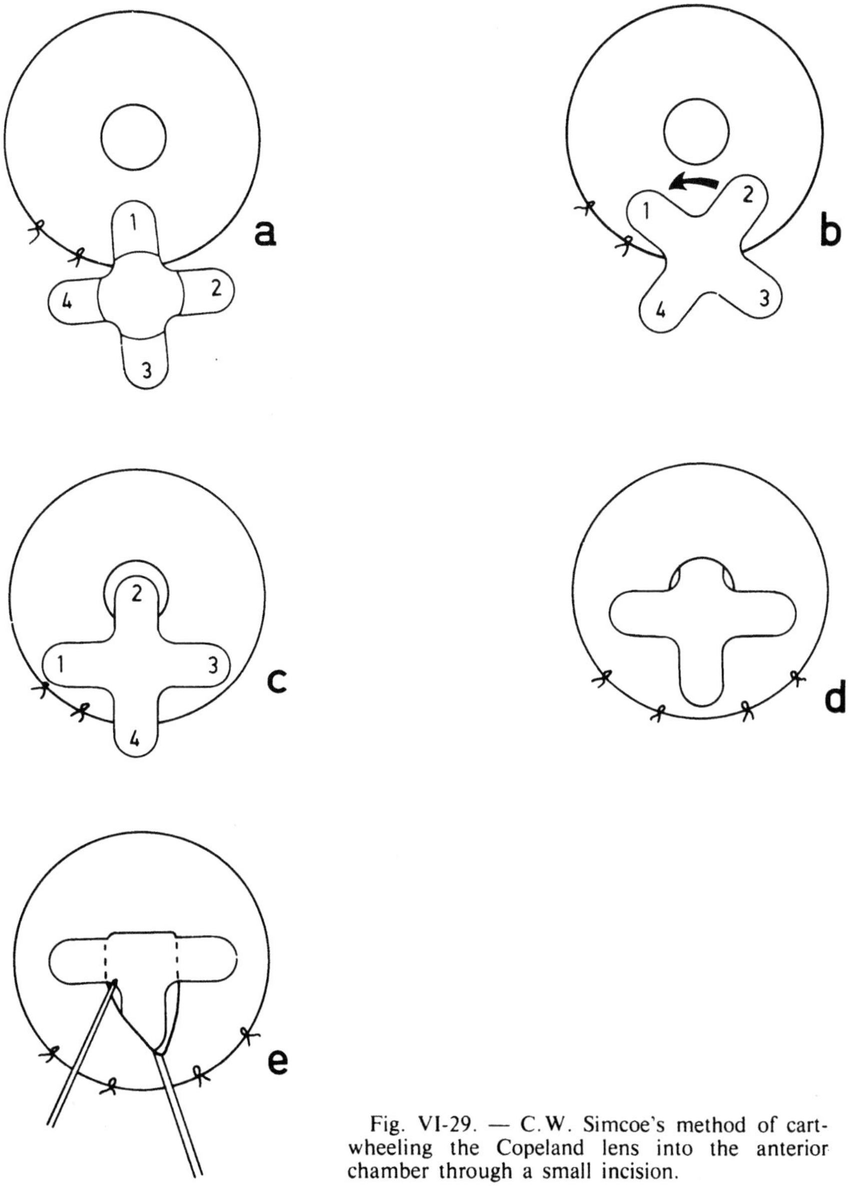

Fig. VI-29. — C.W. Simcoe's method of cartwheeling the Copeland lens into the anterior chamber through a small incision.

As soon as the lens is in the anterior chamber, the incision is closed completely, and the further positioning of the superior support of the lens behind the iris is then done. Two small irrigating instruments are required, one a repositor and the other an iris retractor. Using these instruments, the surgeon simultaneously pushes the lens toward 6 o'clock and slightly depresses it posteriorly toward the vitreous while the iris is hooked and slid in front of the superior haptic.

III. Survey of Early Results

A. Jaffe's Series

The first surgeon to perform a well-documented series of Copeland lens implantations after intracapsular cataract extraction was N.S. Jaffe. In 1968 and 1969, he inserted 81 lens implants. After a two-year moratorium, he began a second series of Copeland implantations in October 1971. The data from these two series were compared (Jaffe and Duffner, 1976). This study is of particular interest since it deals with the experience of one surgeon with a new lens

TABLE VI-14. — *Jaffe's Series of Copeland Lens Implantations*

	Group A	*Group B*
Source	Jaffe and Duffner (1976)	Jaffe and Duffner (1976)
Surgeon	N.S. Jaffe	N.S. Jaffe
Type of Surgery	Intracapsular	Intracapsular
Number of Cases	81	81
Follow-Up	7 mos.-7 yrs, 2 mos.	1 mo.-3 yrs, 9 mos.
Mean age	70.3 yrs.	76.3 yrs.
Corrected Visual Acuity ⩾20/40	65%	79%
Endothelial Corneal Dystrophy		
Central	6%	4%
Partial	2.5%	2.5%
Uveal Reaction		
Iritis	9%	2.5%
Secondary Membranes	9%	10%
Clinical Cystoid Macular Edema	17%	16%
Retinal Detachment	1%	0%
Luxation	0%	7.5%
Glaucoma (persistent)	1%	1%
Hemorrhage	4%	0%
Vitreous Problems	0%	6%
Lens Removal	10%	2.5%

design. Furthermore, all the follow-up examinations were conducted by R. Duffner, who was not involved in the surgery itself. For convenience, the first group will be called Group A and the second Group B.

Comment on Jaffe's Series

Visual Acuity

A corrected visual acuity of ⩾20/40 was initially obtained in about 80% of the cases in both groups. But, later on, the percentage of patients with a visual acuity of ⩾20/40 dropped to 65% for Group A and 79% for Group B. The principal reason for the difference between the groups was the higher incidence of senile macular degeneration in the first group: 12.5% for Group A versus 6% for Group B. In addition, cystoid macular edema and macular pucker resulting in visual acuity ⩽20/40 was twice as frequent in Group A (14% versus 6%).

Endothelial Corneal Dystrophy

A Series:	7 cases = 9%	*B Series:*	5 cases = 6%
Central ECD:	5 cases = 6%	Central ECD:	3 cases = 3.7%
Partial ECD:	2 cases = 2.5%	Partial ECD:	2 cases = 2.5%

For the total series (162 eyes) the incidence of central endothelial corneal dystrophy was approximately 5%. Long term follow-up indicated that the incidence of corneal edema did not increase with time. Lens luxation was not a principal underlying cause. According to Jaffe, corneal edema was frequently associated with recurrent iritis and episodes of elevated intraocular pressure.

Macular Pathology

All types of macular pathology were reported that influenced ultimate visual acuity. As shown on Table VI-15, a fair amount of senile

TABLE VI-15. — *Distribution of Macular Pathology*

	Group A	*Group B*
Number of cases	38 cases (47%)	27 cases (33%)
Senile Macular Degeneration	20 cases (25%)	12 cases (15%)
Clinical Cystoid Macular Edema	14 cases (17%)	13 cases (16%)
Macular Pucker	4 cases (5%)	2 cases (2%)

macular degeneration was present in both groups, which reflects the rather high age distribution of the patients involved. Cystoid macular edema occurred to the same extent in both groups. However, macular pucker following resolution of cystoid macular edema was more frequent in Group A, which indicates that the cystoid macular edema was more serious in this group. Indeed, cystoid macular edema and macular pucker accounted for visual acuity of less than 20/40 for 11 patients (14%) in Group A, but only for 5 patients (6%) in Group B.

Uveal Reactions

Duffner presented his findings on uveal reactions during the early and late postoperative periods in tabular form (see Table VI-16). Recurrent iritis appeared less frequently in Group B (9% versus 2.5%), but this difference could not be traced to changes in surgical techniques or postoperative management. Persistent anterior chamber reaction in both groups occurred in 10% of the patients the mean follow-up period being 4½ years. Jaffe and Duffner considered cystoid macular edema and recurrent iritis to be the most common problems with the Copeland lens.

TABLE VI-16. — *Graded Uveal Reactions*

	Group A	*Group B*
Postoperative		
⩾2+ cells	2.5%	0%
1+ cells	6%	11%
trace cells	5%	17.5%
Recurrent	9%	2.5%
Persistent 1+ cells	10%	10%

Secondary Membranes

The incidence of cyclitic membranes developing on the pseudophakos was vitually the same for both groups (A = 9%, B = 10%). The relation between the high incidence of secondary membrane formation and iritis is not surprising. The presence of cyclitic membranes on the optical portion of the lens was attributed to the following factors:

— the location of the optical portion in the pupillary aperture;

— the extensive contact of the haptics with the pupillary margin;
— the difficulty involved in achieving adequate dilation, which was aggravated by the promptness of synechiae formation.

The membrane were difficult to remove as instrumental access through the pupil is seriously restricted by the Copeland lens.

Luxation

No luxation was recorded for Group A, but there were 6 cases (7.5%) in Group B. This was probably due to reduced use of miotics with Group B during the postoperative period and to a lower incidence of uveal reactions, which resulted in less synechiae formation.

Glaucoma

Although the Copeland lens did not seem to produce persistent elevations in intraocular pressure, recurrent episodes of elevated pressure were reported. They were found to be associated with episodes of iritis.

Lens Removal

The reasons for lens removal are given on Table VI-17. The main reason for lens removal was recurrent episodes of serious iritis associated with glaucoma and corneal edema, especially in Group A. There was one case of recurrent hyphema. Richard Binkhorst has noted that many of the early Copeland lenses were poorly finished and even had sharp edges, which contributed to hyphema and iris irritation in his series (Richard Binkhorst, personal communication, 1978).

TABLE VI-17. — *Reasons for Lens Removal*

	Group A	*Group B*
Luxation	None	1 case = 1.25%
Iritis and Glaucoma plus Corneal Edema	5 = 6%	1 = 1.25%
Corneal Edema	2 = 2.5%	None
Early Recurrent Hyphema	1 = 1.25%	None
Total	8 = 10%	2 = 2.5%

Conclusions from the Early Experience with the Copeland Lens

The degree of uveal reaction was significantly higher for the Copeland lens than for the early iris clip lens. Jaffe and Duffner ascribed this to the extensive contact between the non-fenestrated haptics and the iris tissue. Along with the high incidence of cystoid macular edema (16%), it constituted the most disturbing problem with the early Copeland lens.

Other problems of primary concern were the episodes of elevated intraocular pressure accompanied by corneal edema that were secondary to recurrent uveal reactions.

Adherence of the iris to the optical portion of the lens were common and dilation of the pupil was severely restricted.

Secondary membranes developing on the optical portion of the lens were not infrequent and were difficult to remove.

Even though the Copeland lens was reported to be easier to insert than the other iris supported lenses and had a lower luxation rate, the price paid for these advantages was rather high.

However, as Duffner and Jaffe noted, the data from these two studies do not allow definite conclusions to be drawn for the future, since significant modifications in lens design, surgical technique, and postoperative complication management were introduced during this period. In particular, the quality of the lenses was improved with the tips being rendered smoother and the edges carefully rounded. Thus the intimate contact between the lens and the iris tissue became less aggressive.

B. **The Miami Series**

This study was carried out by L.R. Duffner, W.K. Wallace, and W.R. Stile (1976) on 623 Copeland lens implantations performed by 20 surgeons in the Miami area. It is of particular interest because it deals with the experience of different surgeons using the same lens and because the data were compiled by L.R. Duffner, who had conducted the examinations in Jaffe's series.

The implantations were carried out between 1968 and 1974, with a primary intracapsular procedure being used in virtually all (99.2%) of the cases. During this 6 year period, some changes were introduced in both surgical techniques and in the management of complications, and the lens itself was significantly improved.

TABLE VI-18. — *The Miami Series of Copeland Lens Implantations*

Source	L.R. Duffner, W.K. Wallace, and W.R. Stiles (1976)
Surgeons	20 Miami area surgeons
Type of Surgery	Intracapsular + Primary (99.2%)
Number of Cases	623
Follow-Up	1 to 7 yrs.
Mean Age at Surgery	74.2 yrs.
Corrected Visual Acuity	
≥20/40	63.4%
Endothelial Corneal Dystrophy	
Central	4.9%
Partial	2.2%
Uveal Reactions	
Iritis	2.6%
Secondary Membranes	14.0%
Clinical Cystoid Macular Edema	13.2%
Retinal Detachment	1.0%
Luxation	1.0%
Glaucoma	
Transient	0.3%
Persistent	2.7%
Vitreous loss	3.0%
Lens Removal	4.2%

Comment

Visual Acuity

The reasons for visual acuity of less than 20/40 in 228 patients are given on Table VI-19.

TABLE IV-19. — *Reasons for Visual Acuity ≤20/40 in the Miami Series*

	Number of Cases	*Percentage*
Clinical Cystoid Macular Edema	64	10%
Senile Macular Degeneration	57	9%
Unknown	42	7%
Intraocular Membranes	27	4%
Endothelial Corneal Dystrophy	24	4%
Retinal Disease	11	2%
Optique Nerve Problems	10	2%
Retinal Detachment	6	1%
Vitreous Problems	2	0.5%

Endothelial Corneal Dystrophy

Some degree of endothelial corneal dystrophy was present in 45 cases (7%), with 14 cases of partial ECD and 31 cases of central or total ECD. As in Jaffe's series, Duffner established a correlation between the occurrence of iritis and ECD. Eight lenses had to be removed for this reason. Permanent corneal contact by the implant was not a major problem, with only one lens having to be removed for this reason. Surgical trauma to the endothelium was apparent in 4 cases and produced localized inferior ECD. Duffner and his colleagues suggested that the damage could have occurred by touching the cornea with the interior tip of the lens during the insertion maneuver.

Macular Disorders (Table VI-20)

TABLE VI-20. — *Breakdown of Macular Disorders in the Miami Series*

	Number of Cases	*Percentage*
Cystoid Macular Edema	82	13%
Senile Macular Degeneration	72	11.5%
Macular Drüsen	31	5%
Macular Pucker	9	1.4%

As with Jaffe's series, there is a rather high incidence of cystoid macular edema, 13%. Together with macular pucker, cystoid macular edema was responsible for a definite drop in visual acuity to less than 20/40 in 11.5% of the cases. On the other hand, about a hundred eyes (one out of six patients) had ophthalmoscopic, senile degenerative lesions, which was to be expected in such an elderly population.

Uveal Reactions

As for Jaffe's series, the late presence of cells or flare or both was a common finding. Duffner and his colleagues considered iritis as one of the main postoperative problems. The incidence of cellular reaction is given on Table VI-21. As reported for Jaffe's cases, episodic iritis was frequently associated with corneal decompensation. This was the reason for 8 lens removals.

TABLE VI-21. — *Grade Uveal Reactions*

2+ cells	2.5%
1+ cells	6%
Trace of Cells or Flare or Both	21%

Secondary Membranes

Secondary membranes were present in 14% of the cases, sometimes imparing visual acuity. Of the 623 cases 7% had membranes that did not interfere with vision, 6% had membranes that did interfere, and 0.6% (4 cases) that had to have the lens removed had membraneous structures.

Glaucoma

Pupillary block or transient glaucoma were reported in only 2 cases, which indicates that this problem was minor. According to J.A. Smith and D.R. Anderson (1976), who studied the glaucoma problem with the same patients, 26 (4.3%) of the 606 eyes that did not have glaucoma before implantation developed prolonged pressure elevation. In most of these cases, the onset of the elevated intraocular pressure was concurrent with the onset of iritis.

Luxation

Luxation occurred in 6 eyes or 1%. The report does not indicate whether the luxation was anterior or posterior. In any event, additional surgery was required to reposition 5 lenses.

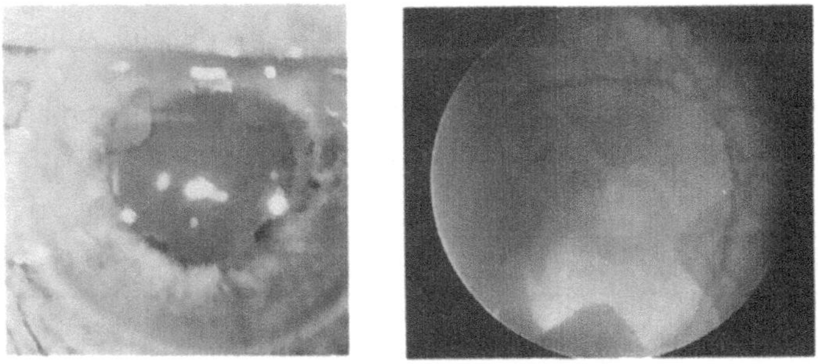

Fig. VI-30. — Left: Posterior subluxation of a Copeland lens. (Courtesy J. Alpar.) Right: Copeland lens dislocated into the vitreous. (Courtesy C. Dyson.)

Lens Removal

Lenses were removed from 26 eyes (4%). The main reasons were:

— Endothelial corneal dystrophy in 16 cases. In 8 eyes, ECD was associated with episodes of iritis, and in only 1 case was corneal contact the reason for explantation.

— Luxation in 6 cases.
— Dissatisfaction without apparent medical reason in 1 case.

Conclusion to the Miami Series

As in Jaffe's series, the postoperative problems included a high incidence of cystoid macular edema, macular pucker, membraneous structures, and persistent uveal reactions. Here, too, corneal dystrophy and glaucoma were frequently associated with episodic iritis. Lens luxation was rare.

IV. Recent Studies

Our attempt to assess the refined Copeland lens and its updated surgical technique was rather frustrating. Only a few studies are available, and they report the results from only a few hundred cases. Since about 30,000 Copeland lenses have been implanted during the last ten years, there is ample reason for concern.

A. Osher's Study

M.S. Osher (1976) reported the favorable results he attained with the implantation of 100 Copeland lenses (see Table VI-22). All patients underwent intracapsular lens extraction, and primary insertion of the lens was performed with the open-sky method.

TABLE VI-22. — *Results Obtained by M.S. Osher with the Copeland Lens*

Source	M.S. Osher (1976)
Surgeon	M.S. Osher
Type of Surgery	Intracapsular + Primary
Number of Cases	100
Follow-Up	3 years maximum
Corrected Visual Acuity	
≥20/40	81%
Endothelial Corneal Dystrophy Central	1%
Uveal Reactions	
Vitreitis	3%
Secondary Membranes	2%
Clinical Cystoid Macular Edema	3%
Retinal Detachment	1%
Luxation	2%
Glaucoma	None

Commentary

Visual Acuity

Osher placed the reasons for visual acuity of less than 20/40 into two categories:

— *Possibly lens related:* 5%
  Cystoid macular edema: 1%
  Vitreitis and possible cystoid macular edema: 3%
  Endothelial corneal dystrophy (implant contact): 1%

— *Non-lens related:* 14%
  Pre-existing macular degeneration: 6%
  Pathology indetermined: 2%
  Retinal detachment: 1%
  Endophthalmitis: 1%
  Trauma, corneal ulcer, hemorrhage, cerebrovascular accident: 4%.

Endothelial Corneal Dystrophy (1 case): 1%

Only one cornea developed localized dystrophy because of endothelial contact by the tip of the implant. In Osher's opinion, corneal edema was avoided primarily because the open sky technique was used and because a shallow anterior chamber was considered a contraindication for lens implantation.

Macular Disorders and Cystoid Macular Edema: 3%

The incidence of clinically apparent and definite cystoid macular edema was 3%, with some cases being associated with vitreitis. According to Osher, the incidence of CME and vitreitis may be decreased by subtenonal injection of 40 mg. Kenalog®, which was not done in the first cases.

Uveal Reactions:

Uveal reactions were insignificant and easily controlled with steroids in the few cases they occurred. Two mild and one severe case of vitreitis were observed. Two cases had membranes that extended beyond the lateral edges of the pupil but did not interfere with visual acuity. These occurred among the earlier cases before Kenalog was introduced.

Luxation: 2%

In one case, luxation was due to the accidental administration of Neosynephrine. In the other case, postoperative miotics had been omitted.

Hemorrhage: 1%

No explanation was suggested for this case of recurrent and massive postoperative hyphema. No late hyphema due to lens chafing occurred.

Discussion: In comparison with the early series reported by Duffner, the results obtained by Osher show improvement in the following respects: iritis was insignificant; the incidence of cystoid macular edema was low; there were no cases of glaucoma being a persistent problem; there were no retrolental membranes that caused visual impairment.

B. Other Studies on the Copeland Lens

1. *Snider's and Taylor's Series: 595 Cases*

The following data on 595 Copeland lens implants were abstracted from publication dealing with the final results of 1000 intraocular implants of lenses of various styles (Snider and McReynolds, 1977; Taylor et al., 1978). Unfortunately, these articles do not give full details about the items we consider significant.

TABLE VI-23. — *Copeland Lens Results from Mixed Statistics*

Source	N.L. Snider and M.U. McReynolds (1977)	D.N. Taylor et al.
Number of cases	399	195
Procedure	ICCE & ECCE, Primary 99%	ICCE, Primary 100%
Follow-up	6 mos. to $1\frac{1}{2}$ yrs.	6 mos. to $2\frac{1}{2}$ yrs.
Visual Acuity	Not available	Not available
Endothelial Corneal Dystrophy	1%	1%
Uveal reaction	Not available	9%
Secondary Membranes	Not available	9%
Clinical Cystoid Macular Edema	4.2%	Not available
Retinal Detachment	1%	0.5%
Luxation	2%	1.5%
Glaucoma	0.5%	Not available
Endophthalmitis	0.25%	Not available

Comment

Endothelial Corneal Dystrophy:
The 1% incidence in both series is concordant and low.

Cystoid Macular Edema:
In the series of Snider and McReynolds, there was a 4.2% incidence of prolonged or severe cystoid macular edema. Taylor et al. reported an incidence of 6% in 500 cases (several lens types), of which one third were persistent. In the latter series, it was impossible to trace the exact incidence of cystoid macular edema for the Copeland lens.

Luxation:
The figures reported, 2% and 1.5%, are remarkably similar. Taylor et al. stated that of the 3 luxations, 1 was anterior and 2 were posterior. The latter cases could be ascribed to sexual activity in the early postoperative period, i.e., on the second and the third day after the operation.

Uveal Reactions:
Taylor et al. make an interesting observation about this. They found recurrent iritis in 24 cases out of the 500 lens implantations (various kinds of lenses). Out of these 24 patients, 18 had received Copeland lenses. The response to corticosteroids was favorable in all cases.

Secondary Membranes:
In this regard, Taylor et al. noted that 19 out of the same 500 patients developed retrolenticular membranes. Copeland lenses were involved in 18 of these instances.

Glaucoma:
Transient glaucoma (pupillary block) occurred in two patients in Snyder's series (0.5%). One case was released by dilatation of the pupil; the other required an additional iridectomy and vitreous aspiration.

2. *Benjamin's Sherman's and Gentry's Series:* 101 Cases

These authors published smaller series of 75 and 26 cases in 1977.

The figures given on Table VI-24 have been abstracted from series of 135 and 100 lens implant cases with different lens types.

TABLE VI-24. — Copeland Lens Results from Mixed Statistics

Source	S.M. Benjamin and O.R. Sherman (1977)	J.H. Gentri (1977)
Number of cases	75	26
Procedure	Intracapsular Primary	Intracapsular Primary
Follow-up	Not available	6 mos. to 2 yrs.
Visual Acuity ⩾20/40	81%	92%
Endothelial Corneal Dystrophy	5.3%	0
Clinical Cystoid Macular Edema	18.6%	11.5%
Luxation	Not available	Not available
Uveal Reactions	5.3%	Not available
Secondary Membranes	1%	Not available
Retinal Detachment	4%	11.5%

Comment

Endothelial Corneal Dystrophy:

For S.M. Benjamin and O.R. Sherman, there is an obvious and close relationship between endothelial decompensation and persistent uveitis, which relationship is also evident in the series reported by L.R. Duffner discussed above.

Cystoid Macular Edema:

Benjamin and Sherman consider the kind of CME that occurs after Copeland lens insertion to be a "malignant form" from which the macula often does not recover. Indeed, more than half the CME cases never cleared.

Retinal Detachment:

Benjamin and Sherman note the possibility that retinal detachment is related to the chronic irritation associated with the use of the Copeland lens.

Conclusion for the Recent Studies on the Copeland Lens

There is a deplorable lack of up-to-date, well-documented, and long-term studies. Combining the data gathered by Osher (1976), Taylor (1978), and Snider (1977), we have short-term results from about 700 Copeland lens insertions after ICCE. The information provided by Benjamin (1977) and Gentri (1977) on a hundred cases has also come to our attention.

The low incidence of 1% of endothelial corneal dystrophy speaks in favor of the Copeland lens because the entire pseudophakos is in the iris plane, well away from the endothelium. The luxation incidence was also low and did not exceed 2% during the two year observation period. But one of the major problems, which was already evident in the early series of Jaffe and Duffner, was still iritis, which seemed to be recurrent (Taylor) and requires aggressive control by extensive and even systemic use of corticosteroids (Osher). The formation of retrolenticular membranes after ICCE is also a continual matter of concern. According to Taylor, both pathological conditions are typical for this particular lens since they were virtually absent in the cases where other lenses were implanted. Clinical cystoid macular edema resulting in a definite loss of useful vision is still a problem, as is reflected in the more recent studies. In 4% of his cases, Snider had to deal with persistent severe macular edema. With reference to his own results, Benjamin considered the macular edema he encountered in 14 eyes out of 75 as a "maglignant form" from which the macular function did not often recover. According to Osher, the severity of cystoid macular edema after ICCE with a Copeland lens can be reduced by routine subtenonal injection of corticosteroids. In any event, to avoid disappointment should cystoid macular edema develop, Osher prefers to operate on patients who will be satisfied with an eventual visual acuity of some 20/50 or 20/70 (Osher, 19778).

V. Conclusions

Because of the monoplanar design of the Copeland lens, the iris is distorted by being stretched in front of and behind the haptics. The resulting intimate contact between the foreign material and the iris aggravates uveal reactions.

In addition, there is constant friction between the iris and the four corners of the cross, which may lead to localized atrophic changes.

In our opinion, there is no solution to these crucial problems.

Uveal reactions can only be reduced by diminishing the contact zones between the lens and the iris for which a biplanar lens seems to be an answer. The problem is, however, that if the surface of intimate contact is reduced, the lens becomes less stable and the rate of luxation will increase. The repositioning of a luxated Copeland lens is fairly difficult and requires skillful surgery.

Even when the best available techniques are applied, surgeons who choose to implant the Copeland lens will have to deal with the specific problems inherent in its design and in its position in the eye.

§3 THE MEDALLION LENS

I. Introduction

J. Worst, of The Netherlands, started to implant the iris clip lens after intracapsular cataract extraction in 1967. He developed various methods for suturing the lens to the iris in order to prevent subluxation or total dislocation (Worst, 1970, 1971).

Because the anterior loops of the iris clip lens lose their stabilizing function when a suture is used, Worst soon developed a lens of his own design without anterior loops. As M.E. Nordlohne (1975) put it, having first adapted the suture to the construction of the iris clip lens, he then conceived the idea of adapting the construction of the lens to the suture.

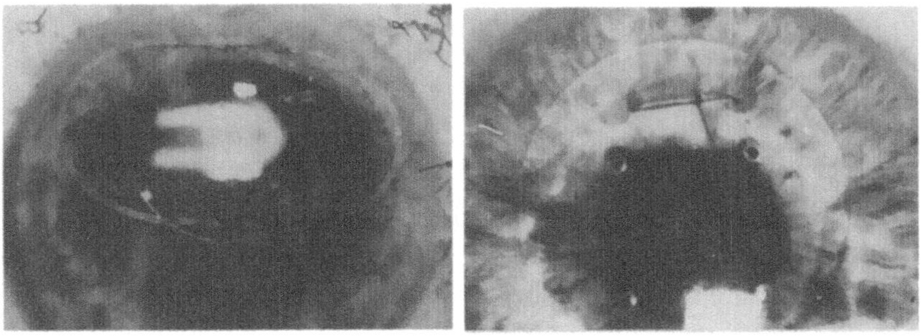

Fig. VI-31. — An iris clip lens and a Worst's medallion lens secured with sutures.

This modified iris clip lens has an optic component 5 mm in diameter surrounded by an eccentric haptic rim with two holes in it to hold the suture. Two posterior loops are attached to the lens body. Worst called his own design the medallion lens and used it for the first time in December 1970.

Within a few years, the medallion lens became very popular. Indeed, according to a survey by K.J. Hoffer (1978) extending to June 1977, at least 16,200 sutured medallion lenses had been inserted, which accounted for 25% of the 70,000 lenses implanted by the members of the American Intra-Ocular Implant Society.

Among the reasons for this widespread popularity was that, while C.D. Binkhorst had already adopted the principle of extracapsular

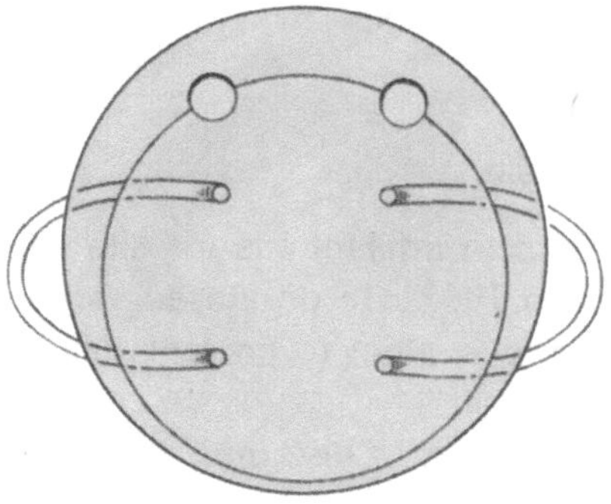

Fig. VI-32. — Schematic presentation of Worst's medallion lens.

lens fixation in the early seventies, the medallion lens remained the only iris supported lens of Dutch origin that was promoted for insertion after intracapsular cataract extraction.

II. Implantation Techniques

A. The Medallion Lens

J. Worst recommends the following procedure (Fig. VI-32):

— The use of a Flieringa ring is advisable.

— After opening wide the anterior chamber (over 180°), a 9-0 or 10-0 polypropylene suture is passed through the iris at 12 o'clock directly behind the sphincter muscle. The bite has to be about 2.5 mm in width. Both ends of the suture are left long and should be kept in the 3 and 9 o'clock meridian.

— The lens is extracted.

— The implant is grasped at the haptic edge with a simple needle holder. Outside the eye, one end of the suture is passed through the corresponding lens perforation from back to front and then from front to back through the other perforation. The suture should be kept carefully stretched by the assistant to prevent it from snaring the posterior loops while the lens is inserted. The cornea is lifted and the two-loop lens inserted. First, one loop is placed behind the iris in the 9 o'clock sector (for right-handed surgeons), and with a sideward movement the other loop is slipped behind the opposite iris sector. A 4-5 mm pupil is ideal for this maneuver. Should it be necessary, the iris may be mechanically pulled over the corresponding loop at 3 o'clock with fine iris forceps in the left hand.

Once the lens is in place, the ends of the iris suture are trimmed long enough to make the knot outside the eye. The knots are slipped into the eye by gently pulling at the ends. The knot is thus placed between the haptic rim and the iris. The suture should be neither too tight nor too loose. The ends of the suture are cut flush with the edge of the haptic rim in order to prevent any contact with the cornea.

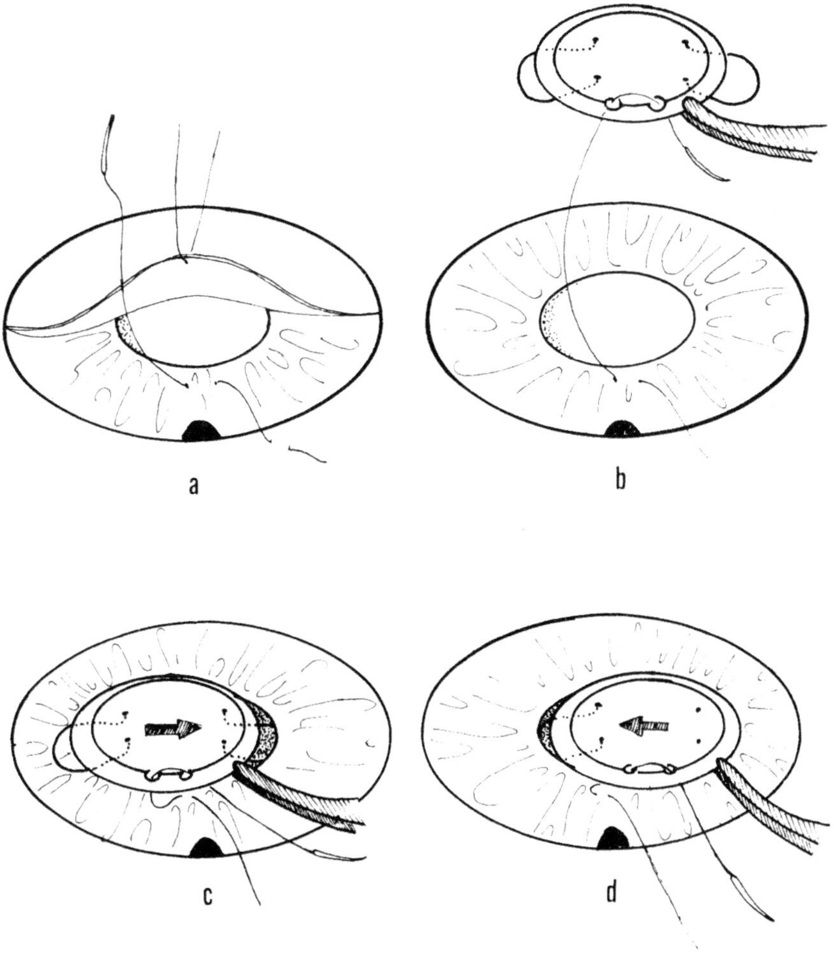

Fig. VI-33. — Steps in the implantation of the medallion lens.

— Two small iridectomies are made either before or after lens insertion.
— The anterior chamber is re-formed with fluid or air.
— The preplaced sutures are knotted.
— The eye is closed watertight. After suturing, the air is replaced by fluid.
— To close the wound, Worst now uses separate stitches of 30 μ steel wire.

Variation

The medallion lens may also be inserted through a smaller corneoscleral incision (120° to 130°), which permits the implant to be placed in a "formed" anterior chamber under an air bubble (J. Alpars' technique). The lens has to be inserted with the loop in a vertical or slightly oblique position and then has to be rotated until the loops are in the horizontal meridian. Preplacement of the iris suture and the tying of the knots are done as described above.

B. The Slotted Medallion Lens

Since 1976, Worst has been using steel sutures instead of Perlon for the fixation of the medallion lens. Therefore, the design of the classic medallion lens had to be modified slightly: two slots connecting the edge with the suture fixation holes were made in the haptic rim to facilitate sliding the steel suture into position (Fig. VI-34).

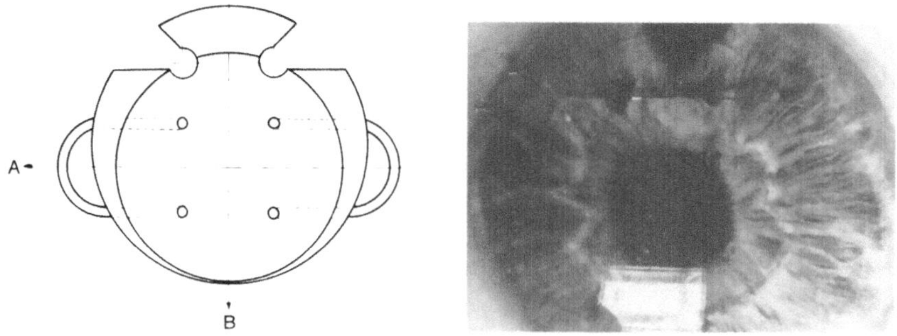

Fig. VI-34. — Worst's slotted medallion lens.

Before delivery of the cataractous lens, the metal thread is passed through the iris at 12 o'clock just behind the sphincter. A 3 mm bite is advisable. As shown in Figure VI-34, a rather large round loop is made with a double throw. This pre-placed metal suture can serve as an iris retractor when cyroextraction is performed.

After cataract extraction, the implant is slid into position. The metal thread ring is passed through the slots and the ends are stretch vigorously. The lens must be steadied by holding it firmly with forceps at its haptic rim while inserting and tightening the suture through the notches, since a "non-supported suture closure" may cause the lens to move dangerously. In contrast to the sutured medallion lens, the knot is placed in front of the lens. Actually, the steel suture is not knotted; the double throw is just pulled tight.

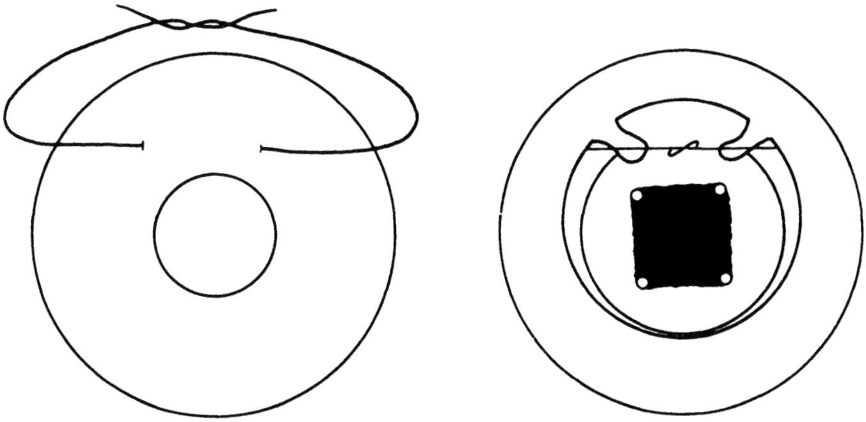

Fig. VI-35. — Slotted Medallion lens techniques: preplaced stainless steel suture forming a large loop and the suture pulled tight.

III. Development of the Medallion Lens

A. Worst's Early Results

As he did for Binkhorst's cases, M.E. Nordlohne (1975) examined the results Worst obtained up until February 1973. Nordlohne's study is of particular interest here because it provides comparative data on the experience of one surgeon with the iris clip lens and the medallion lens.

Unfortunately, the follow-up period for the two lens styles was unequal, being only 1 year at the most for the medallion lens.

TABLE V-25. — *Summary of Results and Complications for 658 Lens Implantations Performed by J.F. Worst between 1967 and 1 February 1973*

Source	M.E. Nordlohne (1975)	M.E. Nordlohne (1975)
Surgeon	J.F. Worst	J.F. Worst
Type of lens	Medallion sutured	Iris clip
Procedure	ICCE + Primary	ICCE + primary
Number of Cases	173	485 238 (49%) not sutured 247 (51%) sutured
Follow-up	8 days to 1 year	Up to $3\frac{3}{4}$ years
Corrected Visual Acuity 20/40	58%	56.5%
Endothelial Corneal Dystrophy	2.9%	2.3% 1.7% not sutured 2.8% sutured
Uveal Reaction (Low Grade)	1.2%	2.0%
Secondary Membrane (Deposit on Lens)	1.2%	1.6%
Clinical Cystoid Macular Edema	3.5%	3.5%
Retinal Detachment	1.7%	1.8%
Dislocation	1.7%	2.7% 3.3% not sutured 2.0% sutured
Glaucoma: Transient	0%	0.6%
Persistent	0%	0%
Lens Removal	1.2%	0.8%
Enucleation	0%	0.2%

Visual Acuity

A corrected visual acuity of ≥20/40 was attained in about 60% of the cases for both lens types. The main reasons for visual acuity of less than 20/200 in 80 cases out of the 658 were:

senile macular degeneration: 24 cases
endothelial corneal dystrophy: 11 cases
retinal detachment: 10 cases
cystoid macular edema: 7 cases

The exact incidence of these complications for the two lens models that resulted in less than 20/200 visual acuity could not be traced.

Endothelial Corneal Dystrophy

In the 658 lens implantations, 17 cases (2.56%) of endothelial corneal dystrophy were encountered. The average interval between the operation and the first detection of incipient endothelial corneal dystrophy was more than one year. The causes were:
— endothelial touching by the implant: 7 cases
— endothelial touching by the iris suture, i.e., the free ends of the suture scratched the cornea: 4 cases
— dislocation: 2 cases
— ocular trauma: 1 case.
For the three remaining cases, the etiology was not clear.

Apparently both sutured lens types have the same incidence. Considering the lower incidence in the non-sutured series, one may conclude that the initial presence of a suture or the extra manipulation required to suture accounted for a slight increase in the incidence of endothelial corneal dystrophy.

TABLE VI-26. — *Incidence of Endothelial Corneal Dystrophy according to Lens Style (Nordlohne, 1975)*

Non-sutured Iris Clip Lens	1.7%
Sutured Iris Clip Lens	2.8%
Sutured Medallion Lens	2.9%

Uveal Reaction

Only low grade uveal reactions were observed for both lens styles. This indicates that the eyes reacted favorably to both the new lens and the suture material (Perlon) used to steady it.

Dislocation

Occurring in 17 cases (2.56%) dislocation was always partial except in one case. The average interval between the operation date and dislocation was 4 months.

TABLE VI-27. — *Incidence of Dislocation according to Lens Type (Nordlohne, 1975)*

Non-sutured Iris Clip Lens	3.3%
Sutured Iris Clip Lens	2.0%
Sutured Medallion Lens	1.7%

As might be expected, the non-sutured lenses luxated more frequently. The slight difference in incidence of subluxation for both sutured lens types seems not to be conclusive since the follow-up period for the medallion lenses was not as long as for iris clip lenses.

From these early short-term results obtained with the medallion lens, we may conclude:

1) The eyes, and particularly the iris, did not have any noticeable reaction to the suture material.
2) This modified iris clip lens without anterior loops has proven to be as stable, at least initially, as the sutured iris clip lens.

B. The Developmental Period

1. *Introduction*

After having performed many hundred insertions of sutured medallion lenses, Worst was confronted around 1973 with a serious problem: iris suture failure. Some of the nylon threads were beginning to break after a few years. The exact incidence of suture failure is unknown but it was large enough for Worst to see the need to develop other ways of securing his medallion lens.

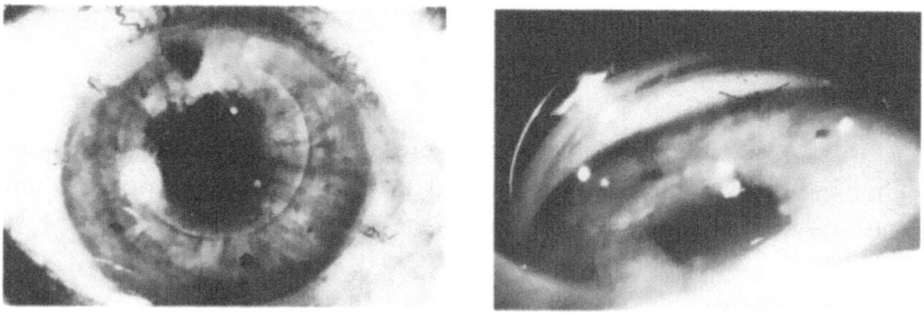

Fig. VI-36. — Medallion lens lacking an iris suture and an iris suture found in the anterior chamber angle below. (Courtesy G. Baikoff.)

Other authors have also reported cases of suture failure. According to B. Drews (1978), the incidence of suture failure increased with time and a failure rate between 2% and 10% could be expected. Among the reasons for nylon suture failure are the following:

— improper γ-ray sterilization;
— the "chafing-through effect" of an occasional sharp edge of a lens rubbing through the suture;

— the biodegradibility of nylon 6 and 6.6 (see chapter III);
— material fatigue (Drews in Boyd 1978).

Another problem Worst wanted to solve was the possibility of subluxation of one or both posterior loops. This was not a major problem (Nordlohne reports an incidence of 1.7% in the first 173

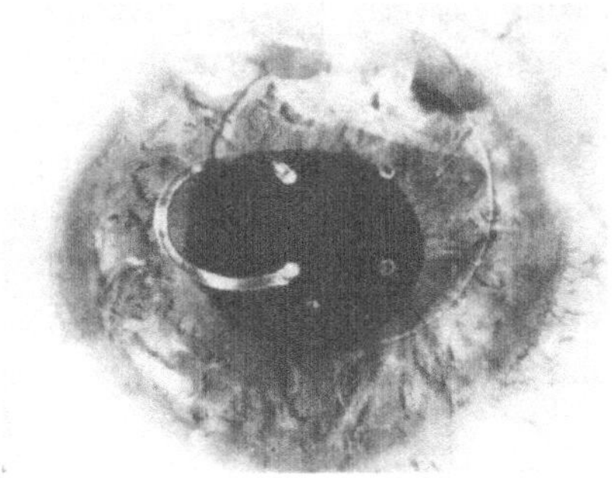

Fig. VI-37. — Anterior dislocation of a medallion lens loop. (Courtesy G. Baikoff.)

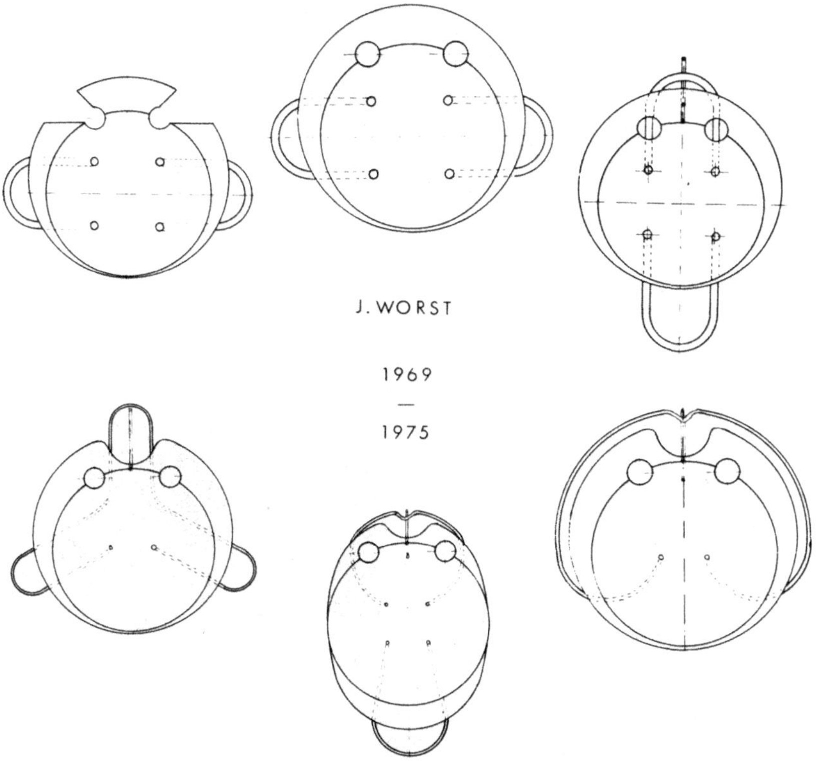

Fig. VI-38. — Lens models developed by J. Worst to enhance lens fixation.

cases), and most of the subluxated loops could be repositioned non-surgically.

In his search for a better method of fixation, Worst's later efforts were primarily focused on finding a type of iris fixation that did not require suturing. Between 1973 and 1975, he developed a whole family of lenses with different "iris fixation devices". At least 12 different lens models were designed with different fixation principles, e.g., clipping through the iris like an earring, hooking through the iris like a coathanger, and slotting through an iridectomy like a safety pin. Like C.D. Binkhorst, he also experimented with capsular support. He finally returned in 1976 to the medallion lens, but now secured with a steel suture through the iris (the slotted medallion lens). These lens is generally implanted after planned extracapsular extraction unless very old patients are involved.

2. *Worst's Modifications of the Medallion Lens*

a. *The Medallion Platinum Clip Lens*

One of the first lenses Worst designed to meet the problems of fixation and stability was the platinum clip lens, which is generally referred to in the literature as the "platina lens".

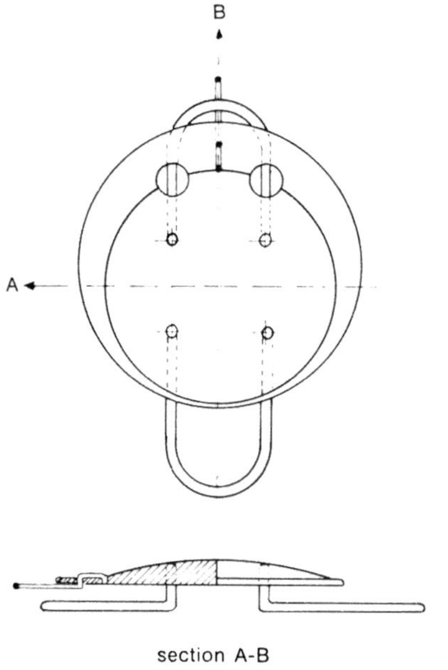

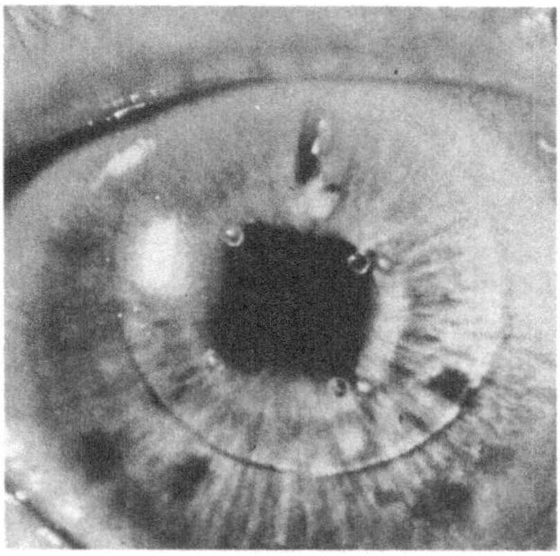

Fig. VI-39. — The medallion platinum clip lens: schematic presentation and photograph showing the lens in situ. (Courtesy J. Worst.)

The lens body is identical to that of the medallion lens, but with the two posterior loops oriented in the vertical meridian. As shown in Figure VI-38, the inferior loop is longer than the superior one, and a small stave (platinum) is embedded in the haptic rim at 12 o'clock. The stave has to be bent through an iridectomy or iridotomy after the lens is put in place. The end of the stave may be bent just enough to meet the superior loop, or more posteriorly so that it can engage the arch of the loop. As the lens is intended to be supported by the pupil, this "trans-iridectomy clip device" is merely a safety device against dislocation and does not play any role in the suspension of the lens. As necessary for any pupil supported lens, the weight of the lens was kept as low as possible, in this case for the model with nylon loops, 11.00 mg in air and 1.80 mg in aqueous.

Initially, the platinum lens was successful, but gradually major and minor problems became apparent.

The proper bending of the stave was not always without risk. If the lens is not steadied firmly enough by the forceps, the bending creates a forward displacement of the lower part of the lens, which can then touch the cornea. Some authors (e.g., Kwitko, 1977) reported that rather firm pressure is needed to bend the stave. Sometimes the closure of the clip device resulted in vitreous loss

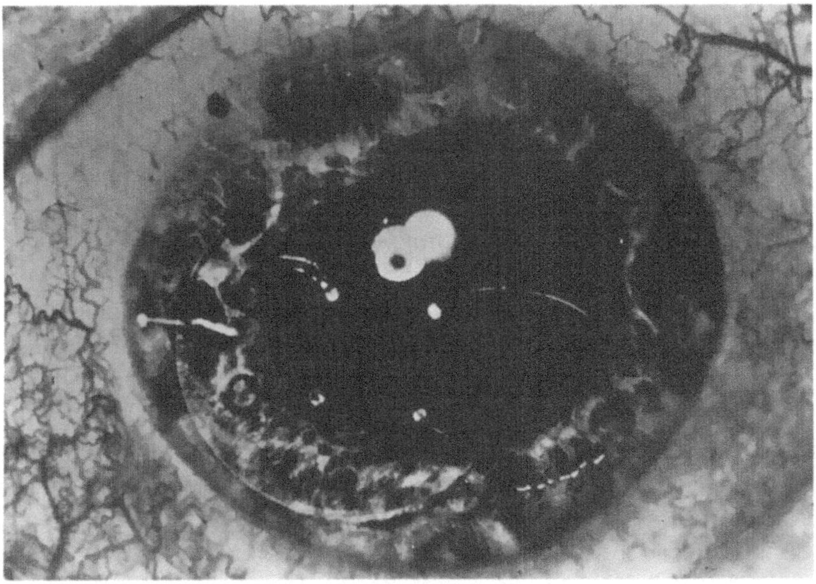

Fig. VI-40. — Rotated platinum clip lens. (Courtesy J. Alpar.)

either through the pupillary aperture or the coloboma (Taylor, 1978). And, according to B. Drews (1978-1979), some of these lenses rotated 180° when the clip was not properly closed or even luxated completely and had to be fished off the retina. But even when the lens was properly inserted, the inferior loop sometimes shifted anteriorly. This complication was the main reason why Worst designed another lens with a large posterior loop.

In Worst's opinion (Boyd, 1978-1979), too many people still continue to insert the platinum clip lens after intracapsular cataract extraction, though he recommends it after extracapsular cataract extraction.

According to K.J. Hoffer (1977) many thousands of these lenses have been implanted.

Since the statistical data on the use of this particular lens after intracapsular extraction are insufficient, we cannot guage the exact incidence of the accompanying problems and complications. The few reports that have been published, moreover, are not all comparable since replicas of the original platina lens with metal loops were used in the United States, which altered both the weight of the lens and the smoothness of the loops. It is known that the metal loops were responsible for a high incidence of chronic iritis, iris atrophy, and cystoid macular edema.

b. *The Single Loop Medallion Lens*

Another lens Worst designed to get around the problem of subluxation was the single or circular loop lens, which was primarily intended for use after ICCE. In contrast to the previous lenses, it was designed to be supported entirely by the iris stroma and not by the pupil, i.e., it was an iridectomy supported lens. For this purpose, a transiridectomy clip had to be devised.

As can be seen in Figure VI-41, the lens body is the same as that of the familiar medallion lens but, instead of a pair of posterior loops, only one large posterior loop, made of titanium, is attached to the optical part of the lens. At 12 o'clock, a thin, malleable platinum wire hook (0.3 mm in diameter) is embedded in the haptic rim. In order to close the transiridectomy device after the lens is put in position, a small iridectomy is made in the superior iris sector and the posterior loop is brought forward through the iridectomy over the metal hook. Owing to its special design, the following advantages were put forward (Worst 1975):

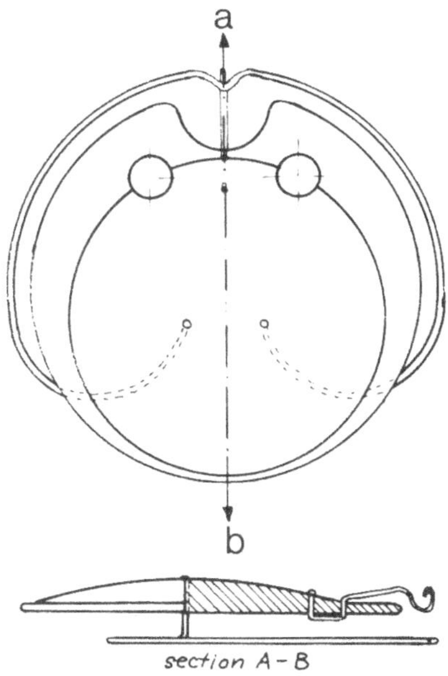

Fig. VI-41. — The single loop medallion lens: schematic presentation.

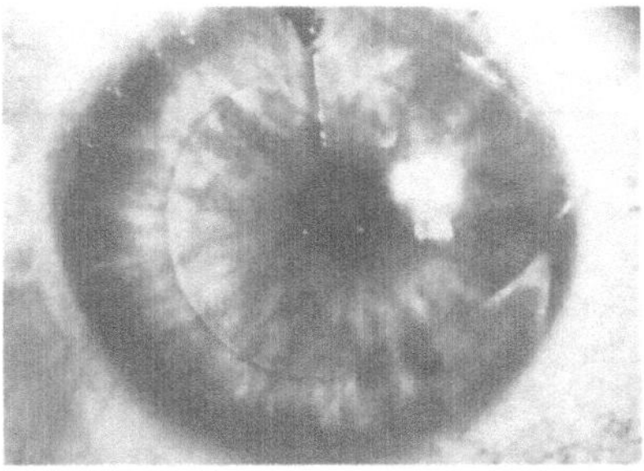

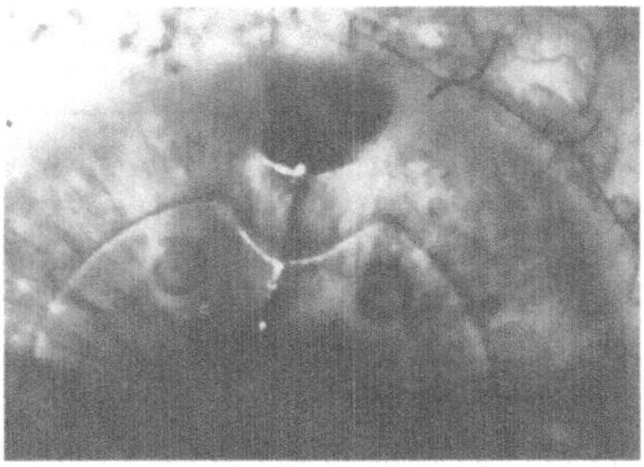

Fig. VI-42. — Left: Single loop lens in situ. Note the presence of steel sutures for the closure of the incision. (Courtesy J. Worst.)
Right: Detail of the closed clip system through a small peripheral iridectomy. (Courtesy J. Worst.)

1. It could be a substitute for the sutured medallion lens.
2. Insertion was found to be easier than that of the other lenses, and the closure of the clip device was reported to be relatively simple provided the proper technique was used.
3. The lens was expected to be unluxatable provided the iridectomy was correctly positioned and the clip device properly closed.
4. The pupil size was the smallest of all the lenses designed (1.2 mm).

In a few years, this lens gained a great deal of popularity, and by 1977 approximately 2500 such lenses were reported to have been inserted (Hoffer, 1978). Even though some surgeons reported good initial results, however, the lens did not live up to expectation.

The surgical procedure turned out to be very demanding: the iridectomy had to be extremely small, and through this aperture the posterior loop behind the lens had to be grasped, lifted, and hooked over the hook in front of the iris, while not making corneal contact, tilting the lens body, or rupturing the vitreous face.

Only a few authors have reported on their experience with this lens. M. Kraff and H.L. Liebermann (1977) dealt with the complications and results obtained with this lens in a comparative study with the medallion lens. According to their findings, the large circular loop lens had an unacceptably high incidence of partial dislocation. On the other hand, A.G. Parelman, who inserted 173 such lenses in one year, and H.N.W. Dethmers, who inserted 50 circular loop lenses, were rather pleased with the results and found the initial complications acceptable.

TABLE VI-28. — *The Medallion Lens vs. the Large Circular Loop Lens (Kraff and Liebermann, 1977)*

Number of Cases	46	254
Mean Age	73 yrs.	74 yrs.
Follow-up	3 mos. to 2 yrs.	3 mos. to 2 yrs.
Lens	Circular loop	Sutured medallion lens
Technique	Intracapsular	Intracapsular
Corrected Visual Acuity ⩾20/40	83%	87.4%
Endothelial Corneal Dystrophy	4.3%	0%
Clinical Cystoid Macular Edema	4.3%	1.2%
Retinal Detachment	2%	0.4%
Glaucoma: Transient	0%	1.6%
Persistent	0%	0.4%
Dislocation (partial)	30.4%	2.5%

The most striking figure is the incidence of partial dislocation: 30% for the circular loop lens versus 2.5% for the sutured medallion lens. In addition, the authors reported recurrent subluxation of the circular loop lens in 17% of the cases.

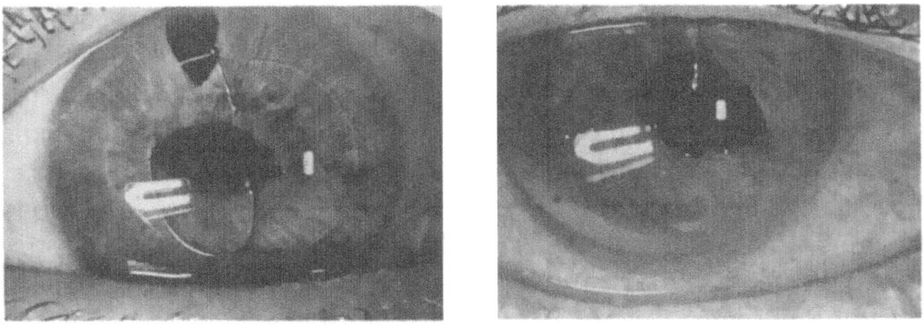

Fig. VI-43. — Left: Subluxated single loop lens. (Courtesy M. Kraff.)
Right: Single loop lens riding low and touching the cornea. (Courtesy M. Kraff.)

Endothelial corneal dystrophy due to contact was ascribed by the authors to the increased mobility of the circular loop lens.

Cystoid macular edema was also found more frequently in the first group. Commenting on their own experience, the authors concluded that the circular loop lens had only disadvantages.

TABLE 29. — *Circular Loop Lens Data*

Source	A.G. Parelman (1976)	H.N.W. Dethmers (1978)
Number of Cases	172	50
Mean Age	≈70	≈70
Follow-up	4 to 15 months	N.A.
Lens Type	Circular loop	Circular loop
Technique	Intracapsular	Intracapsular
Corrected Visual Acuity ⩾20/40	94%	64%
Endothelial Corneal Dystrophy	0%	N.A.
Uveal Reaction (transient)	3%	N.A.
Clinical Cystoid Macular Edema	2.3%	2% (1 case)
Secondary Membranes	1%	2% (1 case)
Dislocation (partial)	13.4%	8% (4 cases)

In Parelman's series, the only relevant figure seems to be the 13.4% of dislocation cases. Parelman stressed that the subluxated portions of the loop could be easily replaced. Recurrent subluxations were not infrequent, occurring in 6% of the cases. Since it did not interfere with vision, most of the patients were unaware of this phenomenon.

In Dethmers's series, the dislocation rate was lower, but still 8%. On the basis of their experience, Parelman and Dethmers concluded that the single loop lens seemed to be a safe, stable, and convenient lens after intracapsular extraction. To prevent lens luxation, however, both authors strongly suggested the use of miotics, which was thought to be beneficial in that it stabilizes the iris diaphragm.

Worst, who built up considerable clinical experience with this lens, recognized the relationship between its excessive mobility and subsequent complications. He noted that even under ideal conditions, there was such a great chance of lateral movement of the lens that the metal feet tended to saw into the iris causing sphincter damage and iris atrophy. Severe iris atrophy occurred when an occasional synechia was formed adhering to one side of the loop. Due to the constant physiologic movement of the pupil, this synechia caused the lens to swing, which was enough for the opposite part of the loop to start sawing through the iris stroma (Worst, 1978). In many of these patients, cystoid macular edema was observed that was frequently associated with a high degree of pseudophakodonesis and iris atrophy. Since the coat hanger principle was not found to be a suitable alternative to fix this lens type after ICCE, Worst decided that it should be withdrawn from the market. Worst, who also used the same lens after extracapsular cataract extraction, remarked that the exact placement of the large circular loop into the capsular bag between the anterior and posterior flaps—necessary in order to improve lens stability—turned out to be technically too demanding. However, the presence of a posterior capsular membrane was found to be a significant advantage in that the lens was more stable and the complications of less importance than with intracapsular aphakia.

3. *Other Lens Designs by Worst*

In addition to the main modifications of the medallion lens described above, a number of other types of lenses were designed. Some were for use after intracapsular cataract extraction (such as the triangle lens), and others only after extracapsular cataract extraction (the cloverleaf lens and the small incision lens). And beginning in 1976, some special lens types were created for use in non-industriaized countries: the Taxilla lens, Mark I, II, and III. These lenses were designed with low cost, mass production in mind.

IV. The Current Situation

After having experimented with various modifications, Worst returned to the medallion lens, which had been slightly altered to facilitate the use of a steel suture. In addition, as noted above, he gradually adopted the practice of combining planned extracapsular surgery and lens implantation. During the period he was introducing major modifications in both lens design and techniques, the original sutured medallion lens was being widely used. Polypropylene (Prolene) sutures, which are thought to be non-biodegradable, became available, thus eliminating the problem of suture failure.

Although K.J. Hoffer (1978) estimated that by 1977 at least 10,000 sutured medallion lenses had been inserted after intracapsular cataract extraction, there are only a few series with a follow-up of more than a few years available.

R. Drews, M.C. Kraff, and H. Lieberman reported on their long-term experience with the sutured medallion lens after intracapsular cataract extraction at the Los Angeles meeting of the American Intraocular Implant Society in March 1978. Other reports combine the results obtained with this lens with those from other lens styles and techniques. Unfortunately, these data do not permit definite

TABLE VI-30. — *Sutured Medallion Lens Follow-Up Studies*

Source	Drews (1978)	Kraff & Lieberman (1978)
Number of Cases	300	500
Procedure	ICCE + primary	ICCE + primary
Follow-Up	6 mos. to $4\frac{1}{2}$ yrs.	max.: $4\frac{1}{2}$ yrs.
Corrected Visual Acuity ⩾20/40	Not available	86%
Endothelial Corneal Dystrophy	0.7% [1]	0.5%
Uveal Reaction	2%	1%
Secondary Membranes	1%	Not available
Clinical Cystoid Macular Edema	2%	3.6%
Retinal Detachment	2%	1.4%
Glaucoma: Transient	Not available	Not available
Late	0.7% [2]	Not available
Dislocation	5%	3%
Endophthalmitis	0.3% [3]	Not available
Hemmorhage	Not available	1.4%

1. Endothelial Corneal Dystrophy: 2 cases (0.7%), one pre-existing Fuchs endothelial corneal dystrophy and one microcornea with a history of acute glaucoma 15 years previously.
2. Late Glaucoma: 2 cases (0.7%), one secondary glaucoma after uveitis in a patient with metastatic cancer; the other $2\frac{1}{2}$ years after surgery because of epithelial downgrowth.
3. Endopthalmitis: good final result.

conclusions on the use of the sutured medallion lens. The results of the experience of Worst in some 2000 cases before 1975 are reported in chapter IX. Additional data on the use of this lens by other authors is also presented in the same chapter.

The incidences of the various complications in these two series of 800 implantations performed by two different surgeons are strikingly similar. The complication rate is quite acceptable with the exception of the incidence of dislocation, which could be ascribed mainly to suture failure.

Drews observed suture failure in 5% of the cases when nylon sutures were used, and he expects an increase in suture failure as time goes by. Both authors switched to polypropylene 9-0 or 10-0 as soon as it became available.

V. Conclusion

We may conclude that the sutured medallion lens has given favorable results. However, it must be noted that these results were obtained by surgeons with a great deal of experience with cataract surgery and lens implantation. Therefore, these results from 800 lens implantations are not representative of the overall incidence of complications with the many thousands of medallion lenses inserted by all other surgeons, the vast majority of whom started to perform lens implantations after 1976. Neither are the results representative of the disasters that occurred in some 6000 eyes before 1977 in the U.S. in which lens replicas with metal loops were inserted mostly after intracapsular cataract extraction (K.J. Hoffer, 1978).

Even when good lenses are used, the sutured medallion lens has its peculiar problems. Indeed, preplacing a suture in the exact position through the iris without damaging the endothelium and preventing this suture from being caught by an instrument or snaring the lens itself is not a simple task.

A possible disadvantage of the sutured medallion lens in the long run may turn out to be its dependence on the suture and on the quality of the part of the iris tissue involved. Should one of these elements fail, the incidence of total lens dislocation may constitute an ever increasing problem. Fortunately, polypropylene seems to be non-biodegradable and the stroma of a normal iris is quite resistant.

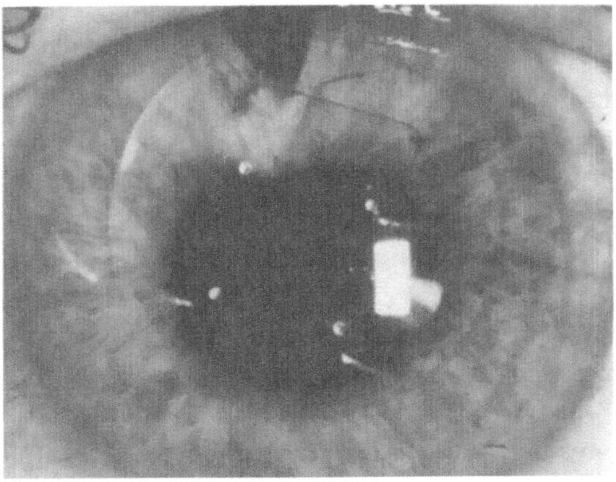

Fig. VI-44. — Disaster with metal looped lenses. (Courtesy B. Drews.) The early complications seen with iris supported lenses made with metal loops include those present in this patient: laceration of the pupil margins, recurrent hyphema, cystoid macular edema, and early corneal dystrophy. This patient also shows a synechia to one of the lens feet and erosion of the nasal foot through the iris from behind. In addition, the nylon suture is broken.

Worst is now building up an impressive series of slotted medallion lens implantations secured with steel sutures. He admits, however, that the correct use of steel wire sutures demands more skill than is the case with polypropylene (Worst, personal communication, January 1979, Leiden). It is still questionable whether the aging iris will be able to tolerate the constant pressure exerted by the suture, especially if well-tightened.

Therefore, the use of this iris supported lens after intracapsular cataract extraction should be limited to those patients with a relatively short life expectancy.

§4 THE SPUTNIK LENS

I. Introduction

After having implanted many iris clip lenses and a modification of it (the Fyodorov Mark I lens), S.N. Fyodorov designed a new lens in 1968. This was the Fyodorov Mark II lens, a lightweight (7.5 mg in air, 0.9 mg in aqueous), iris-supported lens with a biconvex 5 mm polymethylmethacrylate optic (see Fig. VI-45). Three posterior loops extend from the posterior surface, and three antenna-like struts are embedded in the peripheral edge of the optical portion. Both the loops and the struts are made of nylon. Because of its Russian origin and its appearance, it was soon nicknamed the "Sputnik" lens.

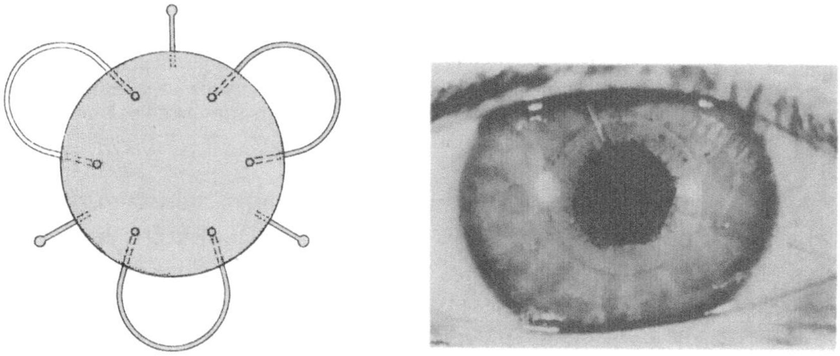

Fig. VI-45. — The Sputnik lens designed by S.N. Fyodorov.

II. Implantation Techniques

The Sputnik lens can be inserted with either the open-sky or the closed chamber technique, with the latter being the preferred method.

A. The Open-Sky Technique

After intracapsular extraction of the cataractuous lens, the iris diaphragm is floated with fluid. The preplaced sutures are carefully looped out in order to keep them from being snared while the implant is being inserted. The lens is best held with a lens forceps, either a Binkhorst forceps or one of its modifications.

The cornea is lifted and retracted. First one loop, usually the inferior, is inserted beneath the iris in the six o'clock position, and then the lens is moved horizontally, medially, and laterally in order to place the remaining two loops in position behind the iris. This maneuver technique requires at least a 6 mm pupil and a concave iris diaphragm, which indicates the absence of vitreous bulge.

B. The Formed Chamber Technique

After delivery of the lens and with direct observation through the cornea, the Sputnik implant is slid into the formed anterior chamber and the inferior loop is positioned behind the iris. Before engaging the two remaining loops behind the iris, the preplaced sutures are closed. Two different techniques are used to position the loops depending on the size of the pupil.

With a 5 to 6 mm pupil, a thin spatula of 0.5 mm in diameter is introduced through the incision and slid anteriorly and perpendicular to one loop. The lens is then slightly depressed and decentered until the loop engages behind the pupillary border as illustrated by Figure VI-46. A similar maneuver is used to position the third loop.

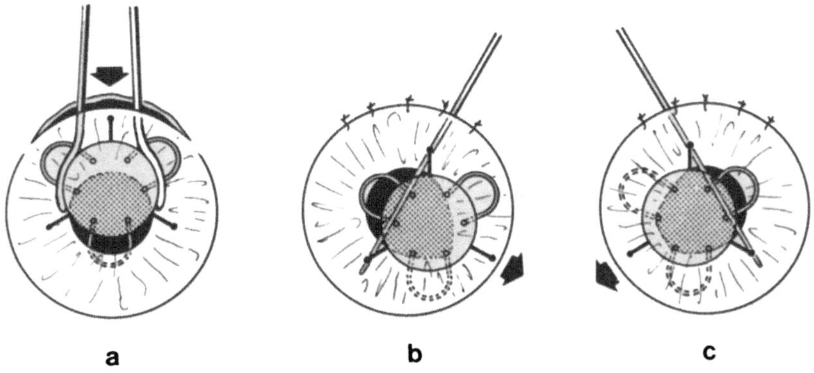

Fig. VI-46. — Steps in the implantation of the Sputnik lens.

When the pupil is rather small, a bimanual technique is indicated. Using a spatula, one of the loops in front of the iris is steadied while the underlying iris sector is pulled in front of the loop by means of either a small iris hook to retract the pupillary border or a fine iris forceps to decentrate the pupil.

Once the lens is in position with the three loops behind and the three struts in front of the iris, the incision is closed in accordance with the general principles of lens implant surgery.

III. Results

There have only been a few reports published on the results obtained with the Sputnik lens. We shall consider those of S. Fyodorov, M. A. Galin, and M. L. Kwitko.

A. Fyodorov's Series

S. Fyodorov had performed some 3000 implantations of various styles of lenses by 1976. In his opinion, the Sputnik lens turned out to be the best in clinical practice. The special design of the lens gives it remarkable stability, and total luxation never occurred. Furthermore, not a single case of endothelial corneal dystrophy was observed during a follow-up period that ranged up to nine years.

TABLE VI-31. — *Sputnik Lens Series of S. N. Fyodorov (1977)*

Source	S. N. Fyodorov (1977)
Surgeon	S. N. Fyodorov et al.
Surgical Procedure	Not available
Number of cases	2000
Follow-Up	1 to 9 years
Corrected Visual Acuity ⩾20/40	96%
Endothelial Corneal Dystrophy	None
Uveal Reactions	
Iritis/Uveitis	0.25%
Secondary Membranes	3.4%
Clinical Cystoid Macular Edema	Not available
Retinal Detachment	2.2%
Luxation	
Total	None
Partial	4%
Glaucoma	
Transient	0.25%
Persistent	None
Hemorrhage	0.33%

As is shown by the data on 2000 Sputnik lenses given on Table VI-31, the complication rate is exceptionally low, with only a 4% incidence of partial luxation and a 3.4% incidence of retrolenticular membranes. Retinal detachment occurred in 2.2% of the cases, and then mainly in patients who had been operated on for traumatic cataracts.

In 1980, S. Fyodorov published updated results from 3000 primary Sputnik style lens implantations for 2614 patients with senile cataracts (1385 cases), complicated cataracts (1516 cases), or congenital cataracts (99 cases). Depending on the type of cataract and the age of the patient, intracapsular, classic extracapsular, or phakoemusification cataract extraction techniques were used.

Examined one month after the implantation, 81.5% of the patients had achieved visual acuity of ⩾20/50 and 92% had regained binocular vision.

Fyodorov noted that the immediate postoperative period was characterized by a response to the surgical trauma and the artificial lens. Frequently a pronounced exudative reaction was observed that could be successfully treated with subconjunctival and topical corticosteroids.

Comparison of complication rates for pseudophakic and aphakic eyes indicates that lens dislocation was the only complication directly attributable to lens implantation (see Table VI-32).

TABLE VI-32. — *Dislocation Rate for 3000 Sputnik Lens Implantations (Fyodorov, 1980)*

In the early postoperative period	
— Lens dislocation	0.8%
Into the posterior chamber	0.3%
Into the anterior chamber	0.5%
— Prong subluxation into the posterior chamber	1.8%
— Loop subluxation into the anterior chamber	6.7%

Fyodorov further observed that the formation of thin synechiae between the posterior loops, the iris, and the anterior hyaloid face prevents postoperative vitreous prolapse and spontaneous rupture of

TABLE VI-33 — *Complication Incidence for 2700 Sputnik Lens Implantations with Follow-Up Periods Ranging from 1 to 11 Years (Fyodorov, 1980)*

Endothelial corneal dystrophy	0.3%
Late uveitis	0.2%
Maculopathy	1.4%
Retinal detachment	1.7%
Dislocation/subluxation	4.0%
Glaucoma (transient)	0.2%
Hemorrhage	0.2%
Secondary cataract	2.7%

the hyaloid membrane. The synechiae also contribute significantly to the stabilization of the iris diaphragm. Table VI-33 gives the late complications that developed in 2700 implantations with follow-up periods ranging from 1 to 11 years.

B. Galin's Series

M. A. Galin gives more details than does Fyodorov on the results and complications of 300 cases of implantations of Sputnik lenses that had been imported from Russia. Six cases in which the cataract extraction was complicated by iridodialysis, sphincter rupture, and vitreous loss were excluded from the series. Also excluded were patients with anterior segment diseases (e.g. iritis, uveitis, corneal abiotrophies), high myopia, malignant diabetes, and glaucoma. Consequently, the data given on Table VI-34 reflect only what can be expected when a Sputnik lens is implanted under the best of circumstances.

TABLE VI-34. — *Sputnik Lens Series of M.A. Galin*

Source	M.A. Galin et al. (1977, 1978)
Surgeon	M.A. Galin
Surgical Procedure	Intracapsular
Number of Cases	300
Follow-Up	5 to 10 years
Mean Age at Surgery	72 years
Corrected Visual Acuity ⩾20/40	88%
Endothelial Corneal Dystrophy	None
Uveal Reactions	
Iritis (sterile hypopion)	2%
Secondary Membranes	11% → 1%
Clinical Cystoid Macular Edema	3%
Retinal Detachment	2%
Total	0.3%
Partial	11% → 5%
Glaucoma	
Transient	8%
Persistent	None

Comment

Visual Acuity:

Patients with pre-existing macular diseases or a history of them were excluded. The causes of corrected visual acuity ⩽20/40 are given on Table VI-35.

TABLE VI-35. — *Causes of Corrected Visual Acuity ≤20/40 in Galin's Series*

Cause	*Number of Cases*	*Percentage*
Cystoid Macular Edema	9	3.0
Senile Macular Choroidal Degeneration	5	1.7
Retinal Detachment	4	1.3
Ischemic Optic Neuropathy	3	1.0
Vein Occlusion	3	1.0
Macular Hole or Pucker	3	1.0
Amblyopia	3	1.0
Diabetic Maculopathy	2	0.7
Unknown	4	1.3
Total	36	12.0

Endothelial Corneal Pathology:

No cases of endothelial corneal dystrophy occurred. Galin occasionally observed small, inconsequential scrolls of Descemet's membrane that resulted from entering the eye. Two significant desinsertions occurred because the incision edge was touched either by the loops or the optical component during lens insertion.

Postoperative striate keratopathy was found to be present in 50% of the cases, with nearly half of them being severe.

Uveal Reactions:

In the first cases, the most serious problem, which required surgical intervention, was membrane formation. It occurred most often when miotics were routinely used postoperatively. With the advent of mydriasis, this problem was reduced, but not eliminated (see Table VI-36). Also, in the early cases, several sterile hypopions were encountered. In Galin's opinion, they were probably caused by inadequate cleaning of the lenses before sterilization.

TABLE VI-36. — *Incidence of Membrane Formation in Galin's Series with the Sputnik Lens*

Year	*Postoperative Treatment*	*Percentage of Cases*
1969	miotics	8
1970	miotics	11
1971	miotics	10
1972	no miotics	4
1973	no miotics	2
1974-76	mydriasis	1

Luxation:

Only one case of total luxation occurred, which certainly reflects the impressive stability of the Sputnik lens. The incidence of subluxation of one or more of the haptic components (loops or struts) was 10% in the early years but then decreased to 5% later on. As shown on Table VI-37, some cases required only medical treatment, others surgical, and some were left untreated.

TABLE VI-37. — *Distribution of Luxations for the Sputnik Lens in Galin's Series*

Year	*Postoperative Treatment*	*Strut or Loop*	*Optic*	*Treated Medically*	*Treated Surgically*	*Untreated*
1969	Miotics	10	1	3	6	2
1970	Miotics	11	0	4	4	3
1971	Miotics	10	0	5	2	3
1972	No miotics	6	0	3	1	2
1973	No miotics	6	0	3	0	3
1974-76	Mydriasis	5	0	2	1	2

Galin reports that most luxations in the first series of patients resulted from decentration of the implant because asymmetrical sphincter adhesions developed on one or more loops. The incidence of this complication was lowered by routine postoperative administration of mild mydriatics and by a slight modification in the lens design: the loops were directed more posteriorly.

Glaucoma:

Transient rises in intraocular pressure during the first postoperative week were not infrequent. In 20% of the cases, increases of more than 6 mm Hg occurred, and in 8%, increases of more than 10 mm Hg were observed. Galin notes that this cannot be ascribed to the use of alpha chymotrypsine for the simple reason that this enzyme was not used. No other reasons are offered.

C. **Kwitko's Series**

As shown on Table VI-38, the incidence of complications in the series by M.L. Kwitko is comparable to those of Fyodorov's and Galin's series. Kwitko, who acquired his initial experience with iris clip lenses, maintains that the advantage of the Sputnik lens is that it provides stable fixation without the potentially dangerous anterior loops of the Binkhorst lenses.

TABLE VI-38. — Sputnik Lens Series of M.L. Kwitko

Source	M.L. Kwitko (1978)
Surgeon	M.L. Kwitko
Surgical Procedure	Intracapsular & Extracapsular
Number of Cases	100
Follow-Up	Maximum of 3 years
Corrected Visual Acuity ⩾20/40	Not available
Endothelial Corneal Dystrophy	1%
Uveal Reactions	
Iritis	Not available
Secondary Membranes	1%
Clinical Cystoid Macular Edema	Not available
Retinal Detachment	Not available
Luxation	
Total	None
Partial	3%
Glaucoma	
Transient	3%
Persistent	0%

In addition to the one case of total endothelial corneal dystrophy, there were two cases of localized endothelial corneal dystrophy. This occurred because of postoperative flat anterior chambers that caused the three end-knobs of the anterior struts to come in contact with the endothelium. Interestingly, the incidence of retrolenticular membrane formation was only 1%. According to Kwitko, secondary membrane formation can be prevented by starting mild pupil dilatation on the second postoperative day.

IV. Conclusion

As is the case for all the previously considered iris supported lenses, the results obtained by these experienced surgeons does not reflect the overall results of the some 7,900 Sputnik lens implants before March 1977 (Hoffer, 1978). But the reports we have do indicate that the Sputnik lens is an interesting iris supported pseudophakos. Indeed, the long term results show that such major complications as endothelial corneal dystrophy and total lens luxation are virtually absent. This advantage is to be attributed to the special configuration of this lens that provides exceptional stability and to the unlikelihood of endothelial corneal contact since the anterior struts are small and lie close to the anterior surface of the iris. Furthermore, it is a lightweight lens (0.9 mg in aqueous) from which adequate long term support by the iris diaphragm has been reported.

From the technical point of view, another advantage certainly is that the Sputnik lens does not rely on suturing or clipping devices for fixation. However, insertion and proper positioning of the three posterior loops and the three anterior struts makes the surgical procedure very demanding. Also during the postoperative period, careful attention and appropriate management are mandatory to prevent subluxation and the formation of secondary membranes.

§ 5 OTHER LENS DESIGNS

I. The Krasnov Extrapupillary Iris Lens

In 1977, M.M. Krasnov from Moscow published a description of the technique for inserting various lens styles of his own design (Krasnov, 1977). In contrast to conventional iris supported lenses, his models are fixed at the periphery of the iris, leaving the pupillary region free. His lenses may be implanted either anterior or posterior to the iris plane.

Krasnov designed two basic types (see Fig. VI-47).

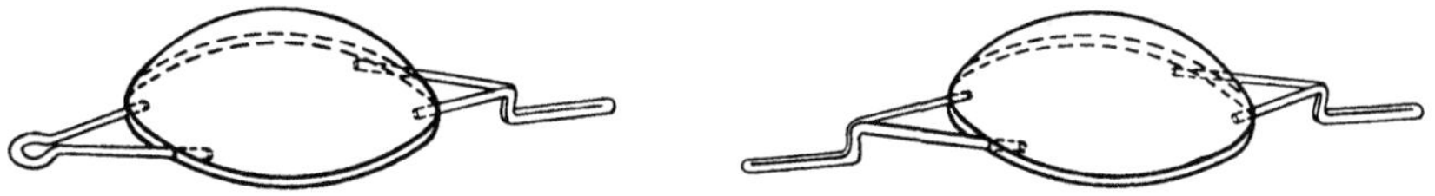

Fig. VI-47. — The Krasnov extrapupillary iris lenses.

To obtain adequate fixation, the bayonet-like fixation prongs are introduced into already made corresponding holes in the iris periphery.

Krasnov, who at that time had performed 189 implantations of this lens type, noted the following advantages: "The pupil is not distorted, so that its form and function remain normal. The danger of dislocation is avoided. The lens may be employed in the presence of an iris coloboma. Since the supporting prongs are made of gold and platinum alloys, good tissue tolerance may be expected."

II. The Sachar lens

In 1978, Sachar introduced an iris supported lens of his own design. As shown in Figure VI-48, the lens has two clip devices for fixation. They are anchored in the peripheral iris stroma. The lens loops are oriented horizontally.

III. The Boberg-Ans Lens

In 1978, J. Boberg-And proposed an iris supported lens with the optical portion located in the posterior chamber (Fig. VI-49).

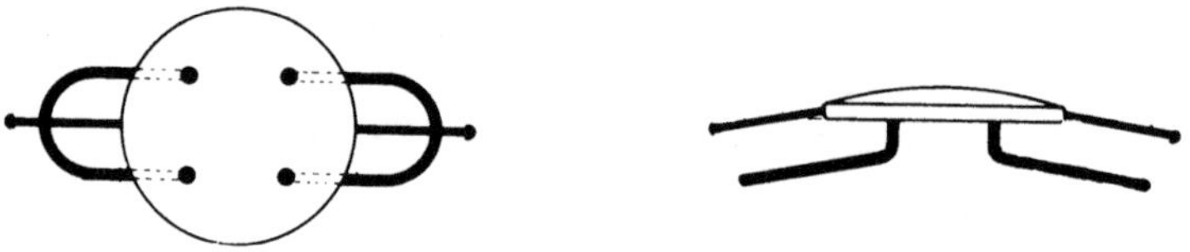

Fig. VI-48. — The Sachar lens.

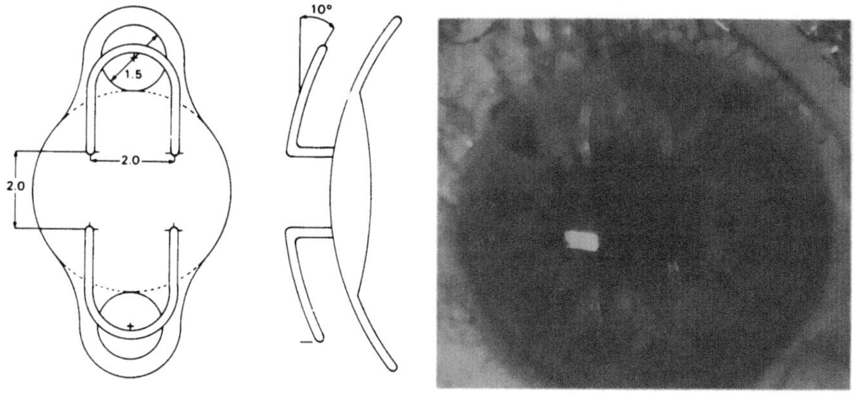

Fig. VI-49. — The Boberg-Ans lens. Note the iris suture around the superior loop.

IV. The Rainin Anchor Lens

At the meeting of the American Intra-Ocular Implant Society at Los Angeles in 1978, A. Rainin presented an iris supported lens of his own design. Having been preceeded by two other models (Mark I and Mark II), the Rainin Anchor Mark III lens seems to have some advantages over other iris supported lenses. No reports have as yet been published on clinical experience with this lens.

V. A Soft Iris Supported Lens

Also in 1978 at the AIOIS meeting, K.R. Mehta proposed a lens of his own design made of HEMA.

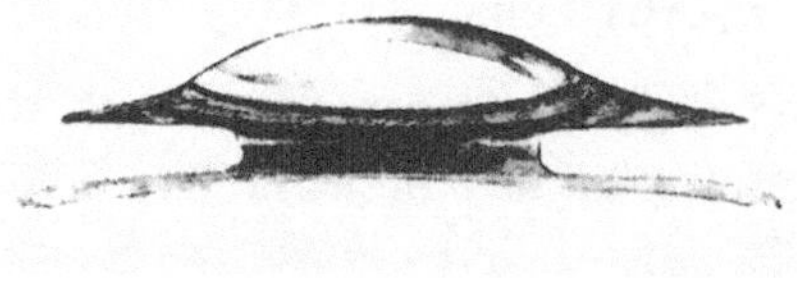

Fig. VI-50. — The soft iris supported lens of K.R. Mehta.

This lens resembles a collar-button. The optic portion is surrounded by a haptic rim, which is placed in front of the iris, and a posterior haptic flange. Thirty-two of these lenses had been inserted.

VI. The Glass Intraocular Lens

K. Barasch and S. Poler (1979) designed an iris supported, one-plane lens having two components: a central optic portion made of glass and the haptic portion of polyimidine.

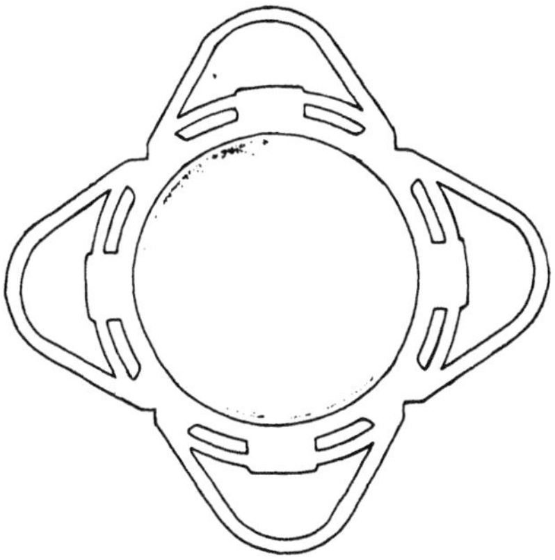

Fig. VI-51. — The one-plane iris supported glass lens of K. Barasch and S. Poler.

The optical portion (0.3 mm thick for a 19 diopter lens) is made of special optical glass that has a refractive index of 1.62. The 4 fenestrated haptic portions are quite thin (0.05 mm). The lens weighs approximately 5 mg in water, and is sterilized in the autoclave. In situ, the optic portion is in the pupillary aperture and one pair of haptics is in front of the iris and the other pair behind.

VII. The Anis Lens

Also at the AIOIS 1978 meeting, F. Anis presented his own iris supported lens. As shown in Figure VI-52, 3 posterior loops are embedded in the optic portion and an anterior loop is added in the superior part. In situ, the tips of both superior loops are provided with a metal staple that is clipped through the coloboma by means of a special micro-staple holder.

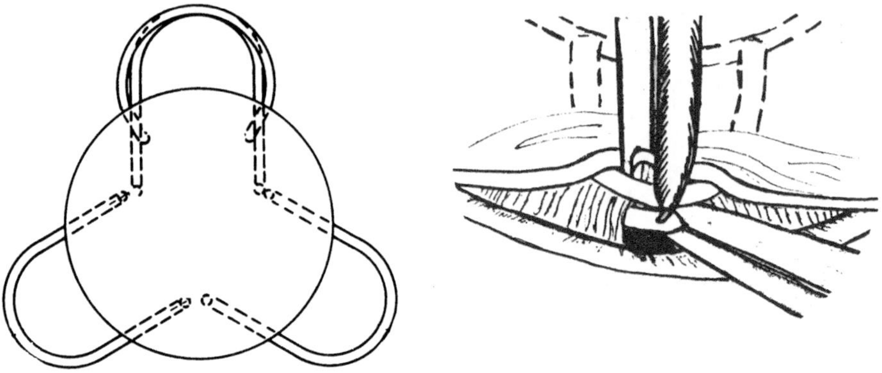

Fig. VI-52. — The Anis lens and the method for clipping the metal staple.

VIII. The Iris Claw Lens

In 1980, J. Worst introduced the "iris claw" lens—a lightweight, single plane, polymethylmethacrylate lens. Fixation is achieved by means of an original device that pinches the iris.

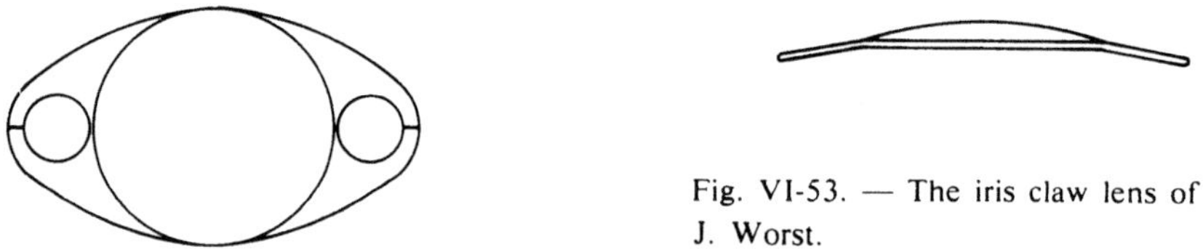

Fig. VI-53. — The iris claw lens of J. Worst.

Also in 1980, L. Amar proposed a posterior chamber lens based on this same fixating principle.

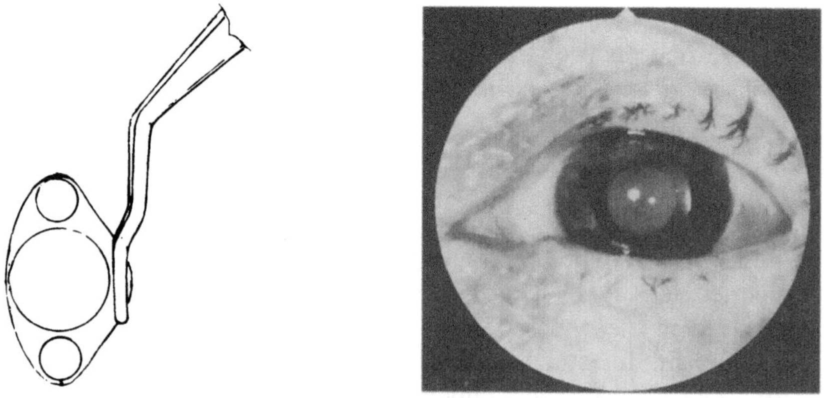

Fig. VI-54. — The iris supported posterior chamber lens of L. Amar.

IX. The Severin Lenses

Also in the late seventies, S.L. Severin proposed two lenses having their optical components behind the iris diaphragm. Both lenstypes are used with intracapsular surgery. As shown in Figure VI-55 one model has three anterior and two posterior loops, and the other model has two posterior loops, two anterior inferior loops, and a stave at the twelve o'clock position, which has to be clipped through the iridectomy to engage the superior posterior loop.

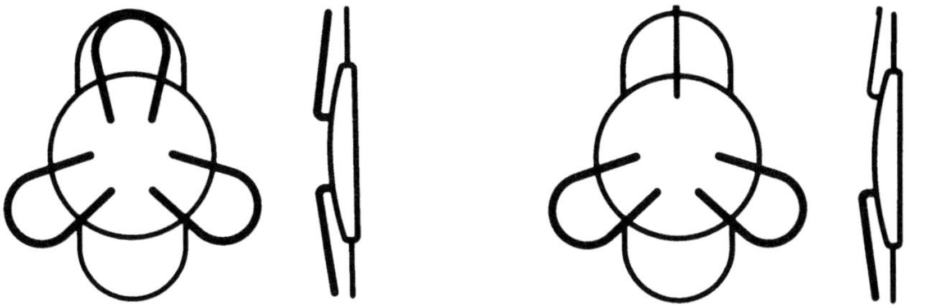

Fig. VI-55. — The Severin lens.

General Conclusion on Iris Supported Lenses

We have reviewed the use of iris supported lenses after intracapsular extraction over a period of 20 years (1958-1978). This period was characterized by the introduction of various modifications in the lens models that eventually led to the modern iris supported lenses.

At the present time, enough experience has been built up to enable us to describe the possibilities and limitations of these lenses after intracapsular extraction.

Since the lens has to be carried by the iris diaphragm, it should be a lightweight lens. Its design must be such that intimate contact between the haptic portions and the iris are minimal so as to avoid continuous iris irritation, which, as has been documented, can have grave consequences. Therefore, for most iris supported lenses, additional measures are necessary to prevent luxation, which leads to more intraocular manipulation. It must also be noted that inserting an iris supported lens after intracapsular extraction always involves the risk of peroperative vitreous problems. These problems may either be cause to abort the procedure or to call for risky peroperative management that leaves the final outcome in doubt. With these reservations, the iris supported lens can give satisfactory results on a short-term basis.

The long-term fate of eyes containing iris supported lenses implanted after intracapsular extraction is still uncertain. On the basis of his vast experience, C.D. Binkhorst (1977) concluded that the iris will never be a suitable long-term carrier. In his opinion, the increasing laxicity of the iris diaphragm as time goes on, and the increasing atrophy of the pupillary border at the contact points with the lens aggravate lens instability. This situation can ultimately lead to accidental subluxation and total dislocation of the lens. Furthermore, in the aphakic eye after intracapsular extraction, there will always be iridodonesis, which in turn causes pseudophakodonesis. In the opinion of Binkhorst, the continuous wobbling of the lens constitutes a permanent source of microconcussions with detrimental effects on the internal structures.

Bearing all these considerations in mind, not so many possibilities remain for dramatic improvement in lens design, technique, or long-term behavior when iris support is intended with intracapsular aphakia.

Therefore, at this stage, the surgeon who considers the use of iris supported lenses after classic total cataract extraction has to limit his case selection to elderly patients with an appropriate iris diaphragm. He should accept the fact that peroperative adverse conditions—particularly vitreous involvement—may constitute a strong indication to abort the implantation. Among, the iris supported lenses, the most suitable, in our opinion, are the iris clip lens with or, possibly, without a suture, and the sutured medallion lens. More clinical experience is necessary with the Sputnik lens to determine whether the results obtained by its promotors are reproducible.

CHAPTER VII

IRIDOCAPSULAR AND CAPSULAR SUPPORTED LENSES

Introduction

The first generation of implant lenses was inserted after planned extracapsular cataract extraction. For fixation, Ridley relied both on support provided by the lens capsule and on additional iris synechiae. Although he was convinced that "the proper place for an artificial lenticulus had to be where nature intended the cristallin to be", iridocapsular fixation was soon abandoned for several reasons such as the difficulty in getting the lens into its proper position, subsequent luxation, delayed iris atrophy and secondary glaucoma. It was some 20 years before interest returned to the idea of capsular fixation. In the mid-sixties, C.D. Binkhorst (1975, p. 185) revaluated this principle and described his first clinical observations as follows:

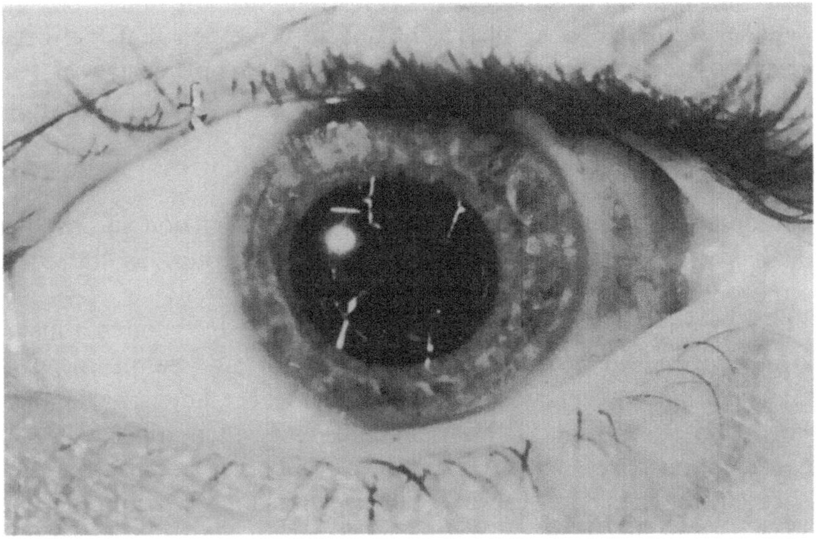

Fig. VII-1. — Iridocapsular lens in situ.

The possibility of capsular support had been forgotten until December 1963, when I inserted an iris clip lens after extracapsular extraction of a traumatic cataract. The posterior loops became embedded in adhesions between iris and capsular membrane. Lenses thus supported could not move around inside the eye; under the circumstances, the anterior loops lost their function. On September the 16th 1965, the first lens with only posterior loops was inserted into a traumatic aphakic eye with an intact posterior capsular membrane. The posterior loops were inserted between iris and capsular membrane after posterior synechiae had been dissected. Afterwards, the loops were found to be firmly embedded in iridocapsular adhesions. This was the origin of the two-loop iridocapsular lens.

In 1972, C.D. Binkhorst reported on the favorable results he obtained with 100 implantations of iris clip and iridocapsular lenses, and in 1976 the results of the first 500 cases.

I. The Advantage of Lens Implantation after Extracapsular Cataract Extraction

Since C.D. Binkhorst began implanting after planned extracapsular surgery in 1965, more and more surgeons have adopted this method. Although the advantages offered by routine extracapsular cataract extraction are still controverted, it is obvious that the shift from the highly perfected intracapsular technique to a method that had been rejected decades earlier must have been based on substantial reasons.

A. Practical Considerations

Adoption of planned extracapsular cataract extraction means that one has a technique that can be used for all age groups, as, indeed, it is the only possible technique for younger patients.

During surgery, the presence of a posterior capsule is often a major advantage. Indeed, if the eye should tense for any reason, the posterior capsule prevents vitreous prolapse into the anterior chamber. Furthermore, insertion of the pseudophakos is often still possible in these circumstances without damage to the cornea because the presence of the posterior capsule allows sufficient deepening of the anterior chamber.

After surgery, fixation and stabilization of the lens are aided by the presence of the posterior capsule, which is an insensitive and avascular membrane that is particularly suitable for holding an implant.

B. Clinical Observations

Having inserted several hundred lenses after both intracapsular and extracapsular procedures, C.D. Binkhorst was in a particularly good position to compare the long term potential of both techniques.

Among his clinical observations, one of the more significant is that extracapsular eyes quieted down sooner after surgery and had less cells and flare in the anterior chamber in spite of the presence of cortical remnants. Binkhorst also noted clearer corneae, less intraocular pressure disregulation, less inflammation, and less cystoid macular edema. To provide an objective basis for his clinical findings, he started in the mid-seventies to take endothelial cell counts with a specular microscope and to assess the behavior of the posterior pole with fluorescein angiography.

Using the specular microscope in a comparative study of 23 patients with bilateral lens implants—intracapsular in one eye and extracapsular in the other—Binkhorst (1978) noted a significantly lower endothelial cell density in the intracapsular eye. The difference averaged 50%. Even though this difference could be partially ascribed to possible toxicity of the supramid used as loop material in the intracapsular cases, it was assumed that continuing endothelial cell loss had occurred in the intracapsular cases.

Another study, in which 120 pseudophakic eyes of 85 patients that had undergone surgery for senile cataracts were involved, established a definite superiority of extracapsular surgery as far as the long term fate of the retina is concerned. Comparable series were chosen. There was no retinal detachment in extracapsular eyes that had never had a posterior capsulotomy.

Indications of previous or existing maculopathy were sought with the usual tests: visual acuity, the Amsler test, and the Haidinger brushes test, the last of which has proved, in the experience of Binkhorst, to be a sensitive means of evaluating macular function. The macular function turned out to have suffered the least after extracapsular extraction without capsulotomy and the most after intracapsular surgery.

C. Theoretical Considerations: The Barrier Deprivation Syndrome

To further explain the superiority of extracapsular cataract extraction, with or without an intraocular lens implant, Binkhorst developed his ideas on what he calls the "barrier deprivation syndrome". According to him, the crystalline lens constitutes a "barrier" separating the anterior from the posterior compartment.

This barrier has a mechanical function; controlling the hydrodynamics of the aqueous humor, the stability of the iris, and the position and dynamics of the vitreous. It also has a membrane function, helping to maintain the biochemical equilibrium that is apparently necessary for the physiology of the eye. Any defect in the barrier, therefore, is likely to have mechanical and biochemical consequences. Complete removal of the barrier in intracapsular surgery obviously has more severe consequences than the incomplete removal that extracapsular surgery involves. In both, changes occur inside the eye that can be grouped under the heading of "barrier deprivation syndrome".

First, there is the lack of iris support, which results in iridodonesis and compromises the physiological aqueous hydrodynamics of the eye. Aberrant aqueous flow causes corneal "turbulence endotheliopathy", which is manifested by pigment uptake of the endothelium and by continual loss of endothelial cells.

Other elements of barrier deprivation are herniation and eventual posterior detachment of the vitreous accompanied by increased vitreous mobility (vitreodonesis) that in turn aggravates iridodonesis and the aberrant character of the aqueous flow.

In Binkhorst's opinion, the concurrence of disturbed aqueous dynamics, increased mobility of the iris diaphragm, and excessive vitreous mobility—together referred to as endophthalmodonesis—may be the common denominator underlying the occurrence of pathological conditions such as the ongoing loss of endothelial cells of the cornea and edema of the retina in the macular area (clinical or subclinical cystoid macular edema) or in the peripheral retina.

In summary, apart from the biochemical disturbance, which has yet to be established, continuous microconcussion from endophthalmodonesis may be considered responsible for alterations in both the anterior and the posterior eye segment.

Thus, the barrier deprivation syndrome has little or nothing to do

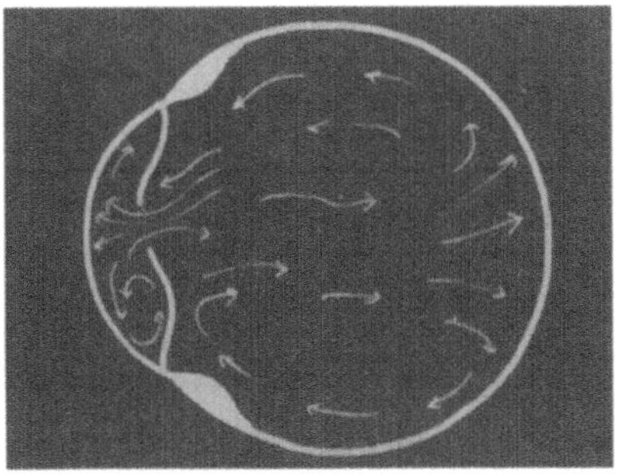

Fig. VII-2. — Schematic representation of endophthalomodonesis. (Courtesy C.D. Binkhorst.)

with intraocular lens implantation as such and concerns primarily intracapsular cataract surgery. Under certain circumstances, however, an intraocular lens could aggravate the consequences of barrier deprivation. As noted above, iris-fixated lenses after intracapsular cataract extraction, and especially a heavy lens with metal loops, increase endophthalmodonesis. Such heavy lenses are known to have caused a high incidence of corneal decompensation and cystoid macular edema. Indeed, Binkhorst considers that all lenses with pronounced pseudophakodonesis involve considerable risk to the cornea and the retina.

II. The Mechanism of Capsular Fixation

The pseudophakos may be stabilized already on the first day after implantation with the iris not involved in the fixation. In such a situation, the loops are located between the anterior and posterior capsules, which seem already to adhere to each other. It may be assumed that this initial adhering mechanism is enhanced by the postoperative increase in protein of the aqueous humor.

The mechanism of definite loop fixation between the lens capsules has been explicated by means of histological examinations that have revealed that capsular fixation is assured when one or more loops are at least partially covered by the anterior lens capsule (Binkhorst and Manschot, 1977). The pseudofibrous adherence of the anterior to the posterior capsule prevents displacement of the enclosed lens. The formation of pseudofibrous tissue seems to be a reaction of the lens epithelium but not, it is thought, to the presence of the implant loop. Indeed, the lens epithelium that lines the inner surface of the anterior capsule has the capacity of producing collagen, and it appears that this pseudofibrous tissue tries to bridge and seel the lumen between

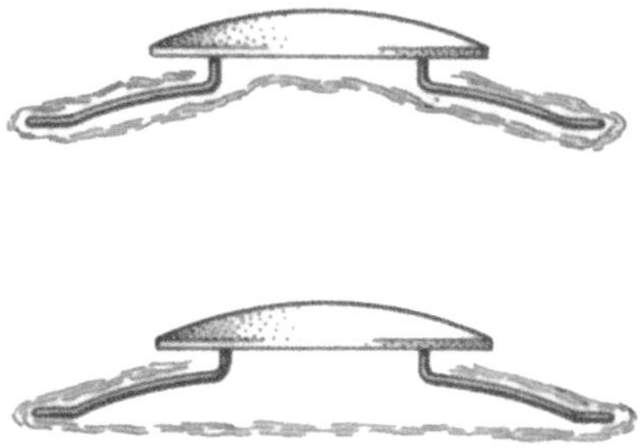

a

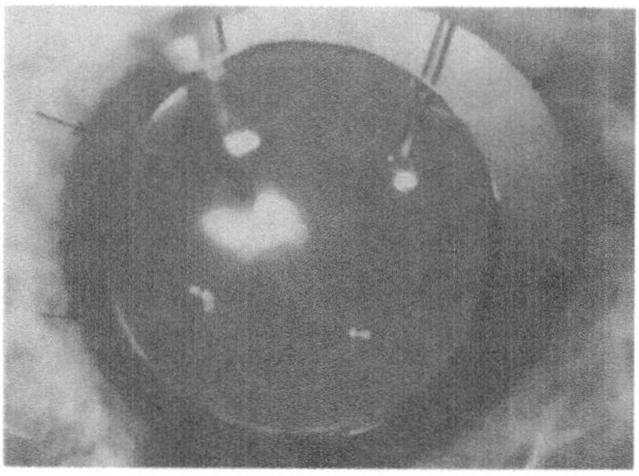

b

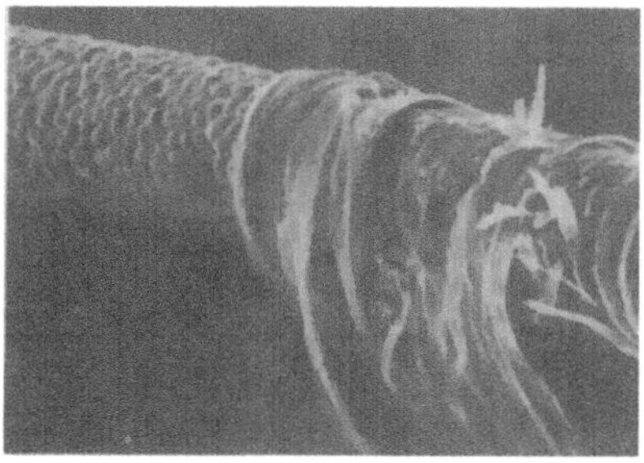

c

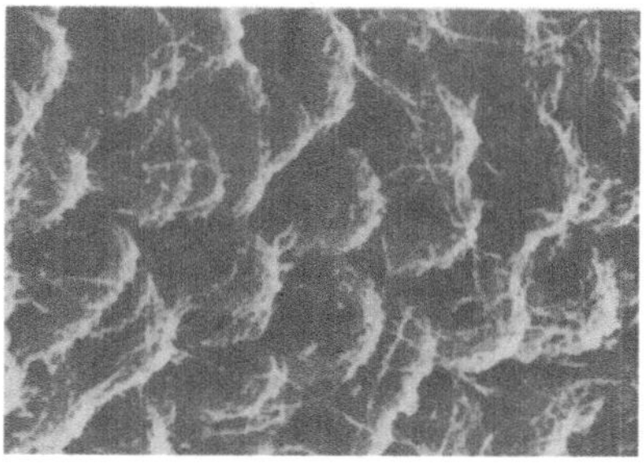

d

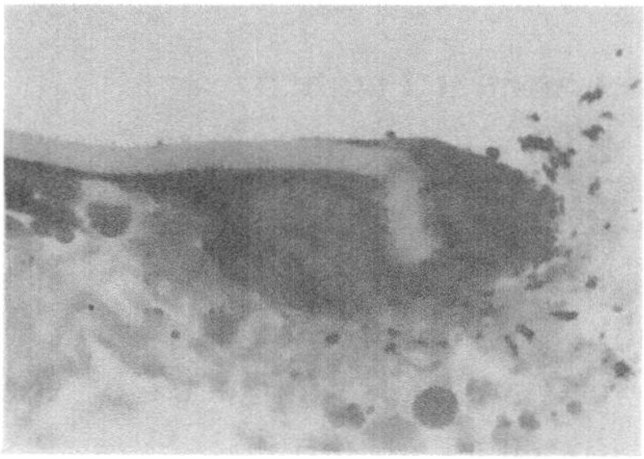

e

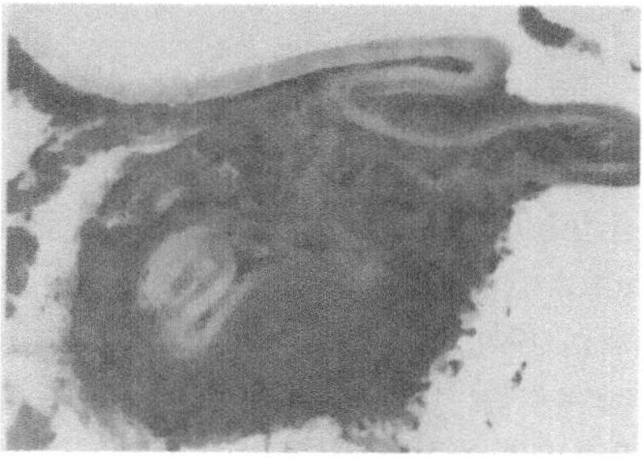

f

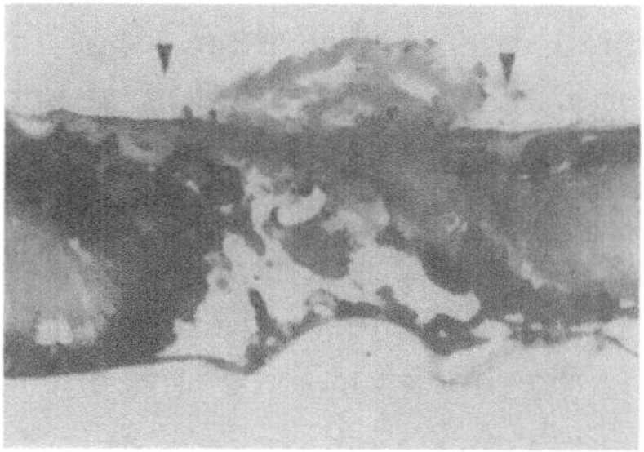

g

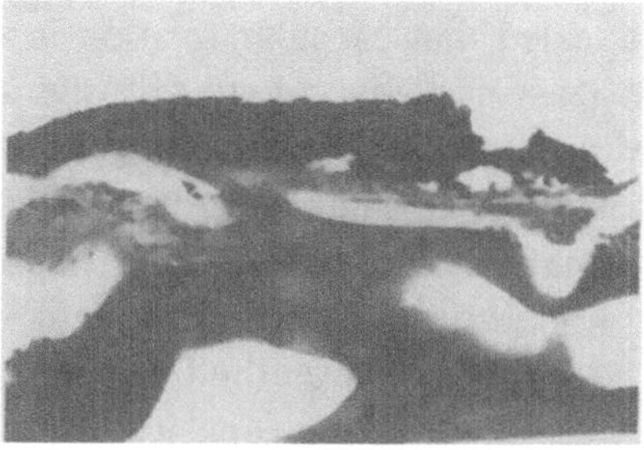

h

the anterior and posterior capsules. This reparative proliferation of epithelial cells is an example of pseudometaplasia, the product of which, according to Manschot, is to labeled pseudofibrous tissue.

The presence of cortical lens remnants plays no part in this fixation mechanism. When a lens loop is surrounded by peripheral lens material, however, the condensation of this material (Soemmering's ring) will provide additional support.

III. Lens Styles Used after Extracapsular Cataract Extraction

The first series of lens types that can be used after extracapsular extraction consists of those lenses for which capsular fixation is not mandatory. These are the familiar iris supported lenses, which can be used after either intra- or extracapsular cataract extraction, for example, the Iris clip lens, the Medallion lens, the Copeland lens, and the Sputnik lens. Neophytes in the field of extracapsular surgery will find these lenses particularly attractive.

The posterior capsule will not only help prevent vitreous from interfering with the lens during insertion, it will also constitute a membrane that stabilize the lens and precludes luxation into the

←

Fig. VII-3a. — Schematic representation of an iridocapsular lens with the loops placed between the anterior capsular flaps and the posterior capsule.

Fig. VII-3b. — Iridocapsular lens in situ. The arrow indicates the margin of the anterior capsular flaps.

Fig. VII-3c. — Scanning electron micrograph of a fragment of the anterior capsule (magnification 450 ×) showing crystallin fibers and epithelial cells. (Courtesy A. Galand.)

Fig. VII-3d. — Scanning electron micrograph of the epithelial cells on the anterior lens capsule (magnification 1550 ×). (Courtesy A. Galand.)

Fig. VII-3e. — Pseudoconnective tissue proliferation around margin of anterior capsule four weeks after extracapsular extraction (H.-E., × 290; Neg. PA 21918 B-7). (Manschot, 1978, p. 465).

Fig. VII-3f. — Pseudoconnective tissue around margin of anterior capsule four weeks after extracapsular extraction (H.-E., × 290; Neg. PA 21918B-3). (Manschot, 1978, p. 465).

Fig. VII-3g. — Pseudoconnective tissue bridging capsular defect, four weeks after extracapsular extraction. The arrows indicate the margins of anterior capsule (H.-E., × 290; Neg. PA 21918 A-3). (Manschot, 1978, p. 466).

Fig. VII-3h. — Pseudoconnective tissue protruding through capsular defect having caused adhesion of capsule with iris four weeks after extracapsular extraction (H.-E., × 290, Neg. PA 22345-1). (Manschot, 1978, p. 466).

vitreous after implantation. Since the technique for inserting these lenses is similar to that used after intracapsular cataract extraction, we shall not discuss it here.

The anterior chamber lenses, which may also be used after planned extracapsular surgery, will be discussed in the chapter on angle supported lenses.

The second series of lens types are those that rely on iridocapsular support. We shall consider first the two-loop iridocapsular lens designed by Binkhorst and then the platinum clip lens and some other iridocapsular lenses designed by J. Worst.

The third series of lens types are intended to be entirely capsular supported. These are the posterior chamber lenses designed by J. Pearce and some other newer lens types that have come out in the late seventies.

Finally, we shall consider the Shearing lens, which is also a posterior chamber lens. It is a modified angle-supported lens that is placed behind the iris, the posterior capsule playing only a secondary role in steadying it.

Evaluation of the advantages and limitations of each of these lens types is difficult since the data available in the literature generally combine the results obtained from different lenses. Moreover, most of the series have only a short follow-up period.

§ 1 IRIDOCAPSULAR LENSES

I. The Binkhorst 2-Loop Lens

As described in Chapter II above, the iridocapsular 2-loop lens has an optical portion 5 mm in diameter made of polymethylmethacrylate in which the posterior loops are embedded. The loops are made out of nylon, metallic alloys, or polypropylene. Since polypropylene is a lightweight material and is reported to be non-biodegradable, it is now being routinely used by Binkhorst and his followers. The weight of the iridocapsular lens with platinum iridium loops is 15 mg in air and 7.5 mg in aqueous; with polypropylene loops, it is 8 mg in air and 1.5 mg in aqueous.

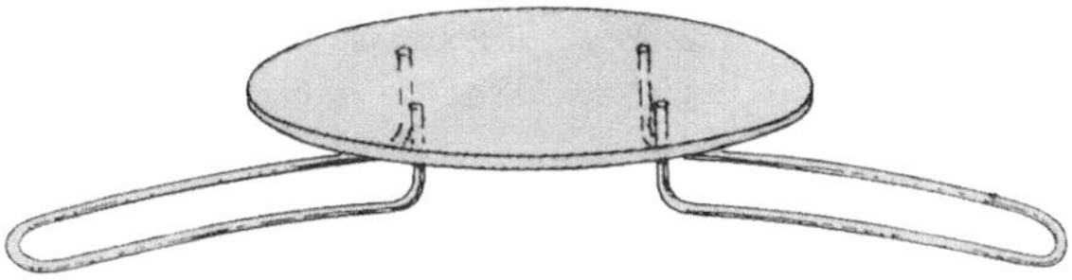

Fig. VII-4. — Schematic representation of the 2-loop iridocapsular lens.

Originally, the lens was intended to be supported by both the lens capsule and the iris, but it turned out that simple capsular fixation without additional iris adhesions could be achieved if the loops were properly placed in the capsular bag. This has the advantage of not disturbing pupil mobility. Generally, however, most lenses have both iris and capsular fixation.

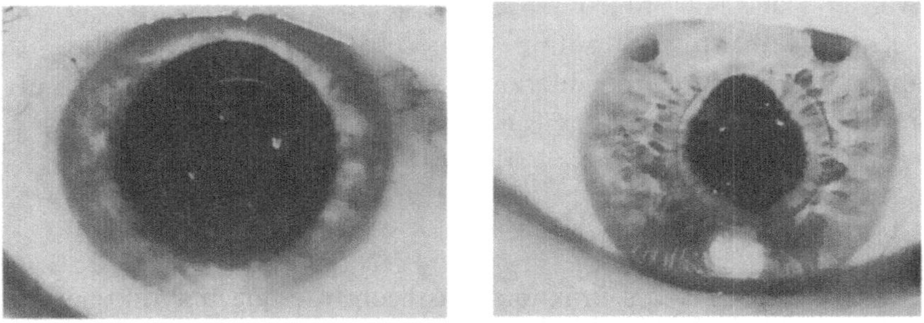

Fig. VII-5. — Capsular (left) and iridocapsular fixation (right) of the Binkhorst 2-loop lens.

Binkhorst's iridocapsular 3-loop lens theoretically offered better capsular fixation. But the insertion of this lens was found to involve increased risk of trauma, and the exact positioning of the three loops in the capsular bag was too demanding.

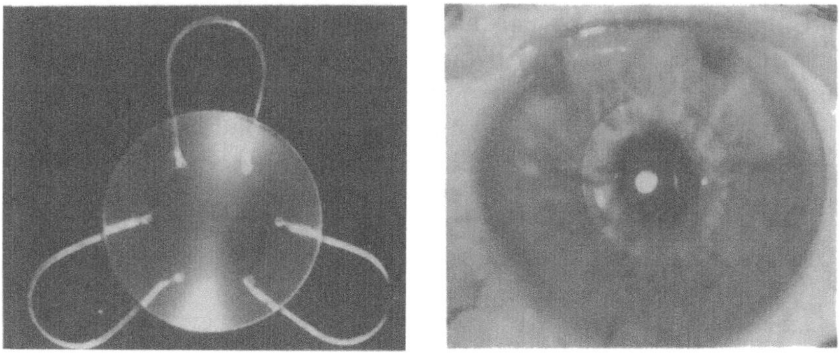

Fig. VII-6. — Binkhorst's iridocapsular 3-loop lens.

Although the iris clip lens was primarily designed to be used after intracapsular cataract extraction, it is also suitable when iridocapsular support is intended. However, this lens should not be used routinely in such cases since the anterior loops have no function in stabilizing the lens itself and may touch the cornea should forward tilting or marked decentration occur. Therefore, this lens is only used after extracapsular cataract extraction if the proper insertion of the posterior loops into the capsular bag is too difficult, for example, when the capsular flaps in the pupillary aperture are hard to identify. Another indication is the presence of a cataract with a liquified cortex (a milky cataract). In this situation, adequate capsular fixation is less likely since most of the epithelial cells have been destroyed. It is note worthy that some surgeons routinely prefer to use the iris clip lens secured with an antiluxating suture. In general, they remove as much as possible of the anterior capsule. This procedure allows early pupildilation and facilitates fundoscopy.

A. **Binkhorst's Technique**

During the 15 years Binkhorst has been inserting his iridocapsular lens after planned extracapsular cataract extraction, he introduced only minor modifications in his basic technique. These refinements involved largely pre- and postoperative management and the elaboration of non-aggressive surgical techniques with modern but simple instruments. In the mid-seventies, Binkhorst slightly modified his standard procedure by implementing the gradual opening and gradual closing technique, a logical extension of his ideas on atraumatic surgery.

1. *Preliminary Steps*

General measures: Antibiotics are routinely given starting 24 hours before the operation. Usually penicillin or streptomycine are the first choice, though sometimes chloramphenicol or ampicillines are used. This medication is continued for five days after the operation.

A hypotonic agent, generally Acetozolamide I.V. 500 mg is given one hour before surgery. Mannitol is not generally added for elderly patients. The anesthesist also orders the premedication for general anesthesia.

Local measures: Antibiotics, corticosteroids (Maxitrol®), and indomethacin eyedrops are administered before surgery. The pupil is dilated with one drop of 1% homatropine two hours before surgery and one drop of 1% Phenylephrine® shortly before surgery.

2. *Implantation Technique*

a. *The Conjunctival Flap*

— A small (3 mm) limbus-based flap allowing good visibility into the anterior chamber is prepared over 170°.
— Dissection is stopped when the clear corneal rim is reached.
— The freeing of this corneal portion is of prime importance for later wound closure.

b. *Keratotomy*

— A 4 mm opening is made in the anterior chamber with a keratome.
— Air is injected with a fine, blunt cannula.

c. *Capsulectomy — Capsulotomy*

— With a special toothed forceps (Vogt type), a central part of the anterior capsule is removed. The micro-forceps has a heeled configuration that allows the jaws to be opened and closed in the anterior chamber without deformation of the incision. Normally, the central part of the anterior capsule is easily removed. Undesirable tearing of the capsule towards the equator in the 12 o'clock area is prevented by cutting it off at the wound edge.

Recently, Binkhorst has been using a Haabs knife to perform a T-shaped capsulotomy. He then separates the anterior capsule from the nucleus by irrigating between them with a small, blunt cannula.

d. *Preplaced Suture and Extension of the Incision*

— Before enlarging the incision with scissors, a suture (10.0 nylon) is preplaced at 12 o'clock.
— If necessary, air is reinjected into the anterior chamber to keep the instruments from touching the endothelium.
— Generally, a 120° incision is made.

e. *Expression of the Nucleus*

— With a Daviel spoon or similar instrument, enough pressure is applied on the scleral part of the incision to cause the superior portion of the pupil to become slightly pear-shaped towards 12 o'clock.
— While maintaining pressure above, counter pressure is then applied with a squint hook in the 6 o'clock limbal area.
— The nucleus is not pushed upwards with the squint hook since then the cornea would fold or wrinkle.

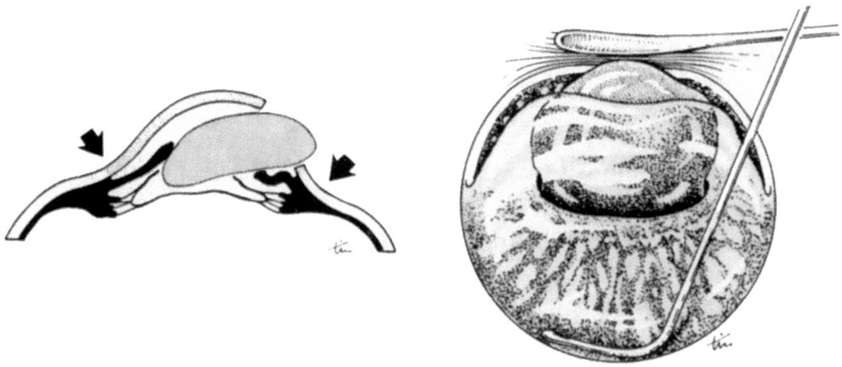

Fig. VII-7. — Bimanual maneuver for the expression of the nucleus.

— It may be helpful to use a sharp needle or similar instrument to pick up the nucleus by harpooning it as soon as the equator of the nucleus presents itself in the incision opening. Use of this technique avoids excessive pressure on the vitreous. If the whole procedure is properly conducted, some air will remain in the anterior chamber even after the delivery of the lens. By a gentle movement, the partly prolapsed iris is repositioned with the olive tip of the irrigating cannula.

What can be done if the nucleus remains in place?

1) If the nucleus is rather large and the incision seems too small, the first maneuver to be considered is enlarging the corneoscleral incision.
2) If the eye is too soft, additional pressure must be exerted by the assistant in the temporal scleral area to raise the vitreous pressure.
3) If the nucleus seems to be trapped by the anterior capsule itself, the capsulectomy has to be enlarged. Irrigating the cortical material between the capsule and the nucleus may be helpful.
4) If the nucleus is obvioulsy retained by a rigid pupil, a sphincterotomy is indicated, which will require adequate suturing afterwards. Forcing a nucleus through a too small and rigid pupillary aperture will result in an overstretched and atonic sphincter.

f. *Removal of Cortical Material*

The appearance of the nucleus can provide a certain amount of useful information about the amount of cortical material remaining. Binkhorst considers a smooth nucleus to be a sign of little remaining cortical material, and an irregular nucleus with several defects a sign of the contrary.

Evacuation of the cortical material is done with small amounts of fluid:

— A *straight cannula* is used to wash out all the loose lens material, both that which is visible in the pupillary aperture and also that which is in the sides and bottom of the capsular bag. The iris surface may be lightly massaged with this instrument to bring hidden cortex material towards the pupil.
— A *backwards bent cannula* (right and left curved) is used to rinse the upper half of the capsular cleft.
— If too much cortical material is still left after irrigation, Binkhorst

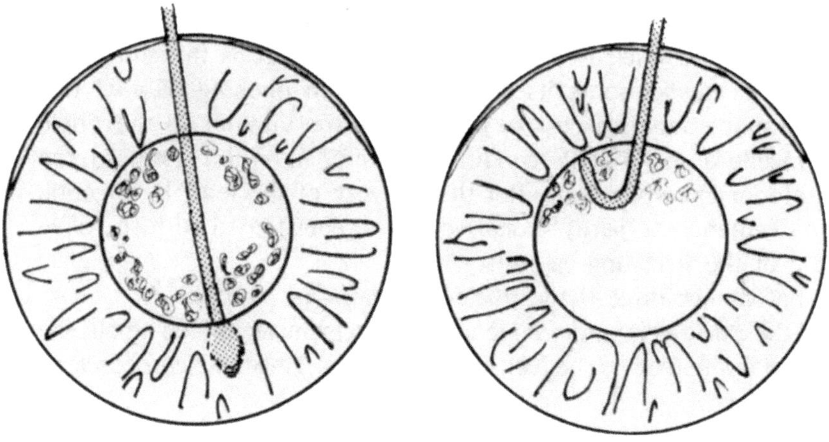

Fig. VII-8. — Evacuation of cortical remnants with straight and backward bent cannulas.

aspirates it with a blunt cannula while the assistant keeps the anterior chamber formed by injecting fluid ab externo.

To a certain extent, subcapsular layers can be removed by irrigation. More adherent cortical membranes or capsular opacities can be handled with a special, sand-blasted cannula, as suggested by Richard Kratz or with his newer cannula with diamond dust on it.

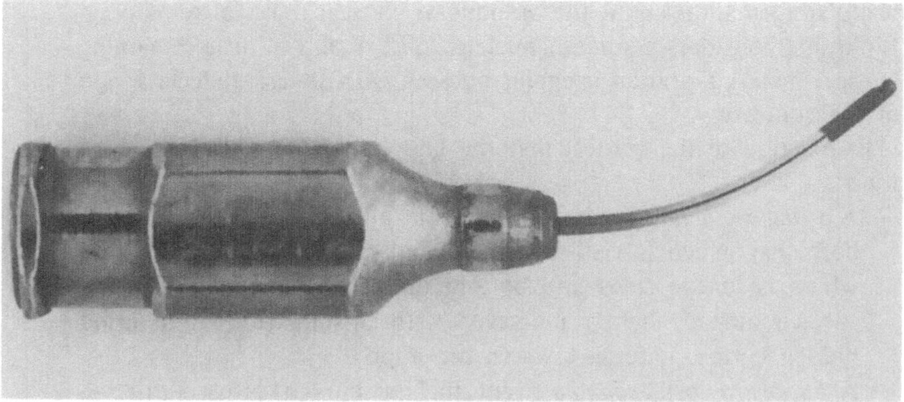

Fig. VII-9. — Roughened cannula for the removal of opacities adhering to the posterior capsule.

Binkhorst prefers an olive cannula roughened by sandpaper, which seems quite suitable in his hands. In Binkhorst's opinion, it is better to end up with an intact, even though opaque, posterior capsule than to clean it excessively since this can rupture the capsule with attendant vitreous loss and an aborted implantation.

g. *Iridectomies*

Two small peripheral iridectomies are made at 10 and 2 o'clock. Later on, after the lens is inserted, it is mandatory to check the patency of the colobomas.

h. *Gradual Closure of the Incision*

In order to maintain the anterior chamber as well-formed as possible during the actual insertion of the lens, two sutures are placed at 10 o'clock and 2 o'clock.

i. *Lens Insertion*

After the lens has been properly rinsed and inspected, it is grasped by the special lens forceps of Binkhorst's own design.

1) *Atraumatic Lens Introduction and Positioning of the Inferior Loop*

— The cornea is lifted gently while the conjunctival flap is held.
— The lens is introduced in close contact with the posterior capsule, and, if necessary, the scleral wound lip and the iris are depressed. A gentle zig-zag motion can help to keep the loops from catching the iris crypts.
— As soon as the inferior loop tip reaches the central pupillary area, it is directed posteriorly to a slight degree to maintain close contact with the posterior capsule.
— Finally, the inferior loop is slipped gently into the inferior capsular cleft and the lens forceps released.

During these maneuvers, the anterior chamber is maintained in two ways:

— Continuous ab externo refilling of the anterior chamber with fluid fed by a rather large cannula connected to a 10 cc syringe;

— Continuous ab interno refilling of the anterior chamber with fluid provided by the special cannula built into the lens forceps.

Note: Air in the anterior chamber during this procedure will interfere with good visibility and may collapse the capsular cleft thus making insertion of the inferior loop more hazardous.

2) *Positioning of the Superior Loop*

In order to maintain a well-formed anterior chamber during this step, further wound closure may be carried out. Additional injection of fluid or even air may be required. The superior loop is inserted by means of a bimanual maneuver as follows:

— The pseudophakos is steadied in the center of the pupil with one hand by means of a repositor.
— In the meantime, with the other hand, the sphincter is engaged with a blunt iris hook and pulled in a circular movement over the upper loop.

At the end of this procedure, the lens is rotated slightly, usually in an oblique position, to situate the superior loops between the anterior and posterior capsules. The anterior chamber is further deepened with air, and the colobomas are checked for patency.

j. *Completion of the Gradual Wound Closure*

With the air bubble still in place, the incision is closed watertight with separated stitches. At least 7 sutures of 10-0 nylon are placed. During this procedure, pilocarpine 4% drops are instilled until good myosis is obtained. Acethylcholine is generally avoided by Binkhorst because of the danger of endothelial toxicity.

Before closing the conjunctiva, the iris root is chekced for peripheral synechiae. If there are any, they are released by stretching the iridectomies with a small repositor or cannula.

Finally, the remaining air is replaced by fluid, and the conjunctiva is closed with three separated sutures.

3. *Post-Operative Measures*

— Before the patient leaves the operating theater, eserine (0.5%) and a few drops of Maxitrol® are administered. Only a protective fenestrated eye shield is used (no patching).

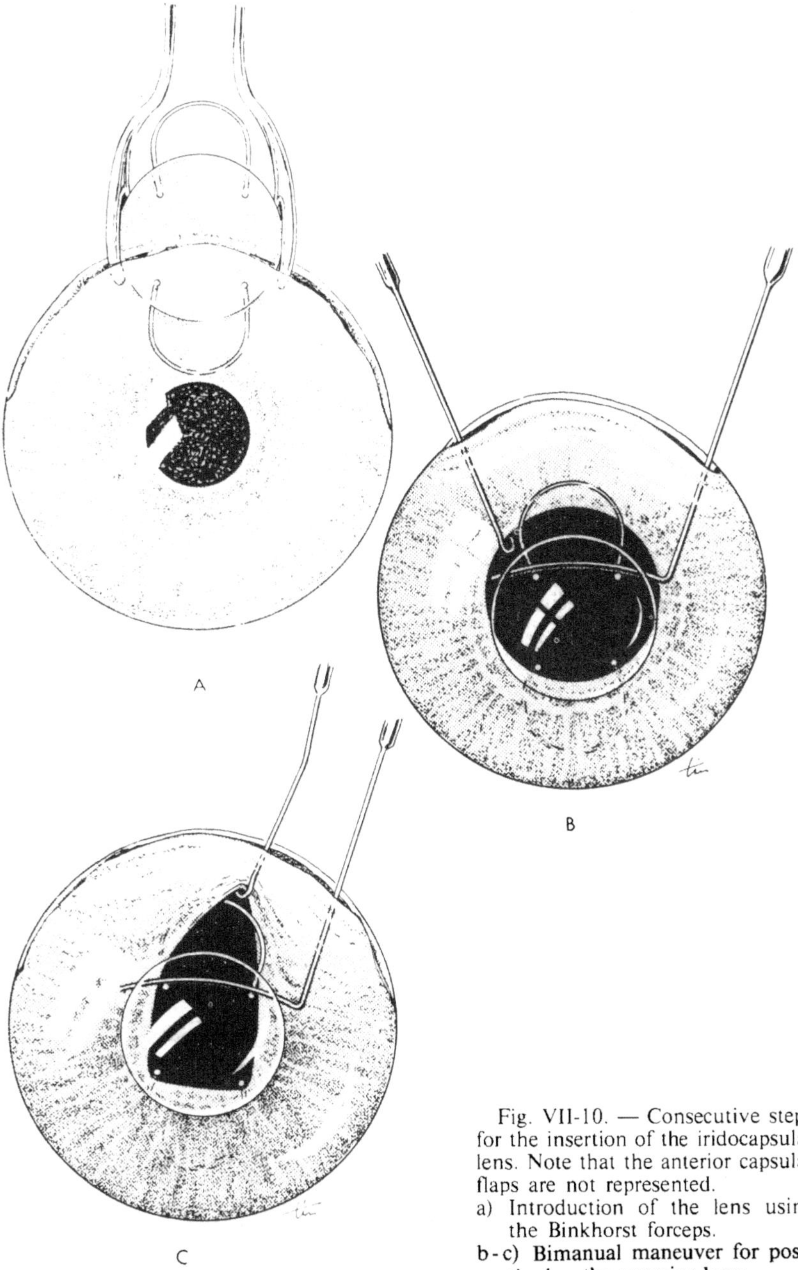

Fig. VII-10. — Consecutive steps for the insertion of the iridocapsular lens. Note that the anterior capsular flaps are not represented.

a) Introduction of the lens using the Binkhorst forceps.

b-c) Bimanual maneuver for positioning the superior loop.

— For five days, the systemic antibiotics are continued, and 3 ml of Irgapyrine® I.M. is administered daily.
— Pilocarpine 2% eye drops are instilled twice a day.
fixation occurs.
— Myotics are usually discontinued after a few days. The behavior of the pupil and the lens are watched carefully: if the lens remains immobile and well-centered even after mild dilation capsular adhesions are most likely to have formed.
— Maxitrol is continued five drops daily, gradually reduced after the first week, and generally stopped after six weeks.

4. *Modifications of Binkhorst's Technique*

A number of modifications in the extracapsular technique have been introduced by various surgeons.
— There is a general tendency to dilate the pupil widely before surgery. This allows a guided anterior capsulotomy to be performed, which favors the correct placement of the lens loop between the anterior and the posterior capsule. Another advantage of good pupil dilation is that it facilitates the removal of cortical material from the periphery.
— Evacuation of cortical remnants is performed with automated irrigating and aspirating devices or with the simple manual methods (described in detail on pp. 121).
— Various suturing techniques to provide extra fixation of the lens have been proposed by Alpar (1977), Gills (1978), and Simcoe (1977).

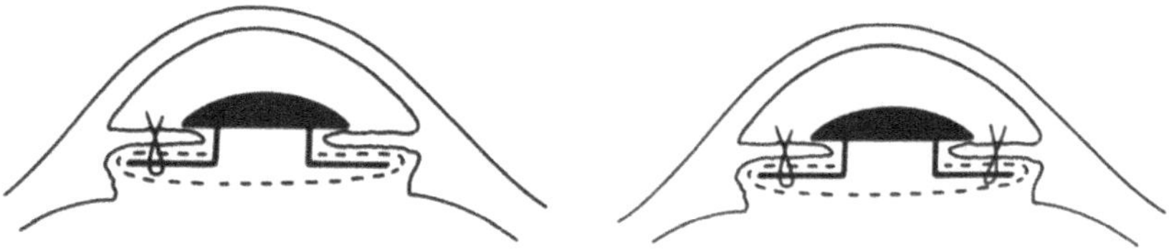

Fig. VII-11. — Additional fixation of the iridocapsular lens.
a) J. Alpar and J. Gills secure the superior lens loop with a suture. The superior capsular flap can be involved in addition to the iris.
b) C.W. Simcoe suggests 2 sutures, one inferior and one superior.

Note: The surgical microscope is useful and may even be essential for the correct execution of these changes in technique.

B. Binkhorst's Results with 500 Implantations after Planned Extracapsular Cataract Extraction

In 1976, Binkhorst reported on his experience and results with his first 500 cases. The follow-up period ranged from 9 months to more than 10 years. The average of the patients was 65.7 years. In about 85% of the cases, the iridocapsular 2-loop lens with metal loops was used, in the rest, an iris clip lens or an iridocapsular 3-loop lens was inserted. Because of the complicated nature of the anterior segment, patients with traumatic cataracts or surgically controlled glaucoma were excluded from the series. (See Table VII-1).

TABLE VII-1. — *Binkhorst's Results with 500 Implantations after Planned Extracapsular Cataract Extraction*

Author	C. D. Binkhorst (1976)
Surgeon	C. D. Binkhorst
Procedure	Extracapsular Cataract Extraction
Number	500
Type of lens: Iridocapsular 2-loop	85%
Iris clip 4-loop	12%
Iridocapsular 3-loop	3%
Age: >50 years	94%
>60 years	72%
average: 65.7 years	
Follow-up	9 months – 10$\frac{3}{4}$ years
Visul acuity $\geq$20/40	83%
Endothelial corneal dystrophy	1.8%
partial	0.4%
total	1.4%
Clinical cystoid macular edema	1.2%
Retinal detachment	1.0%
Dislocation: early	Not available
late	1.8%
After cataract	6.6%
Secondary cataract	35.0%
Tissue reactions: uveitis (transitory)	0.4%
vitritis (mild)	0.2%
Glaucoma (persistent)	1.2%
Hemorrhage	0.8%
Vitreous problems (prolapse)	0.8%
Lens exchange	0.4%
Lens removal	0.2%

Comments and Additional Details

Age at Surgery

The patients were divided into 5 groups as shown on Table VII-2. The first group (those under 50 years old) contains only adults with metabolic cataracts and lens opacities comparable to senile cataracts.

TABLE VII-2. — *Age Groups in Binkhorst's Series*

Age Groups	*Average Age*	*Number of Eyes*	
Under 50	43.3	32	6.4%
50-60	54.8	108	21.6%
60-70	65.1	165	33.0%
70-80	73.8	155	31.0%
Over 80	84.2	40	8.0%
Complete series	65.7	500	100 %

Corrected Visual Acuity

A corrected visual acuity of ≥20/40 was achieved in 83% of the cases. The reasons for a corrected visual acuity ≤20/40 are given on Table VII-3.

TABLE VII-3. — *Reasons for a Corrected Visual Acuity ≤20/40*

	Number of Eyes <20/40, ≥20/200	*Number of Eyes <20/200*
Endothelial corneal dystrophy	1	7
Clinical cystoid macular Edema	5	1
Retinal detachment	2	3
Senile macular degeneration	16	2
Diabetic retinopathy	4	3
Hypertensive retinopathy	1	1
Secondary membrane	14	3
Precipitates on lens	5	—
Glaucoma	1	3
Amblyopia	2	—
Unknown	11	1
Total	62 (12.4%)	24 (4.8%)

Endothelial Corneal Dystrophy

There were 9 cases of endothelial corneal dystrophy: 2 cases of partial endothelial corneal dystrophy and 7 cases of total. Further details of the 9 cases are given on Table VII-4.

TABLE VII-4. — *Details on the 9 Cases of Endothelial Corneal Dystrophy in Binkhorst's Series*

	Number of Eyes
Contact dystrophy with horizontally placed 4-loop lens	3
Severe surgical problems	2
Lens dislocation	2
Decompensation of pre-existing corneal dystrophy	1
No obvious reason	1

Commenting on the underlying reasons for these cases of endothelial corneal dystrophy, Binkhorst noted that the incidence was higher in the first cases. Four cases occured in the first 100 eyes, and the remaining 5 cases were from the last 400. One may conclude that surgical judgment and technique improved as time went on.

It is also instructive to note that 3 cases occurred with iris clip lenses placed horizontally. These were old style lenses for which the loops had not been bent posteriorly.

Two other cases were ascribed to surgical manipulation: in one case serious stripping of the Descemets' membrane occurred, in the other, there was a difficult expression of the nucleus. Lens dislocation accounted for 2 cases and in both, iridocapsular lenses with metal loops were involved.

Clinical Cystoid Macular Edema

All the patients (6) with clinical cystoid macular edema had posterior capsule defects resulting from secondary procedures (needling or aspiration). According to Binkhorst, this striking association points to the important role of the posterior capsule in preventing retinal problems.

Retinal Detachment

Four eyes had a history of a secondary procedure: a capsulotomy (2 eyes) or additional loop suturing (McCannel, 2 eyes). In 1 eye, a lattice-like degeneration was associated with the retinal detachment.

Tissue Reaction

Clinical observation did not sustain the widespread belief that extracapsular cataract extraction causes a higher degree of tissue reaction due to the presence of some cortical material. According to Binkhorst, the eye generally quieted down more quickly after planned classical extracapsular surgery than after intracapsular surgery. Indeed, in only 3 cases of the 500 did Binkhorst note signs of increased postoperative uveitis: 2 cases with a small hypopion and 1 with mild vitreitis. All 3 cases responded promptly to topical corticosteroids and developed full vision.

Occasionally, white or brown precipitates on the lens surface were observed. In Binkhorst's opinion, these precipitates—sometimes falsely referred to as keratic precipitates—are not to be regarded as a product of uveitis. The precipitates were, in all cases, almost completely resorbed in a few months.

Glaucoma

Some transient disregulation of intraocular pressure was present in the immediate postoperative course. The incidence of this feature did not exceed the frequency encountered with intracapsular procedures, and it usually responded favorably to Diamox®. Persistent elevation was noted in 6 cases (1.2%).

— Four eyes with medically controlled chronic glaucoma before implantation decompensated permanently.

— Rubeosis iridis in a diabetic was the cause in 1 case and severe lesions of the Descemet's membrane with endothelial corneal dystrophy the cause in the other.

Note: Patients with a history of glaucoma surgery were excluded from this series.

Hemorrhage

Recurrent iris hemorrhage into the anterior chamber occurred in 4 eyes that had received an iridocapsular lens with platinum loops and had not achieved proper iridocapsular fixation. Three of these patients were using anticoagulants.

Vitreous Problems

During surgery, small vitreous prolapses that could be adequately managed occurred in 4 cases. The lenses were inserted without further complications. There were no instances of substantial vitreous loss in this series of planned extracapsular cataract extraction, so implantation never had to be aborted for this reason.

Lens Exchange

In 2 cases, an iridocapsular lens with platinum loops had to be exchanged for a 4-loop lens with Supramid loops. The underlying reason was a total lack of any form of fixation along with an increasing degree of atrophy of the iris sphincter ("chafing through" effect).

Dislocation

— Firm fixation was observed in 93.4% of the eyes. This was generally achieved within the first weeks, though occasionally it took months.
— Iridocapsular fixation did not develop in 33 eyes (6.6%). In 32 of these 33 cases, a lens with platinum loops was involved. Only once did an iris clip lens fail to achieve good fixation.
— Luxation was observed in 9 of these 33 cases: in 7 cases it was spontaneous, and in 2 it was traumatic.
— Additional fixation was done in 13 cases (2.6%) with the Binkhorst-McCannel technique.

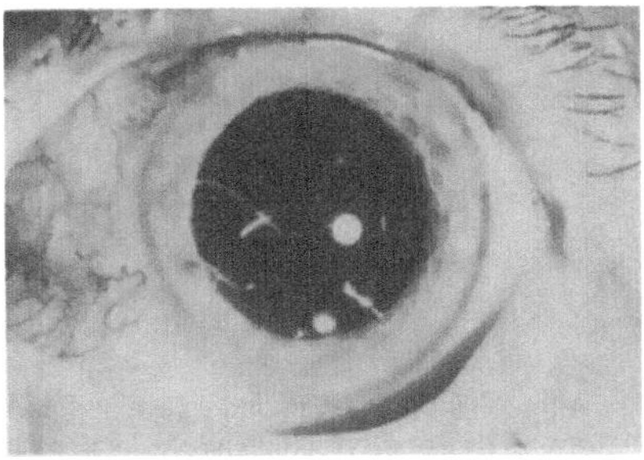

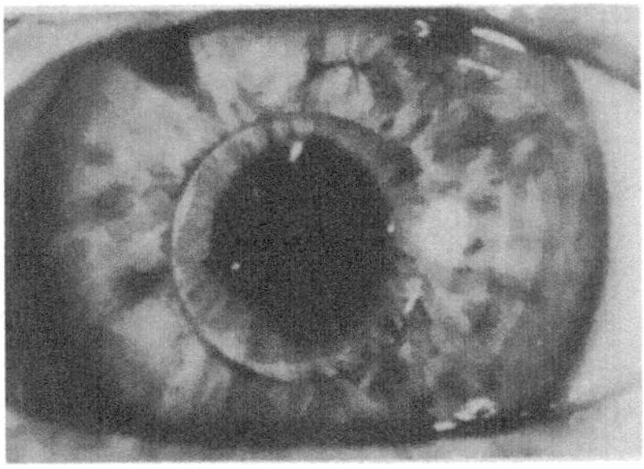

Fig. VII-12a. — A 2 loop lens not stabilized by iridocapsular adhesions.
b. — A Binkhorst-McCannel suture stabilizing the lens.

After Cataract

Aspiration of residual cortical material during the first postoperative week was necessary in 33 eyes (6.6%). The posterior capsule was

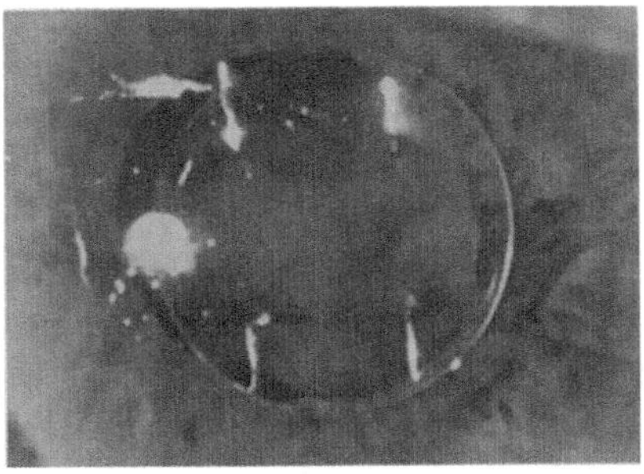

Fig. VII-13. — Cortical remnants in the pupillary area.

inadvertantly ruptured in one case during this procedure, and cystoid macular edema promptly developed.

Secondary Cataract

In 175 eyes, capsulotomies (172 eyes) or capsulectomies (3 eyes) were indicated to improve vision. Capsulotomies were performed once in 156 eyes, twice in 17 eyes, and three times in 2 eyes. Binkhorst succeeded in stripping of the secondary opacities from the posterior capsule without damaging it in 8 cases. At the time of the last follow-up examination, 33.4% of the patients had a posterior capsule defect. The incidence of needling and the average time between surgery and this procedure, however, suggest that the need for secondary capsulotomy increases in time (see Table VII-5).

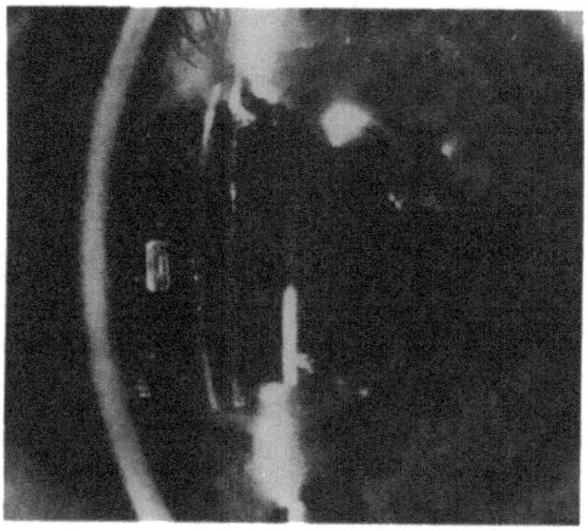

Fig. VII-14. — Secondary opacification of the posterior capsule.

TABLE VII-5. — *The Incidence of Needling Relative to the Observation Time after Surgery*

Hundreds	*Time of Observation*	*Incidence of Needling*
First 100	59-129 months	50%
Second 100	28-59 months	52%
Third 100	35-48 months	30%
Fourth 100	24-35 months	28%
Fifth 100	9-24 months	15%

C. **Results of the Authors**

We started using the Binkhorst lenses in 1967. At first, we used iris clip lenses after intracapsular cataract extraction in elderly patients and iridocapsuar lenses after extracapsular extraction for younger patients. In 1971, we adopted extracapsular extraction and lens implantation as a routine procedure. The technique was initially the same as that outlined by Binkhorst, but minor modifications were later introduced. These will be discussed below. Between 1971 and 1978, we performed over 800 lens implantations after planned extracapsular cataract extraction.

From the total series, we excluded those patients under the age of 55, the cases of traumatic cataract, those cases that underwent previous filtering procedures, and all cases that could not be followed up adequately. Table VII-6 presents our results with these 800 cases.

TABLE VII-6. — *Results of Primary Implantation after Planned Extracapsular Cataract Extraction Obtained by the Authors*

Surgeons	The authors
Type of lens	
Iridocapsular, metal loops	75%
Iridocapsular, polypropylene loops	20%
Iris clip	5%
Procedure	Extracapsular cataract extraction Primary implantation
Number	800
Follow-up	Minimum: 3 years Maximum: 9 years
Mean age	73 years
Corrected visual acuity ⩾20/40	90%
Endothelial corneal dystrophy	None
Tissue reaction:	
Iritis/uveitis (transient)	1.5%
Iritis/uveitis (persistent)	None
Endophthalmitis	None
Iris atrophy (localized)	3%
Glaucoma	
Pupil block	1.8%
Persistent	0.8%
Hemorrhage (late)	0.4%
Clinical cystoid macular edema	1.4%
Retinal detachment	1.2%
Vitreous problems	0.25%
Dislocation	2%
After cataract	6.5%
Capsulotomy	45%
Lens removal or exchange	0.1%
Enucleation	None

Results

Visual Acuity

Corrected visual acuity of ⩾20/40 was obtained in 90% of the cases. The reasons for corrected visual acuity ⩽20/40 were not lens related, for example, senile macular degeneration and other dysfunctions of the retina and the optic nerve.

Endothelial Corneal Dystrophy

There was not one case of total endothelial corneal dystrophy and only one case of superiorly localized dystrophy, which was due to inadvertant partial stripping of Descemet's membrane. The follow-up period for this case was 4 years. Five patients with pre-operative Fuch's guttated corneal disease did not decompensate after the operation. The follow-up period for these patients ranged from 1 to 5 years.

Iritis-Uveitis

Persistent uveal reactions were never a problem. Transient forms of iritis occurred in 1.5% of the cases but were easily managed with topical steroids and mydriatics. In 3 cases, a small hypopion was noticed on the second day after surgery, the underlying cause being contamination during surgery. All three hypopions were cured within 3 days by I.V. administration of antibiotics. The final visual result was not impaired. The presence of cortical remnants, even when excessive, never produced marked inflammatory responses.

Iris Atrophy (Fig. VII-11)

In 3% of the cases, localized atrophy of the iris overlying a metal loop of an iridocapsular lens developed. Although this phenomenon occurred most commonly after a long period of time in the presence

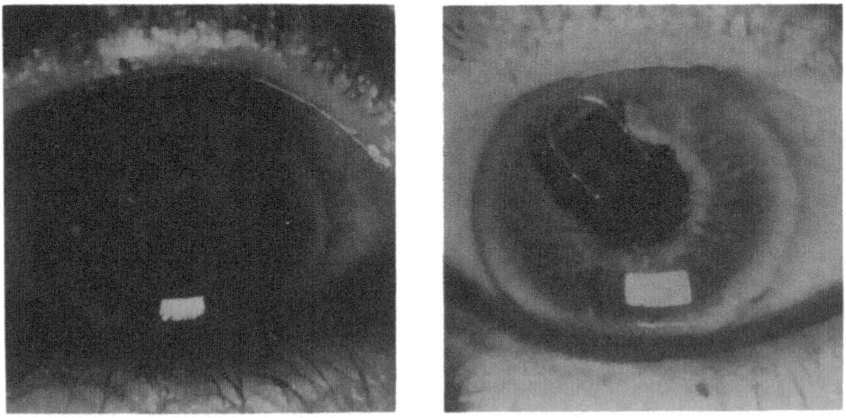

Fig. VII-15. — Localized sector atrophy of the iris overlying a platinumiridium loop that was not fixed in the capsular bag. The pictures were taken 1 and 3 years after implantation.

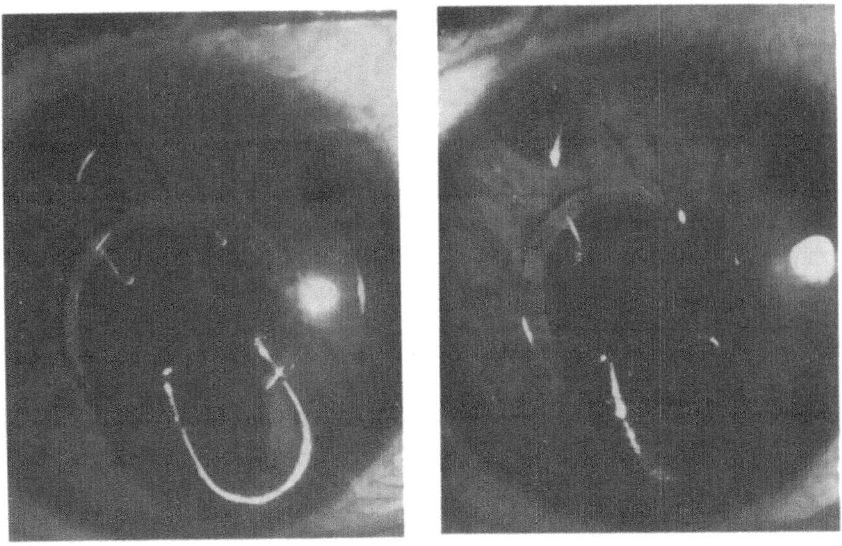

Fig. VII-16. — Left: Iris sector atrophy and subluxation of the inferior loop. Right: Secondary fixation of this loop in peripheral cortical remnants. (Courtesy C.D. Binkhorst.)

of a mobile lens, atrophy was also observed in eyes in which the lens was well-fixed. In these cases, this condition can be ascribed to chafing between the posterior surface of the iris and the metal loop. In no case did this cause the slightest inflammatory reaction.

Glaucoma

Pupillary block was observed in 1.8% of the cases. Early dilation of the pupil cured the situation in all but 2 cases. In these cases, incomplete iridectomies had to be opened surgically. Early post-operative transient rises in intraocular pressure occurred mostly in the first few hundred cases (5%). Later on, routine post-operative administration of Diamox® prevented this complication. Persistent rises in intraocular pressure were uncommon, and only 5 patients are still using pilocarpine or timolol drops to keep the tension under 20 mm Hg. One patient exhibited border-line pressure values before surgery and decompensated after surgery.

Hemorrhage

One patient had a hyphema on the 5th day after surgery but it cleared spontaneously. On three occasions, the late occurrence of a small hemorrhage from behind the iris was noticed in patients with a loose metal looped lens. So far lens exchange has not been indicated.

Cystoid Macular Edema

Clinical cystoid macular edema occurred in 1.4% of the cases. In 8 out of these 10 cases, there was previous needling of the posterior capsule. Whether the clinical cystoid macular edema was initiated by the opening of the capsule could not be established. The relationship is, however, suggestive.

Retinal Detachment

In this group of elderly patients, retinal detachment occurred in 9 cases (1.2%). In 2 eyes with intact posterior capsules, peripheral retinal degeneration was present. The 7 others had undergone previous capsulotomies. Anatomical repositioning was successful in all cases but one. Of the remaining 8 patients, 4 regained visual acuity of $\geq$20/40.

Vitreous Prolapse — Vitreous Loss

In 2 cases where a small vitreous prolapse through a capsular defect was noticed during surgery, an iridocapsular lens was inserted. The final result was not impaired. (Implantation was aborted in 6 cases because of vitreous loss. These cases are not included in the series.)

Fixation and Luxation

Firm fixation was achieved in 92% of the cases. In the remaining 8%, the lenses have only iris support. Spontaneous luxation, either anteriorly or posteriorly, occurred in 16 cases (2%). In 2 cases, the luxated lens settled between the iris and the posterior capsule. Generally, a conservative approach sufficed to achieve repositioning. In 5 cases, the lens was repositioned with a needle knife in an outpatient procedure. Additional fixation with the Binkhorst-McCannel technique was achieved in 2.5% of the cases, which involved iridocapsular lenses with metal loops. In 1 case, a loose metal looped lens was exchanged for a 2-loop lightweight lens because of pupil sphincter erosion.

After Cataract

Because of incomplete removal of either cortical material or subcapsular adhering cortex layers, secondary aspiration of lens remnants from the pupillary aperture was indicated in 6.5% of the cases. The main reasons for incomplete removal of cortical material during surgery were insufficient preoperative pupil dilation and defective surgical technique.

Posterior Capsulotomy

Incision of the posterior capsule to improve visual acuity was indicated in 45% of the cases. In 10%, the capsulotomy had to be performed within the first 6 weeks after surgery. In the remaining cases, it was performed months or even years later. Early post-operative needling procedures were indicated when residual opacifications or irregularities of the posterior capsule were present or because of fibrous deposits on it.

Delayed opacification includes proliferation of lens material resulting in pearl formation or in a thin opaque layer. None of these opacities required anything more than discision with a needle knife in an outpatient procedure.

Comment

The similarity in the incidence of complications between Binkhorst's series and ours shows that Binkhorst's technique is reproducible. The low incidence of most complications is encouraging. Of course, careful pre-operative selection played a major role, since eyes with a history of chronic iritis, borderline intraocular pressure, or peripheral retinal degeneration were rejected.

However, that 8% of the implants did not fix remains a matter of continual concern. As most of the loose lenses have metal loops, we may expect some problems in the future that will require additional suturing (Binkhorst-McCannel technique) or secondary fixation of the loops in peripheral lens remnants. According to C.D. Binkhorst, two opposite pockets are made with a Haab's knife in peripherally located cortical remnants (Soemmering's ring) in which the loop tips are to be positioned.

Latest Results of the Authors

Following the series discussed above, another 200 consecutive implantations (all for senile cataracts) with a follow-up of at least 2 years were carried out with iridocapsular lenses having polypropylene loops (wet sterilized). The most important changes in technique relative to the previous series were more aggressive preoperative pupil dilation, removal of as much cortical material as possible (manual push-pull or microerysiphake technique), and early postoperative mobilization of the pupil. The results are given on Table VII-7.

TABLE VII-7. — *Authors' Series of 200 Iridocapsular Lens Implants*

Surgeons	The authors
Type of lens	Iridocapsular with polypropylene loops
Procedure	Extracapsular cataract extraction Primary implantation
Number	200
Follow-up	Maximum 2 years
Mean age	70
Corrected visual acuity ⩾20/40	92%
Endothelial corneal dystrophy	None
Tissue reaction:	
Iritis/uveitis (transient)	2%
Iritis/uveitis (persistent)	None
Endophthalmitis	0.5%
Glaucoma:	
Pupil block	2%
Persistent	None
Hemorrhage	None
Clinical cystoid macular edema	1%
Retinal detachment	1%
Vitreous problems	None
Dislocation	0.5%
After cataract	1.0%
Capsulotomy	20%
Lens removal or exchange	None
Enucleation	None

Comment

The incidence of after cataract and lens dislocation in this series relative to our previous series shows that the changes in technique were effective. Indeed, the incidence of after cataract dropped from 6.5% to 1% and the rate of dislocation from 2% to 0.5%. Furthermore, firm fixation was obtained in 96% of the cases. Of the remaining 8 lenses, 2 required additional fixation with a Binkhorst-McCannel suture. The other 6 rely on pure iris support. Since the lenses are lightweight and since some iris synechiae are present, not too many problems are foreseen in this regard.

Early, controlled, postoperative pupil dilation generally prevented iris-to-lens synechiae, which provided better visualization of the posterior eye segment. In addition, facilitating the aqueous flow through the pupillary aperture prevents deposition of inflammatory debris on both the posterior capsule and the lens surface. On several occasions, early pupil dilation resulted in a backwards shift of the optic portion of the implant behind the iris plane. So far, these lenses (about 5%), which are thus totally located in the posterior chamber, have behaved extremely well.

In 3% of the cases, various degrees of upward decentration of the lens has occurred. Although in no case is the corneal endothelium in danger, the cosmetic appearance is displeasing, and many of these patients complain of monocular diplopia. This phenomenon only occurred with lenses with polyproplene loops. It could be that these lightweight lenses are drawn up by a shrinkage process involving the remains of the superior anterior capsular flap or some cortical remnants. But a more plausible explanation may be the following. Since the superior part of the iris is more or less traumatized by expression of the nucleus and by the manipulations involved in the positioning of the superior loop of the pseudophakos, adhesions are more likely

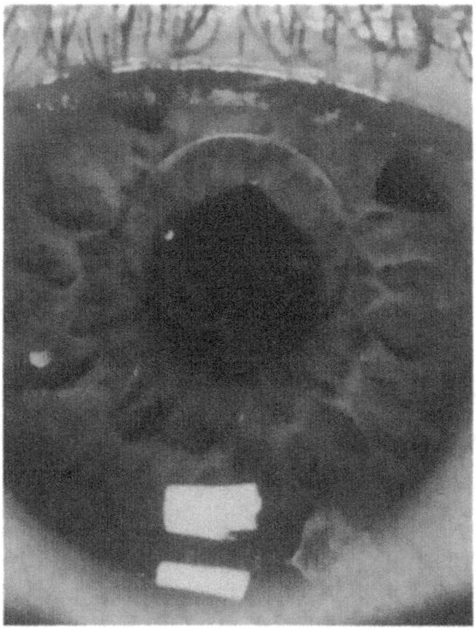

Fig. VII-17. — Upwards decentration of an iridocapsular lens 3 weeks after surgery.

to develop in the early postoperative period between the superior part of the iris sphincter and the superior loop attachments of the lens. These asymmetric adhesions lift the lightweight intraocular lens during pupil dilation and progressively pull the inferior loop upwards. In time, the formation of adhesions between the inferior anterior and posterior capsules prevents the inferior loop from returning to its initial position in the capsular bag, thus ultimately causing permanent upwards lens decentration.

In some cases, excessive decentration could be repaired by pulling the lens downward with a needle knife. Attempts made after the first month after decentration had commenced were usually unsuccessful unless the inferior capsular bag could be reopened. The inferior loop was then slid into the capsular pocket and the lens recentered. The pupil was kept dilated to prevent reformation of asymmetric iris-to-lens synechiae until capsular fixation was achieved.

The preventive measures include proper positioning of both loops in the capsular bag and moderate but sustained pupil dilation commencing in the early postoperative period.

D. **Results from Other Surgeons**

The survey conducted by J. Hoffer (1978) revealed that, up to March 1977, some 13% of all reported lenses implanted were 2-loop iridocapsular lenses after extracapsular cataract extraction. But Hoffer did not include the implants done by Binkhorst or those by H. Hirshman and J. Gills, all of whom performed a great deal of extracapsular surgery while implanting 2-loop lenses.

Incomplete or preliminary reports on the use of iridocapsular lenses confirm that the techniques devised by Binkhorst are reliable. One of the most important problems was learning how to perform the extracapsular technique.

The difficulties encountered in the exact placement of the loops between the capsular flaps constituted another problem. Non-fixation of these heavy lenses, particularly when metal loops were involved, turned out to be a matter of continuous concern. Illustrative in this respect are the data provided by R.P. Kratz et al. (1979). Cataracts were extracted from 320 eyes (average patient age: 72.7 years) by means of phakoemulsification and primary implantation performed. The follow-up time ranged from 3 months to 5 years. The most troublesome complication with the 2-loop iridocapsular lens was subluxation (3.4%). Most of the lenses that subluxated had metal loops. In this series, 3.8% of the lenses had to be removed because of non-fixation, sphincter erosion, or corneal decompensation. Again, in most of these complications, lenses with metal loops were involved.

Conclusions: Iridocapsular Lenses

As did the other lens models, the original iridocapsular lens also underwent modification. Although Binkhorst and others had obtained good results with metal-looped lenses, polypropylene loops were introduced because of the occurrence of iris damage, particularly when adequate fixation had not occurred.

The new, lightweight iridocapsular lens gives very satisfactory results providing the entire surgical procedure is well-conducted: atraumatic extracapsular lens removal and insertion of the pseudophakos in the required position. Another advantage of this lens is that its stability does not rely on sutures or clipping devices, which involve extra intraocular manipulations. Further, since the volume of the lens in the anterior chamber is minimal, it is suitable for use in small anterior eye segments or traumatized eyes with anterior synechiae.

II. The Platinum Clip Lens

The platinum clip lens for use after either intra- or extracapsular cataract extraction (Worst, 1971) has already been described in Chapter VI on iris supported lenses. Worst and many other surgeons, especially in the United States, started using the platinum clip lens in the mid-seventies.

As shown on Figure VII-18, the fixation principle of the platinum clip lens consists of capsular support by the inferior loop while the superior loop and the clip constitue an anti-luxation device. When the inferior loop is not fixed in the capsular bag, the lens can rely on pupil support, and additional fixation is provided by the transiridectomy clip device.

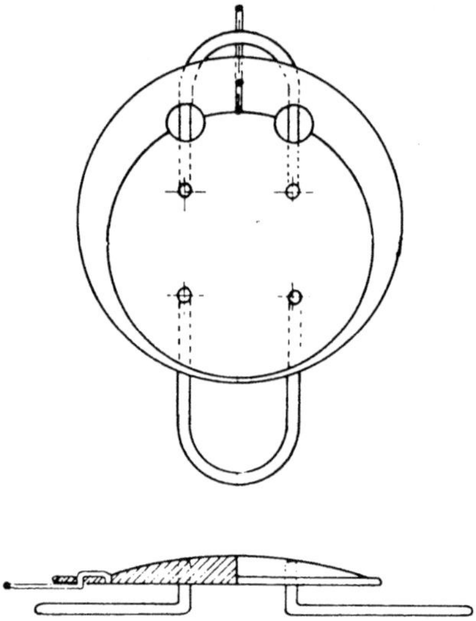

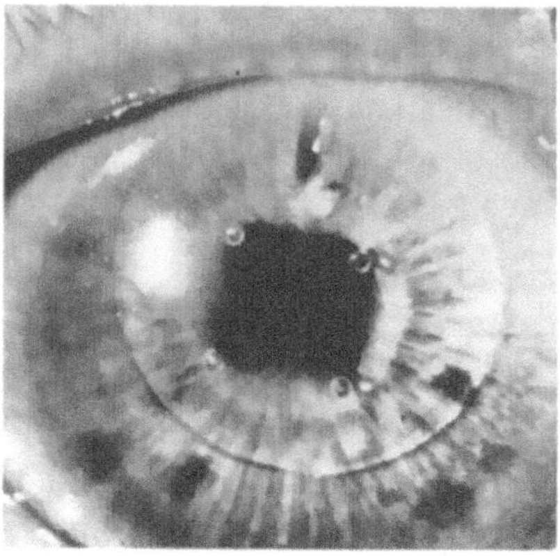

Fig. VII-18. — J. Worst's platinum clip lens.

A. **Surgical Technique**

Of utmost importance for the insertion of this lens are the exact positioning of the inferior loop in the capsular bag and the proper bending of the stave. The main stages of the procedure are as follows:

— Anterior Capsulotomy:
Using a cystotome, a horizontal cut is made 1 millimeter below the center, the upper capsule is sliced up, and its remnants removed.

— Extracapsular Lens Extraction:
The lens is removed either by using the classical method as described for the 2-loop iridocapsular lens or by using automated devices.

— Lens Insertion:
Using a fine forceps, the platinum clip lens is grasped at its haptic rim, and the inferior loop is introduced into the casular bag below. The superior loop is brought behind the upper iris sector by means of either the Binkhorst bimanual spatula and hook technique or pulling with a forceps on the upper iris sector.

— Iridectomy:
An iridectomy is made at 12 o'clock, the lowest part of which must correspond to the clip. An other possibility is to make one

radial iridotomy at the site of the stave and two lateral iridectomies.

— Bending the Stave:
The lens is grasped at the haptic rim with a fine needle holder. The platinum clip is depressed until the olive tip is level with or below the posterior loop.

Several surgeons have modified the technique to facilitate bending of the stave. The lens can be steadied by holding it at the haptic rim with a small forceps, such as a tying forceps (the Shepard modification) or a Bonaculta forceps (J. Sheets, 1977).

It is also possible to stabilize the lens by inserting a spatula between the haptic rim and the iris overlying the superior loop with, for example, a simple flat iris spatula, a Hirshman notched lens spatula, or Kwitko's spatula. In order to bend the platinum stave, some surgeons use a forceps while others use the tip of a Hirshman notched lens spatula or a Bechert bender (G. Knolle, 1980).

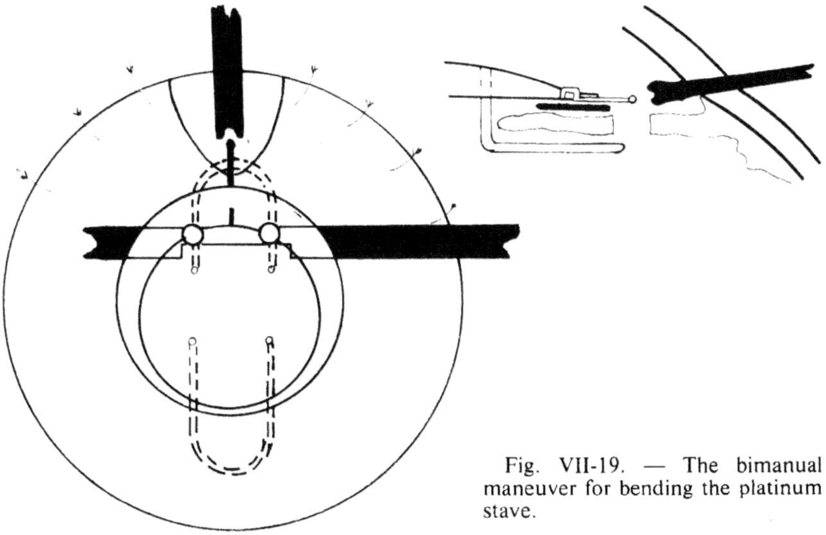

Fig. VII-19. — The bimanual maneuver for bending the platinum stave.

As noted by Jaffe et al. (1978) and Knolle, although the stave is quite malleable, it is still very fragile and may break off after repeated manipulation.

B. Results

As yet, there are no fully documented series available on the use of platinum clip lenses after extracapsular cataract extraction with long-term follow-up periods.

The results obtained by J. Sheets with some 757 platinum clip lens implantations, are probably representative. All the date were compiled by J.W. Maida (1978).

The incidence of corneal edema was 1.5%. There was persistent corneal edema evident 3 months after surgery in 11 out of 757 patients. The luxation incidence was 3%, and Maida noted that this rate decreased as the surgeon gained experience in capsular fixation.

Separate data on other complications were not published. In the opinion of Sheets and Maida, in addition to the advantages of the extracapsular technique (less cystoid macular edema and retinal detachment), the platinum clip lens has an additional advantage over the iridocapsular lens: should the inexperienced surgeon fail to position the inferior loop between the capsular flaps, the transiridectomy clip offers an additional security measure.

Spontaneous postoperative superior decentration and anterior tilting may occur. This phenomenon has also been observed by other surgeons (Knolle, 1980; Jaffe et al., 1978). This is a particularly annoying complication since the superior haptic rim and the stave, even if properly bent, may touch the cornea. Various mechanisms are considered responsible for this upwards migration. Jaffe et al. (1978) saw cortical remnants in the superior cul-de-sac tilt the lens anteriorly and bring the clip into contact with the posterior surface of the superior cornea. Knolle suggested the following as a plausible explanation: "As scarring in the posterior capsule progresses from the inferior portion of the capsular bag upward, the inferior loop is pushed superiorly. Finally, tautening and vertical shortening of the capsule further elevate the Platina lens."

Therapeutic measures include surgical discission of the posterior capsule centrally in order to release the contracture and halt further lens movement (the relaxing incision, Knolle, 1980). When endothelial touch occurs, Sheets recommends making a linear incision in the capsular bag inferior to the lower lens loop. Forceful pressure is then applied to the lens feet with the discission instrument in order to move the lens inferiorly (Knolle, 1980).

In our opinion, a mechanism analogous to that described for the iridocapsular Binkhorst lens may be considered responsible. Indeed, synechiae are likely to develop between the iris and the superior loop with the platina lens since there is no superior capsular flap and since the clipping device tends to immobilize the superior iris sector.

Comment

Although Worst's platinum clip lens is an interesting lens for use after extracapsular cataract extraction, the fixation device has both advantages and disadvantages.

The main advantage is that, should capsular fixation fail, total luxation is unlikely to occur because of the safety clip (the belt and suspenders principle). On the other hand, the proper bending of the stave requires extra intraocular manipulation and is an exacting surgical technique. The occasional postoperative upward decentration and forward tilting of the lens may also be a matter of concern.

Unfortunately, the necessary studies with large series with long-term follow-up periods to determine the potential and limitations of this lens have yet to be done.

C. Modifications of the Platinum Clip Lens

Several versions of the platinum clip lens have been designed, especially in the United States. These versions include lenses with smaller diameters, other loop materials (e.g., metal or polypropylene), and polypropylene staves instead of platinum.

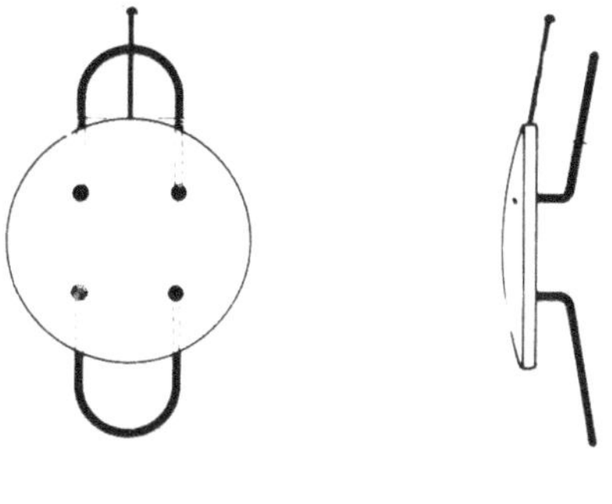

Fig. VII-20. — Modified platinum clip lens without a haptic rim.

Typical of these modified platinum lenses is the one designed by R. Sinskey in which the haptic rim was eliminated and the platinum stave was replaced by a polypropylene one. This peg has to be bent posteriorly through an iridectomy and placed within the superior loop.

III. Other Iridocapsular Lenses

A. The Small Incision Lenses

Two other lenses have been designed by J. Worst that are intended to be used after extracapsular cataract extraction either in primary or secondary procedures. These are the so-called small incision lenses.

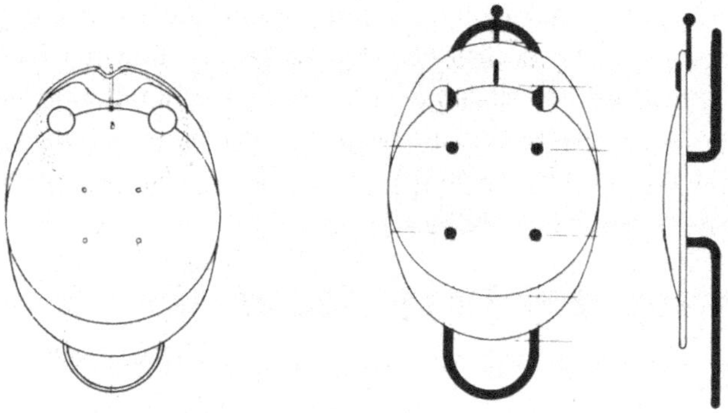

Fig. VII-21. — J. Worst's small incision lenses.

As shown in Figure VII-21, both lenses have a transiridectomy clip device. The clipping principle of the left model differs from that of the platinum clip lens. The horizontal diameter of these lenses was reduced to 5 mm to allow it to be inserted through a small incision.

Crucial aspects of the implantation of these lenses are the proper positioning of the inferior loop in the capsular bag and the closure of the transiridectomy clipping device.

Since no data are available on the results obtained with these two lens styles, it is impossible to weigh their advantages and disadvantages.

B. The Medallion Cloverleaf Lens

Worst also designed the Medallion cloverleaf lens. As shown in Figure VII-22, it is a Medallion lens with 3 posterior loops and a transiridectomy clip device. It was intended to be used exclusively

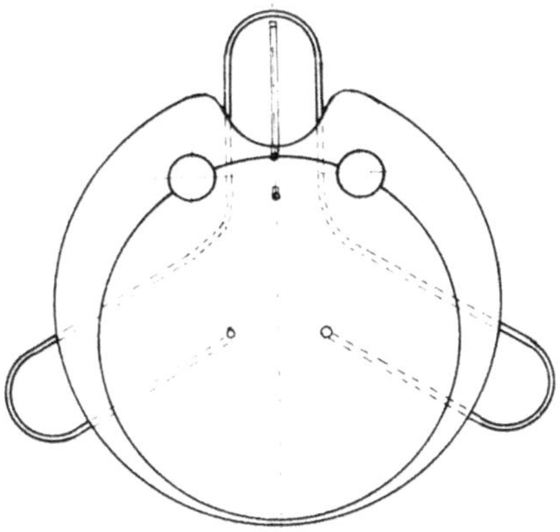

Fig. VII-22. — J. Worst's medallion cloverleaf lens.

after extracapsular cataract extraction. The Medical Workshop has informed us that this lens is no longer available, so we shall not go into the technical details. We do not know how many of these lenses have been implanted.

C. The Medallion Slotted Boomerang Lens

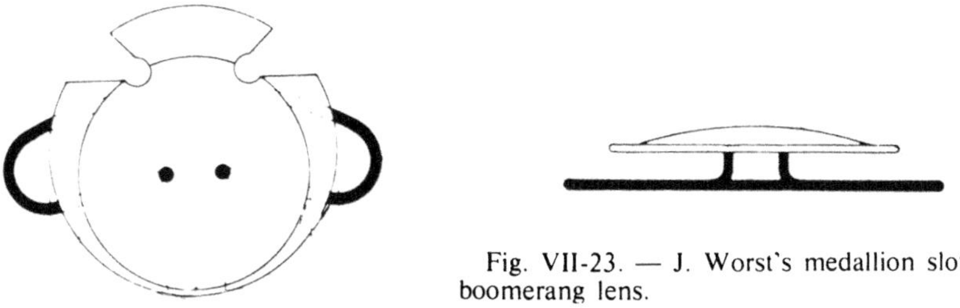

Fig. VII-23. — J. Worst's medallion slotted boomerang lens.

J. Worst also designed the "Boomerang Lens" for primary implantation after extracapsular cataract lens extraction. As shown by Figure VII-23, the large horizontal loop has only two posterior loop attachments. Fixation relies on both a steel suture through the iris and capsular support. Worst advises a T-shaped incision in the anterior capsule that allows the horizontal loop to be placed in the two lateral capsular bags.

§ 2 POSTERIOR CHAMBER LENSES

Theoretically, the best position for a pseudophakos is in the posterior chamber from which, after all, the original lens has been removed. The following advantages are being claimed by surgeons who have begun to use these lenses (Pearce, 1978; Shearing, 1978; Praeger, 1978; Kratz, 1979):

— Cosmetic: The eyes are normal looking since no part of the pseudophakos is visible in the anterior chamber and the pupil size is not affected.
— Optical: As the implant is in the position of the natural lens, i.e. virtually at the nodal point, aniseiconia may, theoretically, be eliminated. Providing the lens is well-centered in the pupillary aperture, there will be no bothersome light reflections.
  Furthermore, the pupillary function is not disturbed, so there is normal adaptation to light and dark conditions.
— Anatomical: No part of the implant lies in the anterior chamber, so postoperative damage to the endothelium by contact is impossible. This is certainly a primary advantage when corneal grafting is considered or filtering procedures are indicated.
  The pupil can be constricted and dilated at will, since the lens does not rely on pupil support, and posterior synechiae are less likely to develop. There is also less of a tendency to pupillary block glaucoma.

The disadvantages of posterior chamber pseudophakoi are as follows:

— All posterior chamber lens implantations require extracapsular cataract extraction, which is a fundamentally different approach than the classic and standard intracapsular technique.
— Depending on which type of lens is used, the presence of well-designed anterior capsular flaps may be mandatory. Furthermore, the problems of intraocular suturing of some lenses must be taken into account.
— Should decentration of the optical portion occur, monocular diplopia may develop, especially in those lenses with a small optical portion. This also applies for cases in which, for one reason or another, the pupil becomes eccentric.
— Secondary opacification of the posterior capsule may constitute a complex problem, since access to the central part of the posterior capsule is difficult.

— Some types of posterior chamber lenses are reported to be extremely difficult to remove without massive destruction of the anterior eye segment.

I. The Pearce Posterior Chamber Lens

John Pearce, who entered the field of lens implantation in 1967, first implanted about a thousand Binkhorst 2-, 3-, and 4-loop lenses. He soon began to appreciate the advantages offered by extracapsular fixation and worked out different methods to improve extracapsular surgery without recourse to expensive and sophisticated devices. As a logical extension of his ideas on intraocular lens fixation, he started performing posterior chamber implants relying on both capsular and iris fixation. The first lenses he used, therefore, were 4-loop Binkhorst iris clip lenses from which the posterior loops had been cut off. He inserted 15 such lenses, into the posterior chamber after planned extracapsular cataract extraction and, in addition, sutured them to the iris. Encouraged by good functional results, he first developed a one-piece, bipedal lightweight posterior chamber lens with fenestrated haptic feet allowing iris suture placement (Figure VII-24). The lens was made entirely of polymethylmethacrylate. Capsular adhesions were facilitated by roughening the haptic feet. The bipod lens is now recommended for secondary insertion through a small incision after prior extracapsular extraction. It can also be used combined with penetrating keratoplasty with double Pearce iris stitch suturing.

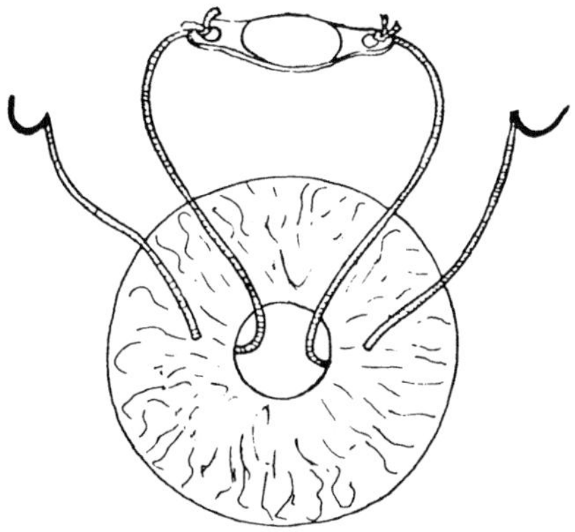

Fig. VII-24. — J. Pearce's bipedal posterior chamber lens allowing iris suture placement.

Later on, to improve lens stability, a tripod lens was designed that proved more extensive capsular fixation (Fig. VII-25). With this lens, too, a suture through the superior fenestrated haptic was found to promote exact centration. Furthermore, the iris stitch fixates the lens while capsular adhesions become effective in about 2 weeks.

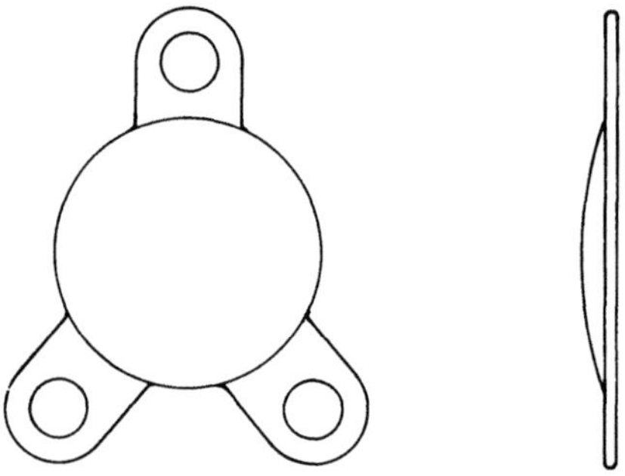

Fig. VII-25. — J. Pearce's tripedal posterior chamber lens. For extra fixation, the haptic is sutured to the iris.

A. **Pearce's Surgical Technique**

The main steps in the insertion of the tripod lens are as follows:

— Anterior capsulotomy: Using a cystotome, multiple small radial incisions are made in the anterior capsule, leaving sufficient capsule below (D-shaped capsulotomy).

— Extraction of the nucleus: With a special irrigating vectis, the nucleus is dislodged in the anterior chamber and removed. The capsular bag is cleaned thoroughly. The removal of the cortical material is begun at 12 o'clock.

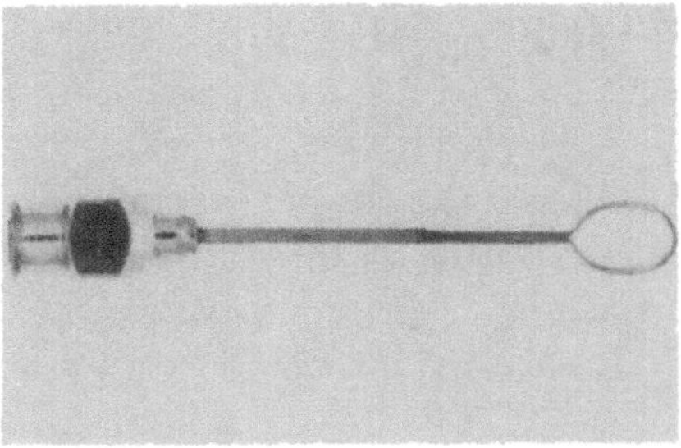

Fig. VII-26. — J. Pearce's irrigating vectis for the removal of the nucleus.

— Lens insertion and fixation: The iris sphincter is grasped at 12 o'clock and the polypropylene suture is passed through the pupil behind the iris to emerge some 2 mm from the limbus in the 12 o'clock area.

Outside the eye, the loose end of the iris stitch is inserted through the fenestration of the superior haptic foot and tied.

The lens is than introduced with the inferior feet down in the capsular bag.

The iris above is pulled over the upper haptic portion of the lens, the iris stitch is pulled tight, and another bite of the iris is taken circumferentially just behind or in front of where the stitch emerged from behind the iris. A small loop remains that is then tied and the ends cut.

B. Pearce's Results

Table VII-8 gives the results obtained by J.L. Pearce with the tripod iris sutured posterior chamber lens.

TABLE VII-8. — *Results of the Series of J.L. Pearce*

Surgeon	J.L. Pearce
Source	J.L. Pearce (1979, personal communication)
Type of lens	Tripod iris sutured posterior chamber lens
Procedure	Extracapsular cataract extraction Primary implantation
Number	444
Follow-up	Maximum 4 years
Mean age	>70 years
Corrected visual acuity ⩾20/40	93.5%
Endothelial corneal dystrophy	0.45%
Tissue reaction:	
Iritis	2%
Endophthalmitis	None
Glaucoma:	
Pupil block	None
Persistent	1.8%
Hemorrhage	None
Cystoid macular edema (clinical)	0.45%
Retinal detachment	None
Vitrous problems	6.8%
Dislocation (partial)	1.4%
Decentration	4.5%
Capsulotomy	9%→16%

Visual Acuity

The reasons for visual acuity <20/40 in 21 of these cases were:

— Senile macular degeneration: 11

— Opacities of the posterior capsule: 7

— Optic nerve pathology: 2

— Amblyopia: 1

Endothelial corneal dystrophy

Although marked post operative striate keratitis occurred in 17 eyes (4.1%), bullous keratopathy developed in only 2 cases. One was superimposed on a known Fuch's dystrophy.

Iritis

In 9 eyes (2%), the presence of iritis required intensive steroidal treatment soon after the operation. Pearce is convinced that postoperative surgical uveitis has been reduced by the use of an antiprostaglandin: oral fluorbiprofen that was started 3 days prior to surgery and continued for 6 weeks thereafter.

Glaucoma

Despite the absence of peripheral iridectomies in most cases, there were no pupil block glaucomas. In Pearce's opinion, peripheral iridectomies can be omitted providing the angle is open on preoperative gonioscopy, most of the cortex is removed, and the posterior capsule is mainly intact.

In 8 eyes (1.8%), glaucoma therapy was necessary to keep the intraocular pressure under control.

Cystoid Macular Edema

Clinical cystoid macular edema was observed in 2 eyes. This low incidence is thought to be related to the high proportion of intact posterior capsules.

Dislocation and Decentration

One of the inferior feet dislocated in front of the iris in 6 eyes (1.4%). This subluxation caused no concern, however, since the dislocated feet were well away from the endothelium.

In 20 eyes (4.5%), the optic decentered out of the visual axis. In 9 eyes (2%), a Binkhorst-McCannel stitch was found necessary.

Capsulotomy

In Pearce's opinion, the low incidence of capsulotomies (9%) may be attributed to atraumatic extracapsular extraction, the use of physiological irrigating solutions, and the removal of most of the anterior capsule. Since the need for capsulotomies will increase as time goes on, he expects that the incidence will finally be some 16%. As long as this figure does not markedly increase, Pearce does not favor routine opening of the posterior capsule at the time of surgery.

Discussion and Conclusion

The visual results obtained in this series are certainly very satisfactory. The low incidence of complications—endothelial corneal dystrophy, iritis, glaucoma, and cystoid macular edema—is also remarkable along with the absence of pupil block. The 4.5% incidence of lens decentration, which is an annoying problem with posterior chamber lenses, may seriously affect visual performance. To prevent this, a lens with a 5 mm instead of a 4 mm optic portion has recently been designed.

Another point of concern is the iris stitch. Although for Pearce this technique only adds 5 minutes to the surgical procedure, it is questionable if the intraocular manipulations will remain innocuous when other surgeons employ this method. Pearce himself has recognized this problem and so he devised a new tripod lens with a 5 mm optic without an iris stitch but with a larger superior haptic. The haptic is manifactured in 2 lengths: 6.5 mm, which is recommended when the horizontal corneal diameter measures more than 11.5 mm, and 6 mm for when the horizontal corneal diameter is 11.5 mm or less. In situ, the superior haptic foot lodges behind the iris with the tip resting in the zonular region. Although implantation is simplified, it remains to be seen if the stitchless lens with an enlarged superior haptic will yield a lower complication rate.

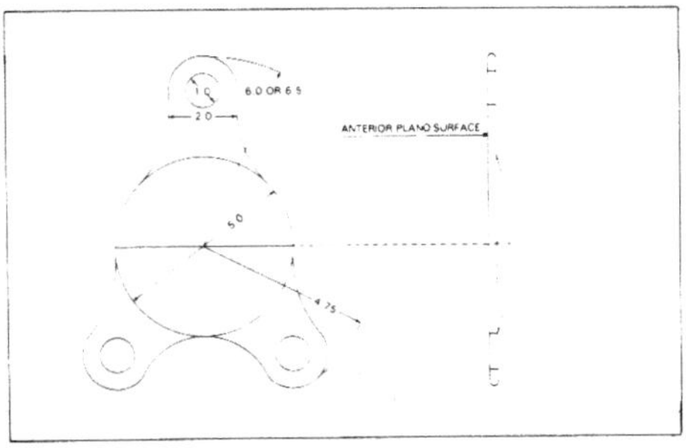

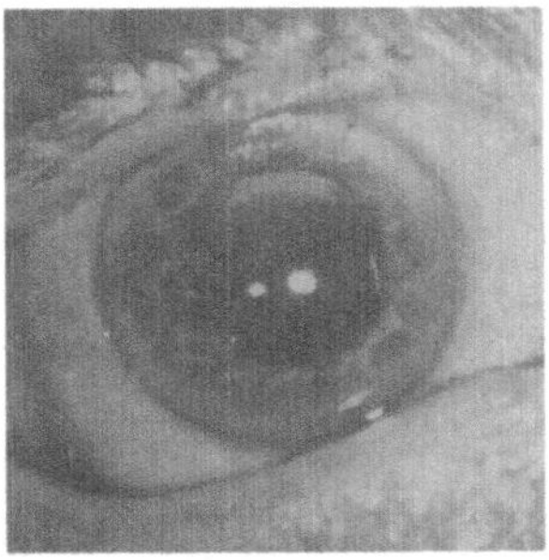

Fig. VII-27. — J. Pearce's tripedal stitchless posterior chamber lens.

R.C. Drews (1980), reviewing 138 cases of which 39 had the superior haptic sutured to the iris, came to the conclusion that these lenses yield excellent results in expert hands.

II. Other Posterior Chamber Lenses

A. The Iridocapsular Lens as a Posterior Chamber Lens

On occasion, it was noticed by C.D. Binkhorst and ourselves that the iridocapsular lens may become a posterior chamber lens when mydriatics are used in the early postoperative period (Fig. VII-28). Only a few iridocapsular lenses will become true posterior chamber lenses, since this seems to depend on the space available between the iris diaphragm and the posterior capsule. At present, Binkhorst is experimenting with a 2-loop lens with the optic enlarged from 5 mm to 6 mm in diameter and with flatter posterior loops and also with another type that has 4 loops (Fig. VII-29). During surgery the short anterior loops of the 4 loop posterior chamber lens are placed in front of the iris and the posterior one in the capsular bag. When capsular fixation is achieved in the postoperative period, pupil dilation allows the anterior loops to disappear behind the iris in the posterior chamber.

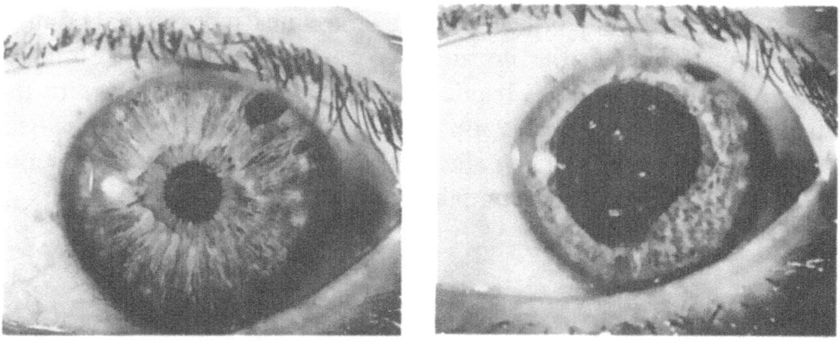

Fig. VII-28. — C.D. Binkhorst's 2-loop iridocapsular lens located behind the iris, before and after pupil dilation.

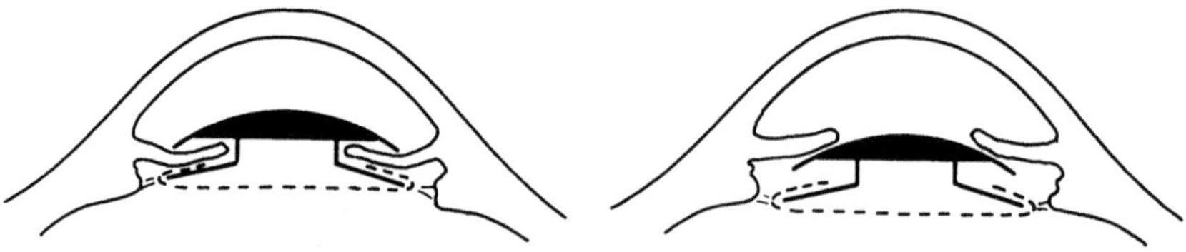

Fig. VII-29. — Experimental 4-loop posterior chamber lens of C.D. Binkhorst.

B. The Little-Arnott Lenses

The first lenses (Mark I) were quite similar to the tripod lens designed by J.L. Pearce, with only slight variations in length. The actual lens (Mark III) is a bipod posterior chamber lens with anterior loops.

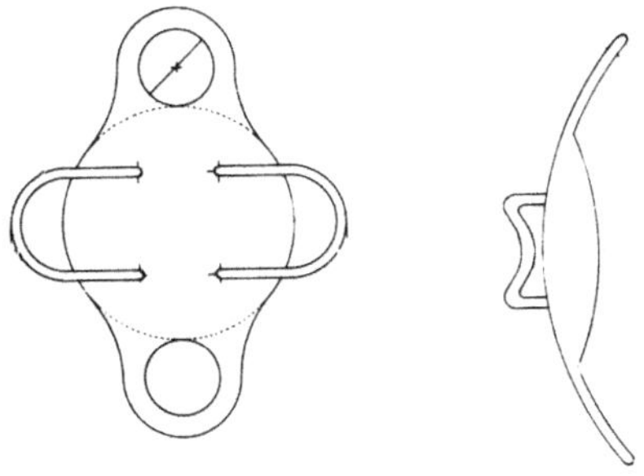

Fig. VII-30. — The Little-Arnott posterior chamber lens.

C. The Harris Lens

W. Harris's lens does not require suturing and achieves rather good fixation, provided that good anterior capsular flaps are prepared. In 1979, the results of 365 cases were reported. But since this series included different types of posterior chamber lenses, it is impossible to come to any conclusions with regard to this lens.

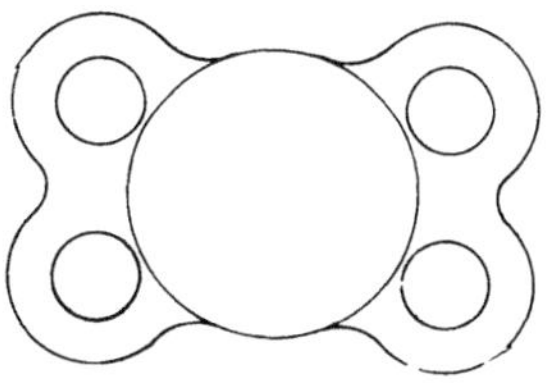

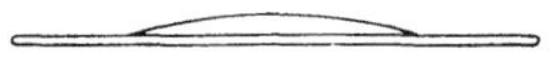

Fig. VII-31. — W. Harris's posterior chamber lens.

D. The Coleman-Taylor Lens

The Coleman-Taylor lens, which was proposed at the 1978 AIOIS meeting, has a 6 mm optic, 3 posterior loops and one anterior loop; it is intended to be inserted between the posterior capsule and the anterior capsular flaps after extracapsular cataract extraction. In order to prepare adequate anterior capsular flaps, an anterior capsulotomy in the form of an inverted " Y " is suggested. Additional stability and centration is provided by suturing the anterior loop to both the anterior capsule and the iris diaphragm.

Since long-term results are not available from this lens type, no definite conclusions can be drawn on its ultimate value.

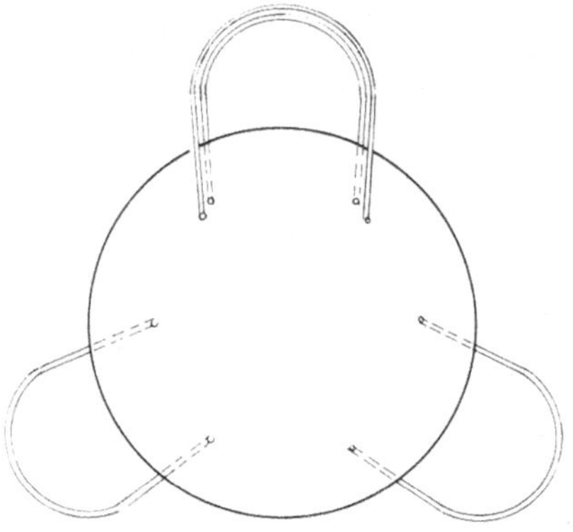

Fig. VII-32. — The Coleman-Taylor posterior chamber lens.

E. The Anis Lens

A. Anis in the late seventies proposed a posterior chamber lens to be placed in the original lens capsule. The optic portion carries two large, opposing, and flexible semicircular loops. For correct positioning of the lens A. Anis proposed the use of a doulbe lens glide, which is delivered with the implant.

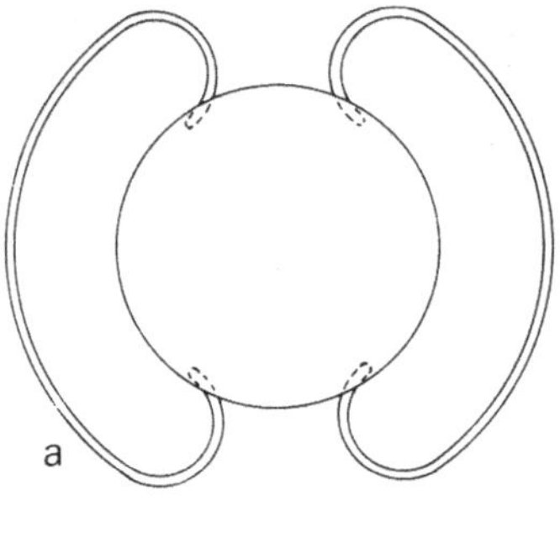

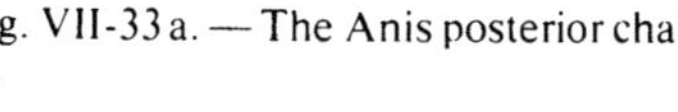

Fig. VII-33a. — The Anis posterior chamber lens.

F. The Ong Capsular Lens

The lens devised by T. S. Ong has an overall diameter of 11 mm and two asymmetrical haptic loops that are placed in the capsular bag.

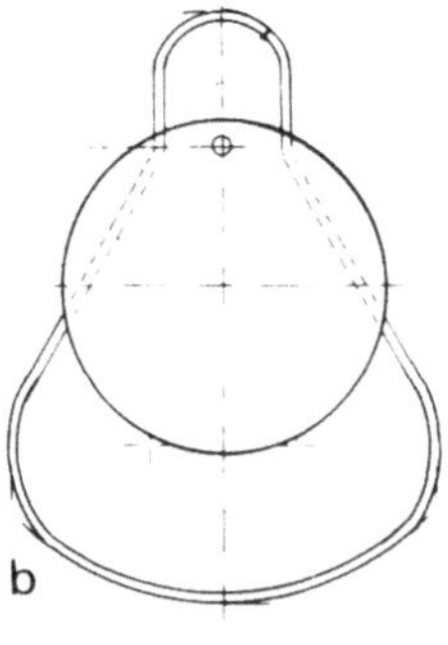

Fig. VII-33b. — The Ong capsular lens.

G. The Sheets Lens

This posterior chamber lens has been developed to fit entirely in the capsular bag. It has two loops that provide four arcs of fixation.

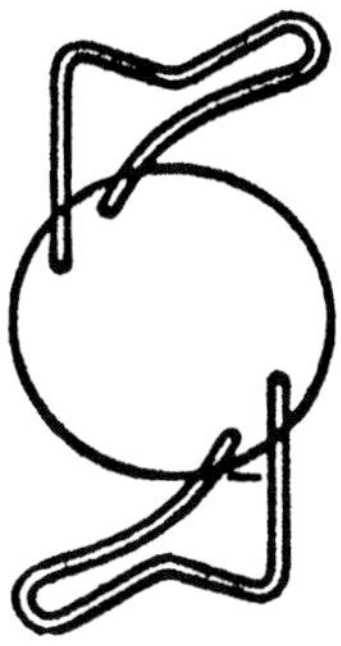

c

Fig. VII-33c. — The Sheets lens.

III. The Shearing Lens

S. P. Shearing first implanted his posterior chamber lens in 1977, and reported on his clinical experience with some 100 cases the next year. Because this lens gained considerable popularity in the late seventies, we shall treat it in detail.

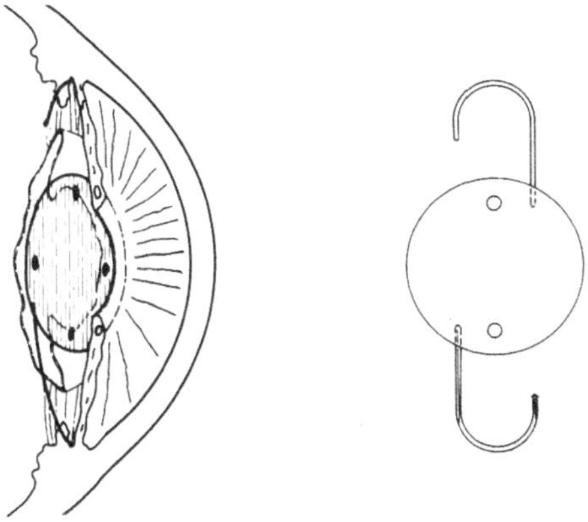

Fig. VII-34. — The Shearing posterior chamber lens.

As shown on Figure VII-34, this lens resembles the original Barraquer angle supported lens designed in the 1950's and consists of a planoconvex optic (5 or 6 mm in diameter) and 2 incomplete loops of 4-0 polypropylene suture material extending from the optic disc in the same geometrical plane. The standard overall length is 13 mm.

The loops are treated to spring back to their original shape after being compressed during lens insertion. The centration and fixation of the lens are provided by the loops extending within the "ciliary sulcus" behind the iris diaphragm. While the lens does not depend on adhesions to the posterior capsule for primary fixation, adhesions generally do develop and serve as a secondary form of fixation. The Shearing lens can be used in both primary and secondary procedures.

A. Shearing's Surgical Technique

After extracapsular cataract extraction is performed in which as much anterior capsule as possible is removed, the lens is grapsed by one of the haptic loops with an angled forceps. Using the so-called closed chamber technique, the inferior loop is introduced between the lips of the incision and slipped under the iris in the 6 o'clock position. The open tip of the superior loop is then grasped with forceps and carried down toward the 6 o'clock position until the superior border of the pupil is cleared. The superior loop is then released. The loops spring back to their normal shape, automatically centering the lens and fixing it. After the incision is closed, a central opening in the posterior capsule is made. In order to facilitate access to the retrolenticular space, the cystotome is passed through the iridectomy. Shearing notes that the margins of the capsules may adhere to the posterior lens surface after a capsulotomy is performed. Even if the seal is incomplete vitreous is still prevented from coming forward.

B. Results of Shearing's First Cases

In 1978, Shearing reported on the short-term results he obtained with his lens. Most of the cases he selected had rather poor vision, so they had "less to lose" if the lens did indeed turn out to cause unforeseen complications. Six lenses were implanted secondarily after extracapsular cataract extraction. Four metal-looped lenses inserted after extracapsular extraction were replaced with Shearing lenses. The remaining 90 cases were primary insertions.

As shown on Table VII-9, no serious complications occurred in this short follow-up period, the only problem of concern being lens decentration, which occurred with a lens with a 5 mm optic. An

TABLE VII-9. — *Results of J.P. Shearing's Implantation of 100 Shearing Lenses*

Surgeon	J.P. Shearing
Source	J.P. Shearing (1978)
Type of lens	Shearing lens
Procedure: ECCE Primary	90%
Secondary	10%
Follow-up	Maximum 15 months
Corrected visual acuity ⩾20/40	78%
Endothelial Corneal Dystrophy	None
Tissue reaction: Iritis (transient)	4%
Glaucoma: transient	9%
persistent	None
Hemorrhage (hyphema)	1%
Cystoid macular edema (clinical)	None
Retinal detachment	1%
Dislocation	None
Decentration	1%

attempt to move the lens was unsuccessful because the loops were "frozen". So the loops were cut and the 5 mm lens replaced with a 6 mm one. So far, no lens dislocation has been observed.

C. Results Obtained by Other Surgeons

Similar promising results were obtained by Kratz et al. who inserted 756 Shearing lenses. As originally suggested by Shearing, incision of the posterior capsule was routinely performed (Kratz et al., 1979).

As Table VII-10 shows, the major complications of endothelial corneal dystrophy, iritis, glaucoma, and cystoid macular edema were nearly absent. In the view of Kratz et al., these results lend credence to the reliability of the Shearing lens. With respect to other lens styles, such as the 2-loop and 4-loop Binkhorst lens and the Choyce Mark VIII, a major advantage is the absence of any foreign body in the anterior chamber. And, unlike the angle supported lenses, the flexible haptic extending into the so-called ciliary sulcus did not give rise to any complaints of soreness upon touching or blinking. It also appears that the Shearing lens has the lowest overall complication rate.

In the view of these authors, this particular posterior chamber lens also has advantages over other types of posterior chamber lenses. Insertion was found to be particularly simple. And since no intrao-

TABLE VII-10 — *Results of Kratz, Mazzocco, Davidson and Maloney with 756 Shearing Lenses*

Surgeon	R.P. Kratz et al.
Source	R.P. Kratz et al. (1979)
Procedure	ECCE Primary
Number of Cases	756
Follow-up	3 months-18 months
Age	>70 years
Corrected visual acuity ⩾20/40	91%
Endothelial Corneal dystrophy	None
Tissue Reaction:	
Iritis (transient)	3.3%
Endophthalmitis	0.1%
Glaucoma	0.4%
Hemorrhage (hyphema)	0.1%
Cystoid macular edema (clinical)	2.1%
Retinal detachment	1.3%
Subluxation	0.4%
Lens removal	0.3%

cular suturing is required, intraocular manipulation is kept to a minimum. Owing to the spring-like action of the loops extending into the ciliary sulcus, excellent centration of the optic portion is achieved, which makes the presence of anterior capsular flaps unnecessary. So far, subluxation has rarely occurred.

R. Drews (pers. comm. 1979) reported that around 8000 Shearing lenses were implanted in the United States, which indicates the increasing popularity of this new design. It is not yet known, of course, whether the results obtained by surgeons in general will match those obtained by Shearing and Kratz.

Of interest here are the occasional problems that have been reported. During lens insertion, the most serious problem that may occur is inadvertent rupture of the posterior capsule or zonule by the inferior loop. This complication may go undetected at the time of surgery, and the lens may dislocate inferiorly soon thereafter. Surgical intervention is then necessary. Shearing (1979) notes that a hook introduced into the positional lens hole can be used to rotate the lens over an intact portion of the capsule. If this is impossible, lens loops may be sutured to the iris with McCannel sutures, or the surgeon may attempt iris plane fixation by lifting the lens optic into the anterior chamber. Should the surgeon know of a ruptured zonule or capsule at the time of surgery, another style of lens should be implanted.

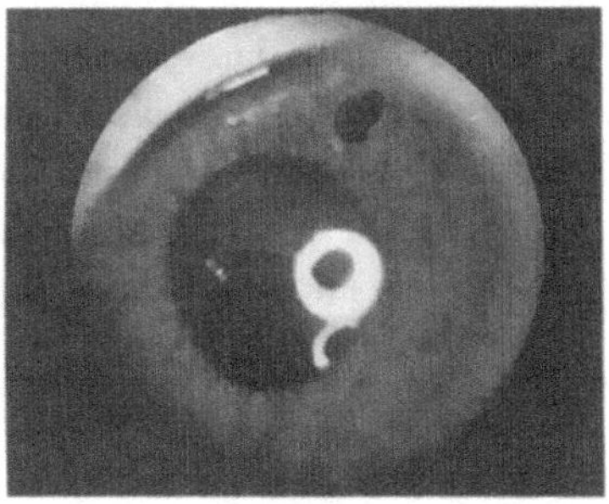

Fig. VII-35. — The Shearing lens partially dislocated into the vitreous. (Courtesy J. Alpar.)

In the opinion of C.W. Simcoe (1979), the stiff, straight loops of the Shearing style lenses resist compression during insertion, and the tip of the loop exerts focal concentrated pressure on the ciliary body and the zonule. To reduce the risk of zonule rupture, Simcoe compresses the lens loops with a forceps before implantation.

R.M. Sinskey (1979) advises that the zonular integrity be checked after the lens is brought into position. If pressure applied to one side of the lens causes it to spring back, the zonular fibers are intact.

Except when the capsule or zonule is ruptured, decentration of the lens is rare. Kratz noted that decentration is more likely to occur with secondary implantation since adhesions with the posterior capsule are less likely to develop. In these cases, the routine use of a McCannel suture is indicated (personal communication, 1979). According to G.D. Faulkner (1979), the standard Shearing lens with an overall diameter of 13 mm is too short to "lock" into the "ciliary sulcus" in large anterior eye segments. So he now measures the horizontal corneal diameter from "white-to-white" and does not implant this particular lens when it equals or exceeds 12,5 mm.

Another complication peculiar to posterior chamber lenses is "pupil capture" in which part of the iris is trapped behind the lens optic

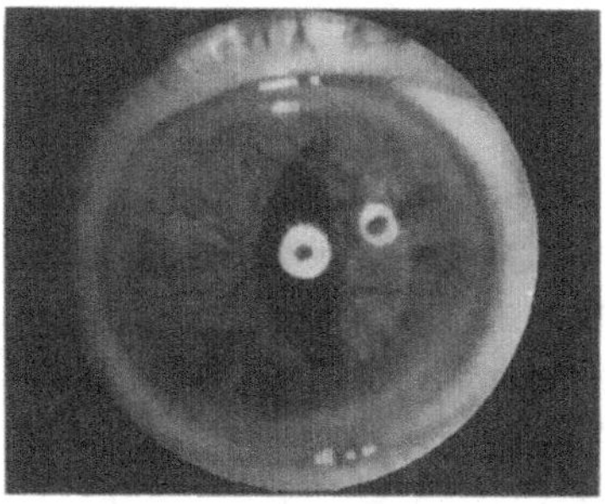

Fig. VII-36. — Pupil capture with the Shearing lens resulting in an oval pupil.

causing an oval pupil. According to Shearing, pupil capture can be caused by frequent or vigorous dilations in the immediate postoperative period, or it can be a response to pressure from a large air bubble in the anterior chamber. This condition may respond to conservative therapy: with the patient in the supine position and the pupil dilated, the lens may sink back, which will allow the pupil to contract in front of the lens.

D. **Modifications of the Shearing Lens**

1) R. Kratz (1978) proposed that the loops of the Shearing lens not be constructed in the same geometrical plane as the optic disc but rather be tilted slightly anteriorly (15°) (fig. 31). This moves the optic portion posteriorly which favors capsular adhesion formation and decreases the possibility of pupil capture.

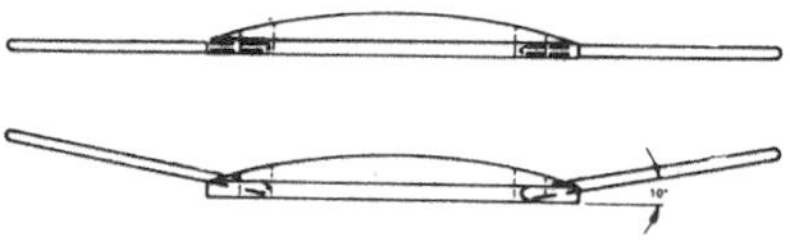

Fig. VII-37. — Kratz's modification of the Shearing lens: the orientation of the loops has been changed.

2) K. Hoffer (1979) uses Shearing-style lenses with a ridge around the posterior lens surface, which is intended to inhibit formation of Elshnig's pearls and deposition of inflammatory debris on the central posterior capsule.
3) C.W. Simcoe (1979) has designed 2 and 3-loop posterior chamber lenses that have easily compressible loops, non-perpendicular loop orientation, and loop ends curved to fit either the "ciliary sulcus" (13 mm model) or the capsular fornices (10.5 mm model). Simcoe contends that the well-rounded, compressible loops prevent inadvertant zonular rupture during insertion.
4) Shearing style lenses with shorter loops to be inserted in the capsular bag.

Although the short follow-up period does not permit definitive conclusions about the long-term behavior of the Shearing lens, the low complication rate speaks in its favor. Many ophthalmologists may see the need for extracapsular surgery as a serious limitation. Whether or not the fixating principle of loops extending into uveal tissue will prove to be innocuous in the long run is also a matter of speculation. Shearing argues that the polypropylene loop memory is

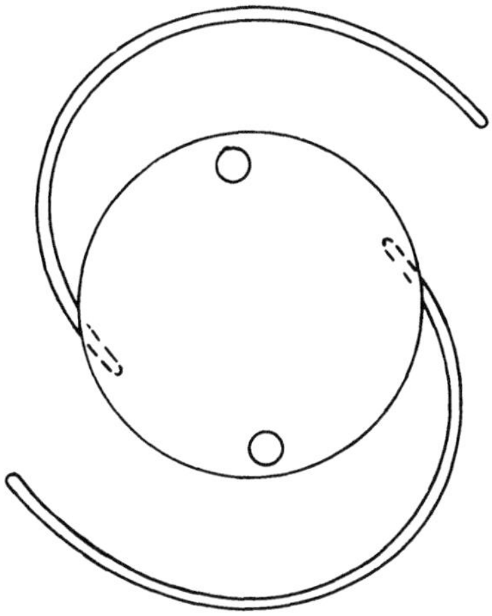

Fig. VII-38. — C.W. Simcoe's modification of the Shearing lens. It has easily compressible loops and a non-perpendicular loop orientation.

not permanent, so the loop will gradually lose its spring, which in turn will eliminate long-term continuous pressure against the ciliary tissue.

Conclusion

The survey we conducted covers a period of 15 years during which the extracapsular method was increasingly perfected. The initial lens designs were also refined and newer models came on the market. The series we analyzed seem to confirm the idea of Binkhorst that extracapsular cataract extraction combined with lens implantation provides a wide range of substantial advantages. The idea to reevaluate the capsular membrane, which is avascular and insensitive, as a means of fixation for a pseudophakos certainly seems to have been sound. Indeed, it is reassuring that this fixation mechanism has shown no signs of failure over the long term.

CHAPTER VIII

ANGLE SUPPORTED LENSES

Introduction

Angle supported lenses have two components: an optical component from 4 to 6 mm in diameter made of polymethylmethacrylate and a haptic portion of polymethylmethacrylate or flexible material that provides a bridge-type support between the optical component and the angle of the anterior chamber.

Typical of these two fixating mechanisms are:

— the original rigid Strampelli anterior chamber lens (1954);

— the original Dannheim anterior chamber lens with flexible nylon supports (1956).

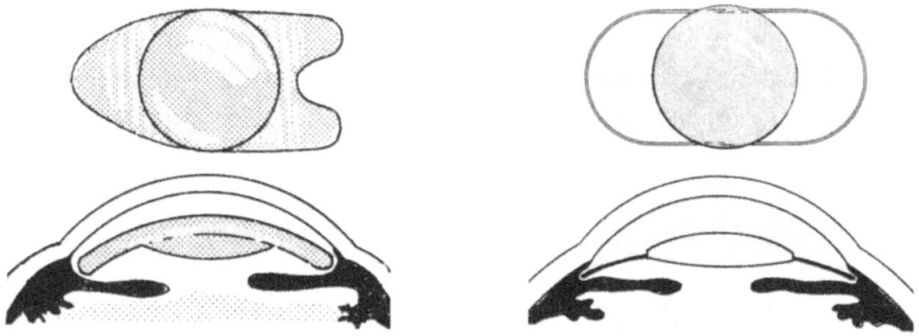

A B

Fig. VIII-1a. — The Strampelli lens.
b. — The Dannheim lens.

According to K. Morcher (personal communication, 1979), the Dannheim lens is still being used by some surgeons. Unfortunately, no long-term results have ever been published.

In the first ten years after their introduction, some of these lenses gained rapid popularity. Relative to the original capsular supported

Ridley lens, which was introduced in 1949, they had the following advantages:

— They could be used after both extra- and intracapsular cataract extraction.

— It was easier to insert them.

Although some authors reported remarkable initial results, the use of all these early models had to be suspended since the long-term results were poor, the main complication being an unacceptably high incidence of endothelial corneal dystrophy.

The catastrophic experience with angle supported lenses in these first ten years—they were implanted not only in aphakic eyes but also in phakic eyes to correct myopia—brought implantation into general disrepute and severely retarded further development. Even now, some prominent European surgeons continue to censure lens implantations because of the results of this period.

Nevertheless, D.P. Choyce, after having used the early anterior chamber lenses, decided to pursue the idea of angle supported lenses. Between 1957 and 1978, he designed nine different models, each being a response to a specific problem. The purpose of his effort was to find an innocuous lens to be located in the anterior chamber that would have long-term stability without harming either the corneal endothelium or the uveal tissue. In Choyce's opinion, his Mark IX lens, which came out in 1978 satisfies both criteria.

In contrast to iris supported, iridocapsular supported, and capsular supported lenses, most of Choyces' lenses were intended to be inserted into an already aphakic eye in a secondary stage procedure. Since 1976, however, Choyce's angle supported lenses have been implanted in primary procedures, particularly in the United States.

I. Secondary Implantation

A. The Developmental Period: Choyce Mark I – Choyce Mark VII

Choyce reported on the developmental period during which major changes in his lens design were introduced in his monograph, "Intraocular Lenses and Implants" (1964). The data reproduced below concerning types I through IV have been largely taken from this monograph.

1. *Choyce Mark I: The First 100 Cases*

Choyce's Mark I was his first modification of the Strampelli triangular lens with a fixed length. Though very similar to Strampelli's lens, it differed in the following respects:

— It was made of Perspex CQ (as used by H. Ridley), whereas Strampelli used polymethylmethacrylate from another source.
— The radius of anterior curveture was changed from 12 to 14 mm, thus flattening it in order to keep it away from the posterior surface of the cornea.
— The thickness of the haptic portion was reduced from 1 mm to 0.9 mm.

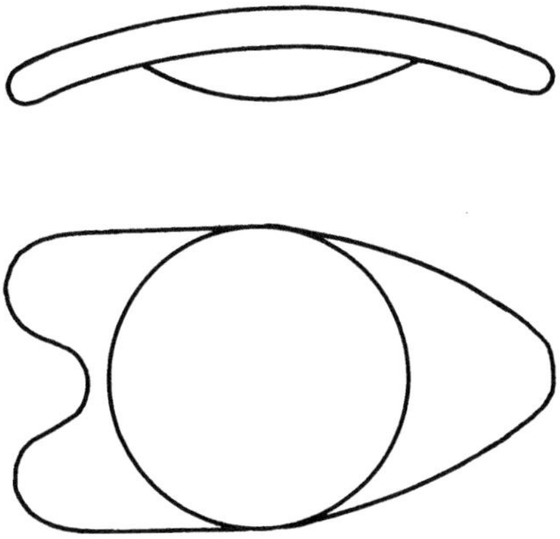

Fig. VIII-2. — The Choyce Mark I lens.

Choyce selected unilateral aphakics for his first cases, and reported on his first 100 cases in 1964 and again in 1976 (see Table VIII-1).

Commentary

Visual Acuity

After two years, 58% of the patients had a corrected visual acuity of 20/40 or better. But before implantation, 76% of the aphakics had a corrected visual acuity of 20/40 or better. Thus, secondary implantation of the Mark I lens resulted in a significant decrease of visual acuity.

TABLE VIII-1. — *The Results of Choyce's First 100 Cases of Mark I Implants*

Author	D.P. Choyce (1964)
Surgeon	D.P. Choyce
Lens Type	Mark I
Surgical Procedure	Secondary, Intracapsular
Number of Cases	100
Follow-Up	5 years
Corrected Visual Acuity	
⩾20/40	58%
Endothelial Corneal Dystrophy	10% (after 5 years)
	28% (after 19 years)
Macular Changes	N.A.
Retinal Detachment	N.A.
Internal Iris Prolapse	8%
Iritis	6%
Dislocation (posterior)	1%
Glaucoma	7%
Lenses Removed	4%
Exchanged	5%
Enucleation	8%

N.A. = Not available.

Endothelial Corneal Dystrophy

By the end of the first year, the incidence of endothelial corneal dystrophy was 5%; after 5 years, 10%, and after 19 years, 28%. According to Choyce, at least 5% of the cases were due to improper sterilization (Cetremide), other reasons being contact between implant and cornea, unsuitable eyes, and presence of vitreous in the anterior chamber.

Iris

Iritis leading to secondary glaucoma occurred in 6 cases.
There were 8 cases of internal iris prolapse, a forward ballooning of the iris diaphragm (as with an iris bombé). This condition occurred mostly in the early postoperative period and was attributed either to wound dehiscence or to iris-lens adhesions (pupillary block). On occasion, this problem required surgical treatment, i.e., a peripheral iridectomy.

Iris atrophy was not infrequent and started within a few weeks. It was ascribed to excessive contact between the moving iris and the implant and occurred particularly when the lens was too long.

Dislocation

Only one implant dislocated. This was a posterior dislocation into the vitreous in a case of subtotal traumatic aniridia in which the support provided by the residual iris was insufficient.

Glaucoma

The cases of glaucoma were considered to be caused primarily by recurrent iritis.

Lens Removal

No reasons were given for the removal that was necessary in 4 cases.

Lens Exchange

In 5 instances, the lenses turned out to be too short and were replaced by longer ones.

Enucleation

The causes of the loss of these eyes were given as follows:
- A shallow anterior chamber resulting from preexisting aphakic glaucoma.
- Cetrimide induced iridocyclitis: secondary glaucoma.
- Implant too short and not removed in time: secondary glaucoma.
- Iridocyclitis and secondary glaucoma in a diabetic patient.
- Thrombosis of the central retinal vein.
- Epithelialization of the anterior chamber: secondary glaucoma.

Conclusion

Although the majority of these unilateral aphakic patients were rehabilitated and although the new design was stable enough, the method had to be improved because of:
- Inadequate sterilization.
- Gradual deterioration of the cornea.
- Too many iris problems.
- The difficulty in determining the proper lens length.
- Enucleation.

2. *Modifications of the Choyce Mark I Lens*

The Choyce Mark II Lens (1958) (Fig. VIII-3)

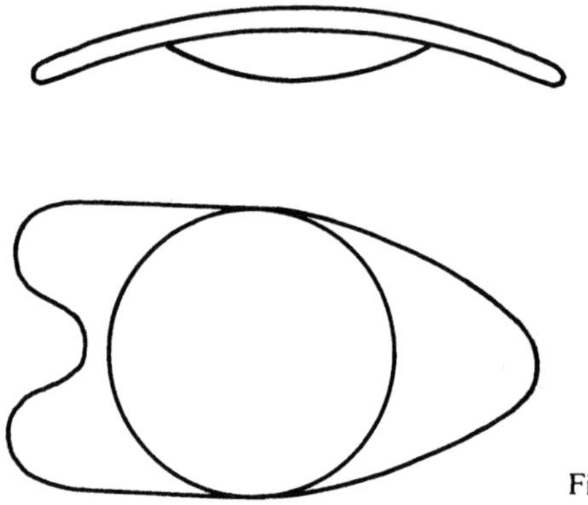

Fig. VIII-3. — The Choyce Mark II lens.

In this model, the thickness of the haptic portion was reduced from 0.9 to 0.5 mm. This modification was made because of a pathological study of an eye containing a Mark I lens. This eye showed marked distortion of those parts of the angle that were in contact with the tip and the feet of the implant (Ashton and Choyce, 1959). One hundred thirty Mark II lenses were implanted.

The Choyce Mark III Lens (1959) (Fig. VIII-4)

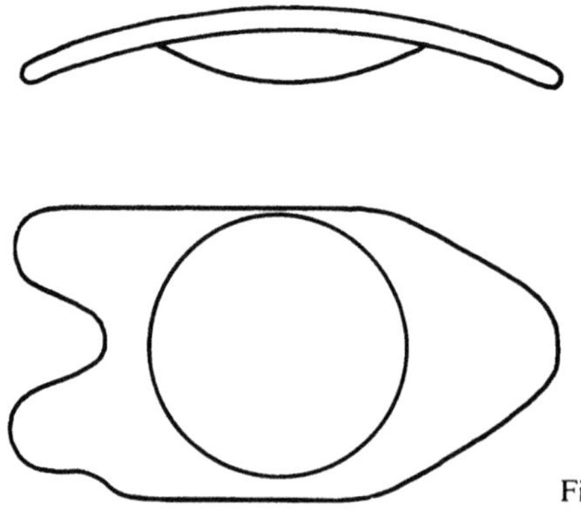

Fig. VIII-4. — The Choyce Mark III lens.

Because internal iris prolapse especially in the 6 o'clock area remained a major problem, a 0.5 mm inferior ledge was added to the Mark II model. One hundred twenty of these lenses were implanted.

The Choyce Mark IV Lens (1961) (Fig. VIII-5)

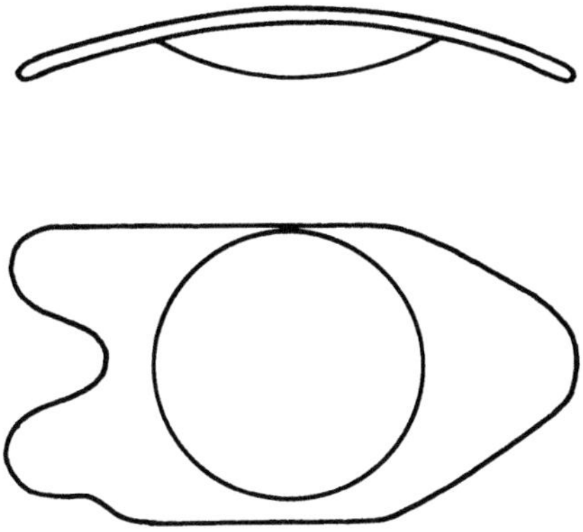

Fig. VIII-5. — The Choyce Mark IV lens.

In this model, the thickness of the haptic was further reduced from 0.5 mm to 0.25 mm. Choyce considered the advantages of this lens to be greater ease of insertion, a deeper anterior chamber, and less danger of endothelial corneal dystrophy. Twenty such lenses were implanted.

The Choyce Mark V Lens (1962) (Fig. VIII-6)

Because internal iris prolapse remained a bothersome factor, three small holes, 0.5 mm in diameter, were drilled in the haptics to facilitate free circulation of aqueous through the implant, especially during the immediate postoperative period. One hundred thirty Mark V lenses were implanted.

Two years after the Mark V modification was introduced, Choyce published the results of his first 500 implantations of Mark I through

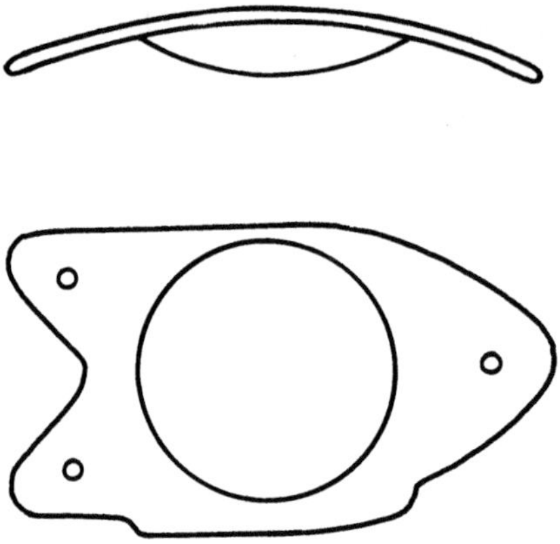

Fig. VIII-6. — The Choyce Mark V lens.

Mark V lenses. Since the data is incomplete and since the follow-up period for the Mark V lens was too short, we shall only comment on the complications that are representative for this developmental period.

TABLE VIII-2. — *Modifications of the Original Strampelli Lens by D.P. Choyce To Prevent Endothelial Corneal Dystrophy, Angle Atrophy, and Internal Iris Prolapse*

	Thickness of haptic	*Inferior ledge*	*Perforations*	*Number implanted*
Mark I	0.91 mm	NO	NO	100
Mark II	0.50 mm	NO	NO	130
Mark III	0.50 mm	YES	NO	120
Mark IV	0.25 mm	YES	NO	20
Mark V	0.25 mm	YES	YES	130
			Total:	500

Visual Acuity

Figures for visual acuity were given for the first 300 cases on Table VIII-3. Visual acuity improved significantly in the later cases, undoubtedly because of refinements in both lens design and technique.

TABLE VIII-3. — *Visual Acuity before and after Lens Implantation, with a 2 year Follow-Up for the Last Series (Choyce, 1964)*

		Before Implant	*After Implant*
Corrected Visual Acuity ⩾20/40	First Hundred	76%	58%
	Second Hundred	76%	75%
	Third Hundred	72%	80%

Endothelial Corneal Dystrophy

Except for the first hundred cases, ECD was of minor importance during the first few years after lens implantation. Indeed, there was only an incidence of 1.7% (7 cases) in the 400 implantations of Mark II to Mark V lenses. But as with the first hundred cases where the incidence of ECD climbed from 10% to 28% after 19 years, the incidence in the last 400 cases increased from 1.7% to 7% after 15 years (Choyce, 1976). Still, ECD was less likely in the second series since the clearance between the artifical lens and the corneal endothelium had been increased (Table VIII-4).

TABLE VIII-4. — *Depth of the Anterior Chamber, Choyce Mark I-Mark V*

	Number	*Anterior Chamber Depth*
Mark I	100	1.68 mm
Mark II-III	200	1.94 mm
Mark IV-V	100	2.20 mm

Early Internal Iris Prolapse

As we have mentioned, early internal iris prolapse was a troublesome factor (2.75% in the last 400 cases) and was one of the principle reasons for changing the lens design.

Length of the Implant

While in the first hundred cases 5 lenses had to be removed and replaced by longer ones, only 3 out of the following 400 had to be exchanged because they were too short. Not all the short lenses had to be exchanged, however. Some had started to rotate but later became fixed as a result of a local iris reaction. Only when the short implant began to act like a loose foreign body in the anterior chamber did it have to be removed without delay.

Commenting on his first 500 implants, Choyce concluded in 1964 that endothelial corneal dystrophy remained a serious hazard for anterior chamber implant surgery. He believed that it would never be completely banished, though the incidence could be reduced by careful attention to implant design, case selection, surgical technique, and postoperative care.

3. *The Choyce Mark VI and Choyce Mark VII Lenses*

Between 1962 and 1963, Choyce modified the Mark V lens significantly by changing the principle of fixation. Up till then, all the lenses had a single anterior profile, the radius of curvature always being 14 mm. Fixation in these early models was achieved by the three tips of the haptic resting on the angle of the anterior chamber, thus involving the trabecular meshwork and sometimes the endothelium.

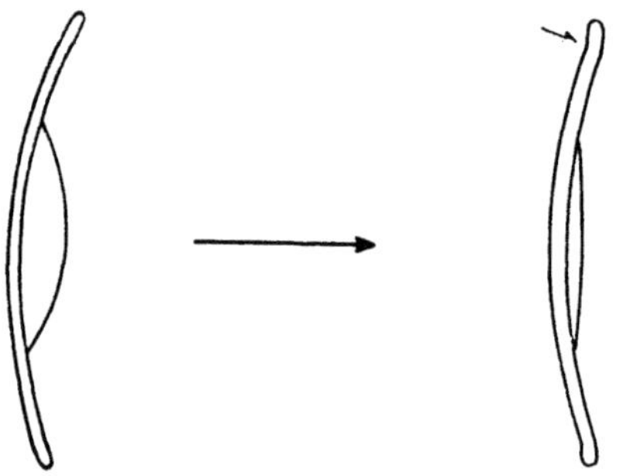

Fig. VIII-7. — Profile change in the early sixties.

To lessen the risk of contact between the lens and the endothelium and also to reduce the pressure on the delicate structures of the angle, the profile of the lens was altered by flattening the tips of the haptics as shown in Figure VIII-7. Consequently, the principle of fixation changed from angle fixation to iris-scleral fixation (Choyce, 1965). As we have noted, in 1960 H. Ridley had modified his tripod anterior chamber lens by flattening the tips of the haptic legs. In his opinion, this flattening would lessen the danger of pressure on the corneal periphery and keep the lenticulus close to, but just clear of, the iris (Fig. VIII-8).

Soon after he had introduced the Mark VI, Choyce designed the Mark VII. The profile remained the same, but the inferior ledge, which had been introduced with the Mark III, was eliminated

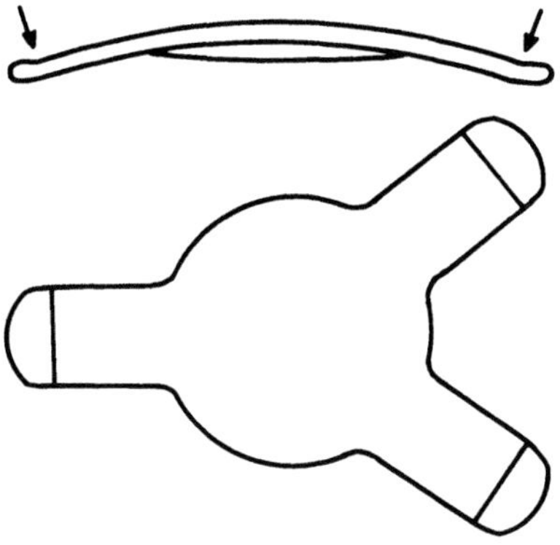

Fig. VIII-8. — The Ridley tripod anterior chamber lens.

(Choyce, 1965). Separate data on the results and complications for these two lenses have not been published.

B. Fifteen Years of Experience with the Choyce Mark VIII Lens (1963-1978)

In 1963, Choyce further modified his lens by changing the shape from triangular to quadrangular in order to increase its stability.

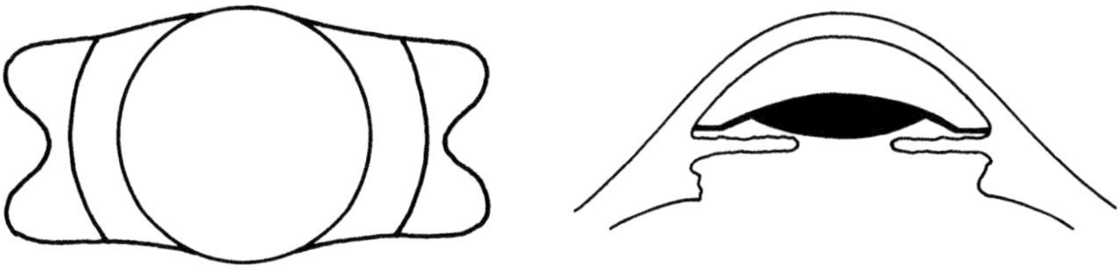

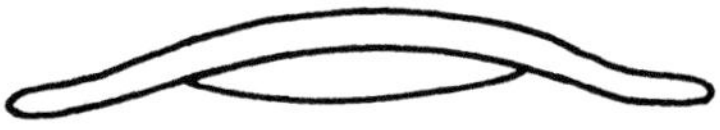

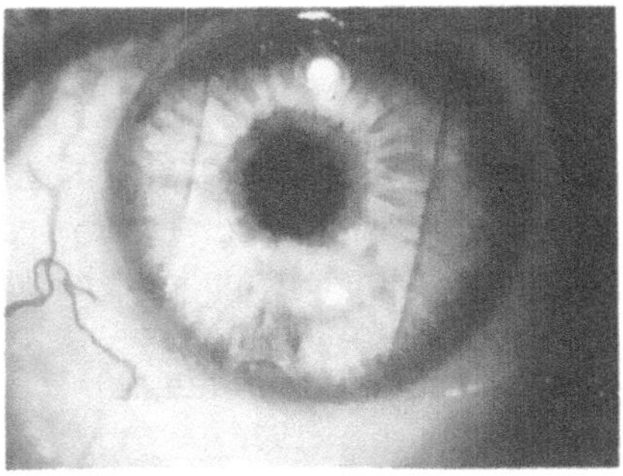

Fig. VIII-9. — The Choyce Mark VIII lens. (Courtesy H.J. Shammas.)

The Mark VIII has four flattened feet intended to be located parallel to the iris plane. The thickness of the haptic is 0.25 mm. The optic is biconvex. Its anterior radius is kept constant at 14 mm, while

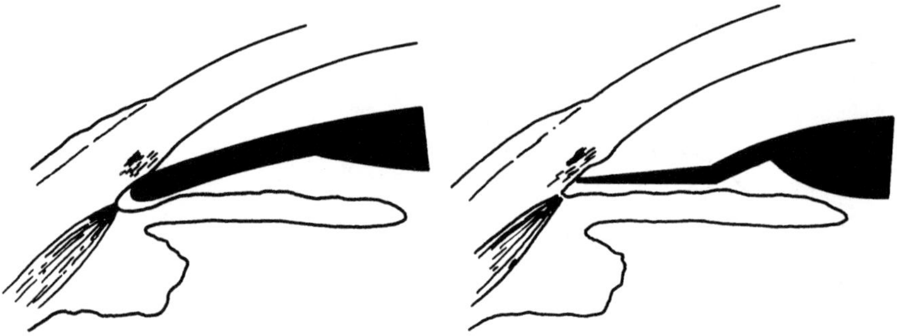

Fig. VIII-10. — The Choyce Mark I lens versus the Choyce Mark VIII lens. Note the differences in thickness and profile.

the posterior varies according to the required power. The length varies from 10.5 to 14 mm, and the width of the central portion is 6 mm (note: the length of an angle supported lens is the diameter of the circle that circumscribes the lens, see Fig. VIII-11). Colored haptics are available, and, for aphakic patients with various degrees of partial aniridia, two-loop external fixation implants can be obtained.

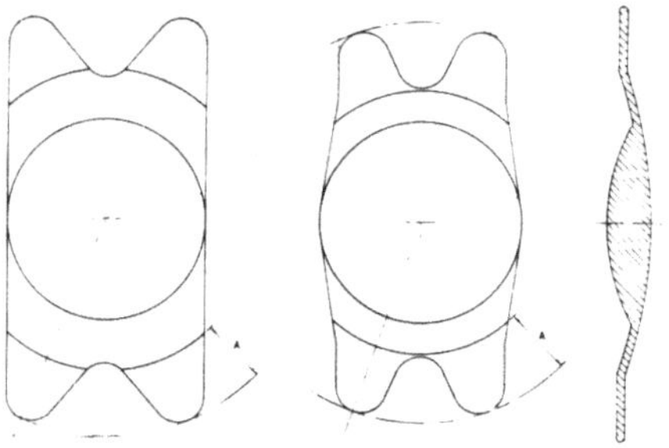

Fig. VIII-11. — The Choyce Mark VIII lens. Note: For angle supported lenses, the length of the lens is taken to be the diameter of the circle that circumscribes the lens.

Between 1963 and 1978, Choyce inserted about a thousand Mark VIII lenses using secondary procedures. In his opinion, the routine insertion of angle supported lenses during a second stage procedure is preferable to a combined procedure, that is, cataract extraction + lens implantation in the same session. He adduces the following reasons for this (1976):

— The refraction can be determined precisely, thus aiding selection of the correct power of the pseudophakos.
— The corrected visual acuity is known, so there is a target to aim at.

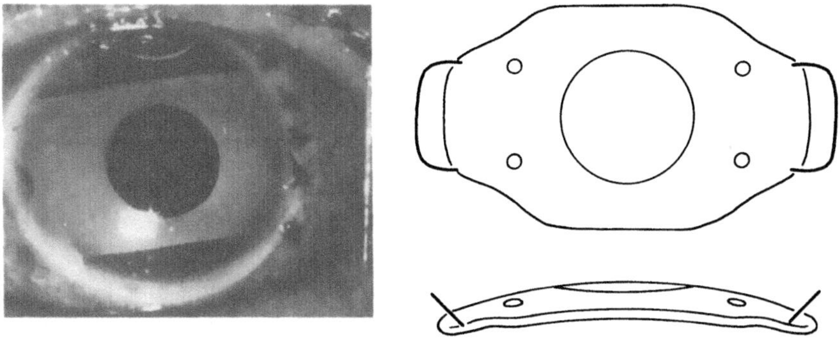

Fig. VIII-12a. — The Choyce Mark VIII lens with colored haptic in situ.
b. — The Choyce Mark VIII lens made for external fixation. (Courtesy D.P. Choyce.)

— The visual fields can be charted.
— Any intraocular pathology can be identified.

1. *Results and Complications with the Mark VIII: Choyce's Series*

Because differentiated data are lacking, we can only comment on the incidence of a few items. Additional data on complications and results had to be compiled from a report dealing with 1000 secondary Mark II—Mark VIII implantations (Choyce, 1977), which does not

TABLE VIII-5. — *Results and Complications in 800 Cases of Secondary Mark VIII Implantations by D.P. Choyce*

Author	D.P. Choyce (1976)
Surgeon	D.P. Choyce
Lens Type	Mark VIII, Choyce
Surgical Procedure	Secondary, Intracapsular
Number of Cases	800
Follow-Up	Average: 6 1/2 years
Corrected Visual Acuity ⩾20/40	N.A.
Endothelial Corneal Dystrophy (Bullous Keratopathy)	1.5%
Clinical Cystoid Macular Edema	N.A.
Retinal Detachment	1.5%
Iritis-Uveitis	N.A.
Internal Iris Prolapse	N.A.
Infection	0.125%
Dislocation	None
Glaucoma	N.A,
Implants removed	1%
Enucleation	None

N.A. = Not available.

enable us to assess properly the Mark VIII lens itself (see Table VIII-5).

Visual Acuity

According to Choyce (1977), the average pre-implantation corrected visual acuity for 1000 consecutive Mark II—Mark VIII implantations was 20/20. After secondary lens implantation, the average corrected visual acuity was 20/30. Comparing pre- and post-operative visual acuity, we may conclude that secondary implantation of an angle supported lens resulted in an average drop in visual acuity of 30%. About 3% of the eyes ended up with a visual acuity of less than 20/200.

Endothelial Corneal Dystrophy

Bullous keratopathy was reported to be 1.5%. This very low figure Choyce attributed to the special design of the Mark VIII lens, since the average anterior chamber depth is 2.85 mm. As shown on Table VIII-6, the Mark VIII lens has the lowest incidence of bullous keratopathy.

TABLE VIII-6. — *Endothelial Corneal Dystrophy Incidence for the Mark I to the Mark VIII Choyce Lenses (Choyce, 1976)*

	Number	*Average Follow-Up (Years)*	*Average Anterior Chamber Depth*	*Endothelial Corneal Dystrophy (bullous keratopathy)*
MarkI	100	19	1.68 mm	28%
Mark II-Mark VII	328	15	2.15 mm	7%
Mark VIII	800	6½	2.85 mm	1.5%

Iritis—Uveitis—Pupil Block

The exact incidence of these complications is unknown. We do know that the 3% incidence of lens removal of the thousand implantations (Mark II-Mark VIII) was due to hyphema or iritis (Choyce, 1977). Choyce (1978) noted that even after the Mark VIII was introduced, iritis, internal iris prolapse, and pupil block occasionally were problems.

Glaucoma

The average postoperative tension recorded in the thousand cases was 19 mm Hg and ranged from 8 to 40 mm Hg.

Cystoid Macular Edema

The exact incidence of this complication is not known, though it was reported as having occurred in some 6% of the 1000 lens implantations (Choyce, 1977).

Vitreous Loss

The exact incidence of vitreous loss in the 800 implantations of Mark VIII lenses is not known, but it was reported to have occurred in 7% of the 1000 Mark II-Mark VIII implantations.

On the basis of his extensive experience, Choyce reported that, although vitreous loss is always more likely to occur when a aphakic eye is reopened, this event is of minor importance. Indeed, in his opinion, the vitreous of an aphakic eye after intracapsular cataract extraction seems to change its character after being exposed to aqueous: it loses much of its tendency to adhere to adjacent structures and to cause persistent iritis. When vitreous loss did occur, it was not necessary to do a vigorous vitrectomy as in primary cases: cutting off the vitreous at the wound edge and inserting the lens proved to be all that was required to manage the situation.

Lens Removal

No reasons have been given for the 8 cases of removal of Mark VIII lenses.

2. *Evaluation by J. Pearce*

As he did in his study of C.D. Binkhorst's iris clip lens implants, J. Pearce examined 79 of Choyce's implants selected at random (see Table VIII-7). He published his results in February, 1975. This study of 11 Mark V-Mark VII lenses and 68 Mark VIII lenses is of major importance for the proper assessment of Choyce's results. Indeed, Choyce himself has often cited this report as representative of his own series.

TABLE VIII-7. — *Results of Pearce's Study of Lens Implantations Done by D.P. Choyce*

Author	J. Pearce (1975)
Surgeon	D.P. Choyce
Lens Types	11 Mark V-Mark VII 68 Mark VIII
Procedure	Intracapsular, secondary
Number of Cases	79
Follow-Up	Average: 5.5 years
Corrected Visual Acuity ⩾20/40	85%
Endothelial Corneal Dystrophy	
— Partial	13.2%
— Total (bullous)	1.3%
Clinical Cystoid Macular Edema	5.9%
Retinal Detachment	None
Tissue Reactions	
Uveitis	3%
Secondary Membrane	1.5%
Glaucoma (persistent)	9%
Vitreous Loss	7.3%

Visual Acuity

Corrected visual acuity of 20/40 or better was recorded in 58 cases (85%). Before implantation, the average visual acuity of the aphakic patients was 20/20; after, it was found to be 20/30. Thus the secondary implantation of a lens resulted in an average decrease of visual acuity of 30%, which confirms what was noted above.

Endothelial Corneal Dystrophy

Excluding 2 cases of Fuch's dystrophy and 1 case of pre-existing corneal dystrophy, Pearce noted an incidence of 1.3% (1 case) of total or bullous keratopathy, and 13.9% (9 cases) of partial keratopathy. Further deterioration into generalized ECD was expected in 2 cases.

Pearce observed that:

— The duration of the implantation seemed to be a common denominator in the cases of corneal change.

— The changes usually seemed to be related to an area overlying the feet of the implant (see Fig. VIII-13), although there was no corneal endothelial contact with the implant.

— Four cases had 1 or 2 tips of the implant lodged in the ciliary body.

— Three cases had free vitreous in the anterior chamber touching the endothelium and, in these cases, the average amount of peripheral anterior synechiae was 46%, well above the average of 30% for the entire series.

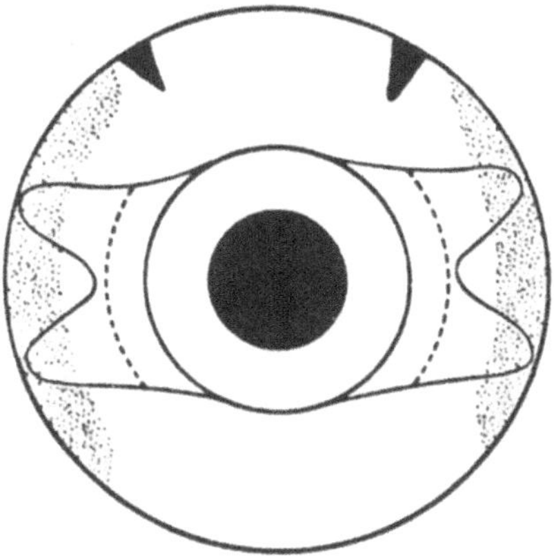

Fig. VIII-13. — Localized corneal dystrophy overlying the feet of a Choyce angle supported lens. (Courtesy J. Pearce.)

Macular Disorders

Senile macular degeneration was noted in 4 eyes and clinical macular edema in 4 others (6%).

Uveitis

Two eyes (3%) had suffered from severe uveitis, requiring systemic and topical steroids. In both cases, visual acuity was severely impaired.

Pathology of the Angle and Glaucoma

Using a gonioscope, Pearce found an average obturation of the angle by goniosynechiae of 30% (120°) resulting from both the lens extraction and the secondary implantation. The average intraocular pressure was 19 mm Hg and ranged from 8 to 40 mm Hg. Six cases evinced a persistent rise in intraocular pressure. In 5, more than 50% of the angle was found to be obturated by peripheral anterior synechiae. This figure is strikingly higher than the average of 30% of goniosynechiae over the entire series, which suggests a probable relationship between high intraocular pressure and angle pathology. Pearce suggested that implantation in a secondary procedure was probably responsible for additional formations of peripheral anterior synechiae.

Distortion of the Pupil

Oval pupils or elliptical distortion of the pupil in the meridian of insertion of the implant was noted in 17 eyes (21.5%). According to Pearce, such distortion was caused by pulling the iris over while inserting the implant. Apart from affecting the pupillary reaction to light and miotics, however, it has little visual significance.

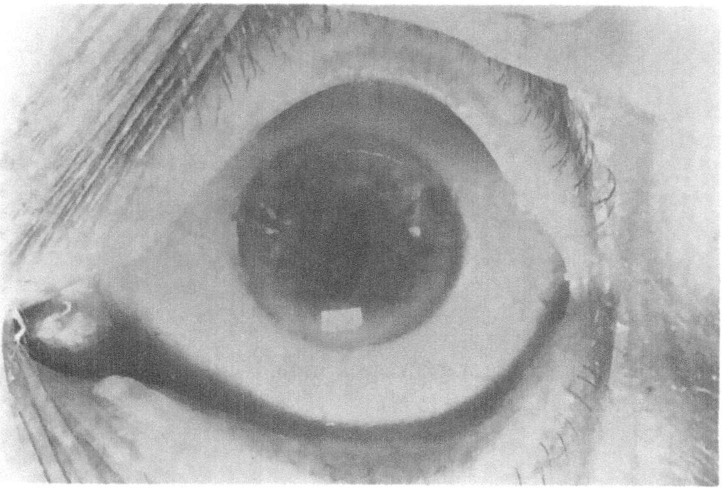

Fig. VIII-14. — Oval pupil with Choyce Mark VIII lens.

Although the small number of cases studied by Pearce does not permit statistical evaluation, we may conclude the following:
- Secondary implantation involves a considerable risk to visual acuity.
- The incidence of endothelial corneal dystrophy, partial and total, is significant.
- Reopening the anterior chamber and insertion of an anterior chamber lens enhances peripheral anterior synechiae formation, which may contribute to secondary glaucoma.
- Lens stability was good, no dislocations being reported.

3. *Conclusion*

After the developmental period during which many changes in the basic lens design were introduced, the Mark VIII was Choyce's preferred lens for 15 years. Provided the implant was of the proper length, the stability of the Mark VIII lens was significantly better than that of the earlier models. The incidence of bullous keratopathy was reduced and was reported to be 1.5%. The presence of vitreous in the anterior chamber before or during lens insertion never constituted a major problem.

Secondary implantation did involve risk to the final visual result, however, and, unfortunately, the exact underlying reasons for this could not be traced. Although the incidence of bullous keratopathy was only 1.5%, localized endothelial corneal dystrophy, mostly overlying the haptic feet, was reported in 13.5% of the cases (Pearce, 1975; Choyce, 1977). Another problem of major concern seems to have been the occurrence of clinical cystoid macular edema, which was probably present in 6% of the cases. No etiological information was reported. The presence of postoperative iritis and the occurrence of pupil block associated with internal iris prolapse were also occasional matters of concern.

After 15 years of experience with the Mark VIII lens, Choyce decided to improve the Mark VIII design, the primary reasons being the search for less iris tissue involvement, especially in a small anterior eye segment. So in order to provide more clearance between the lens surface and the iris, in 1978 Choyce designed the Mark IX, in which the central portion was moved forward. This decreased the depth of the anterior chamber slightly. We shall list the principal advantages of the Mark IX lens at the end of this chapter.

C. Secondary Implantations of the Choyce Mark VIII Lens by Other Surgeons

Although insertion of the Mark VIII lens in already aphakic eyes was not then considered a routine procedure, S. Harrison started using the Choyce lens in the United States in the early seventies. In 1978 at the American Intra-Ocular Implant Society meeting in Los Angeles, he reported on his long-term experience with 63 secondary implantations in both intracapsular and extracapsular aphakic conditions. J. Tennant (1977) also reported on 37 cases with a 1 year follow-up.

Even though some essential data are lacking, the following aspects of these two series (100 cases) deserve comment. The absence of endothelial corneal dystrophy is remarkable, especially in view of relatively long observation periods. The incidence of uveitis was

TABLE VIII-8. — *Results of Secondary Implantation of the Mark VIII Lens Obtained by Harrison and Tennant*

Author	S. Harrison *	J. Tennant (1977)
Surgeon	S. Harrison	J. Tennant
Type of Lens	Choyce Mark VIII	Choyce Mark VIII
Surgical Procedure	Intracapsular & Extracapsular Secondary	Intracapsular Secondary
Number of Cases	63	37
Follow-Up	7½ years maximum	1 year
Mean Age	N.A.	53
Corrected Visual Acuity ≥20/40	78%	67.8%
Endothelial Corneal Dystrophy	None	None
Cystoid Macular Edema (Clinical)	8% (5 cases)	2.7% (1 case)
Retinal Detachment	1.6% (1 case)	None
Tissue Reactions		
Iritis/Uveitis	1.6% (1 case)	None
Endophthalmitis	N.A.	None
Glaucoma (pupil block)	3% (2 cases)	None
Hemorrhage (hyphema)	N.A.	10.8% (4 cases)
Vitreous loss	N.A.	5.4% (2 cases)
Lens Removal	N.A.	None
Enucleation	N.A.	2.7% (1 case)

* Tape recorded, March 1978, Los Angeles meeting of AIOIS.
N.A. = Not available.

quite low, and the 4 cases of hemorrhaging that Tennant had were ascribed to initial errors in technique. In the opinion of these surgeons when secondary implantation after intracapsular cataract extraction is indicated, an angle supported lens may be recommended.

II. Primary Implantation

A. Primary Implantation of the Choyce Mark VIII Lens by D.P. Choyce

Since he was satisfied with the results he obtained with secondary implantation, it was only in 1970 that D.P. Choyce performed his first primary implantation. Seven years later, he reported on his first 50 primary Mark VIII implants (Choyce, 1977) (Table VIII-9).

The following points deserve comment. There was only 1 case of bullous keratopathy, 2 cases of clinical cystoid macular edema, and 3 cases where the lens had to be removed—once because of an error in refraction and twice because of iritis or hyphema.

Comparing the average times for recovery of the eye after primary versus secondary implantation, Choyce noted that after secondary

TABLE VIII-9. — *Results of Primary Implantation of the Mark VIII Lens*

Author	D.P. Choyce (1977)
Surgeon	D.P. Choyce
Type of Lens	Mark VIII
Surgical Procedure	Intracapsular (45) Extracapsular (5) Primary
Number of Cases	50
Average Follow-Up	3 years
Corrected Visual Acuity ⩾20/40	81%
Endothelial Corneal Dystrophy (Bullous Keratopathy)	2% (1 case)
Cystoid Macular Edema (Clinical)	4% (2 cases)
Retinal Detachment	N.A.
Tissue Reactions	
Internal Iris Prolapse	N.A.
Iritis/Uveitis	2% (1 case)
Glaucoma	N.A.
Hemorrhage	N.A.
Vitreous Loss	2% (1 case)
Lens Removal	6% (3 cases)

N.A. = Not available.

implantation the eye recovered more rapidly (8 weeks vs. 14 weeks). This led Choyce to conclude that, although no really significant difference in the final results was observed, in his hands secondary implantation of the Mark VIII lens is to be preferred.

B. Growing Interest in Primary Implantation of the Choyce Mark VIII Lens

The possibility of implanting the Choyce Mark VIII lens in a primary procedure attracted much attention since it had often been reported to be exceptionally stable and also suitable for implantation after the familiar technique of intracapsular cataract extraction.

In 1970, S. Harrison and J. Giovinco started primary implantation of the Mark VIII lens on a moderate scale in the United States. A national survey conducted by the American Intra-Ocular Implant Society revealed that, up to September 1975, only 18 Choyce anterior chamber lenses were reported to have been implanted, which was 0.15% of the 12,167 lens implantations that had been performed. At the Dallas meeting in 1975 of the AIOIS, J. Tennant, an enthusiastic proponent of Choyce's ideas, reported on the favorable results he had obtained with the Mark VIII lens. In view of his experience with Medallion lenses, he considered the anterior chamber lens much superior. The popularity of the Mark VIII lens grew.

To resolve a bothersome early postoperative complication—pupil block and internal iris prolapse—Tennant modified the original Mark VIII design. The new design had a forward-placed optic with a plano-convex configuration to minimize postoperative glaucoma and iris-lens synechiae (Fig. VIII-13) (Tennant, 1976).

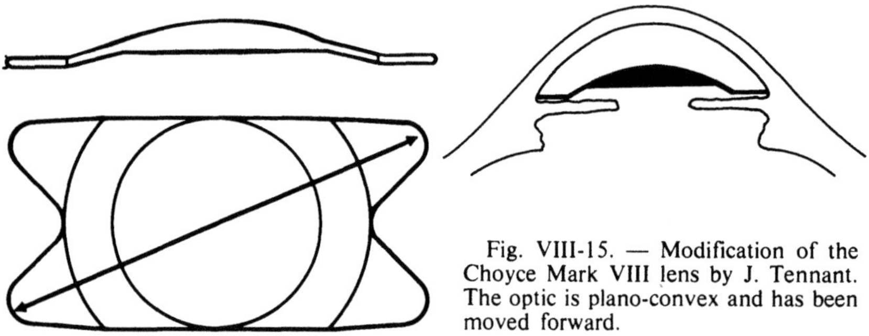

Fig. VIII-15. — Modification of the Choyce Mark VIII lens by J. Tennant. The optic is plano-convex and has been moved forward.

In 1976, Tennant published a manual, *A Lens for All Seasons,* describing all the aspects of inserting the Mark VIII lens. A demand subsequently developed that the original manufacturer of the Mark VIII lens, Rayner, could not meet. American implant manufacturers entered the market and began mass production of these lenses, using different processes and even different raw materials.

Most of the postoperative complications that then developed from these "Choyce-style" lenses could be attributed to improper manufacturing. These problems were a high incidence of recurrent hyphema, severe uveitis with possibly related cystoid macular edema, and secondary glaucoma.

C. **Data on Primary Implantation of the Choyce Mark VIII Lens by Other Surgeons**

We have compiled the results published by R. Azar (1978), J. Tennant (1976), and S. Harrison (1978) and so have data on over a thousand primary implantations of the Mark VIII lens. Most of them were supplied by Rayner's, the original manufacturer.

As can be concluded from the figures given on Table VIII-10, endothelial corneal dystrophy was never a problem, and the incidence of uveal reactions was low. The rate of internal iris prolapse was reported only by Azar, and this at 3%. Even though Tennant often referred to the problem of internal iris prolapse in his manual, and even though it was the main reason for producing a modified

TABLE VIII-10. — *Results of Primary Implantations of the Mark VIII Lens*

Author	J. Tennant (1976)		R.F. Azar (1978)	S. Harrison (1978) *	
Surgeon	J. Tennant		R.F. Azar	S. Harrison	
Type of Lens	Mark VIII		Mark VIII	Mark VIII	
Origin	Rayner		Rayner	N.A.	
Surgical Procedure	Primary		N.A.	Primary	
	Intracap.	Extracap.		Intracap.	Extracap.
Number of Cases	133	27	800	63	39
Average Follow-Up	1 year	1 year	3 years	$7\frac{1}{2}$ years maximum	
Corrected Visual Acuity ⩾20/40	79%	67%	N.A.	86%	
Endothelial Corneal Dystrophy	0.75%	None	None	None	
Cystoid Macular Edema (clinical)	0.75%	3.7%	2.5%	5%	
Retinal Detachment	N.A.	N.A.	None	None	
Tissue Reactions					
Iritis/Uveitis	0.75%	11%	2%	2%	
Endophthalmitis	None	None	None	N.A.	
Dislocation	0.75%	None	None	N.A.	
Glaucoma	None	None	0.7%	3%	
Hemorrhage	3%	3.7	2%	3%	
Vitreous Loss	6%	14.8%	N.A.	N.A.	
Lens Exchange	None	None	N.A.	N.A.	
Removal	0.75	None	0.3%	N.A.	
Enucleation	None	None	N.A.	N.A.	
Internal Iris Prolapse	N.A.	N.A.	3%	N.A.	

* Tape recorded at the March 1978 meeting of the AIOIS at Los Angeles.
N.A. = Not available.

version of the Mark VIII lens, he did not give the exact incidence in his series. The reasons for the 2% to 3% incidence of postoperative hyphema were not given. All three authors found it to be a stable lens, provided the exact length was chosen. It would perhaps be gratuitous to conclude that these surgeons were wholly pleased with the Mark VIII, since Tennant modified it to reduce the postoperative incidence of iris-lens synechiae and glaucoma, and Azar introduced a tripoid angle supported lens that, in this opinion, is easier and safer to insert as well as being more stable.

In 1979, R.P. Kratz et al. (1979) reported on the results they obtained with 215 Choyce-Rayner Mark VIII anterior chamber lenses. They were inserted in primary procedures in about an equal proportion of intracapsular and extracapsular cataract extractions. The follow-up periods ranged from 3 months to 5 years (see chapter IX). There were no cases of endothelial corneal dystrophy nor were there any problems with lens stability.

There was an incidence of postoperative uveitis of more than 5%, which could be adequately managed with steroids. Clinical cystoid edema occurred in 8.4% of the cases, and hyphema was observed in 6.4%. The authors ascribe the hemorrhaging not to poorly finished or to long lenses, but to minimal trauma inflicted on the trabecular meshwork at the time of insertion (4.7%) or in the late postoperative period (1.4%).

Comparing these results with those obtained with other lenses (iris clip, iridocapsular, Shearing), Kratz et al. noted that, in spite of its remarkable stability, the Mark VIII does have a number of problems that do not encumber other lens designs.

III. The Principal Problems with the Choyce Mark VIII Lens as Reported between 1976 and 1978

In late 1976, sporadic cases of severe uveitis were reported to the American Intra-Ocular Implant Society by a considerable number of surgeons who had implanted Mark VIII lenses manufactured by McGhan, an American implant manufacturer.

In May 1977, several cases of severe complications were reported for Mark VIII lenses that had been made by another American manufacturer, Surgidev. The complications reported to the AIOIS included early and late iritis, uncontrolled high intraocular pressure

(30-77 mm Hg), recurrent sputtering hyphema, and massive hyphemas as late as 6 to 8 months after the operation (Ellingson, 1977; Azar, 1978).

Gradually, these unusual findings were recognized as being part of a typical syndrome, the UGH syndrome: uveitis, glaucoma, and hyphema. In the literature, this is sometimes referred to as the Ellingson syndrome. Its exact incidence remains unknown.

The severity of the UGH syndrome after insertion of Mark VIII style lenses supplied by various manufacturers can be determined from the data given on Table VIII-11. Out of a total of 493 implants, the UGH incidence was 15%. In more than half of the UGH cases, the lenses had to be removed.

TABLE VIII-11. — *Uveitis-Glaucoma-Hyphema Syndrome with the Mark VIII lens by Surgeon and Manufacturer*

Surgeon	*Manufacturer*	*Number Implanted*	*UGH Syndrome*	*Lenses Explanted*
Choyce (1977)	Rayner	50	≥2	2
(1978)	Surgidev	16	≥2	2
	McGhan	30	≥4	4
Ellingson (1978)	Surgidev	11	9	7
	Iolab	47	5	2
Azar (1978)	Surgidev	27	≥4	4
Kratz* (1978)	Surgidev	40	11	5
	Rayner	220	12	2
Brodstein (1978)	Surgidev	23	15	7
De Haven (1978)	Iolab	29	11	4
	Total	493	75	39
	Percentage	100%	15%	8%

* Tape recorded at AIOIS Meeting, March 1978, Los Angeles.

A. Clinical Findings Concerning the UGH Syndrome

The onset of the clinical picture has been reported to occur at about 10-12 weeks after the implantation, though some cases were reported to commence as much as 6 months later.

Iris changes were noted along the course of the lens, especially along the posterior edges. These changes varied from mild erosion of the superficial layer to fairly deep grooves. Ragged tufts and strands of stroma were occasionally observed partially floating in the anterior chamber. When iris vessels were involved, blood seepage, even followed by intractable hemorrhaging, was often observed (Keates and

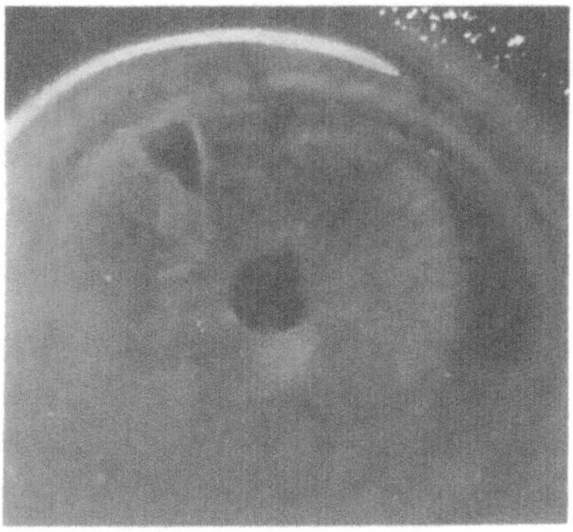

Fig. VIII-16. — Erosion of the iris stroma by the posterior edge of a Choyce-style lens, afterwards removed. (Courtesy R. Kratz.)

Kratz, 1978; Brodstein, 1978; Gowan, 1978; De Haven, 1978; Kline, 1978; Moore and Steller, 1978; Keats, 1979).

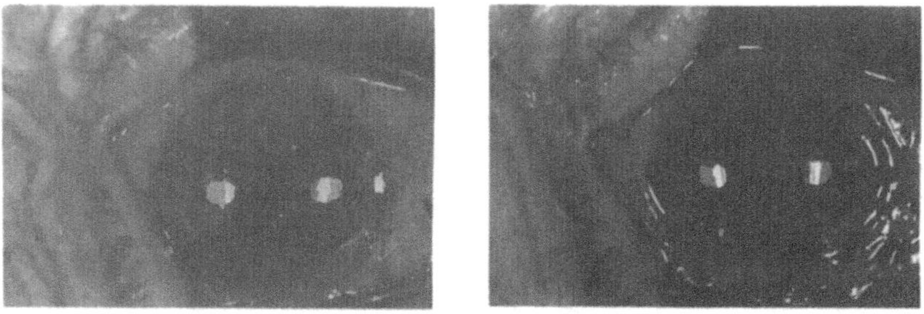

Fig. VIII-17. — Hyphema caused by a Choyce-style lens. (Courtesy J. Alpar.)

Gonioscopic examination revealed that sometimes the footplates of the lens were no longer behind the scleral spur but had warped out. When the warped footplates impinged on the angle structures, the resulting irritation of the sensitive vascular structure was often followed by hemorrhaging. In addition, chronic postoperative uveitis associated with precipitates on the lens surface became apparent when the footplates distorted the iris or the ciliary body (Ellingson, 1977, 1978; Azar, 1978).

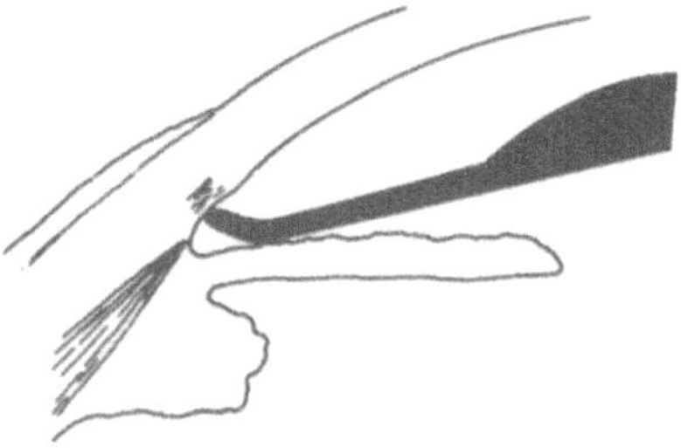

Fig. VIII-18. — Warped footplate of a Choyce-style lens impinging on the angle structure.

Cystoid macular edema was frequently associated with the UGH syndrome (Ellingson, 1978). Vitritis was also observed (Moore and Steller 1978).

Cases of severe secondary glaucoma were reported in association with uveitis or hemorrhaging.

B. Treatment of the UGH Syndrome

In mild cases, a conservative approach sufficed (specific treatment of the uveitis or hypertension). However, in severe cases of recurrent hyphemas, recalcitrant uveitis, and intractable glaucoma, the lens had to be removed (see Table VIII-11). This was reported to be very effective. Ellingson reported that all of his cases of UGH syndrome were reversed and the eye quieted down without medication after about 2 months after the removal of the offending lens. Similar observations by other surgeons are common. Choyce stated in his 1978 Ridley Lecture, however, that once the UGH syndrome is well established, lens removal was not always sufficient to bring it under control.

C. Etiology of the UGH Syndrome

1. *The Lens*

Table VIII-12 gives the defects discovered in lenses that had to be removed because of the UGH Syndrome.

TABLE VIII-12. — *Manufacturing Defects in Mark VIII Lenses Removed because of the UGH Syndrome*

Surgeon	*Lens Origin*	*Number Removed*	*Lens Defect*
Ellingson	Surgidev	7	Significant warpage
	Iolab	2	Rough edges in the middle portion of the optic
	McGhan	1	Warpage
Kratz	Surgidev	5	"Razor blade" sharp posterior edges
De Haven	Iolab	4	The posterior edges of lens around the optic area were very rough and sometimes almost sawtoothed
Brodstein	Surgidev	7	Irregularities in the posterior edges
Shepard	Surgidev	1	Warpage

a. *Warpage*

The first mechanism suggested by Ellingson (1977) as a cause of the UGH syndrome was warpage of the tips of the footplates: one or more of the tips curled forward. This was the case with the 7 lenses that Ellingson removed. It has been suggested (Hubbell, Tennant, Roy, personal communications, 1978) that the warped lenses could have been delivered that way from the manufacturer. However, several lenses that had been carefully inspected before surgery and did not show any warpage did manifest this defect after removal from the eye. Therefore, the warping must have occurred in situ.

Precisely how a warped footplate induces UGH is still a matter of speculation. Tilting of the lens, which may alter the iris-lens relationship, pressure upon the angle structures with subsequent distortion, and irritation or atrophy of adjacent structures such as the iris base, the ciliary body, and the trabecular meshwork, are possibilities that have yet to be confirmed by anatomopathological studies.

The cause of the warpage is also controverted. Ellingson (1977) has suggested that the cause could be molecular stress within the lens. And there could have been residual internal strain, especially in injection molded lenses. Such deformation is common in plastic materials in certain conditions. However, polarized light studies of 7 lenses failed to confirm this hypothesis (Ellingson, 1978). Another possible explanation for warpage in situ is that the footplate is deformed by the continuous pressure exerted on the lens by the sclera.

b. *Improper Finishing*

There is evidence that sharp edges and poorly polished areas along the posterior surface of the lens were responsible for iris erosion (Table VIII-12). Keates and Kratz have postulated that the superficial shaving of iris tissue caused by the sharp posterior lens edges induced uveites, and deeper shaving into the iris stroma brought on hemorrhaging. Kratz also noted that the shaving effect was more pronounced in intracapsular cases than extracapsular ones, and, on the basis of his experience with 313 anterior chamber lens implantations, stressed the influence of iridodonesis in the UGH syndrome (Kratz, 1978). In his judgment, the lens capsule contributed a great deal to stabilizing the iris diaphragm. After extracapsular extraction, excessive rubbing against the sharp edges would be markedly reduced, thus accounting for the significant decrease in the incidence of UGH.

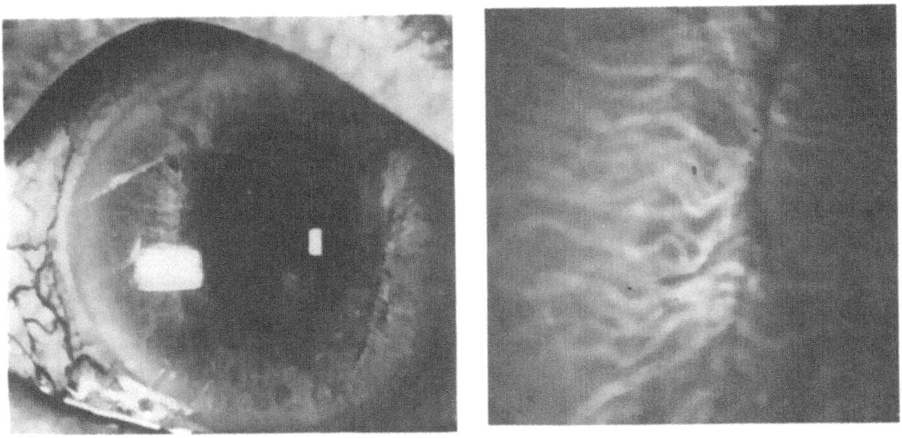

Fig. VIII-19. — View of a lacerated iris caused by a Choyce-style lens (removed): low magnification (left) high magnification (right). (From *AIOIS J.* IV 189, 1978).

Choyce has always insisted on the vital importance of properly finishing anterior chamber lenses. The smoothness and roundness of the feet and edges are crucial lest the eye be injured. Injection-molded lenses may had particular problems in this regard. With this particular manufacturing process, special care has to be taken in polishing the lens perimeter lest sharp edges and various other irregularities such as lips and nipple-like projections remain on the lens.

c. *Materials and Sterilization*

This is the most uncertain of the hypotheses. Some authors have suggested that the material itself degrades, i.e., depolymerization occurs subsequent to injection molding, or that there is a toxic effect caused by decomposition of the additives, such as the azocatalyst used as initiator in the Rohm and Haas polymethylmethacrylate. But the presence of toxic elements has not yet been demonstrated (Choyce, 1978).

Unlike the original Mark VIII lenses manufactured by Rayner, which were sterilized by Ridley's wet method, most of the lenses involved in the UGH syndrome were dry-packed and sterilized with ethylene oxide.

Choyce classified the different Mark VIII lenses to clarify the manufacturing defects. This classification is given on Table VIII-13. From the reports on the faulty lenses, the Type C lenses had the highest incidence of involvement in the UGH syndrome (see Fig. VIII-20).

TABLE VIII-13

	Type A	*Type B*	*Type C*
Material	Perspex CQ	Perspex CQ	Rohm & Haas
Catalyst	Peroxide	Peroxide	Azo catalyst
Raw Material	Sheets	Sheets	Pellets
Processing	Milled Compress. molded Hand polished	Milled Compress. molded Hand polished	Injection molded
Sterilization (up to 1978)	Wet (Caustic Soda)	Dry (ethylene oxide)	Dry (ethylene oxide)
Manufacturer	Rayner	Cilco Precision-Cosmet Intermedics	McGhan Surgidev Iolab

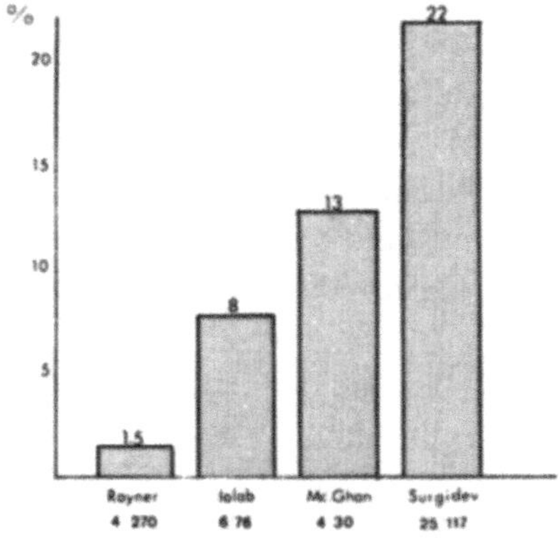

Fig. VIII-20. — Percentage of lenses removed because of the UGH syndrome in relation to the number of lenses implanted produced by various manufacturers.

2. *Poor Surgical Judgment and Poor Surgical Technique*

Insertion of a lens that is too long can cause trauma in the eye. C.J. Zobian and J.W. Beem (1977) demonstrated with gonioscopy that the supports of an overlong lens push the iris back and rest on the ciliary body. Such patients have a high incidence of uveitis and require more steroids. In a few cases, these authors discovered red cells in the anterior chamber, but so far they have not encountered a case serious enough to warrant removal of the lens.

D.L. Praeger (1977) reported that if the lens is even slightly longer than necessary, a sharp haptic portion will erode through the iris and probably cause recurrent microhyphema with persistent uveitis that require removal of the lens.

The footplates of the lens should be placed on the sclera just behind the scleral spur where they will remain parallel to the iris. If they are placed into the trabecular meshwork, progressive dialysis of the angle may be followed by hemorrhaging. If they are placed into the iris or the ciliary body, recurrent postoperative uveitis will occur (Ellingson, 1977).

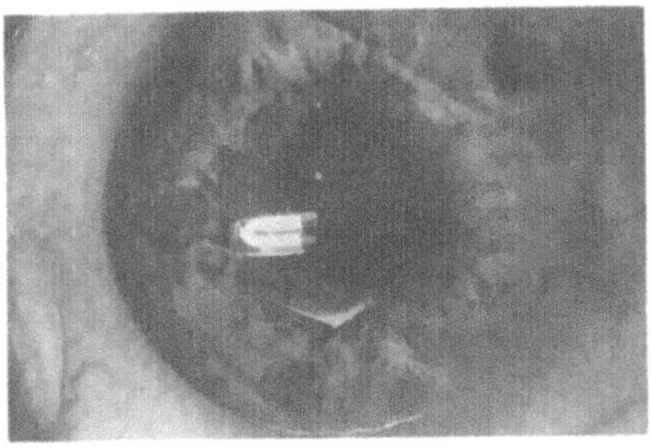

Fig. VIII-21. — Iridodialysis with an angle supported lens resulting in subluxation of the implant. (Courtesy M. Kraff.)

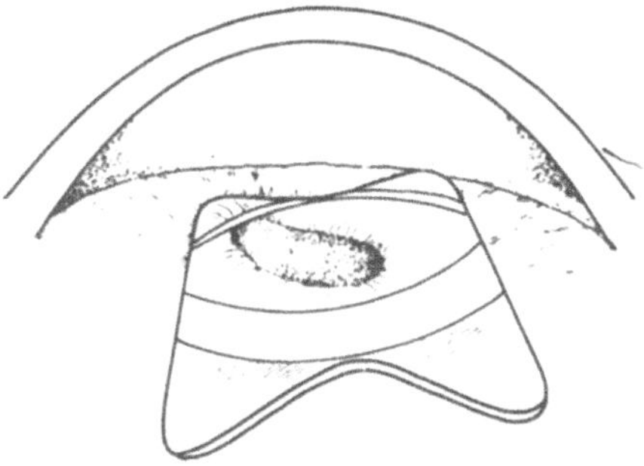

Fig. VIII-22. — Schema illustrating the tip of an angle supported lens impinging on the iris root.

Among the local adverse conditions predisposing to excessive iris contact is a shallow anterior chamber. Some general factors, such as diabetes and hemorrhagic diathesis, also predispose to sputtering hyphema (Azar, 1978).

Conclusion on the UGH Syndrome

There is sufficient evidence to suspect that manufacturing flaws are the primary cause of the UGH syndrome. But poor surgical judgment and faulty technique, even when the lens has been well-designed and properly manufactured, may give rise to minor or major postoperative complications that develop into uveitis, glaucoma, and hyphema.

IV. The Choyce Mark IX Lens

In 1978, D.P. Choyce launched the Mark IX lens as the successor to the Mark VIII. The following discussion is based largely on the Ridley Lecture delivered by Choyce in Japan in 1978.

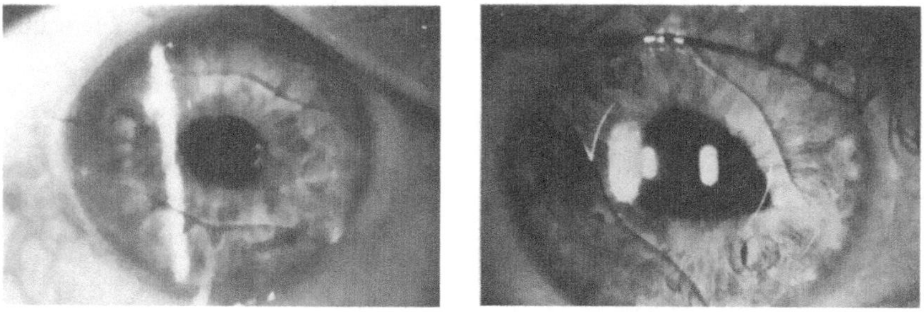

Fig. VIII-23. — The Choyce Mark IX lens. (Courtesy D.P. Choyce.)

A. Limitations of the Mark VIII

— The Mark VIII was not as stable in children's eyes as was expected. Later trauma can shift the implant fractionally and tear the iris root causing serious bleeding into the anterior chamber.
— It was also found to yield less favorable results than expected in small anterior eye segments.
— Problems occurred when the Mark VIII was inserted in a primary procedure following planned extracapsular cataract extraction or phacoemulsification.
— Other occasional complications were:
  - Pupil block causing prolapse of the iris in front of the implant;
  - Slight decentration from the visual axis;
  - A foot getting trapped in one of the iris openings.
— Finally, maintaining a stock of anterior chamber lenses of different lengths was felt to be an expensive nuisance.

B. Description of the Mark IX Lens

Like the Mark VIII, the Mark IX lens is a one-piece, one-material (Perspex CQ), quadripedal, anterior chamber lens. It differs from the Rayner-Choyce Mark VIII model in the following respects:

1. Two widths are available: 4 mm and 5 mm.
2. The top and bottom edges are smoothly scalloped to a maximum depth of 0.5 mm between the tips of the feet and the widest portion of the optic.
3. The indentation (dovetail or crotch) between each pair of feet is 0.5 mm for all lengths.
4. There are two holes 1 mm in diameter in the vaulted area between the foot portion and the optic.
5. The four feet are flattened, the extent being
   1.75 mm for the 11.0, 11.5, and 12.0 mm lengths;
   2.00 mm for the 12.5 and 13.0 mm lengths;
   2.25 mm for the 13.5 and 14.0 mm lengths.
6. The optic comes in 3 configurations: biconvex, convexo-plano with a plane posterior surface, and plano-convex with a plane anterior surface. As with the Mark VIII, the lengths range from 11.0 to 14.0 mm in 0.5 mm steps, and the optical powers in aqueous range from +14 to +24 D in 2 D steps.

There are no plans for making the Mark IX with colored haptics.

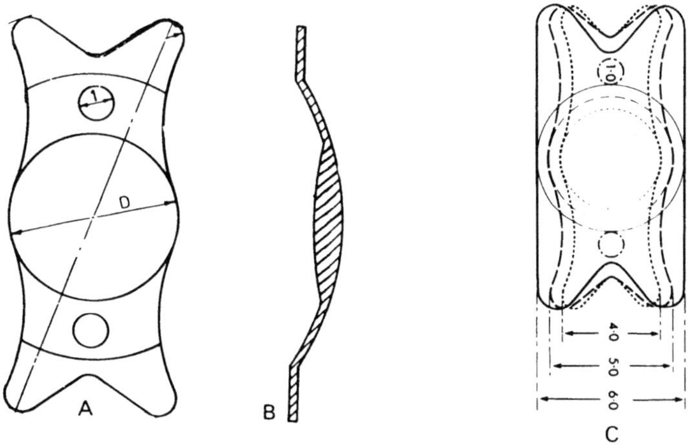

Fig. VIII-24. — The Choyce Mark IX lens.

C. Advantages of the Mark IX over the Mark VIII

1. The internal opening of the incision required for lens insertion is smaller: 5 and 6 mm for the 4 and 5 mm widths respectively.

2. The narrower width is intended for extracapsular extraction particularly after phacoemulsification (small incision)—and for eyes with a small anterior segment.
3. Access to the posterior capsule to perform a capsulotomy is easier.
4. Maintaining the anterior chamber with air is easier with the smaller incision.
5. Insertion of the lens is easier because of the decreased danger of "spearing" the iris.
6. The two 1 mm diameter holes in the haptic have several functions:
   a. They facilitate circulation of aqueous.
   b. They make centration of the lens easier as the tip of a spatula can be inserted into a hole in order to guide the lens.
   c. Translimbal fixation sutures can be placed through them (Fig. VIII-25).

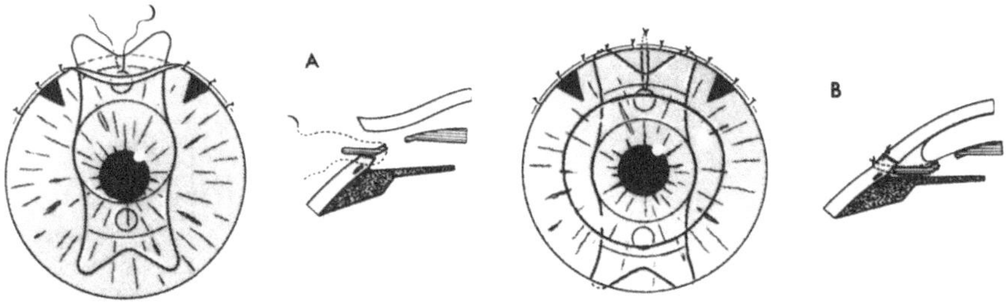

Fig. VIII-25. — Translimbal fixation of the Choyce Mark IX implant.

7. The scalloping of the upper and lower edges reduces the risk of pupil block.
8. While some degree of postoperative dilation of the pupil is still necessary, it need not exceed 5/6 mm and may be discontinued sooner.
9. Less foreign material is introduced into the eye: the implant takes up less room and weighs less.

Pilot studies have indicated that both the 4 mm and the 5 mm versions are just as stable as the Mark VIII. As already mentioned, the Mark IX might well be better for young children, and also adults if there are large iridectomies close to the resting place of one or more feet. Indeed, in these cases lens stabilitv can be enhanced by using translimbal fixation (8/0 nylon). In addition if during surgery it is found that a lens 0.5 mm longer than the one available is needed, the short lens may be sutured without ill effect.

Since only preliminary reports on the Mark IX are available at this time, we cannot evaluate the results and expected advantages.

V. Surgical Technique

A. Choyce's Method of Secondary Implantation
(Choyce 1976, 1977, 1978)

The pupil is routinely kept in miosis with 4% Pilocarpine eyedrops starting the night before surgery. Before opening the anterior chamber, a light cautery barrage is laid down to seal off the limbal incision. A corneal scleral section is made with a Graefe knife from 7 to 11 o'clock in the right eye and from 1 to 5 o'clock in the left eye. If necessary, the anterior chamber is reinflated with saline or air, and any peripheral anterior synechiae are separated with a blunt spatula. The lens is held with the special forceps at the haptic portion and slipped into the anterior chamber. During this maneuver, it is prudent to point the tip of the implant slightly towards 6 o'clock to keep it away from the pupil. When the distal feet of the implant have passed towards the nasal limbus, the assistant should place the tip of a repositor between the proximal feet of the implant to steady it while the forceps are removed. To introduce the proximal feet into the angle, the outer scleral lip of the incision is gently grasped with fine-toothed forceps and pulled outwards and slightly upwards while gentle pressure is applied on one foot of the implant with an iris repositor. The same procedure is repeated for the other foot. It is usually obvious when the feet are safely inside the anterior chamber and resting snugly in the angle.

Then, if no adverse conditions are present, the incision is closed. Should the iris bulge, it is released by additional iridectomies either between the proximal feet of the implant or inferiorly in the 6 o'clock iris sector.

Choyce routinely orders 40 mg triamcinolone I.M. prior to surgery and administers a sub-conjunctival injection of Gentamycine after.

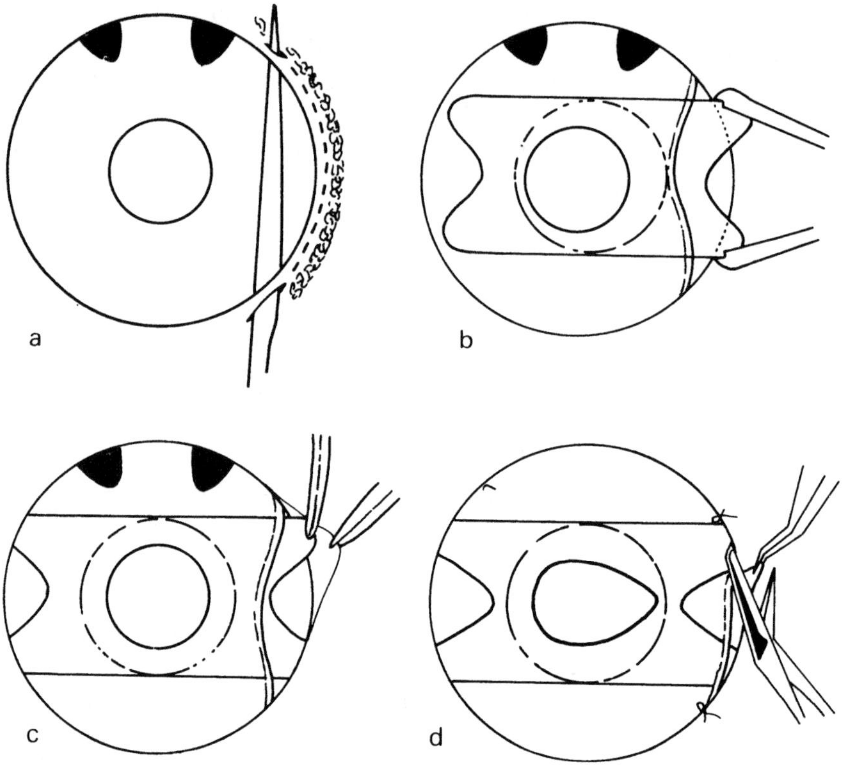

Fig. VIII-26. — Steps in the secondary implantation of the Choyce Mark VIII lens:

a) temporal incision with a Graefe's knife;
b) insertion of the lens using the Choyce 135° forceps;
c) maneuver for inserting the proximal foot;
d) additional iridectomy between the proximal feet.

Choyce strongly recommends a temporal incision and a horizontal or slightly oblique positioning of the implant for the following reasons:

— Ease of access: vertical insertion is more difficult because of the upper eyelid and the eyebrow.
— Astigmatism resulting from the conventional, 3 to 9 o'clock cataract incision usually leaves a degree of with-the-rule astigmatism which will be largely canceled out by a temporal incision.
— It is desirable to avoid reopening the previous cataract incision.

B. Choyce's Method of Primary Implantation

A 180° section is made diagonally from 10:30 to 4:30 o'clock in the left eye or from 7:30 to 1:30 in the right eye. A Graefe knife is used and, if necessary, the incision is enlarged with a corneal scissors. No conjunctival flaps are cut. Two peripheral iridectomies or, if the circumstances indicate, a sector iridectomy may be performed. Usually, two sutures are placed at 11 and 1 o'clock.

After delivery of the lens, either intracapsularly or extracapsularly, the incision is partially closed leaving an 8 mm opening temporally, and pilocarpine 4% drops are started on the cornea. The insertion of the implant either horizontally or diagonally is done in the usual manner. A clear haptic implant is used if a round pupil extraction has been performed, and an implant with a colored haptic is used with a sector iridectomy. The anterior chamber is kept reformed while the incision is closed. Tennant, along with most of the surgeons who use angle supported lenses, inserts the implant vertically from 12 to 6 o'clock, making peripheral iridectomies at 10 and 2 o'clock.

C. Additional Guidelines on the Proper Technical Management of Angle Supported Lenses

1. *Lens Inspection*

Before the lens is inserted, it must be inspected for the following:

a. *Length*

To confirm the length on the label, the implant is measured with a ruler and the overall diagonal length is noted.

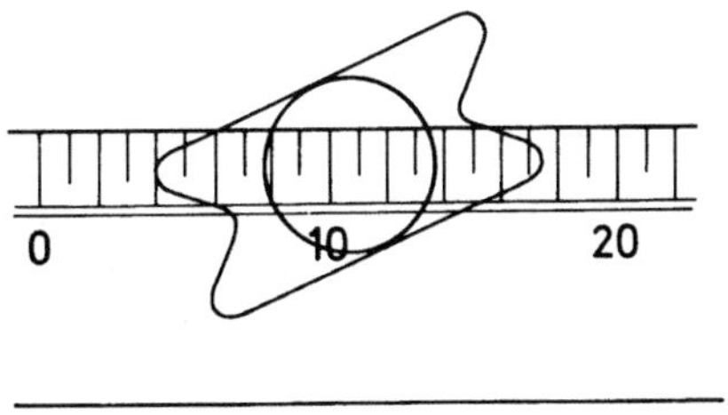

Fig. VIII-27. — Method for checking the overall length of the implant.

b. *Defects in Manufacture*

The Rocking Test (Ellingson, 1977): The lens is placed on a flat surface and each of the four feet is pressed in turn with a blunt instrument. If all four feet are in the same plane, the lens will not rock. If there is any warpage, it will.

Fig. VIII-28. — The rocking test.

The Edge Finish (Ellingson, 1978): Each lens should be inspected with the operating microscope set at large magnification. All the edges must be smooth and well-rounded.

Any defective lens should, of course, be rejected.

2. *Determination of the Lens Length*

Determining the length is a matter of special concern for a rigid, fixed length, anterior chamber lens. Indeed, if it is too short, it will spindle around and damage the endothelium; if it is too long, pressure will be exerted on the angle structures and cause distortion of the pupil and possible iridodialysis, hemorrhaging, uveitis, and pain.

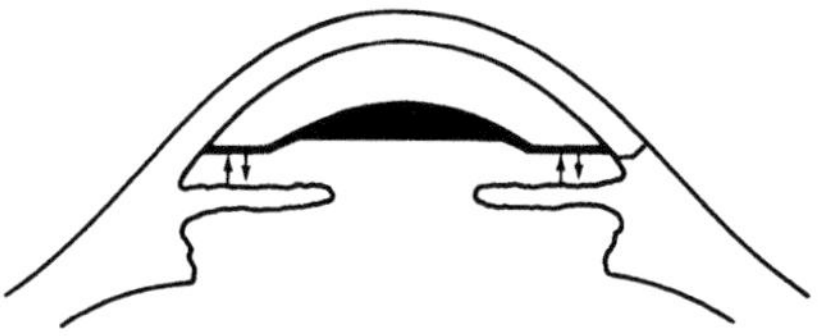

Fig. VIII-29. — Illustration of lens mobility when the lens is too short. (Based on J. Tennant, 1976.)

a. *Preoperative Estimation of the Length*

The Mark VIII lens is designed to fit behind the scleral spur. From experience, it has been found that the proper length for the lens is the diameter of the scleral spur plus approximately 1 millimeter. It has been demonstrated anatomically (Kasner, 1976) and goniometrically in vivo (Worst, 1976) that the scleral spur is directly under the limbus at 3 and 9 o'clock. Therefore, the diameter of the scleral spur can be determined by measuring the horizontal diameter of the cornea from white-to-white. A lens 1 mm longer than this is the proper size in over 90% of the cases. Even though the anatomy of the external limbus is oval, the internal limbus is circular. Theoretically, therefore, the lens may be placed on any axis.

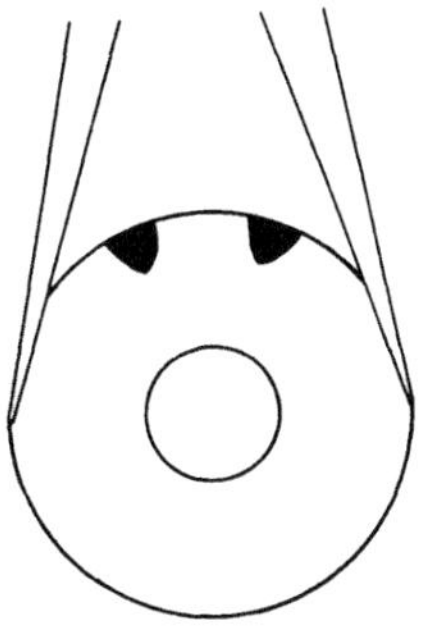

Fig. VIII-30. — Measurement of the horizontal corneal diameter from white-to-white.

K. Buol Heslin (1979) dissected 20 cadaveric eyes and reported some variation between the real diameter of the internal scleral ring and the predicted value according to the white-to-white plus one millimeter rule. As shown on Table VIII-14, the predictions tend to fall slightly short.

TABLE VIII-14. — *Variation of Direct Cadaver Measurements from White-to-White Plus One Estimates of Anterior Chamber Diameters (K- Buol Heslin (1979))*

Number of Cases	*Variation in mm*
1	−0.25
1	−0.10
7	0.00
1	+0.10
2	+0,20
2	+0,40
3	+0,50
1	+0,70
1	+0,80
1	+1.20
20	

Analyzing the length of a hundred of his last implants and excluding 4 congenital cataract cases associated with microphthalmia, Choyce calculated the frequencies given on Table VIII-15. Thus the 12.0, 12.5, and 13.0 mm lengths are used roughly in the proportion of 1:2:1.

TABLE VIII-15. — *Lens Length Frequencies for 100 Mark VIII Implants (Choyce, 1978)*

Number of cases	*Length in mm*
2	11.5
25	12.0
50	12.5
22	13.0
1	13.5

In Choyce's opinion, any surgeon who finds that he is using more of the longer implants than this should examine his technique very closely, the suggesting being that he is erring on the side of excessive length. Choyce considers the ideal length to be just not too short, and he decries what he sees as the current tendency to implant longer lenses.

C. Kelman (personal communication, 1979) and J. Worst (personal communication 1979) are investigating the possibilities to construct an optical device to measure the internal diameter of the scleral ring prior to surgery. This device will probably be of help in solving one of the major problems of fixed length angle supported lenses.

b. *Peroperative Estimation of Lens Length*

Dip Stick Method of C. Kelman

An irrigating spatula graduated in 0.5 mm intervals is used as a dip stick to measure the internal anterior chamber diameter.
After delivery of the lens, the spatula is moved across the anterior chamber to the opposite angle until resistence is met. The reading is taken at the point of the pupillary aperture that is estimated to be the center. This reading is then doubled to obtain the diameter of the internal anterior chamber diameter.

Unfortunately, small measurement errors are always possible because of parallax and false estimates.

K. Buol Hesling (1979) compared peroperative dip stick measurements with preoperative white-to-white plus one estimates in fifty

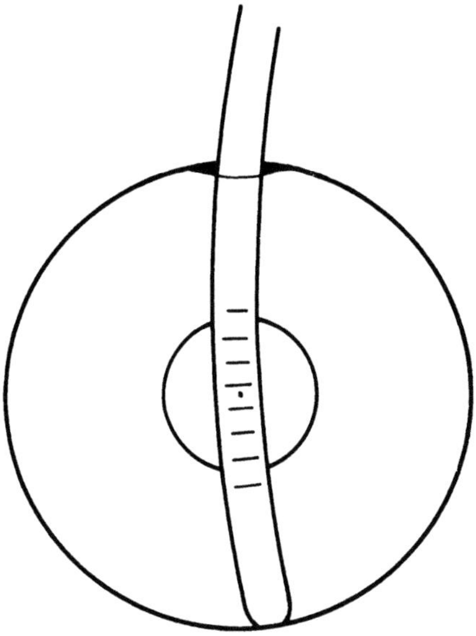

Fig. VIII-31. — The dip stick method for determining the length of the implant.

cases. As shown on Table VIII-16, he found a tendency for the dip stick method to produce slightly longer measurements than could be predicted with the white-to-white plus one rule.

TABLE VIII-16. — Variations of Dip Stick Measurements from White-to-White Plus One Estimates of the Anterior Chamber Diameter (K. Buol Heslin (1979))

Number of Cases	*Variation in mm*
1	−1.00
1	−0.75
1	−0,50
3	−0.20
1	−0,10
20	0.00
3	+0.20
1	+0,30
9	+0.50
1	+0.60
2	+0.70
5	+1.00
1	+1.10
1	+1.50
50	

Clearance of the Scleral Arch

If the incision is made at the junction of the white and the blue, about 1 mm of the proximal lens feet should extend from the wound after the distal feet are inserted.

An additional guide is offered by the scleral arch that is formed when the sclera is pulled back to allow the insertion of the proximal foot. Indeed, this arch should just circumscribe the foot so that only minimal pressure is required to insert the tip of the lens. If the lens is too long, the sclera cannot be pulled hard enough to bring the arch over the foot. If the lens is too short, the foot will drop too easily into the scleral arch.

Nudge Test (Tennant, 1976)

The nudge test indicates whether the lens is too short or not. Before the eye is closed, the cornea is lifted and a small instrument is placed into the crotch of the lens. When the lens is nudged gently, it should only move very slightly. If it is too short, the proximal foot will come into view from beneath the edge of the incision, and it must be replaced by a lens 1 mm longer.

Rotation test (Shepard, personal communication, 1978; Keates, 1979)

With the anterior chamber already restored with fluid, the lens is rotated over a half an hour of circumference. If it remains in the new position, it is too short and will later spin in the anterior chamber. If it returns to its original position, the length is correct.

Tap Test (Tennant, 1976)

The tap test indicates whether the lens is well fixed or not. After the eye is closed and the anterior chamber refilled with fluid, tapping on the sclera perpendicular to the axis of the lens will cause the iris to move. If the lens also moves, it is too short and must be replaced by a lens 1 mm longer. The test is then repeated. Tennant considers this test very reliable: it will identify a lens that is too short more than 99% of the time.

Choyce feels that these tests are very valuable for the neophyte Mark VIII implanter, but they are not really necessary after one has acquired sufficient experience.

c. *Postoperative Controls*

Blink Test (Tennant, 1976)

The purpose of the test is to see if the lens is stable and fixed. When the patient blinks, the lens should not move.

Gonioprism Test

Gentle pressure is exerted on the cornea with a small, flat, contact gonioprism, such as a Zeiss prism. If the counter-pressure of the vitreous body forces the foot of the lens to move in front of the scleral spur, the lens is too short and must be replaced to avoid corneal dystrophy.

3. *Remarks on the Incision*

Choyce states that the incision should be corneal enough and beveled enough to make a definite ledge or shelf behind which the feet of the implant can be tucked. This prevents the troublesome tendency of the lens to move out while the sutures are being placed when the incision is closed.

The section should also be large enough to provide an internal opening 1 mm larger than the maximum width of the lens. This allows the lens to be easily inserted without danger of stripping Descemet's membrane and enables one to make two iridotomies or, preferably, two iridectomies on either side of the proximal feet.

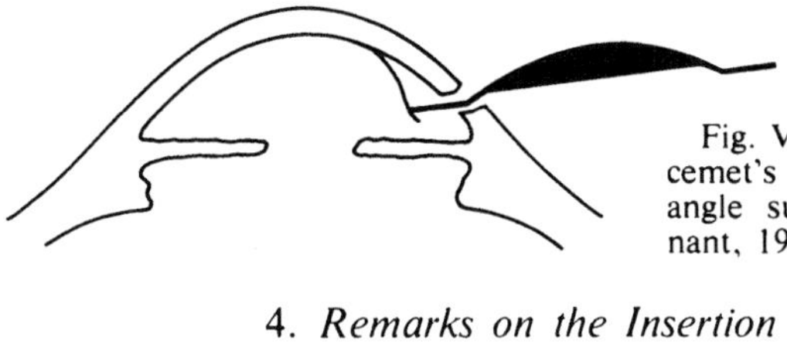

Fig. VIII-32. — Desinsertion of Descemet's membrane while inserting an angle supported lens. (From J. Tennant, 1976.)

4. *Remarks on the Insertion Technique*

a. *The Pupil and the Anterior Chamber*

Before the lens is inserted, the pupil must be constricted and the anterior chamber reformed by air or fluid.

A dilated pupil increases the risk of engaging either the vitreous with subsequent vitreous loss or a peripheral roll of the iris and then tucking it between the feet of the implant and the scleral spur.

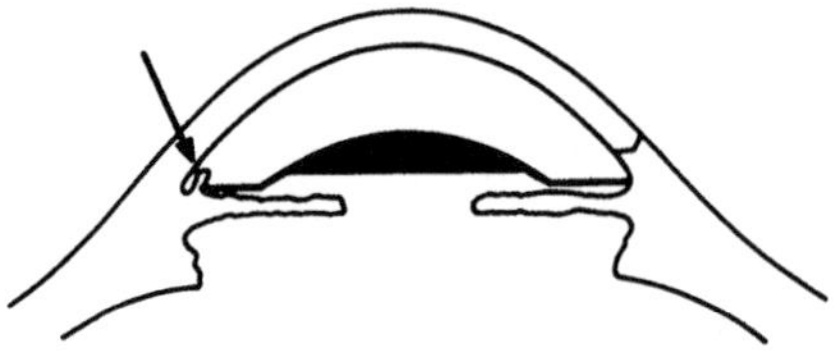

Fig. VIII-33. — Representation of iris tuck. (From J. Tennant, 1976).

A reformed anterior chamber helps in gliding the lens across the chamber without touching the iris or the endothelium. It also keeps the lens from slipping into an iridectomy, with subsequent tearing of the iris root. But if there is too much air in the anterior chamber, the lens will drop and the distal feet will engage the body of the iris and cause tucking.

b. *Insertion Forceps*

Normally, the lens is held with the special Choyce Forceps, which have ridges for gripping the fine lateral edges of the lens. Tennant advocates a special titanium needle holder of his own design, and Shepard uses his Shepard I Forceps.

c. *The Sheets Glide*

A plastic glide almost as wide as the corneoscleral incision is prepared. The glide is introduced very carefully, not touching the endothelial surface. If the iris vitreous face moves forward, the lateral track sutures can be tied temporarily to permit better retention of the air bubble in the anterior chamber. The glide can then be more easily slid beneath the air bubble, across the pupil, and into the opposite angle. The Sheets glide prevents inadvertant catching of an iridectomy, the pupillary border or an iris colloret crypt by one of the advancing feet. And with the glide in place and an air bubble above it, the lens can be introduced without trauma to the cornea. Removing the glide helps to withdraw the peripheral iris from the opposite angle, thus permitting the distal lens feet to rest against the scleral spur.

d. *Placing the Distal Feet*

When the distal feet reach the opposite angle, the lens is released. Special care must be taken to replace the distal feet in the angle if they drop from the angle down onto the iris. Otherwise the lens will tuck the iris when the proximal feet are inserted. Therefore, in order

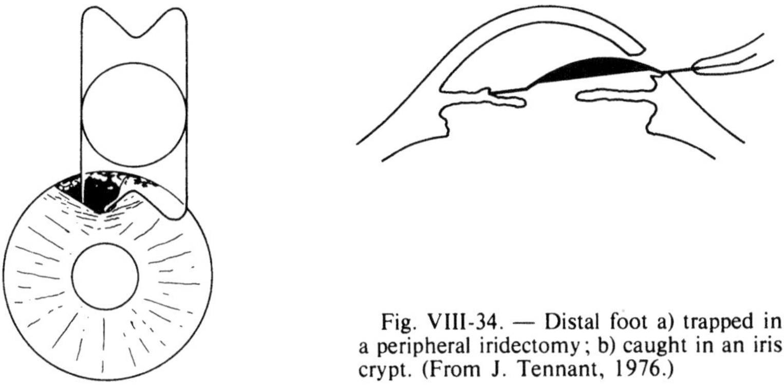

Fig. VIII-34. — Distal foot a) trapped in a peripheral iridectomy; b) caught in an iris crypt. (From J. Tennant, 1976.)

to prevent the lens from dislodging or displaying, the assistant places an iris spatula between the proximal feet. His only mission is to steady the lens and prevent it from slipping out. During this maneuver, the assistant has to be very careful not to exert pressure on the implant or to push it into the opposite iris root and perhaps even into the ciliary body beyond it thus tearing these delicate blood vessels and causing operative hyphema (Choyce in Boyd 1975-1976).

With Tennant's technique, however, the lens need not be steadied. Tennant feels that if the lens is introduced with a closed system technique with the anterior chamber maintained, the lens does not have a tendency to slip out of the incision.

e. *Placing the Proximal Feet*

Once the forceps are removed, all that remains is to introduce the two proximal feet into the angle of the anterior chamber. This is best achieved by gently catching the part of the outer scleral lip of the incision lying between the proximal feet with a fine-toothed forceps and retracting it outwards and slightly upwards while pressing gently on one foot of the implant with the tip of an iris repositor or needle holder. The lens is held gently in position with a smooth forceps resting against the center recess. The scleral lip is then grasped with a toothed forceps immediately beneath one of the lens feet and is rolled peripherally to permit the foot to drop into the angle posterior to the scleral lip of the wound. The second foot is dropped into place in the same way.

During the insertion of the distal and proximal feet, it is of utmost importance to avoid pushing the lens in the distal direction, since this may lead to serious bleeding of the iris.

f. *Gonioscopic Control*

When the operation is finished, gonioscopic control is indicated to make sure the feet are in the right place. If the surgical technique is faulty, the footplates end up in the angle or in the tissue of the iris or the ciliary body.

If the footplates are placed in the angle, the resultant dialysis of the angle structures will promptly be followed by hemorrhaging, which may be massive (Ellingson, 1977).

R.F. Azar (1978) has noted that torque forces occurring while the proximal feet are being placed may push properly placed distal feet into the angle structures. And Harrison (1978) pointed out that the same torque effect on the footplates develops if the tip of the opposite footplate slips into the iridectomy.

If the footplates enter the iris or the ciliary body below the scleral spur, pupillary distortion will be apparent. This may result in chronic postoperative uveitis accompanied by precipitates on the lens surface (Ellingson, 1977). Whether iris tuck should be released at this stage is a disputed question (Panel Discussion on Anterior Chamber Lenses, March, 1978, AIOIS Meeting in Los Angeles). Some surgeons hold that postoperative low-grade iritis and ocular tenderness are associated with iris tuck, but others maintain that the only consequence of an iris tuck is cosmetic, namely, an oval pupil. Therefore the latter do not recommend any untucking maneuvers, since untucking one tip may tuck the other.

5. *Vitreous Loss*

Choyce has often stressed the significant difference between postoperative complications resulting from vitreous loss occurring during primary implantation and that occurring during secondary implantation. The vitreous that escapes on reopening an aphakic eye is a mixture of aqueous and anterior vitreous and does not have the same jelly-like consistency as formed vitreous, which may escape at the time of primary cataract extraction. Nor does its escape from the eye in small quantities involve the same pessimistic prognosis (Choyce, 1978).

If vitreous loss occurs after primary implantation, it all must be removed from the anterior chamber with whatever vitrectomy technique one favors. If vitreous is present during primary lens insertion, it is likely to cause adhesions between the iris and the lens, which may result in prolonged iritis and decreased optical clarity.

But vitreous loss after secondary implantation need not deter the surgeon from carrying on and completing the operation. The most effective method of dealing with vitreous prolapse is by running a damp swab along the incision: the vitreous will adhere to the swab, and it can be cut off flush with the section. Vitreous present on completion of the section should be cut off before the implant is inserted, again after insertion, and also after the corneal sutures have been tied so that none is present between the lips of the incision.

6. *Prevention of Iris Bulge and Pupillary Block*

During the early postoperative period, close and extensive contact between the anterior iris surface and the lens may occur and disturb the aqeuous flow through the pupillary aperture. If the iridectomies function improperly, pupillary block develops and a typical forward ballooning of the iris will occur on one or both sides of the lens (internal iris prolapse).

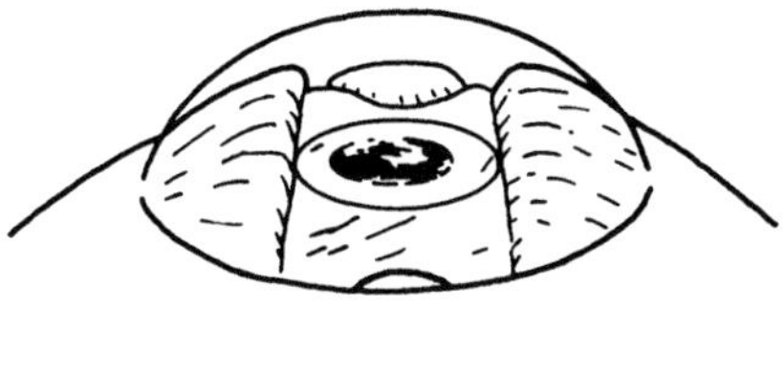

Fig. VIII-35. — Internal Iris prolapse with a Choyce Mark VIII lens. (From J. Tennant, 1976.)

Different measures are to be considered during and after lens implantation to prevent or cure iris bulge or pupillary block.

a. Adequate iridectomies: There must be adequate openings in the iris—in practice at least 2 iridectomies on either side of the proximal feet—that are far enough apart so that the implant does not engage them. Special care must be taken in positioning the lens since a lens foot may occlude the iridectomy.

b. If the extraction is extracapsular, either planned or unplanned, all of the cortex must be removed. If any is left behind the iris, it will swell and push the iris forward against the implant and synechiae and possibly pupillary block will develop.
c. Perfect wound closure: The iris will hermiate around the body of the lens any time fluid is lost from the anterior chamber. It follows that a wound leak may give rise to an iris bombé.
d. Postoperative dilation of the pupil: A widely dilated pupil with the margins extending slightly beyond the optic portion of the lens prevents synechiae formation between the iris and the lens in the postoperative edema period.
e. Aggressive and quick control of any form of iritis: To prevent iris edema and iritis, postoperative inflammation of the eye should be vigorously controlled with steroids, either topical or general of both. This keeps the iris from touching the lens and thus prevents pupillary block.

7. *The Sore Eye Syndrome*

During the first 3 to 6 postoperative months, most patients complain of soreness or tenderness when the eye is touched or rubbed, without there being any form of iritis. Choyce recommends that codeine be used routinely for relief. According to Kratz et al. (1979), tenderness upon touching or blinking may persist up to 3 years. Although the etiology remains obscure, this syndrome was found to be frequently associated with misplaced footplates or iris tuck (Kratz and Shepard, 1978).

VI. Summary and Conclusions

From 1957 to 1978, D.P. Choyce introduced nine modifications of the original Strampelli lens, each new design being the answer to a specific problem. Major steps in this evolution were:
— The change in the profile by the flattening of the haptic supports, which provided scleral rather than angle fixation (1963);
— The shift from a triangular to a quadrangular configuration (1963);
— The introduction of the Mark IX lens in 1978 with the optic shifted forward.

In view of the data presented above, anterior chamber lenses have these advantages:

1. The lens is made from the same material throughout (Perspex CQ) which has been proven over the long term to be well tolerated by the eye.
2. If the lens is the proper length, good stability may be expected.
3. Insertion is relatively easy.
4. It can be inserted after both intracapsular and extracapsular cataract extraction either as a primary or a secondary procedure.
5. Fixation does not depend on either pupil or iris integrity, which is an advantage when there are large iris defects.
6. Funduscopy after intracapsular cataract extraction is easy.
7. Should the lens have to be removed, it can be done without great risk of damaging intraocular structures.

These advantages have contributed to the increase of popularity of these lenses. Modern angle supported lenses occupy an important place in the range of intraocular lenses according to the latest survey conducted in the United States.

However, in our opinion, there are limitations that may not be overlooked in the use of rigid, fixed length, anterior chamber lenses. Since Choyce does not consider anterior chamber lenses with compressible extremities as a viable alternative to his lens, some major problems will remain. One continuing matter of concern is the selection of the length, since the lens must fit snugly behind the scleral spur.

In view of the present state of the art, the long term fate of these eyes with artificial lenses, which are, after all, surrounded by vital and delicate structures may be problematic. In this regard, there is always the possibility that one ore more of the tips of the footplate may be dislodged by an external force that deforms the anterior eye segment. A slight subluxation of the lens caused by a minor trauma may displace a footplate and bring it into contact with the iris root or the trabecular meshwork. And the displacement of one footplate may produce a torque effect on the opposite one.

As we have noted in our discussion of the UGH syndrome, only very well finished lenses may be used.

Finally, case selection is crucial for both primary and secondary implantation. One has to be extremely cautious if the eye has a narrow anterior segment or if the patient has diabetes, extensive goniosynechiae, or hemorrhagic diathesis.

The ultimate judgment on rigid, angle supported lenses has yet to be made. Certainly, the Mark VIII lens and its variants occupy an important place in the implant repertoire and have proven to be of value for implantation in long-standing aphakic eyes after intracapsular cataract extraction.

VII. New Lens Designs

A. The Azar Pyramid Mark III Lens

After having implanted a large number of Choyce Mark VIII lenses, R.F. Azar (1978) introduced his own design. The Azar Mark III angle supported lens has a triangular configuration with the optical component moved forward.

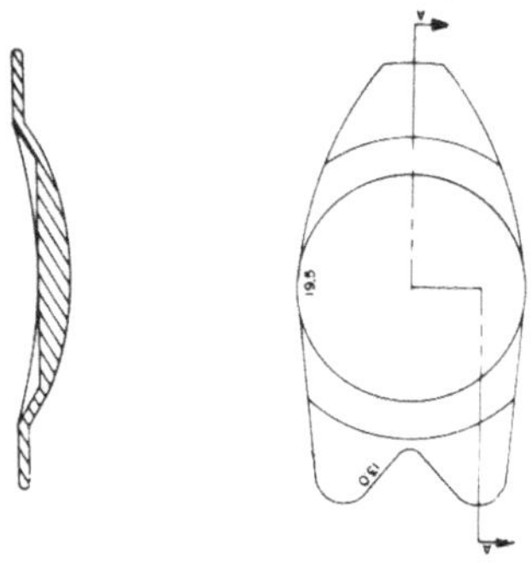

Fig. VIII-36. — The Azar Pyramid Mark III lens.

Azar maintains that the triangular shape of the distal foot makes insertion easier and safer: twisting or torque effects on the distal foot while the proximal feet are being put in place are prevented; iris tuck is less likely to occur; and postoperative tenderness is decreased. Although the support is only tripodal, stability is reported to be satisfactory.

B. The Kelman Anterior Chamber Lens

The Kelman Anterior Chamber Lens (1977) has a triangular configuration resembling a figure seven with a centrally placed 4 mm optic. It is thin (optical zone: 0.42 mm, haptic zone: 0.2 mm), flexible, lightweight (2 mg in aqueous), and made entirely of polymethylmethacrylate.

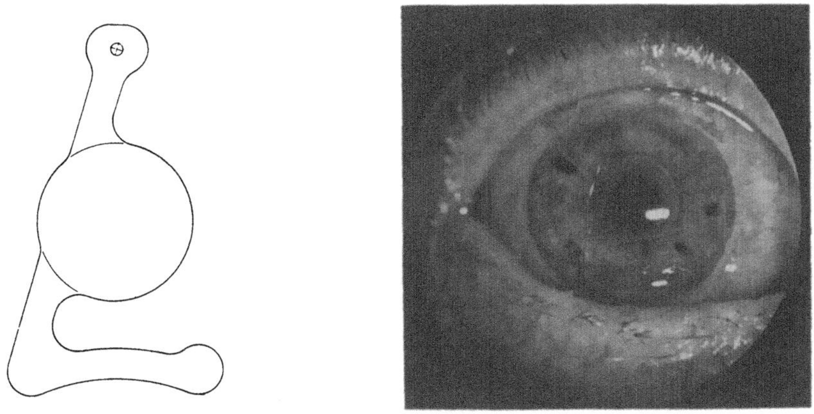

Fig. VIII-37. — Schema of the Kelman anterior chamber lens and photography showing the lens in situ.

Kelman's lens can be used after intracapsular cataract extraction both as a primary or a secondary procedure. It is particularly suited for use with phacoemulsification techniques since it can be inserted through a 4 mm incision. Good stability is provided by its wide, 3-point fixation. A few hundred such lenses have been inserted (Fig. VIII-33) (Kelman, at Cannes, 1979). Although the follow-up period is too brief to draw definite conclusions, the postoperative course has been reported to be satisfactory: the eyes are quiet and the subjective discomfort that is peculiar to angle supported lenses is almost totally absent.

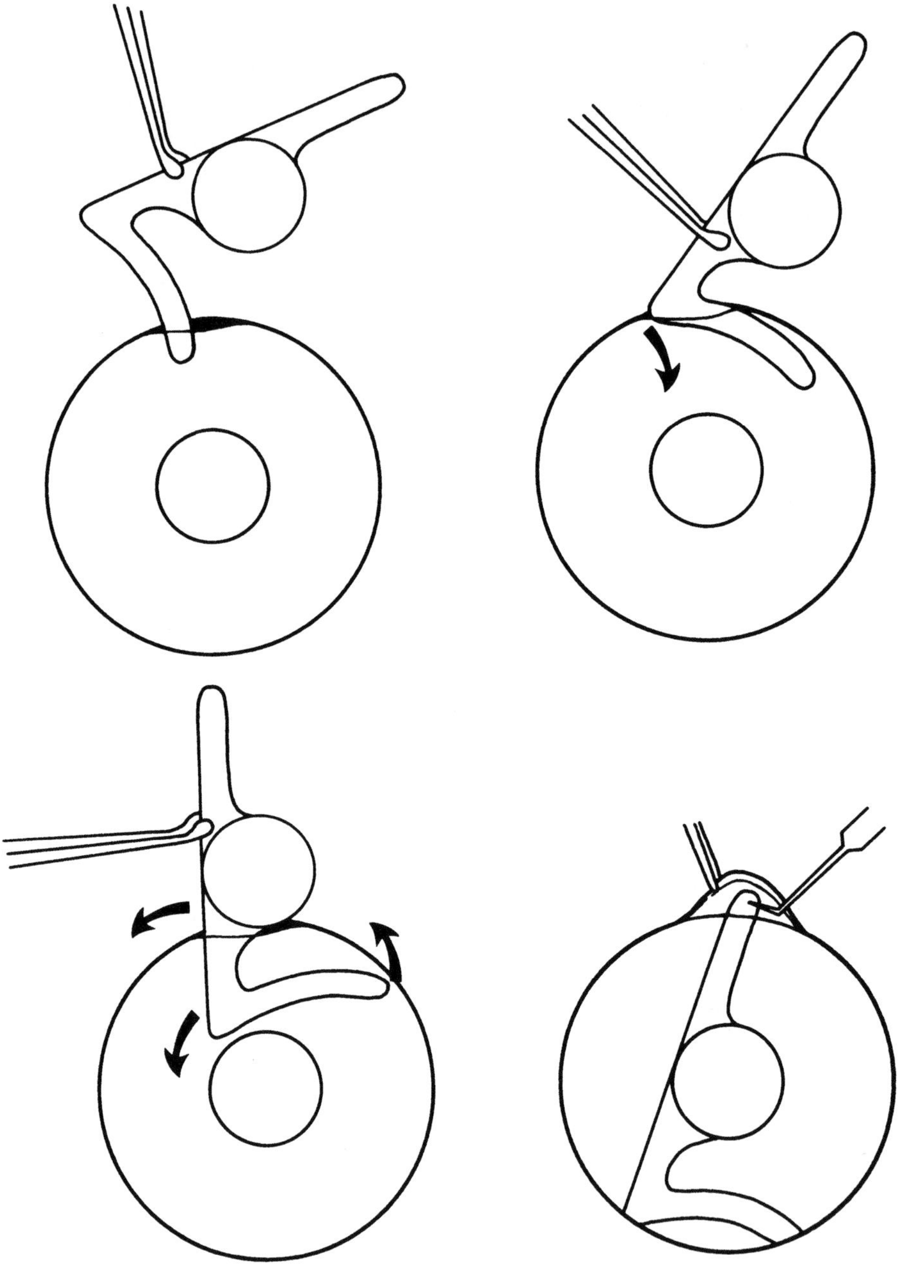

Fig. VIII-38. — Steps in the insertion of the Kelman lens through a small incision.

C. The Tennant Anchor Lens

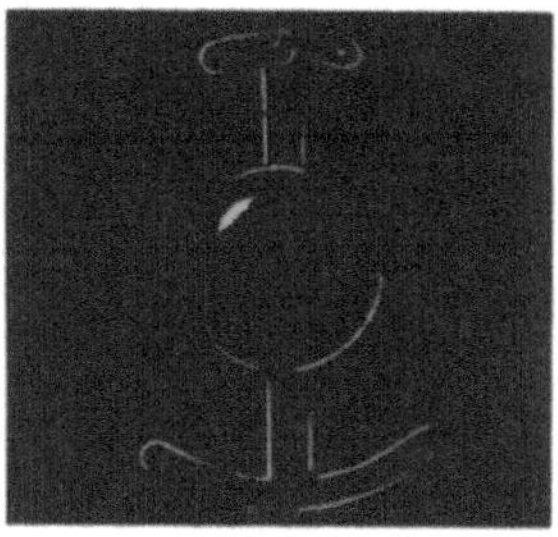

Fig. VIII-39. — The Tennant anchor lens.

At the 1980 meeting of the International Implant Club, J. Tennant presented a new lens of his own design, which is made entirely of polymethylmethacrylate and is slightly flexible. No clinical results are as yet available.

D. The Leiske Angle Supported Lens

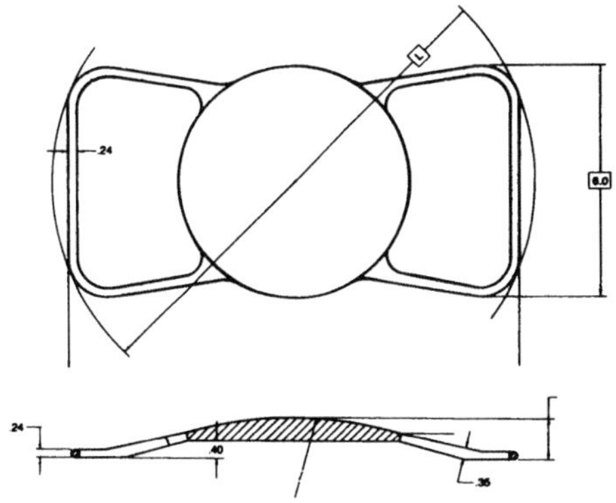

Fig. VIII-40. — The Leiske Angle Supported lens.

The lens resembles the Dannheim lens, but the loops are made of polymethylmethacrylate. This lens is under investigation.

CHAPTER IX

MIXED RESULTS AND COMPARATIVE STUDIES

Presented here are a number of extensive series compiled from the results obtained with a variety of lenses. Though we have had occasion to refer to some of these studies already, we thought it useful to present here the most characteristic data from them by way of summary.

Also presented are several comparative studies concerned with intracapsular versus extracapsular extraction and lens implantation as well as the behavior of the pseudophakic versus the aphakic eye.

I. Results Obtained with Various Lenses by the Same Surgeon or Surgical Team

1. **J. Worst et al.** (see Table IX-1)

Endothelial Corneal Dystrophy (2.4%)

This figure reflects the incidence of irreversible total corneal dystrophy. Minor forms of corneal edema were dealt with by means of loop amputation or correction of the position of the lens, which was usually sufficient to stop the edematous process.

Vitritis (3.5%)

In Worst's opinion, this is a disconcertingly high figure. In many cases, vitritis and cystoid macular edema were found to be associated.

Cystoid Macular Edema (4%)

There was a tendency to spontaneous recovery, and 58% of these cases regained useful vision of >20/60.

TABLE IX-1. — *Results of 1813 Lens Implantations by J.C. Worst et al.*

Source	J.C. Worst et al., 1977		
Surgeon	J.C. Worst et al.		
Lens types	Medallion 2-loop	1003	55%
	Binkhorst 4-loop	523	29%
	Medallion transiridectomy clip	207	11.5%
	Medallion small incision	70	4%
	Binkhorst iridocapsular	6	0.3%
	Fyodorov	4	0.2%
Surgical Procedure	Primary ICCE: 1519		
	Secondary ICCE: 19		
	Primary ECCE: 199		
	Secondary ECCE: 76		
	Total series: 1813		
Follow-up	6 months to 8 years		
Age of patients	50-70 years: 34.5%		
	Over 70 years: 56.5%		

	Total Series	*Primary ICCE*	*Primary ECCE*
Corrected visual acuity ⩾20/40	68.2%	68.5%	74.8%
Endothelial corneal dystrophy	2.4%	2.5%	3%
Clinical cystoid macular edema	4.0%	4.1%	1%
Retinal detachment	2.0%	2.1%	1.5%
Dislocation	4.3%	N.A.	N.A.
Iridocyclitis	0.9%	N.A.	N.A.
Vitritis	3.5%	3.9%	1%
Infection	0.5%	N.A.	N.A.
Secondary Membranes	4.8%	0.8%	25.6%
Glaucoma, transient (pupillary block)	0.1%	N.A.	N.A.
Lens removal	0.9%	N.A.	N.A.
Enucleation	0.2%	0.1%	0.5%

N.A. = Not available.

TABLE IX-2. — *Distribution of Complications relative to Type of Cataract*

Total series of 1813 cases	*Traumatic Cataract*	*Congenital Cataract*	*Senile, Mature, and other Cataracts*
Complications	76 cases	15 cases	1722 cases
Endothelial corneal dystrophy	3.9%	0%	2.3%
Retinal detachment	2.6%	0%	2.0%
Vitritis	2.6%	0%	3.6%
Lens luxations	9.2%	13.3%	4.0%
Infections	1.3%	0%	0.5%
Cystoid macular degeneration	2.6%	0%	4.1%
Secondary cataract formation	25.0%	26.6%	3.7%
Evisceration/Enucleation	1.3%	0%	0.2%
Lens removal	9.2%	13.3%	0.4%

Complications in Relation to the Type of Cataract

Comparison of the complication rates associated with traumatic cataracts, congenital cataracts, and senile, mature, and posterior polar cataracts reveals a significant divergence in the number of lens luxations, lens removals, secondary cataract formations, and other complications. Evidently, anatomically disrupted or congenitally underdeveloped eyes are poorer prospects for lens implantation.

Complications after Secondary Lens Implantation

In Worst's experience, secondary implantation after intracapsular cataract extraction is a dubious procedure since 7 out of the 19 cases developed cystoid macular edema.

TABLE IX-3. — *Complications after Secondary Lens Implantation*

	ICCE Secondary	*ECCE Secondary*
Complications	19 cases	76 cases
Corneal dystrophy	1-5.3%	0
Retinal detachment	1-5.3%	0
Vitritis	1-5.3%	2-2.6%
Cystoid macular degeneration	7-36.8%	1-1.3%
Secondary membrane formation	2-10.5%	21-27.6%

Lens Removal

The reasons for lens removal in the 16 cases are given on Table IX-4.

TABLE IX-4. — *Reasons for Lens Removal in 16 out of the 1813 Cases*

Number of cases	*Complication*
1	Multiple complications
6	Lens luxation
5	Corneal dystrophy
1	Trauma (with sharp object) 3 weeks after implantation
1	Secondary cataract formation, membranectomy. Child of 4 years old
2	Lens implantation caused high myopia $\approx$ 13 D. The lens power has not been pre-determined

Enucleation/Evisceration

The indications for enucleation/evisceration in 4 out of the 1813 implantations are given on Table IX-5.

TABLE IX-5. — *Indications for Enucleation/Evisceration in 4 of the 1813 Cases*

Case 1:	Male, 62 years, traumatic cataract, secondary implantation after extracapsular cataract extraction. Complications: Vitritis, secondary glaucoma leading to absolute glaucoma, lens removal followed by enucleation (same year).
Case 2:	Female, 78 years, senile cataract, intracapsular extraction. Preexisting retinopathia hypertonica. Complications: Hemorrhagic glaucoma because of central venous thrombosis, rubeosis iridis, followed by enucleation 2 years after implantation.
Case 3:	Female, 64 years, senile cataract, extracapsular extraction. Corneal transplant had been performed on some eyes before lens implantation. Complications: Infection, panophthalmitis, followed by enucleation.
Case 4:	Female, 86 years, senile cataract, intracapsular extraction. Complication: One year after implantation (very successful) a severe blunt trauma led to enucleation.

2. H. Hirschman

The incidence of endothelial corneal dystrophy, clinical cystoid macular edema, and uveitis is given only in those cases in which the final visual result was less than 20/40.

TABLE IX-6. — *Results of 1784 * Lens Implantations by H. Hirschman*

Source	H. Hirschman, 1978	
Surgeon	H. Hirschman	
Lens types	Worst Medallion 2-loop	34.4%
	Binkhorst 2-loop iridocapsular	23.9%
	Worst platinum clip	19.9%
	Binkhorst 4-loop iris clip	10.0%
	Fyodorov-Binkhorst	7.4%
	Fyodorov Sputnik	1.7%
	Other	2.7%
Surgical procedure	ICCE	49.4%
	ECCE	22.6%
	Phakoemulsification	19.6%
	Primary	95%
	Secondary	5%
Follow-up	3 months to 10 years (46.6% of the cases, 1 year or less)	
Age	<20 years	0.3%
	>60 years	73.3%
Corrected visual acuity $\geqslant 20/40$		83.4%
Endothelial corneal dystrophy		3.2%
Clinical cystoid macular edema		2.5%
Retinal detachment		2.1%
Dislocation (50% required surgical repositioning)		5.9%
Uveitis		0.8%
Secondary membranes (discission required in 10.8%)		12.6%
Glaucoma		
transient (pupillary block) (in 55.6% with platinum clip lenses)		1.1%
Vitreous loss		9.6%
Lens removal		1.8%

* The data is incomplete or irretrievable for 124 patients, thus the percentage base is 1660.

Retinal Detachment (2.1%)

About half of the cases (43.7%) of retinal detachment were associated with vitreous loss during surgery, and three-fourths of the retinal detachments occurred within the first year after implantation.

Dislocation (5.9%)

The incidence of dislocation was nearly equally distributed over the eyes implanted with intracapsular cataract extraction and those with extracapsular cataract extraction. Surgical repositioning was necessary in half of these cases.

Suture failure occured with 4.7% of the Medallion lenses. The incidence of iris sphincter erosion was 1.7%, the majority of these cases involving metal-looped iridocapsular lenses.

In the majority of the cases, secondary pupillary membrane formation followed extracapsular cataract extraction or phacoemulsification. The reasons for the 1.8% incidence of lens removal are as follows: corneal touch, 0.6%; inflammation, 0.7%; and dislocation 0.5%. In half of the cases of corneal touch, the cause was dislocation due to peroperative vitreous loss.

3. N.S. Jaffe

TABLE IX-7. — *Results of 800 Lens Implantations by N.S. Jaffe*

Source	N.S. Jaffe, 1978		
Surgeon	N.S. Jaffe		
Lens types	Binkhorst 4-loop Binkhost 2-loop		
Surgical procedure	ICCE ECCE	698 102	87% 13%
Follow-up	6 months to 3½ years		
Age	From 54 to 94 years Mean age: 73.86 years		
Corrected visual acuity ⩾20/40			90.3%
Endothelial corneal dystrophy			0.6%*
Clinical cystoid macular edema			1.5%*
Retinal detachment			0.5%*
Dislocation			2.9%
Tissue reaction			N.A.
Secondary membranes			3.5%
Glaucoma			0.1%*
Hemorrhage			N.A.
Vitreous problems			7.1%
Loss (peroperative)			2.5%
Loss (during implant manipulation)			3.7%
Bulge (with preventive aspiration)			0.85%
Lens exchange			0.12% (1 case)
Lens removal			0.25% (2 cases)

* Incidence of endothelial corneal dystrophy, clinical cystoid macular edema, and retinal detachment in those cases in which the final visual result was ⩽20/40.
N.A. = Not available.

The causes of visual acuity of less than 20/40 (incidence: 78/100, 9.8%) are as follows:

Senile macular degeneration	4.1%
Clinical Cystoid macular edema	1.5%
Endothelial Corneal dystrophy	0.6%
Retinal detachment	0.5%
Hypertensive retinopathy	0.4%
Diabetic retinopathy	0.3%
Secondary membranes	0.1%
Amblyopia	0.8%
Others	0.8%
Unknown	0.6%

For the determination of the dislocation rate (2.9%), the series of 800 Binkhorst implants was expanded to 939 cases. After ECCE, the incidence was 4/108 (3.7%); after ICCE, 23/831 (2.8%). The breakdown of dislocation cases is given on Table IX-8. Three implants without sutures in the ICCE series dislocated completely into the vitreous.

TABLE IX-8. — *Breakdown of Dislocations*

	Number of cases	*Dislocations*	
ECCE			
Iridocapsular lenses	33	3	9.1%
Iris clip without suture	17	1	5.9%
Iris clip with suture	58	0	0.0%
ICCE			
Iris clip without suture	402	13	3.2%
Iris clip with suture	429	10	2.3%

Surgery had to be performed for secondary membranes in 28 eyes (3.5%) in order to improve vision: after ECCE: 15/102 (14.7%), after ICCE: 13/698 (1.9%).

Vitreous problems occurred in 57 of the 800 cases (7.1%):

During ICCE: 11/698 (1.5%)
During ECCE: 10/102 (9.8%)
During lens insertion: 19
During transiridectomy suture: 10
During aspiration for vitreous bulge: 7

The high incidence of vitreous loss during ECCE was due to inexperience with automated devices. The vitreous could be satisfactorily managed, and in no case did the implantation have to be aborted. There was a higher incidence of clinical cystoid macular edema in cases with an operative vitreous disturbance: 2/57 (3.5%) in cases with vitreous problems, 1/743 (1.3‰) in cases without vitreous problems.

4. D.D. Shepard

TABLE IX-9. — *Results of 500 Lens Implantations by D.D. Shepard*

Source	D.D. Shepard, 1977	
Surgeon	D.D. Shepard	
Lens Types	Binkhorst-Worst	44.6%
	Binkhorst-Fyodorov	37.2%
	Copeland	5.2%
	Platina style	5.2%
	Medallion style	4.0%
	Other	3.8%
Surgical procedure	ICCE	95.4%
	Primary	96.2%
	Secondary	3.8%
Follow-up	4 months to 57 months	
Age	⩾45 years	
Corrected visual acuity ⩾20/40		79%
Endothelial corneal dystrophy		1.8%
Clinical cystoid macular edema		15.4%
Retinal detachment		3.6%
Dislocation		
Partial		7.6%
Total		0%
Iridocyclitis		2.4%
Vitritis		4.6%
Secondary membranes		2.6%
Endophthalmitis		0%
Glaucoma		
Transient (pupillary block)		0.8%
Persistent		1.0%
Hemorrhage, anterior chamber		1.6%
Lens removal		2.2%
Enucleation		0.2%

The incidence of clinical cystoid macular edema can be broken down according to lens type as follows:

Copeland lens	3.9%
Iris-supported lens with supramid loops	13%
Iris-supported lens with metal loops	33%

The incidence following secondary implantation was 21%.

The following reasons were given for lens removal:

— The pseudophakos was pulled up by an updrawn pupil, usually because of iris or vitreous incarceration in the wound, or superior peripheral anterior synechiae.

— The pseudophakos sagged because of the cutting of the inferior pupillary margin by heavy metal posterior loops (sphincter erosion).

— The pseudophakos was displaced because the posterior loops became fouled in bands of residual cortex remaining after inflammed extracapsular cataract extraction.

The one case of epithelial downgrowth requiring enucleation was due to persistent wound leak around loose silk sutures. The pseudophakos itself was not a causal factor.

5. N.L. Snider and W.U. McReynolds

TABLE IX-10. — *Results of 500 Lens Implantations by N.L. Snider and W.U. McReynolds*

Source	N.L. Snider and W.U. McReynolds, 1977	
Surgeons	N.L. Snider and W.U. McReynolds	
Lens types	Copeland	79.8%
	Binkhorst 2-loop capsular fixation	6.4%
	Worst platina	6.2%
	Worst Medallion circular loop with clip	5.4%
	Worst Medallion iris suture	1.6%
	McGhan 4-strut iris diaphragm	0.6%
Surgical procedure	ICCE	64%
	ECCE	36%
	Primary	96.6%
	Secondary	1.4%
Follow-up	6 months to 1½ years	
Age	≥60 years	90%
Corrected visual acuity ≥20/40		83%
Endothelial corneal dystrophy		0.4%
Clinical cystoid macular edema		7.4%
Retinal detachment		1%
Dislocation (Binkhorst-McCannel suture 0.8%)		3.8%
Iridocyclitis		N.A.
Vitreitis		N.A.
Endophthalmitis		0.2%
Secondary membrane		2%
Glaucoma		
Transient (pupillary block)		0.4%
Persistent		N.A.
Hemorrhage, anterior chamber		0.6%
Vitreous loss		2.5%
Lens removal		N.A.
Enucleation		0%

N.A. = Not available.

Clinical Cystoid Macular Edema (7.4%)

In 3.8% of the cases, the cystoid macular edema was transient and recovery of the visual function was complete. In the remaining 3.6%, the edema was prolonged and/or severe. In all but one of the cases, the Copeland lens was involved, the majority of them having been inserted after intracapsular cataract extraction.

Clinical Cystoid Macular Edema and Retinal Detachment in function of the Status of the Posterior Capsule

Of the 181 extracapsular cataract extraction cases, 97 had an intact posterior capsule. There was 1 case of retinal detachment in this group. Of the remaining 84 cases in which the capsule had been opened, 3 cases of retinal detachment and 3 cases of severe cystoid macular edema occurred.

6. R. Kratz, T. Mazzocco, B. Davidson, and W. Maloney

TABLE IX-11. — *Results of 1146 Lens Implantations by R. Kratz, T. Mazzocco, B. Davidson, and W. Maloney*

Source	R. Kratz et al., 1979		
Surgeon	R. Kratz et al.		
Lens types	Binkhorst 2-loop	308	27.9%
	Binkhorst 4-loop	332	28.0%
	Choyce Mk VIII (Rayner)	215	18.8%
	Shearing posterior chamber	291	25.4%
Surgical procedure	ECCE (phakoemulsification in the majority of the cases)		
Follow-up	3 months to 5 years		
Age	Average 75 years		

	Binkhorst 2-loop	*Binkhorst 4-loop*	*Choyce VIII (Rayner)*	*Shearing*
Corrected visual acuity ⩾20/40	82%	81%	80%	91%
Endothelial corneal dystrophy	2.3%	0.9%	0%	0%
Clinical cystoid macular edema	4.2%	7.5%	8.4%	2.4%
Retinal detachment	1.3%	1.2%	3.1%	0.5%
Subluxation	3.9%	3.5%	0%	0.7%
Iritis (temporary)	2.3%	4.2%	6.5%	2.1%
Hyphema	0%	0.3%	6.4%	0%
Lens removal	2.6%	0.3%	0.5%	0.3%

Complications were most frequently encountered with the 2-loop lenses when metal looped lenses were involved. R. Kratz et al. concluded that the Shearing lens has the lowest complication rate relative to the Binkhorst and Choyce lenses. Telling against the Shearing lens is the relatively short follow-up time it has, having been implanted first only in 1977. Furthermore, it is not suitable for intracapsular surgery and the pressure it exerts on the ciliary body may cause damage in the long term.

II. Intracapsular Cataract Extraction (ICCE) & Lens Implantation versus Extracapsular Cataract Extraction (ECCE) & Lens Implantation

1. J.G.C. Renardel de Lavalette *

TABLE IX-12. — *Results of 328 Lens Implantations by J.G.C. Renardel de Lavalette: ICCE + Implantation versus ECCE + Implantation*

Source	J.G.C. Renardel de Lavalette, 1978				
Surgeon	Surgical team of the Rotterdam Eye Clinic				
Lens types	Iridocapsular	96		96 ECCE	29%
	Medallion	88	73 ICCE	15 ECCE	27%
	Iris clip	81	79 ICCE	2 ECCE	25%
	Clover leaf	48		48 ECCE	15%
	Circular loop	15	15 ICCE		4.5%
Surgical procedure	ICCE + Implantation 167				51%
	ECCE + Implantation 161				49%
Follow-up	From 1 to 5 years				
Age	<50 years				4.5%
	>75 years				49%

	ICCE + Implantation		*ECCE + Implantation*	
Corrected visual acuity ⩾20/40	73.8%		85.7%	
Endothelial corneal dystrophy	11	6.6%	5	3.1%
Clinical cystoid macular edema	17	10.2%	5	1.9%
Retinal detachment	2	1.2%	0	
Dislocation	14	8.4%	9	5.6%
Decentration	9	5.4%	5	3.1%
After cataract	4	2.4%	42	26.1%
Tissue reaction				
Iritis (hypopion)	4	2.4%	2	1.2%
Uveitis	11	6.6%	10	6.2%
Endophthalmitis	0		3	1.9%
Vitreous problems				
Vitreous loss	8	4.8%	3	1.2%
Lens removal	5	3%	3	1.2%
Enucleation	0		0	

J.G.C. Renardel de Lavalette concluded that in lens implant surgery extracapsular cataract extraction is safer than intracapsular cataract extraction, especially if late complications are involved. The figures cited for the incidence of endothelial corneal dystrophy, clinical cystoid macular edema, and retinal detachment are relevatory in this respect.

* Communication to the authors.

TABLE IX-13. — *Causes for Visual Acuity <20/40: Renardel de Lavalette's Series*

	ICCE 43/167 (26%)	*ECCE 23/161 (14%)*
Endothelial corneal dystrophy	10	4
Clinical cystoid macular edema	15	2
Senile macular degeneration	9	3
Endophthalmitis	0	3
After cataract	0	3
Other	6	3
Unknown	3	5

2. R. Kern

TABLE IX-14. — *Comparative Study of Iridocapsular Lenses after Extracapsular Cataract Extraction versus Iris Clip Lenses after Intracapsular Cataract Extraction by R. Kern*

Source	R. Kern, 1977		
Surgeon	R. Kern		
Lens types		Iridocapsular lens (metal loop)	Iris clip lens (without suture)
Surgical procedure		ECCE	ICCE
Follow-up		1-25 months (mean 12 months)	1-43 months (mean 27 months)
Age		5-86 years (mean 62.8 years)	42-91 years (mean 71.6 years)
Number		100	100
Corrected visual acuity ⩾20/40		86%	87%
Endothelial corneal dystrophy		0%	0%
Clinical cystoid macular edema		1%	2%
Retinal detachment		0%	2%
Dislocation		6%	1%
After cataract			
Aspiration of cortical remnants		17%	
Discission of secondary cataracts		4%	
Uveitis		Mild and rare	Mild and rare
Glaucoma			
Persistent		1%	2%
Lens removal		1%	2%

TABLE IX-15. — *Operative Complications, Kern's Series*

	Iridocapsular group	*Iris clip group*
Implantation aborted because of:		
— Imminent vitreous prolapse	4	4
— Vitreous loss	4	0
— Extremely narrow pupil	2	1

Note: The 4 cases of vitreous loss occurred in patients with traumatic cataract.

TABLE IX-16. — *Primary Causes of Visual Acuity <20/40, Kern's Series*

	Iridocapsular group	*Iris clip group*
Corneal scars due to keratitis scrophulosa or injury	6	2
Vitreous hemorrhage	0	1
Maculopathy		
Dry	5	2
Edematous	1	6
Central vein thrombosis	0	2
Retinal detachment	0	2
Preexisting amblyopia	2	0

TABLE IX-17. — *Aniseikonia *, Kern's Series*

	Iridocapsular group	*Iris clip group*
No. aniseikonia	15	10
0.1-1%	10 = 34 out of 38	21 = 52 out of 64
1.1-2%	5	19
2.1-3%	4 = 89%	8 = 81%
3.1-4%		4
4.1-5%	2 = 4 out of 38	4 = 12 out of 64
5.1-6%	1 = 11%	3
over 6%	1 = 11%	1 = 19%
not measured or not measurable	62	36

* Measured with the *Phasedifferenzhaploskop*, difference of image-size in %.

III. Pseudophakia versus Aphakia

1. N.S. Jaffe et al.

N.S. Jaffe et al. have published a retrospective study of 2 groups that were matched as closely as possible according to surgeon, surgical technique, time interval of the study, and ocular status. The cases were selected from 512 consecutive intracapsular cataract extractions followed by the insertion of a 4-loop iris clip lens and from 653 consecutive intracapsular cataract extractions without implantation.

The reasons for the ommission of 12 lens implantation cases and 153 routine intracapsular cataract extraction cases are given on Table IX-18.

TABLE IX-18. — *Reasons for Exclusion of Patients from the Series of Jaffe et al.*

	Routine ICCE	*ICCE with Implantation*
Patients less than 60 years old	74	3
Myopia (aphakic refraction +6.00 D or less)	31	0
Follow-up period too short	22	3
Glaucomatous optic atrophy	11	1
Previous repair of retinal detachment	3	0
Combined surgery	7	5
One-eyed patient	5	0
Total	153	12

The authors note that the figures for the incidences of endothelial corneal dystrophy, clinical cystoid macular edema, and retinal detachment only concern those cases in which the complication was responsible for a visual acuity $\leqslant 20/40$.

TABLE IX-19. — *Comparison of Binkhorst Iris Clip Lens Implantation with Routine Intracapsular Cataract Extraction*

Source	N.S. Jaffe et al., 1978	
Surgeons	N.S. Jaffe et al.	
Surgical procedure	ICCE	ICCE with Implantation (primary)
Lens types	—	Iris clip (Binkhorst)
Number	500	500
Age	Average 73 years	74 years
Follow-up	6 months to 3 years	6 months to 3 years
Corrected visual acuity $\geqslant 20/40$	85.4%	89%
Endothelial corneal dystrophy	0.4%	1.2%
Clinical cystoid macular edema	2.2%	1.4%
Retinal detachment	0.8%	0.6%

N.S. Jaffe et al. concluded that the visual acuity results were comparable for the two groups: 89.0% of the implant group and 85.4% of the routine intracapsular group achieved 20/40 or better visual acuity.

TABLE IX-20. — *Causes of Visual Acuity <20/40, Series of Jaffe et al.*

	ICCE *Nr.*		*ICCE + Implantation* *Nr.*	
Senile macular degeneration	38	7.6%	21	4.2%
Clinical cystoid macular edema	11	2.2%	7	1.4%
Corneal edema	2	0.4%	6	1.2%
Retinal detachment	4	0.8%	3	0.6%
Vein thrombosis	0		4	
Diabetic maculopathy	3		1	
Vitreous hemorrhage	2		0	
Macular pucker	1		1	
Macular hole	0		1	
Retinitis pigmentosa	1		1	
Optic atrophy	0		1	
Glaucomatous atrophy	0		1	
Ischemic optic neuropathy	1		2	
Amblyopia	2		3	
Congenital nystagmus	1		0	
Secondary membrane	1		2	
Expulsive hemorrhage	1		0	
Unknown	4		1	
Total	73		55	

The rates of complications were also comparable for both groups except for corneal edema, which was higher in the implant group (1.2%) than in the routine intracapsular group (0.4%). The rate of clinically significant cystoid macular edema was higher in the routine intracapsular group (2.2%), however, than in the implant group (1.4%).

2. **B.S. Prokop**

B.S. Prokop has compared two consecutive series of patients operated upon in approximately the same time period (≈40 months), each comprising 200 patients. The first series consists of intracapsular cataract extractions without implantation, and the second with implantation.

Because of preoperative case selection the two series cannot be considered as being perfectly matched. Prokop excluded from the implant series those patients with known preoperative glaucoma and longstanding, severe diabetes. Consequently, these patients underwent routine intracapsular cataract extraction. On the other hand, patients with macular degeneration were considered good candidates for intraocular lens implantation.

TABLE IX-21. — *Comparative Study on Intraocular Lenses versus Routine Cataract Extraction, B.S. Prokop's Study*

Source	B.S. Prokop, 1977	
Surgeon	B.S. Prokop	
Surgical procedure	ICCE	ICCE + Implantation
Lens types	—	Copeland 139 Medallion (sutured) 61
Number	200	200
Age	Average 70 years	Average 73 years
Follow-up	Maximum 40 months	Maximum 40 months
Corrected visual acuity ⩾20/40	79%	88%
Endothelial corneal dystrophy	0%	0%
Clinical cystoid macular edema	0.5%	2%
Retinal detachment	3%	0.5%
Dislocation		1.5%
Iridocyclitis		
Mild	0%	5%
Severe	0.5%	1%
Endophthalmitis	0%	0.5%
Glaucoma	1%	3%
Hemorrhage	0%	0.5%
Lens removal		1%

3. D.E. Williamson

TABLE IX-22. — *Comparative Study of Pseudophakia versus Aphakia by D.E. Williamson*

Source D.E. Williamson, 1977		
Surgeon D.E. Williamson		
Surgical procedure	ICCE	ICCE + Implantation (primary)
Type of lens		Medallion sutured
Number	200	200
Age	Not available	Not available
Follow-up	6 months	6 months
Corrected visual acuity ⩾20/40	79%	71%
Endothelial corneal dystrophy	0%	1.5%
Clinical cystoid macular edema	6%	5.5%
Retinal detachment	1.5%	0%
Dislocation		6%
Tissue reactions		
Uveitis (mild)	0.5%	1%
Secondary membranes	0%	1%
Glaucoma		
Transient (pupillary block)	0.5%	1%
Vitreous loss	0.5%	2% (lens related)
Lens removal		0%

Surgical reinterventions in the pseudophakic group were carried out for the following reasons:

— Dislocation (1.5%).

— Endothelial corneal dystrophy (grafting) (1.5%).

— Discissions (1.5%).

Since the follow-up period for these cases was at the most six months, the value of these data is restricted.

4. R.F. Azar

TABLE IX-23. — *Comparative Study of Pseudophakia versus Aphakia by R.F. Azar*

Source R.F. Azar, 1976			
Surgeon R.F. Azar			
Surgical procedure	ICCE 91% ECCE 9%	ICCE + Implantation ECCE + Implantation (primary)	82% 18%
Number	200	200	
Types of lens		Medallion sutured Iridocapsular 2-loop Binkhorst 4-loop Medallion circular loop	88% 6% 3% 3%
Age ⩾65	93%	78%	
Follow-up	Max 2 years	Max 1 year	
Corrected visual acuity ⩾20/40	94%	81%	
Endothelial corneal dystrophy	0%	2.5%	
Clinical cystoid macular edema	12%	9%	
Retinal detachment	1%	0.5%	
Dislocation		5.5%	
Iritis	2%	1.5%	
Endophthalmitis	0%	0%	
Glaucoma, pupillary block	0%	1.5%	
Hyphema	1%	1%	
Vitreous loss	1.7%	2.5%	
Lens removal		0.5%	

5. **W.J. Stark et al.**

The cases were age-matched, and the eyes were selected following identical criteria. Excluded were:

- patients under 65, one-eyed patients and patients with poor motivation;
- eyes with diabetic retinopathy, high myopia, a history of retinal detachment or uveitis, Fuch's dystrophy, or glaucoma.

TABLE IX-24. — Comparative Study of Pseudophakia and Aphakia by W.J. Stark et al.

Source	W.J. Stark et al., 1977	
Surgeons	W.J. Stark and L.W. Hirst	
Surgical procedure	ICCE	ICCE + Implantation (primary)
Number of cases	100	100
Type of lens		Binkhorst iris clip and transiridectomy suture (prolene 10.0)
Average age	70 years	67 years
Follow-up	12 months	12 months
Corrected visual acuity ⩾20/40	93%	93%
Endothelial corneal dystrophy	0%	0%
Clinical cystoid macular edema	3%	3%
Retinal detachment	3%	2%
Dislocation		1%
Uveitis persistent (mild)	0%	4%
Endophthalmitis	0%	1%
Secondary membrane	0%	1%
Glaucoma		
Pupillary block	0%	1%
Persistent	0%	0%
Hemorrhage	0%	0%
Vitreous problems	1%	12%
Loss	1%	9%
Aspiration	0%	3%
Removal		1% (endophthalmitis)

Note: Six patients of the implantation group underwent a second operative procedure because of complications. As the author observe, this underscores the increased risk potential of lens implantation.

6. M.A. Galin

In 1977, M.A. Galin et al. published the results obtained from a selected group of 300 eyes (Table IX-25). Some of the data were updated the following year (Jaffe et al., 1978).

Although the series are age matched and most preexisting pathology excluded, they are not perfectly comparable: patients with preoperative corneal diseases and maculopathological conditions were excluded from the implant series but not from the control group.

TABLE IX-25. — *Comparative Study of Pseudophakia versus Aphakia by M.A. Galin et al.*

Source M.A. Galin et al., 1977, 1978.		
Surgeons M.A. GALIN et al.		
Surgical procedure	ICCE	ICCE + Implantation (primary)
Number of cases	300	300
Type of lens		Sputnik
Average age	72	72
Follow-up	5-10 years	5 years
Corrected visual acuity ⩾20/40	Unavailable	88%
Endothelial corneal dystrophy [1]	0%	0%
Clinical cystoid macular edema	3%	3%
Retinal detachment	2%	2%
Dislocation		
Partial		10%
Total		0.3%
Tissue reactions [2]		
Chronic iritis	0%	0.3%
Endophthalmitis	0%	0%
Secondary membrane formation	0%	10%
Glaucoma		
Transient [3]	5%	8%
Pupillary block	0%	0%

Additional data

[1] Striate keratopathy

Striate keratopathy	Non-implant	Implant
Severe	3 cases	20 cases
Moderate	5 cases	30 cases
Mild to none	92 cases	50 cases

[2] Sterile hypopion: 2% in the implantation series versus none in the non-implant series. In Galin's opinion, this was probably because of inadequate cleaning of the lenses before sterilization.

[3] Incidence of transient rise in intraocular pressure in the immediate postoperative period:

Rise in pressure	Non-implant	Implant
>6 mm Hg	15%	20%
>10 mm Hg	5%	8%

7. D.M. Taylor et al.

TABLE IX-26. — *Comparative Study of Pseudophakia versus Aphakia by D.M. Taylors et al.*

Source D.M. Taylor et al., 1978		
Surgeons D.M. Taylor et al.		
Surgical procedure	ICCE	ICCE + Implantation (primary)
Types of lens	—	Worst Platina 48%
		Copeland 39%
		Worst single loop 5%
		Worst Medallion 5%
		Fyodorov Sputnik 2%
		Others 1%
Number	500	500
Age	>50 years 98%	>50 years 98.5%
Average	71.8 years	73.2 years
Follow-up	>2½ years	>6 months
Correced visual acuity ⩾20/40	83%	86.5%
Endothelial corneal dystrophy	0.4%	0.4%
Clinical cystoid macular edema	2%	6%
Retinal detachment	2.8	0.2%
Dislocation		
Partial		3.2%
Total		0.4%
Tissue reactions		
Iritis (mild)	1.2%	4.8%
Vitreitis	0%	0.4%
Endophthalmitis	0%	0.4%
Retrolenticular membranes	N.A.	3.8%
Glaucoma		
Transient (pupillary block)	0%	0.4%
Persistent	0%	0%
Vitreous loss	3%	3%
Hemorrhage		
Hyphema	3.2%	11.8%
Vitreous (severe)	0.8%	1.2%
Lens removal		0.2%

Note: In the lens implant series, the incidences of clinical cystoid macular edema, iritis, and retrolenticular membranes are striking. Most of these complications occurred with the Copeland lens.

CHAPTER X

SECONDARY LENS IMPLANTATION

"Secondary lens implantation" means the implantation of an artificial lens in an eye from which the lens had been removed in a previous surgical session.

The pioneers of this procedure in the fifties considered that secondary implantation was indicated for a unilateral aphakic patient who needed binocular vision for occupational, mental, or physical reasons. Also candidates were children with unilateral aphakia resulting from a traumatic cataract. As observed by many, the capacity of implanted lenses to prevent amblyopia and restore binocular vision was striking.

These indications are still considered valid, but there is no general agreement about case selection, the kind of pseudophakos to be implanted, or the risk-benefit ratio involved.

I. Incidence

During the last 20 years, secondary implants constituted only a small proportion of the total number of implants performed (see Tables X-1, X-2, and X-3). Even though there were, and are, a large number of aphakic patients, most surgeons did not favor the secondary procedure with the exception of D.P. Choyce. Darin notes that Choyce accounted for more than half of the secondary procedures performed during this period.

TABLE X-1. — *Incidence of Secondary Implant Procedures (Darin, 1977)*

Number of Surgeons	*Total Implants*	*Secondary Implants*	%
41	25,234	2164	8.6

In a later study done at the request of the American Intra-Ocular Implant Society, K.J. Hoffer (1978) reported an incidence of secondary procedures of only 4% of the 70,000 implants surveyed. These

TABLE X-2. — *Secondary Implant Procedures Reported by Surgeons Who Had Performed More Than 1000 Implants (Darin, 1977)*

Surgeon	*Total Implants*	*Secondary Implants*	%
C.D. Binkhorst	2000	150	7.5
D.P. Choyce	1250	1200	95.1
M.A. Galin	1800	12	0.6
J.C. Worst	2250	50	2.2
H. Hirschmann	1800	83	4.1
N.S. Jaffe	1500	1	0.06
R.W. Barnet	1000	101	10.1
J.H. Little	1350	36	2.8
J.H. Sheets	1200	23	1.9

TABLE X-3. — *Distribution of Secondary Implant Procedures according to the Type of Preexisting Aphakia (Darin, 1977)*

Number of Secondary Implants	*After Intracapsular Cataract Extraction*	*After Extracapsular Cataract Extraction*	*Unknown*
2164	1224	574	366
Percentage	56.6%	26.5%	17%

2608 implantations were performed by only a third of the 734 surgeons who participated in the study. In general, most of the surgeons who had performed more than 200 implantations had done some with secondary procedures. The types of lenses implanted were not indicated in the survey report.

II. Secondary Implantation of Iris and Iridocapsular Supported Lenses

A. Indications

In the early fifties, C.D. Binkhorst started to implant lenses with a secondary procedure in unilateral aphakics in order to restore binocular vision. At first, he used the anterior chamber lenses available at the time and implanted at least 35 lenses with rigid supports and several with elastic supports (Dannheim lens). In 1958, he started to use his iris clip lens. After having performed 70 secondary implants of his lens, he reported that the final visual result was poor in about 10% of the cases, even though binocular vision was restored in 89% of the cases and there was remarkably little inflammatory response.

Poor results were ascribed mainly to a number of unfavorable conditions resulting from the cataract extraction such as corneal damage, anterior or posterior synechiae, and free vitreous in the anterior chamber. The last two conditions in particular required complex surgical procedures that enhanced the risk of postoperative complications such as cystoid macular edema and endothelial corneal dystrophy.

Later, Binkhorst (1967) came to the conclusion that secondary insertion of an iris clip lens after intracapsular cataract extraction should not become a standard procedure because better results had been attained with primary implants. Eyes containing a capsular membrane after extracapsular cataract extraction, however, were still considered by Binkhorst to be good candidates.

Therefore, he restricted his secondary implantations to those cases where the vitreous was separated from the anterior eye segment by a capsular membrane and to the rare cases of intracapsular aphakics for which rehabilitation of binocular vision was of prime importance and could not be achieved by contact lenses. In the latter cases, however, Binkhorst would only reopen an eye if no vitreous was present in the pupillary aperture.

Not all surgeons completely agree with Binkhorst. For example, Jaffe et al. (1978), while admitting that secondary implant surgery is easier when a posterior capsule is present, do not consider the presence of vitreous in the pupillary aperture to be a strict contraindication, though these surgeons do regard a substantial amount of free vitreous in the anterior chamber to be a contraindication.

According to Eichenbaum (1977), if adequate measures are taken to prevent vitreous escape, its occasional occurrence should not deter the surgeon from inserting a lightweight iris clip lens, providing this complication is properly managed (vitrectomy). If this is done, the presence of an iris clip lens of itself will not increase the risk of cystoid macular edema or retinal detachment. However, as Jaffe et al. (1978, p. 130) note, "both the surgeon and the patient should realize that there is a possibility that the procedure may make the patient worse."

Nor is J. Worst a proponent of lens implantation for intracapsular aphakia. His early experiences in 19 cases resulted in a 36.8% incidence of clinical cystoid macular edema. For secondary implantation, he recommends two lenses of his own design: the Small Incision Lens and the Iris Claw lens.

Note: It is possible that, with the use of Hyalon® (a viscous solution containing 1% sodium hyaluronic acid) or similar viscous agents, there will be fewer restrictions for secondary implantation after intracapsular aphakia. Indeed, such agents allow the maintenance of a formed anterior eye segment and thus prevent endothelial damage and vitreous involvement. The innocuosity of these agents is not yet fully established, however.

B. Binkhorst's Fixation Modalities for Secondary Implantation in Extracapsular Aphakia

1. When capsular fixation is impossible, the use of an iris clip lens is to be considered providing the iris diaphragm and the pupil width are suitable. Depending on the local situation, additional sutures may help to steady the lens.

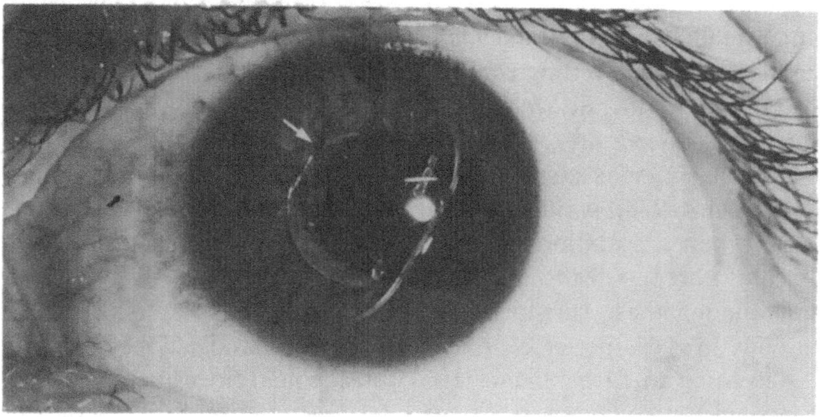

Fig. X-1. — Secondary implant of an iris clip lens; a suture (arrow) was used to steady the lens. (Courtesy C.D. Binkhorst.)

Secondary implantation of an iris clip lens may also be appropriate when there are large iris colobomas. One or more sutures will provide adequate reconstruction of the pupil and keep the lens in the required position.

2. When there are posterior synechiae present, posterior lens loops should be inserted into the iridocapsular cleft. Good fixation can be achieved by placing a loop between two adjacent posterior synechiae. Special attention should therefore be paid to the location of posterior synechiae during the preoperative examination. If extensive posterior synechiae are present, release of these adhesions should be consid-

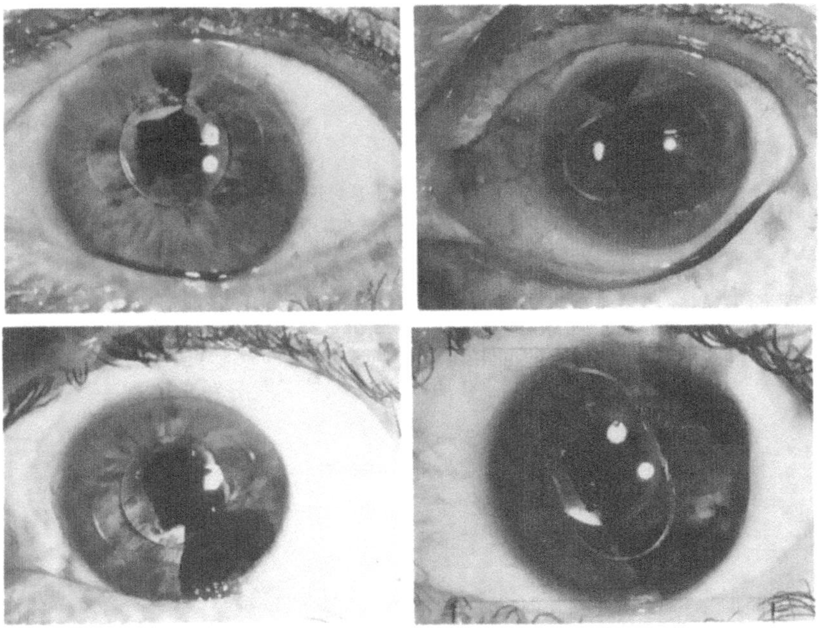

Fig. X-2. — Reconstruction of the pupil with sutures to hold an iris clip lens. (Courtesy C.D. Binkhorst.)

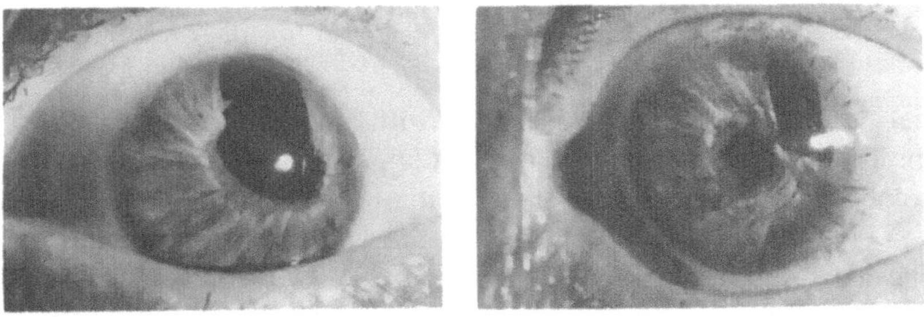

Fig. X-3. — A lightweight iridocapsular lens was used in this case instead of an iris clip lens. Since capsular fixation was unlikely to occur, the coloboma was closed with a suture. (Courtesy C.D. Binkhorst.)

ered. Binkhorst has noted that new synechiae, which will then provide firm fixation for the embedded loop, are likely to develop in that area.

3. There is also the possibility of forming a new pocket in peripheral areas containing some cortical lens remnants (e.g. a Soemmering's ring) to insert a loop. For this the peripheral cataractous mate-

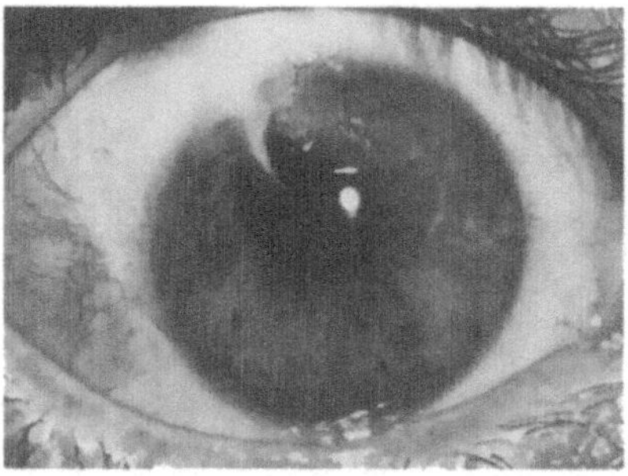

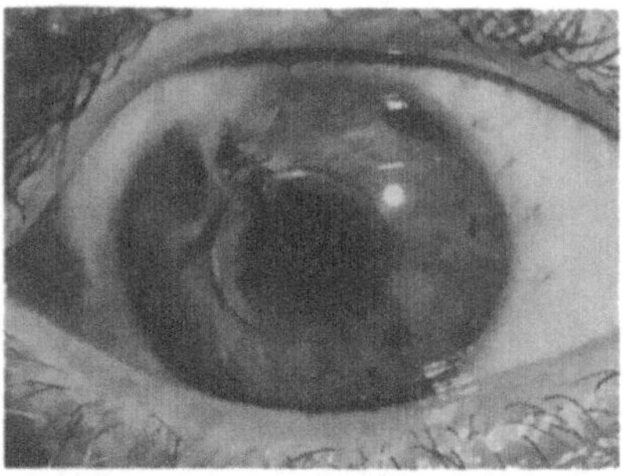

Fig. X-4. — Here, an iridectomy was performed to loosen the anterior synechiae. The iatrogenic coloboma thus obtained was closed with 2 iris sutures to stabilize the lightweight iridocapsular lens. (Courtesy C.D. Binkhorst.)

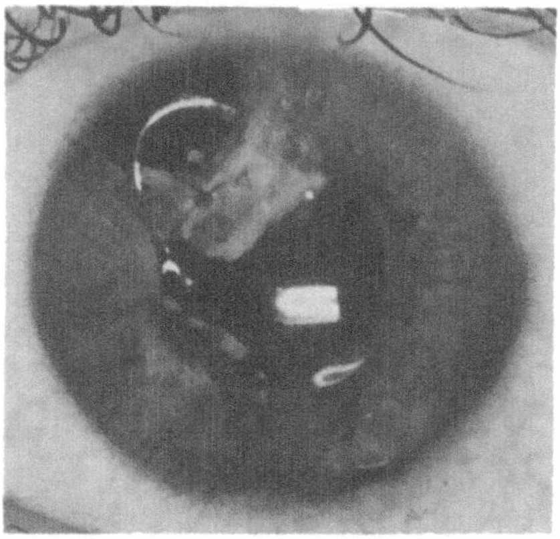

Fig. X-5. — Iridocapsular lens with the loops fixed by posterior synechiae that reformed after being released.

rial has to be carefully dissected with an instrument such as a discision knife. This kind of fixation is primarily of value if large iris colobomas prevent iridocapsular fixation.

4. If these possibilities are exhausted, which is rare, the posterior capsule itself can be used as a support. A two-loop lens has to be introduced inversely and the optic portion passed through a capsulotomy like a collar button.

→

Fig. X-6. — Binkhorst's technique for fixation of a 2-loop lens in peripheral lens remnants. With a sharp knife, 2 opposing pockets are formed in which the tips of the loops have to be placed. (Courtesy C.D. Binkhorst and L. Loones.)

Fig. X-7. — In this case, the lower lens remnants had to be dissected to allow the positioning of the lower posterior loop of an iris clip lens. (Courtesy C.D. Binkhorst.)

Fig. X-8. — This 2-loop lens has been placed with the optic portion slipped through the posterior capsule like a collar button. The schema illustrates a similar situation.

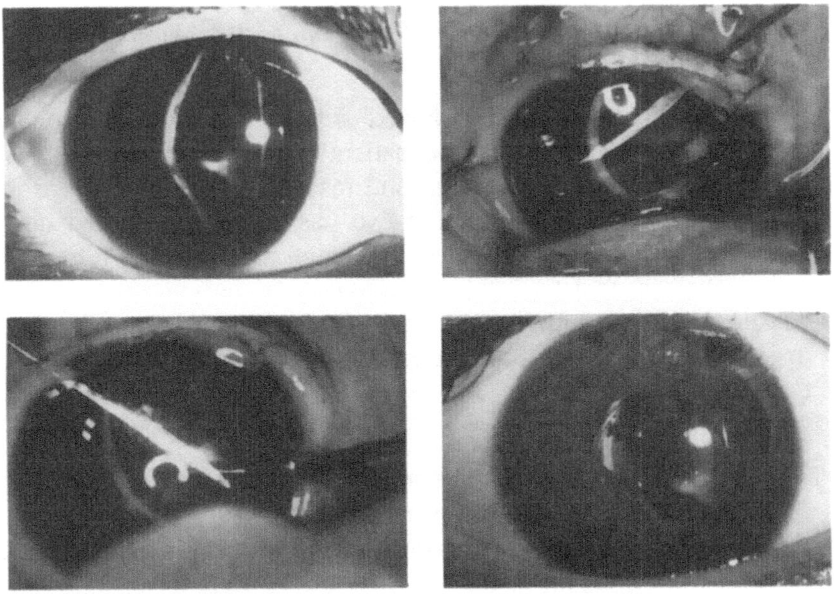

Fig. X-6.

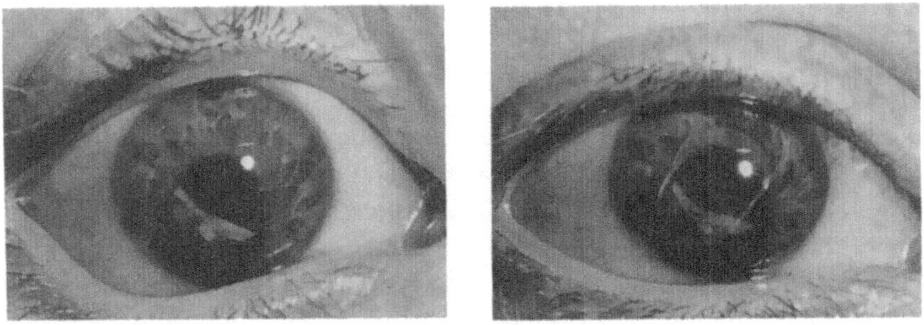

Fig. X-7.

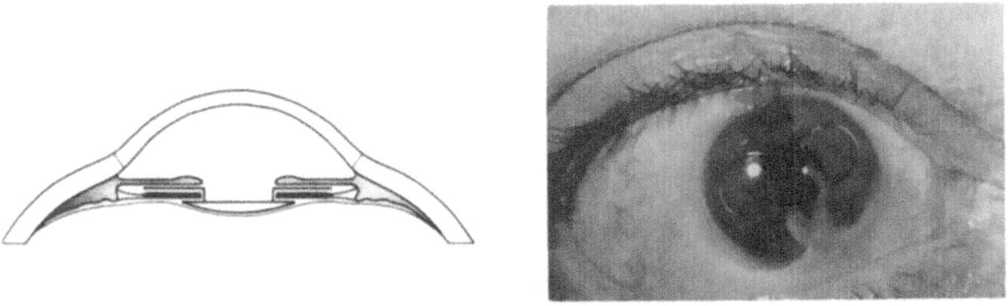

Fig. X-8.

III. Secondary Implantation of Angle Supported Lenses

A. Indications

Unlike Binkhorst, D.P. Choyce still favors routine secondary implantation. He removes the patient's own lens, generally with intracapsular cataract extraction, and inserts the pseudophakos some weeks or months later after the eye has completely settled down. Choyce considers long-standing, uncomplicated aphakic patients to be excellent candidates for his lens type.

Choyce (1976) summarized some of the advantages and disadvantages of the two-stage procedure as follows:

Advantages

— The refraction can be determined precisely, thus aiding in the correct choice of a pseudophakos.
— Since the corrected visual acuity is known, there is a target to aim at.
— The visual fields can be charted.
— Any additional intraocular pathology can be identified.

Disadvantages

— Peripheral anterior synechiae can interfere with the proper positioning of the haptics into the scleral rim.
— Reopening the eye can involve increased risks for the corneal endothelium.

Note: Even though vitreous loss is more likely to occur in secondary implantation, Choyce does not think that it will affect the final result. Indeed, he observed that vitreous loses much of its tendency to adhere to adjacent structures and to cause persistent iritis after it has been exposed to aqueous. In his experience, management of vitreous loss during a secondary implantation can be limited to cutting off the modified vitreous at the wound edge and need not involve a vigorous vitrectomy.

B. Results

Choyce has performed more than 1200 angle supported implants with secondary procedures to date. Table X-4 gives the kind of aphakics for which Choyce found that the insertion of his angle supported lens was indicated. Choyce considers this distribution typi-

TABLE X-4. — *Causes of Cataracts in 100 of D.P. Choyce's Patients (Choyce, 1975)*

Senile	67
Traumatic	17
Congenital	7
Following uveitis	4
Following filtration surgery for glaucoma	3
Following heterochromic cyclitis	2
Total	100

TABLE X-5. — *Short-Term Complications of 100 of D.P. Choyce's Patients (Choyce, 1975)*

Endothelial corneal dystrophy (the contralateral eye showed cornea guttata)	1
Uveitis, persistent	5
Hyphema, persistent	1
transient	2
Glaucoma, transient (pupil block)	1

cal. With regard to his own postoperative problems, he found the distribution of early complications given on Table X-5 also typical.

The average recovery time after secondary implantation is reported to be eight weeks (Choyce, 1977).

It was necessary to remove the implanted lens in 3 of these 100 cases: one lense because of an hyphema that kept reforming, and the other two because of uveitis that did not settle down (one patient was diabetic).

Long-term complications that developed in 1000 secondary Mark VIII implantations were reported in 1977 and are here given on Table X-6. As these figures show, the results are good except for the incidence of clinical cystoid macular edema and the number of implants that had to be removed because of hyphema or iritis. The

TABLE X-6. — *Long-Term Results of 1000 Secondary Mark VIII Implantations (Choyce, 1977)*

Visual acuity ⩾20/40	81%
Endothelial corneal dystrophy (bullous keratopathy)	1.5%
Clinical cystoid macular edema	6%
Implant removed because of hyphema or iritis	3%
Vitreous loss	7%

1.5% incidence of endothelial corneal dystrophy refers only to the cases of bullous keratopathy. As already noted, J. Pearce found an additional 13.5% incidence of partial endothelial corneal dystrophy in a random selection of 73 of Choyce's patients. By clinical observation, Choyce has determined that this partial endothelial corneal dystrophy is non-evolutive (Choyce, 1977).

Corrected visual acuity ⩾20/40 was attained for 81% of the patients. Since we do not have sufficient data on preoperative visual acuity, we cannot evaluate the risk-benefit ratio as regards visual acuity. As stated above, Pearce found an average drop in visual acuity of 30% when comparing the values from before and after implantation.

Over the last few years, angle supported lenses have become more popular. Particularly in the United States, many surgeons have been attracted to the Choyce Mark VIII, which Choyce considers the most suitable lens for secondary implantation. J. Tennant (1976), J. Sheets (1977), B. Boyd (1978), and S. Harrison (1978) have published their results. These reports cover 143 secondary lens implantations mainly after intracapsular surgery. There was not one case of endothelial corneal dystrophy and the incidence of other complications such as iritis, cystoid macular edema, and secondary glaucoma was quite low, except when defective lenses were used. Although the figures given for visual acuity are satisfactory, no comparisons were made between preoperative and postoperative visual performance.

Surgeons who have used angle supported lenses consider its advantages over the various types of iris-supported lenses to be as follows:

1. It can be inserted through a small incision (the Mark IX, for example, needs only a 5 mm opening).
2. Insertion disturbs the configuration of the incision very little, so a "closed chamber" technique is possible.
3. Intraocular manipulations to close a coloboma or to steady the lens are not necessary.
4. When large colobomas are present, an anterior chamber lens (Mark VIII) with colored haptics can be used.
5. In Choyce's experience, as already noted, vitreous in the pupillary aperture is not a matter of concern, and even substantial vitreous prolapse into the anterior chamber does not seem to affect the final result.
6. Extraction of the implant is easy.

IV. Secondary Lens Implantation Series of Various Lens Types

Secondary insertion of an intraocular lens involves, as we have often had occasion to note, at least the risk of decreasing visual acuity. Nevertheless, there are many aphakics who ought to be rehabilitated, especially monocular patients. There is no agreement on which lens type is best, nor is there a lack of controversy around the problem of case selection. Some prominent surgeons consider implantation only for extracapsular aphakia while others perform secondary implantation also for intracapsular aphakia. For the future, prudence will probably require compromises with regard to the different lens types, their choice depending on the specific situation. The experience of F. Hardenberg (1977) and H.J. Shammas and C.F. Milkie (1978) with 135 cases is representative to a degree in that it reflects the results of secondary implantation of various lens types after both intracapsular and extracapsular cataract extraction. Again, we must add the caveat that larger series with longer follow-up periods are necessary to draw valid statistical conclusions about the risk-benefit ratio involved.

A. Hardenberg's Study

F. Hardenberg (1977) published a well-documented study of 64 secondary implantations of both Binkhorst and Choyce lenses after intra- and extracapsular aphakia. His indications for considering secondary implantation were:

1. Unilateral aphakia with developing strabismus or subjective contact lens intolerance;
2. Unilateral aphakia with corneal decompensation from contact lenses;
3. Unilateral or bilateral aphakia with occupational requirements that cannot be met by spectacle or contact lens correction;
4. Bilateral aphakia with inability to adapt to spectacle or contact lens correction;
5. Aphakia in one eye and pseudophakia in the other in special situations.

The guidelines Hardenberg uses for the choice of the lens are given on Table X-7.

Hardenberg's results are given on Tables X-8 and X-9. On the basis of this series, he concluded that a candidate for secondary implantation had roughly one chance in four of losing some central

TABLE X-7. — **Guidelines for Lens Selection** *for Secondary Lens Implantation (F. Hardenberg, 1977)*

Condition	*Lens Type*
Extracapsular aphakia	All types
Intracapsular aphakia with free vitreous face	Alle types
Intracapsular aphakia with ballooning vitreous	All types (after vitreous section or manipulation)
Subsequent discission anticipated	Iris-supported lens
Pupillary reconstruction required	Iris-supported lens
Insufficient iris	Angle-supported lens
Iris tenting vitreous tenting	Angle-supported lens

TABLE X-8. — *Visual Acuity with Secondary Implantation, Hardenberg's Series (1977)*

Preoperative Visual Acuity	*Number of Patients*	*Postoperative Visual Acuity < Preoperative Visual Acuity*	*Postoperative Visual Acuity ≥ Preoperative Visual Acuity*
20/25 or better	37	11 or 30%	26 or 70%
20/40 or better	55	17 or 31%	38 or 69%
All cases	63	18 or 29%	45 or 71%

TABLE X-9. — *Complications in Hardenberg's Series (1977)*

Complications	*Number of Patients*	*Percent*
Cystoid macular edema	4	6
Lens dislocation	3	4
Hyphema	3	4
Bullous keratopathy	2	3
Discission	2	3
Vitrectomy (unplanned preoperative)	2	3
Severe iritis (hypopyon)	1	1
Secondary glaucoma	1	1
Lens removal	1	1
Retinal detachment	0	—
Flat chamber	0	—
Intraocular infection	0	—

visual acuity in the process and roughly one chance in three of increasing his central visual acuity. Postoperative visual acuity was equal to or better than preoperative acuity in three-fourths of the cases.

B. Shammas's and Milkie's Study

H.J. Shammas and C.F. Milkie (1978) reported on the results they obtained with the implantation of 36 Choyce Mark VIII "lathe cut" lenses, 21 Worst platinum-clip lenses, and 13 Worst Medallion lenses. There were 53 intracapsular and 17 extracapsular aphakics, with phakoemulsification having been used in the latter cases. The series does not include either patients with preexisting macular changes or patients in which phakoemulsification was combined with incision of the posterior capsule. Also excluded were eyes in which injection molded angle supported lenses had been implanted. The follow-up ranged from 9 to 41 months, with an average of 19 months. During the surgical procedure itself, the most serious problem was vitreous loss in 7 cases (10%). Significant postoperative problems were endothelial corneal dystrophy (1 case), retinal detachment (1 case), cystoid macular edema (3 cases), and dislocation of 3 of the Worst lenses.

The one case of endothelial corneal dystrophy was ascribed to the use of an open-sky technique and the surgical manipulations required to insert a Medallion lens. Such corneal changes were not encountered when the Choyce Mark VIII lens was implanted.

The 3 cases of cystoid macular edema occurred after intracapsular cataract extraction and when the anterior hyaloid face was intact. The final visual acuity improved in 2 of these cases to ≥20/40, but remained at 20/60 in the third case. All 3 of these cases involved intracapsular cataract extraction. In a later study (1979), Shammas and Milkie again emphasized the higher incidence of cystoid macular edema in secondary procedures relative to primary procedures.

Surgical repositioning was indicated in the 3 cases of dislocation, all of which were of Medallion lenses.

Relative to the aphakic condition, final visual acuity remained the same or improved in 91% of the cases. Decreases in visual acuity were attributed to endothelial corneal dystrophy, high astigmatism, and cystoid macular edema. In the opinion of Shammas and Milkie, final visual acuity was not influenced by the presence of vitreous in the anterior chamber (27 cases, 39%).

In this study the authors concluded that the Choyce Mark VIII was the superior lens.

Conclusion

When considering secondary lens implantation, the surgeon must carefully weigh the risks and the benefits. As we have shown, there is a price to pay for the patient's rehabilitation regardless of which type of lens is used.

Aphakia, of itself, is never a sufficient indication for the implantation of an artificial lens. It should be considered only when visual rehabilitation is very important.

Extracapsular aphakia undoubtedly involves the least amount of risk for the eye, and it may also be considered for various types of lenses. With intracapsular aphakia, iris supported lenses are not indicated because of their lack of long-term stability. For these cases, lenses that rely on angle support have proven to be superior.

CHAPTER XI

LENS IMPLANTATION IN CHILDREN TRAUMATIC AND INFANTILE CATARACTS

Encouraged by the good results obtained with lens implantation in adults particularly with regard to binocular vision, some surgeons have corrected traumatic and congenital cataracts in children with lens implants. Anterior chamber lenses were first used in conjunction with secondary procedures.

I. Early Reports

A. Traumatic and Infantile Cataracts: D.P. Choyce

D.P. Choyce (1964) has reported on some cases of traumatic and congenital cataracts that led him to conclude that lens implantation in these cases matched and even exceeded the advantages of contact lenses. In a few cases, he used anterior chamber lenses in phakic children for optical correction of uniocular and binocular myopia, for functional rehabilitation of phakic eyes with albinism, and for cosmetic improvement of blind eyes with ugly cataracts.

1. *Traumatic Cataract*

D.P. Choyce's experience with his first traumatic aphakic cases can be summarized as follows.

The age at which the trauma occurs is of prime importance: the younger the patient, the greater the chance of amblyopia.

The interval between injury and treatment is also crucial since delay can put the final result at risk.

This encouraged Choyce to deal expeditiously with traumatic cataracts when the patients were under 10 years old. In some cases, he judged that implantation had to be performed even before the eye had time to settle down completely.

Traumatic cataract surgery on children is always more demanding than on adults, and, since no two injuries are exactly alike, Choyce could not lay down many rules for surgical management.

Because of the special fixating principle of anterior chamber lenses, large traumatic colobomas did not interfere with lens insertion provided that adequate peripheral support remained. This made ample excision of prolapsed iris tissue and iris to cornea adhesions possible. Lenses with external fixation were sometimes used to achieve greater stability, and lenses with colored haptics were implanted when large sections of the iris were missing that had to be covered (Fig. XI-1).

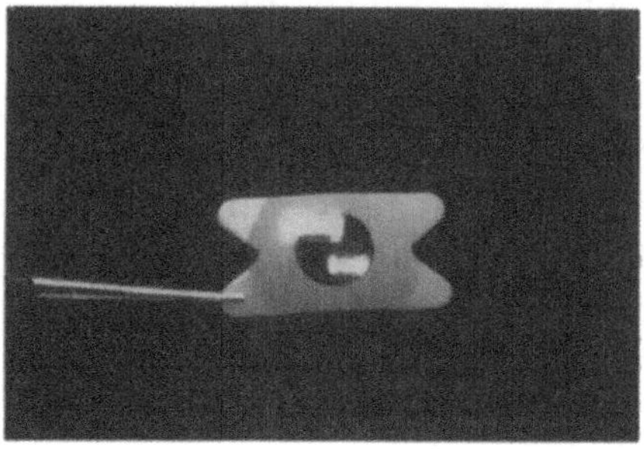

Fig. XI-1. — The Choyce Mark III with colored haptic.

Choyce considers unabsorbed soft lens matter, epithelialization of the anterior chamber, and extensive anterior synechiae to be contraindications. But the suggestion that it would be unwise to implant a fixed length anterior chamber lens in a young child because of the possibility that it might become too short has not been confirmed in practice. Choyce's own analysis of the different lengths used supported the opinion of Wolff (1950) and Duke Elder and Wybar (1961) that the cornea reaches adult size at the age of 2 or 3 years. In any case, Choyce felt that a margin of safety was provided by the ease with which an implant that had become to short in the growing eye could be replaced.

TABLE XI-1. — *Correlation between Mean Horizontal Corneal Diameters and Age (Choyce, 1964)*

Age in Years	*Mean Corneal Diameter, 3-9 o'clock (in mm)*
0-4	11.63
5-14	11.75
15-24	11.69
25-34	11.89
35-44	11.61
45-54	11.65
55-64	11.50
65-74	11.57
75-84	11.62

Results

We have detailed results of 4 traumatic cases. In Cases 7 and 8, the injuries occurred at the ages of 8 and 4 years old respectively. For both, capsulotomies had to be performed 4 months and $1\frac{1}{2}$ years after the secondary lens implantation respectively.

For Case 7, the follow-up period at the time of publication was 6 years. The visual acuity was 6/12 unaided and 6/5 with −2.00 sph.: −0.75 cyl. Full binocular vision could be demonstrated.

For Case 8, the implant inserted by another surgeon was exchanged to allow better access for a capsulotomy. The replacement lens had a colored haptic in anticipation of the tendency for the iris to atrophy and for the pupil to enlarge or displace with the passage of time (erosion of the pupillary border). Visual acuity was 6/9 and there was full binocular vision.

In the other two cases, Cases 11 and 12, the patients were respectively 13 and 14 years old at the time of injury and the follow-up times were respectively 7 and $3\frac{1}{2}$ years.

For Case 11, an anterior chamber lens was implanted in a secondary procedure. Visual acuity was 6/5 with −1.50 sph., −3 cyl. Binocular vision was 80% on the Wirt Stereo Test and residual aniseikonia was 1%.

For Case 12, a capsulotomy was performed 3 months after the secondary implantation of an 11.5 mm anterior chamber lens. Visual acuity was 6/12 unaided and 6/6 with +1.50 sph., −3.00 cyl. Full binocular vision was obtained. Although the clearance between the implant and the endothelium was only 1.6 mm, no signs of corneal dystrophy were apparent after $3\frac{1}{2}$ years.

2. *Congenital Cataract*

D.P. Choyce also reported his experience with 20 cases of congenital cataract in children. The results are encouraging since 12 of the 20 cases attained a visual acuity of better than 20/200 though binocular vision could not be demonstrated in any of them.

- There were great difficulties in ruling out associated pathology, which was considered a contraindication for lens implantation. Choyce warns particularly against any degree of microphthalmia.
- The surgical procedures were notoriously difficult, and dense membranes, which formed behind the lens and which resisted all attempts at surgical division, prejudiced the visual results.

TABLE XI-2. — *Results from Treating Congenital Cataract with Anterior Chamber Implants (Choyce, 1964)*

Good surgical and fair visual result	12
Good surgical but poor visual result	5
Epithelialisation' of anterior chamber leading to glaucoma and enucleation	1
Accidental trauma leading to phthisis bulbi	1
Intracapsular extraction: later removal of implant	1

— Amblyopia also contributed to poor results, expecially in the unilateral cases.

At that time, Choyce concluded that the results of treating congenital cataracts with intraocular implants were not as satisfactory as those with traumatic cataracts.

To our knowledge, Choyce has not published the results of any other series with children after this initial period, and he mentions the use of his later lens models for children only occasionally. In his opinion, the Mark IX lens seems to have some advantages over the previous models, since it is better suited for small anterior eye segments and permits relatively easy access to the retropupillary space.

B. Traumatic and Infantile Cataracts: C.D. Binkhorst

1. *Traumatic Cataract*

C.D. Binkhorst performed his first implantation for a traumatic cataract in a child in 1959 and 6 others in 1962; he published his results in 1964 (Tables XI-3 and XI-4). Dannheim anterior chamber lenses with elastic supports were inserted in two-stage procedures. In

TABLE XI-3. — *Visual Acuity and Binocular Vision in 7 Children with an Intraocular Lens following Traumatic Cataract: Binkhorst and Gobin (1964)*

Case Nr.	*Age at Injury in Years*	*Injury/Aphakia Interval in Months*	*Aphakia/Pseudophakia Interval in Months*
1	8	16	2
2	3	16	5
3	2	24	12
4	3	1/4	12
5	9	10	4
6	3	$2\frac{1}{2}$	$1\frac{1}{2}$
7	8	$3\frac{1}{2}$	$1\frac{1}{2}$

TABEL XI-4. — *Injuries to the Eye: Binkhorst and Gobin (1964, p. 174)*

Case-no.	*Visual acuity*	*Position of eyes*	*Simultaneous perception*	*Fusion*	*Stereoscopic vision*
1	0.67	parallel	+	from −4° to +35°	+
2	0.5	unknown	?	?	?
3	0.5/60 excentric fixation	5° convergent	—	—	—
4	1.0	5° divergent	+	+ without amplitude	?
5	0.25	parallel	+	from −5° to +6°	?
6	1.0	parallel	+	from −4° to +6°	probably
7	1.0	2° convergent	+	from +6° to +20°	?

Binkhorst's opinion, this particular lens seemed apt to cause fewer complications than the other anterior chamber lenses with fixed length in use at the time.

Eight more Dannheim lenses were inserted over the following years (Binkhorst and Gobin, 1967). After these, all subsequent cases were provided with iris clip or iridocapsular lenses. The updated results of Binkhorst's total experience in 26 cases with these 3 different lenses were published in 1969 (see Table XI-5 and XI-6).

With regard to the management of traumatic cataracts in children, we shall concentrate on the problem of the prevention of amblyopia and on some aspects of the surgical technique as outlined by Binkhorst in the publications cited above.

a. *Measures for the Prevention of Amblyopia and the Loss of Binocular Vision*

It soon became obvious that too much time was elapsing between the injury and the lens insertion. At first, it was thought that children with unilateral aphakia should first try contact lenses (Binkhorst and Gobin, 1964), but this practice caused a considerable waste of time, which promoted amblyopia. Indeed, in the aphakic children Binkhorst treated with contact lenses, eye deviation was never cured, either spontaneously or after muscle surgery, as long as the contact lens was worn. And in some cases, the contact lens itself was suspected of causing squinting. Therefore, it was concluded that contact lenses should not be routinely prescribed in these cases. In fact, the need to reduce the interval between injury and implantation made the one-stage procedure more and more attractive.

TABLE XI-5. — *Results in 26 Children with Unilateral Post-Traumatic Pseudophakia Binkhorst et al. (1969)*

Case no.	*Age at injury (yrs)*	*Interval between injury and implantation (yrs)*	*Corrected visual acuity*	*Residual deviation (°)*	*Binocular vision (Fusion)*				
					First degree	*Second degree (°)*	*Third degree*		
							Synoptophore	*Fly test*	*Wirt test*
1	Two	3	0.01 *	+5	—	—	—	—	—
2	Two	4/12	0.8	+13	—	—	—	—	—
3	Three	1½	0.1	+2 L/R_3	—	—	—	—	—
4	Three	1	1.0	0	+	−6 to +6	+	+	0.1
5	Three	4/12	1.0	0	+	−3 to +2	+	+	0.6
6	Three	5/12	1.25	0	+	0 to −2	—	—	—
7	Three	4/12	0.6	0	+	—	—	—	—
8	Four	3/12	0.6	0	+	−6 to +3	+	+	0.5
9	Five	3	0.3	−5	+	—	—	—	—
10	Six	3/12	0.8	0	+	−4 to +6	+	+	0.8
11	Six	1	0.5	0	+	+3 to +17	—	—	—
12	Seven	1½	1.0	0	+	−7 to 0	−	+	0.7
13	Eight	1½	0.8	0	+	0 to +30	+	+	0.5
14	Eight	5/12	1.25	0	+	−2 to +8	+	+	1.4
15	Eight	12	1.0	0	+	+3 to +7	+	−	−
16	Nine	1	0.3	0	+	−3 to +8	−	−	−
17	Ten	2	0.6	0	+	−2 to +7	+	+	−
18	Ten	1	0.8	0	+	0 to +15	+	+	0.6
19	Ten	9	1.0	0	+	−4 to +8	−	+	0.6
20	Ten	1	1.25	0	+	−4 to +9	−	+	0.3
21	Eleven	3	1.6	0	+	−2 to +10	+	+	0.7
22	Twelve	2/12	2.0	0	+	−8 to +15	+	+	0.8
23	Thirteen	6	1.6	0	+	−6 to +20	−	+	0.7
24	Thirteen	6	0.6	0	+	−3 to +10	+	+	−
25	Fourteen	3	1.25	0	+	−4 to +4	−	−	−
26	Fourteen	6/12	1.6	0	+	−7 to +16	+	−	0.5

TABLE XI-6. — *Visual Acuity Measured by Snellen's E-test in 26 Children with Unilateral Lens Implants, Injured at Ages Ranging from 2 to 14 Years (Binkhorst et al., 1969, p. 524)*

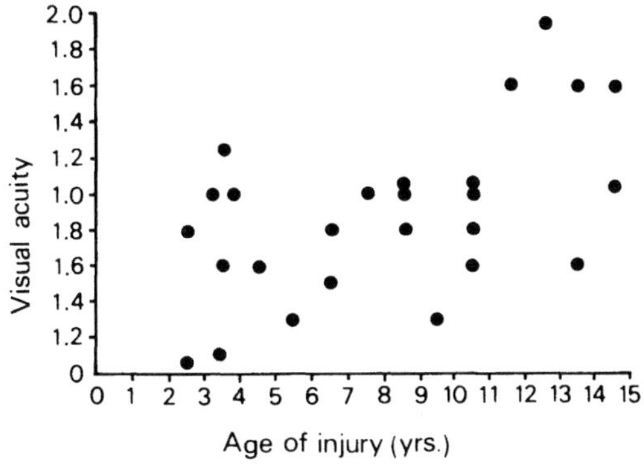

Other important measures were taken to regain visual acuity and to restore binocular vision after implantation:

— In the postoperative period, sustained occlusion of the fellow eye was advocated until maximal visual acuity was regained. Once optimal vision was achieved, careful binocular re-education was accomplished by gradual reduction of occlusion. Indeed, the achievement of binocular vision was always considered the best guarantee against suppression and thus against amblyopia and squint development.

— If deviation was present and unlikely to heal spontaneously, muscle surgery was indicated. Fortunately, in 9 out of the 21 children with squint, the condition cleared up spontaneously after lens implantation without any orthoptic training. It was also observed that long-standing deviation needed surgery sooner than did recently developed squint.

— Finally, periodic testing of visual acuity was required for a number of years for timely detection of secondary cataracts and incipient amblyopia.

b. *Some Technical Considerations*

C.D. Binkhorst has observed that lens implantation in a child is always an extremely demanding task. Despite all the measures taken to provide a soft eye with a deep anterior chamber, the surgery was often hampered by a forward bulging of the iridocapsular diaphragm. It was not always possible, therefore, to avoid touching the endothelium. In this regard, insufflation of air into the anterior chamber proved useful.

As a rule, a 4-loop lens was used in those cases where synechiae were not likely to develop, and the iridocapsular lens in those cases where firm iridocapsular or capsular fixation could be expected.

In the one-stage procedure, the posterior loops of the iridocapsular lens were buried in the iridocapsular cleft. In the two-stage proce-

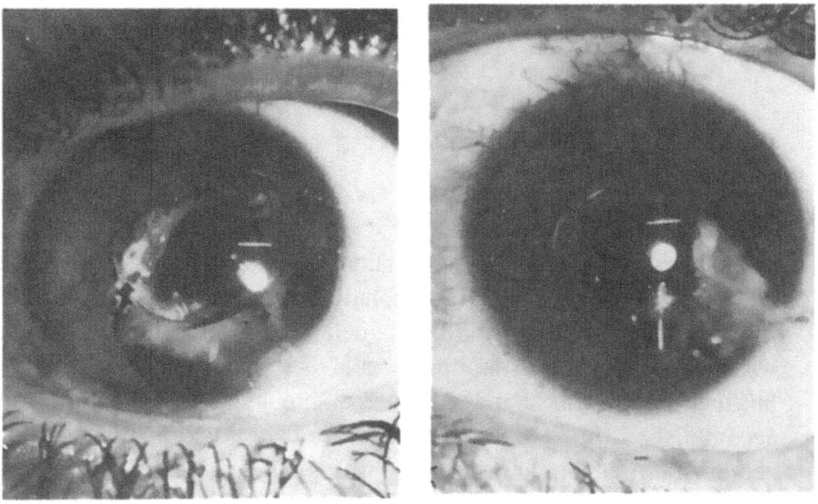

Fig. XI-2a. — Eyes with a large iris coloboma in which an iridocapsular lens has been implanted. The lens loops were placed in the iridocapsular cleft, and the presence of a large coloboma did not interfere with lens stability. (Courtesy C.D. Binkhorst.)

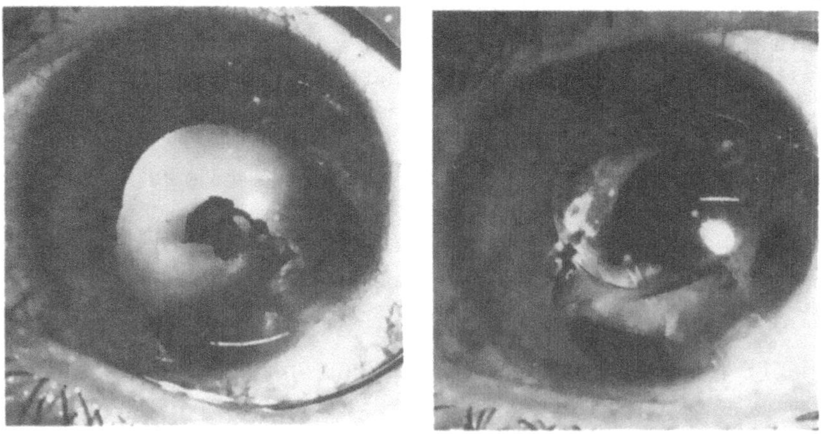

Fig. XI-2b. — In this case, firm capsular support was obtained in spite of a large coloboma. The upper and lower loops were placed in the original lens capsule. (Courtesy C.D. Binkhorst.)

dure, they were placed exactly where the adhesion had been cut to ensure that efficient iridocapsular adhesions embedded them. Because of the firm fixation that develops in the iridocapsular cleft, the iridocapsular lens could be used in cases with iris coloboma. Suturing iris tissue to steady the lens or to close colobomata was not considered necessary.

When peripheral anterior synechiae were present, the following practices were adopted:

— No attempt was made to loosen small peripheral synechiae even if many were present because of their natural tendency to reform and because they do not interfere with a pre-pupillary positioned capsular supported lens.

— Large and extensive anterior synechiae incarcerated in the wound were not dissected from corneal scar tissue, but just separated from the iris diaphragm by two radial cuts on each side of the adhesion to allow the iris diaphragm to fall back to its natural position.

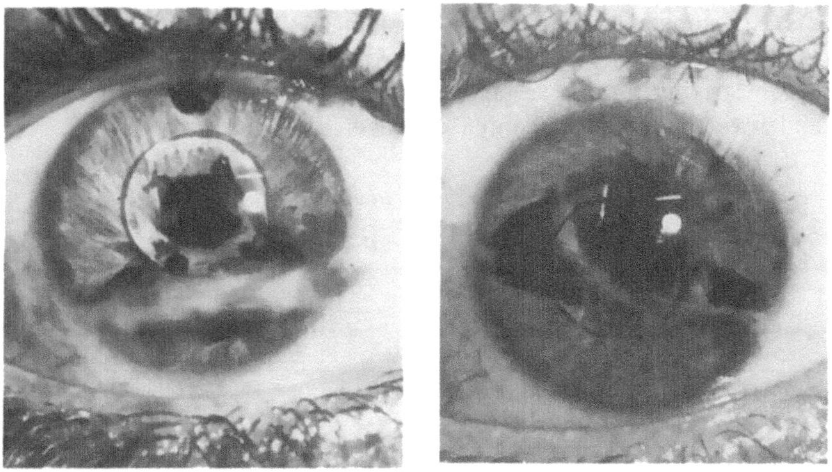

Fig. XI-3. — Examples of radial iridotomies performed to deepen the anterior chamber when extensive anterior synechiae are present. (Courtesy C.D. Binkhorst.)

— When an aphakic eye had an intact but opaque posterior capsule, no attempt was made to perform a capsulotomy before lens insertion as this would create far less favorable conditions for a secondary implant since the formed vitreous could bulge into the anterior chamber. Therefore, when a capsulotomy was indicated,

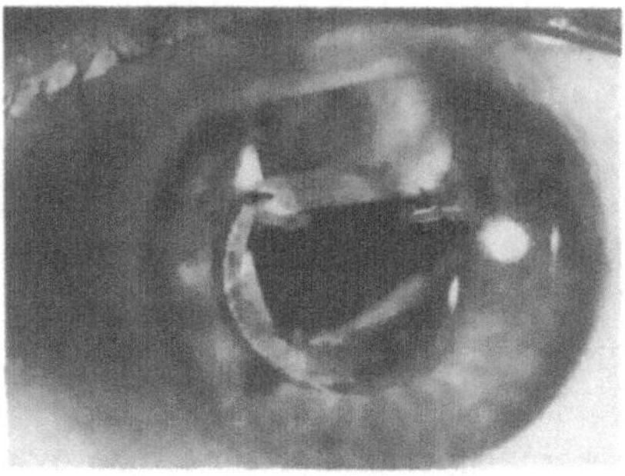
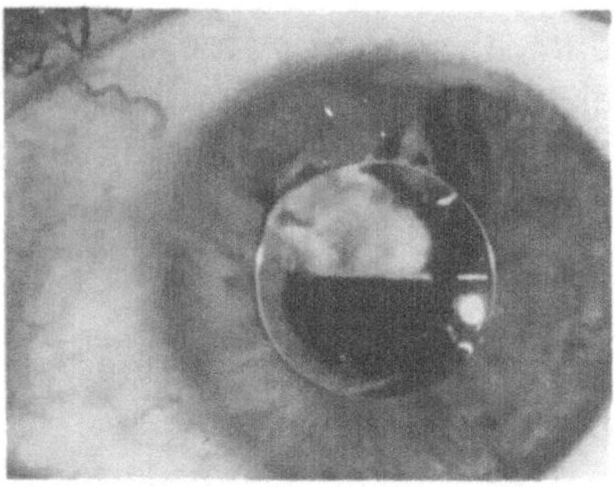

Fig. XI-4. — In these cases the thick posterior membrane had to be cut immediately after the lens was implanted. (Courtesy C. D. Binkhorst.)

this was carried out immediately after wound closure in a well-formed anterior chamber.

2. *Congenital Cataracts*

In 1970 and 1972, C.D. Binkhorst published the results of the first cases of congenital and infantile cataracts that he had treated with implantation, and, in 1975, M.E. Nordlohne reviewed them. There was a striking difference between the results obtained with bilateral and with unilateral congenital cataracts.

TABLE XI-7. — *Visual Acuity and Binocular Vision in Patients with Congenital Cataracts Treated with Lens Implantation: Unilateral versus Bilateral Cases (Nordlohne, 1975, p. 135)*

	Number of		*Average Visual*	*Binocular Vision*			
	Patients	*Eyes*	*Acuity*	*Absent*	*Simult. Percep.*	*Fusion*	*Steropiss*
Unilateral	23	23	20/200	4	—	—	1
Bilateral	14	20	20/40	3	—	—	6

As shown on Table XI-7, the visual acuity of the patients with unilateral cataracts was very low. Most of these eyes suffered from deep amblyopia that, along with the presence of associated pathological conditions often precluded good results.

In the 23 cases of unilateral cataracts, there were 11 instances of various degrees of microphthalmia, 5 of nystagmus, and 1 case each of microcornea, persistent primary vitreous, and retrolental membrane.

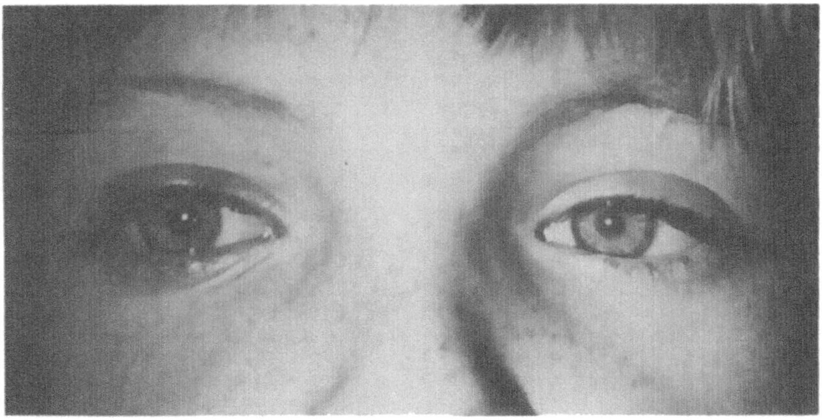

Fig. XI-5. — Bilateral congenital cataract with asymmetric evolution. The right eye began to squint at the age of 5, and a lens was then implanted. The photograph was taken when the child was 11 years old, the lens having been in place for 6 years. (Courtesy C. D. Binkhorst.)

More encouraging were the results with bilateral congenital cataracts in which the worst eye was generally the one operated on. Although some of these eyes already suffered from amblyopia and some showed strabismic deviations, the visual improvement was more rewarding (Fig. XI-5).

From the technical point of view, the following points are of interest. Lens implantation under the age of 1 year was never performed. In the majority of the cases, the cataract removal and the lens implantation were done with a one-stage procedure, with preliminary needling performed for most of the cases an average of 7 days prior to the implantation. As already noted for the cases of traumatic cataract in children, one of the major difficulties during surgery was the tendency of the anterior eye segment to collapse, which sometimes made atraumatic placement of the lens impossible. Nordlohne note that there were no serious postoperative complications, though postoperative capsulotomies were frequently necessary.

II. Later Reports

A. Binkhorst's Latest Data on Traumatic Cataracts in Children

Between 1966 and 1976, a total of 81 children suffering from unilateral traumatic cataracts or aphakia were operated on by Bink-

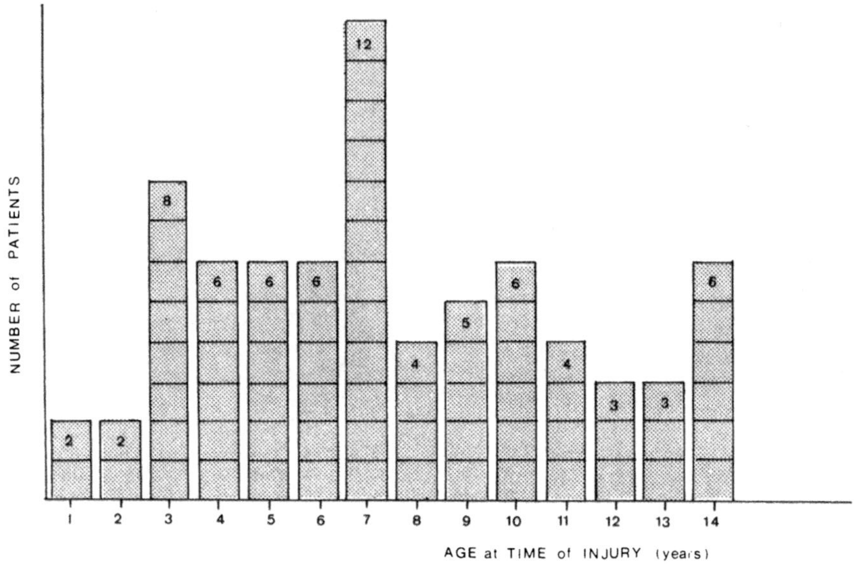

Fig. XI-6. — Age distribution at the time of injury. (Binkhorst et al., 1978).

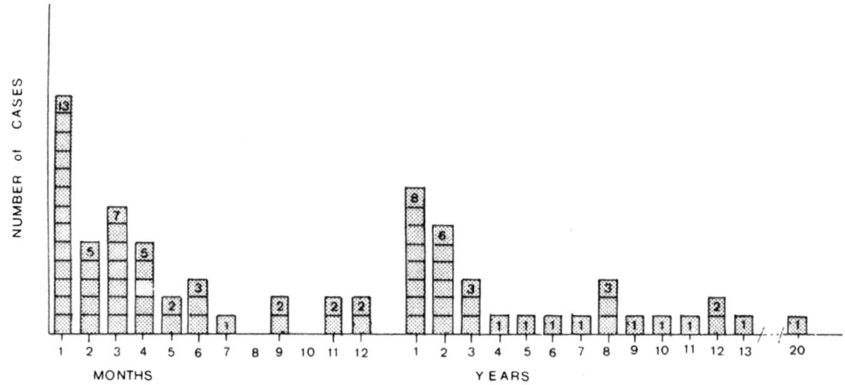

Fig. XI-7. — Number of cases relative to the intervals between injury and lens implantation (Binkhorst et al., 1978).

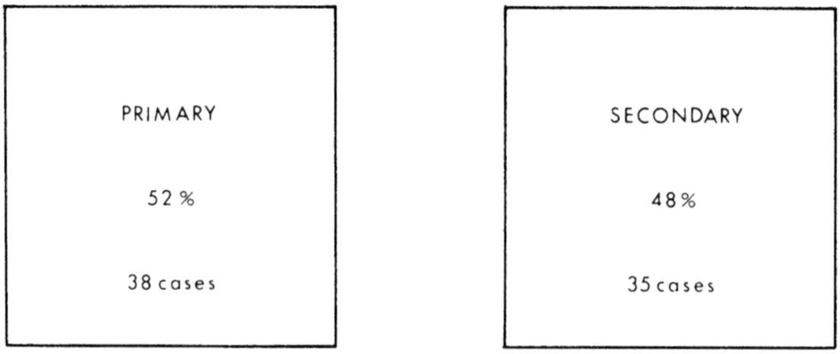

Fig. XI-8. — Procedural distribution.

horst and given 2- and 4-loop lenses. In 1978, Binkhorst published the results of 73 of them. The follow-up ranged from at least one year to a maximum of 12 years with an average of 6.5 years.

1. *Functional Results*

As Binkhorst has stressed, the functional results are generally dependent on such factors as case selection, degree of functional loss, rapidity of treatment, and efficacity of monocular and binocular re-education.

a. *Visual Acuity*

The figures given on Table XI-8 are impressive (57% attained 20/30 or better) and confirm Binkhorst's 1964 judgment that the prognosis for eye injuries with lens opacity in young children need not be as pessimistic as was generally supposed if sustained and adequate management is provided.

TABLE XI-8. — *Corrected Visual Acuity of 72 Pseudophakic Eyes. The Visual Acuity was Impossible to Determine for One 2-Year Old Child*

Corrected Visual Acuity	*Complete Series*
⩾20/40	56 eyes (78%)
⩾20/200	67 eyes (93%)
<20/200	5 eyes (7%)

Age et Injury: 1-14 years
Number of eyes: 72

The average visual acuity without correction was 20/60. That emmetropia was rarely achieved reflects Binkhorst's opinion that iseikonia in unilateral pseudophakia should take precedence over emmetropia. Spectacle correction was three times more often a minus correction than a plus. The plus correction ranged from +0.25 to +2.25 diopters (average: +1.25 diopters) and the minus correction from −0.25 to −7.75 diopters (average −2.50 diopters). The average spectacle correction for all pseudophakic eyes was −1.25 diopters. This slight myopia is also of importance because it favors visual training without additional spectacle correction when the fellow eye is occluded.

Again, as can be seen on Table XI-9 and XI-10, visual acuity increases with age. The low visual acuity of the youngest group can

TABLE XI-9. — *Average Visual Acuity in Three Groups According to Age at Injury (Binkhorst et al., 1978)*

	Age at Injury	Corrected Visual Acuity
Group I	1 to 4 years (17 eyes)	0.4
Group II	5 to 7 years (24 eyes)	0.7 –
Group III	8 to 14 years (31 eyes)	0.7 +

TABLE XI-10. — *Corrected Visual Acuity in Three Groups according to Age at Injury (Binkhorst et al., 1978)*

Corrected Visual Acuity	Group I 1 to 4 years 17 eyes	Group II 5 to 7 years 24 eyes	Group III 8 to 14 years 31 eyes
≥20/40	10 eyes (59%)	20 eyes (83%)	26 eyes (84%)
≥20/200	13 eyes (76%)	24 eyes (100%)	30 eyes (97%)
<20/200	4 eyes (24%)	0 (0%)	1 eye (3%)

be ascribed to the higher incidence of amblyopia and to some poor surgical results.

TABLE XI-11. — *Causes of Visual Acuity of Less Than 20/40 and Less Than 20/200 (Binkhorst et al., 1978)*

	Corrected Visual Acuity <20/40		Corrected Visual Acuity <20/200	
	Number	Percent	Number	Percent
Amblyopia	6	8.4%	2	2.8%
Retinal Detachment	2	2.8%	2	2.8%
Siderosis Bulbi	1	1.4%	1	1.4%
Corneal scar	3	4.2%	—	
Macular Lesions	4	5.6%	—	
Total	16	22%	5	7%

Table XI-11 gives the distribution of the reasons for less than good visual results. Some of these complications will be considered separately below.

TABLE XI-12. — *Visual Acuity and the Type of Procedure (Binkhorst et al., 1978)*

	Average Corrected Visual Acuity
Primary Procedure	0.71
Secondary	0.58

Table XI-12 shows that the average corrected visual acuity was better for those patients operated on with a one-stage procedure, which supports Binkhorst's opinion that one-stage surgery is preferable when not contraindicated.

b. *Binocular Vision*

The binocular status and position of the eye of 66 of the 73 patients could be assessed (7 were not available for examination).

Forty-eight patients (73%) had no deviation in the primary position, 11 (17%) had exodeviation, and 7 (10%) had esodeviation. Four patients with a small exodeviation and the 48 without any deviation demonstrated stereopsis with the Fly and Wirst stereo test (see Table XI-13).

TABLE XI-13. — *Binocular Status and Position of the Eye of 66 Patients*

Number	*Percent*	*Deviation*	*Cases with Stereopsis*
48	73%	Ortho	48
11	17%	Exo	4
7	10%	Eso	0

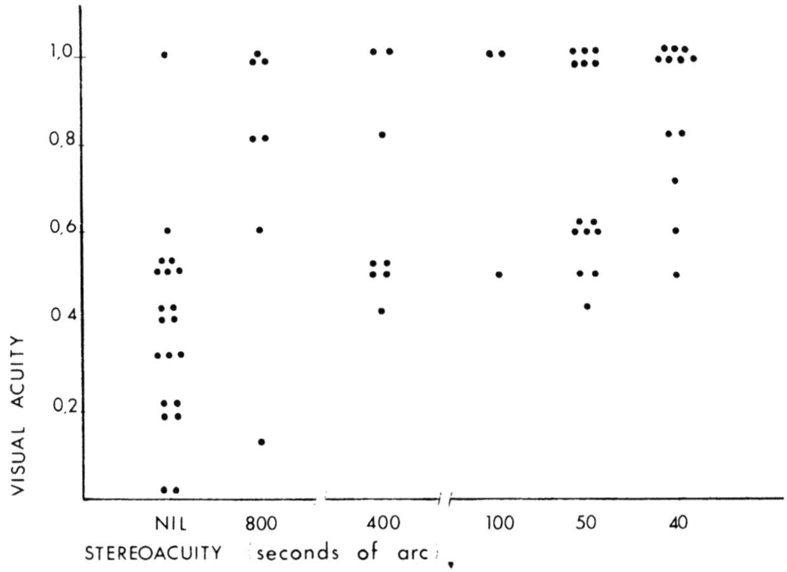

Fig. XI-9. — Stereoacuity of 66 patients in relation to visual acuity.

Thus, as of the last examination, 52 patients (79%) had useful binocular vision. This demonstrates the high degree of rehabilitation that can be obtained with implant lenses. Several deviations cured spontaneously after lens implantation, although it sometimes took years of obstinate occlusive therapy to achieve a satisfactory result.

2. *Complications*

In children with cataracts, it is almost impossible to distinguish the sequelae of the injury, of the cataract surgery, and of the lens implantation. Serious complications were encountered in 8 cases (10%), in 2 of which the eye was ultimately lost. Fair to good vision was preserved for the other 6 cases.

a. *Behavior of the Cornea*

Corneal problems developed in 2 cases, both times because of endothelial contact by the implant.

A minor corneal problem occurred when a four-loop lens, inserted in a secondary procedure, failed to develop capsular fixation. Pupillary mobility repeatedly brought one of the anterior loops in contact with the cornea so that the loop had to be removed.

A more serious problem occurred when one implant caused an internal corneal lesion with subsequent thickening and vascularization. The lens was removed.

Endothelial cell counts were performed on 34 patients chosen at random. On the average, there were 38.3% fewer cells in the injured eye than in the healthy fellow eye. There can be no doubt that cell destruction occurred because of the combination of injury, cataract surgery, and lens implantation. Cell densities of less than $1000/mm^2$ were found in two eyes, which was taken to be an ominous sign for the future transparency of these corneas when the aging process brings on further cell loss.

b. *Behavior of the Uvea*

Serious uveal reactions were uncommon, and mild surgical iritis could always be managed with topical corticosteroids. Pigmented deposits on the lens were frequently observed in the early postoperative period but they disappeared almost completely over the years. Significant iris atrophy due to iridolenticular contact was not encountered, even over the long term. Only localized patches of iris atrophy were observed at those points where the bare iris was in constant friction with the metal loops (fig. 9). In Binkhorst's opinion, immobilization of both the lens and the iris prevents significant iris atrophy.

c. *Intraocular Pressure*

In 2 cases, the intraocular pressure was disregulated. Further antiglaucomatous surgery was required after implantation for one child who suffered from repeated glaucoma attacks that had been controlled with fistulizing surgery prior to implantation. For the other child, pilocarpine and Diamox® were sufficient to control the elevation of the intraocular pressure after implantation.

d. *Retinal Problems*

There were 3 cases of retinal detachment: one case was repaired (visual acuity: 20/30); the second was treated without success; the third, in which the retinal detachment was suspected before implantation, developed phthisis of the eye after implantation.

In 2 cases, there was ophthalmoscopic evidence of maculopathy having caused significant loss of visual acuity. Sequelae of cystoid macular edema was considered responsible for some loss of central visual acuity in at least 2 other cases.

e. *Lens Luxation*

There was only one case of lens luxation: a two-loop lens inserted into an artificial pupillary aperture luxated into the vitreous. It was exchanged for a four-loop iris-clip lens.

f. *Discisions*

Capsular membrane needling was done for 68% (26 out of 38 eyes) of the patients who underwent one-stage procedures. In 5 cases, the capsulotomy had to be performed twice. In a few instances of injury in very small children, the posterior capsule was needled already at the end of the implant procedure in order to speed up visual recovery.

Of the 35 secondary implant patients, later needling of the capsular membrane was performed in 22 cases (63%) and excision of the capsular membrane in only 1 case. For the other cases, needling or excision were performed at the time of implantation.

3. *Remarks on General Management*

Few changes have had to be introduced into the management of traumatic cataracts in children since Binkhorst outlined it in 1969. The basic ideas are still:

a. Prevention of amblyopia by expeditious rehabilitation of the binocular function with an artificial lens implantation as soon as possible. Binkhorst does not advocate intentional secondary implantation as this is too time-consuming and thus increases the risk of amblyopia and quint. Contact lens correction has too low a success rate to justify this attitude. But this does not mean that treatment was always instituted immediately. Never were cataract extraction and lens implantation performed on a freshly and severely injured eye. The eye was always allowed to recover from the injury, and as soon as it was found to be quiet enough, a one-stage cataract extraction and lens implantation was performed unless there were contraindications. Among the reasons for post-hemophthalmos, and marked disregulation of the intraocular pres-gy, marked post-traumatic iritis, vascular ingrowth, infection, hemophthalmos, and marked disregulaton of the intraocular pressure. During the cataract extraction, the conditions that indicate that the implantation of the lens be postponed or cancelled are mainly vitreous prolapse, choroidal hemmorrhage, and the absence of the anterior chamber.

b. Two important requirements apply with regard to the lens itself:
   - Firm fixation of the intraocular lens to the capsular membrane. Indeed, firm fixation is of the utmost importance for these young patients, who will be participating in active sports and games. Strong and stable capsular membrane fixation is usually obtained for traumatic cataract treated with a one-stage procedure. When the lens is inserted in a secondary stage procedure, every effort should be made to obtain firm capsular or iridocapsular fixation.
   - Immobilization of the iris membrane to prevent iris chafing and late localized atrophy. This can be done by promoting adhesions between the pupillary border and the posterior loop attachment during the early post-operative period by the judi-

cious administration of miotics. Iris membrane immobilization prevents sphincter muscle erosion and stromal atrophy that would otherwise occur during the very long intraocular lens lifetime of these patients.

c. Lens implantation in children is no light matter, for this type of surgery requires exceptional experience and judgment. The problems involved are complex:
   - General rules as to the optimal time for lens implantation and the correct way to perform it cannot be formulated.
   - Young children are always difficult to examine prior to surgery, so it is often necessary to conduct preoperative examinations under narcosis. Frequently, one has to make important decisions during the surgical procedure for which there are no precise guidelines.
   - One has to rely on the cooperation of parents or parental substitutes during the pre- and postoperative periods, which may last for years.
   - The surgeon has to be backed by other experts (anesthesist, retinal surgeon, orthoptist).
   - Finally, the surgeon must be able to make use of advanced techniques such as electroretinography and echography, the latter being of importance for iseiconic correction, one of the keys to binocular recovery.

Therefore, as Binkhorst concluded, only the surgeon who feels a special commitment to this specific problem and to whom enough cases are referred for him to enlarge and maintain his experience should embark on this kind of surgery.

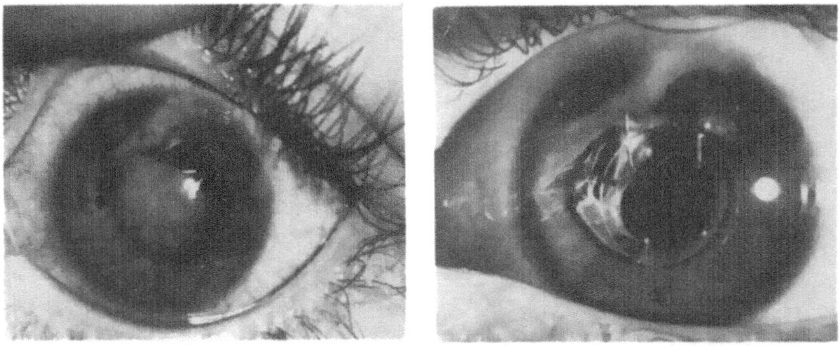

Fig. XI-10. — A moderately mutilated eye. A synechotomy and extracapsular cataract extraction were performed, and an iridocapsular lens was implanted. (Courtesy C.D. Binkhorst.)

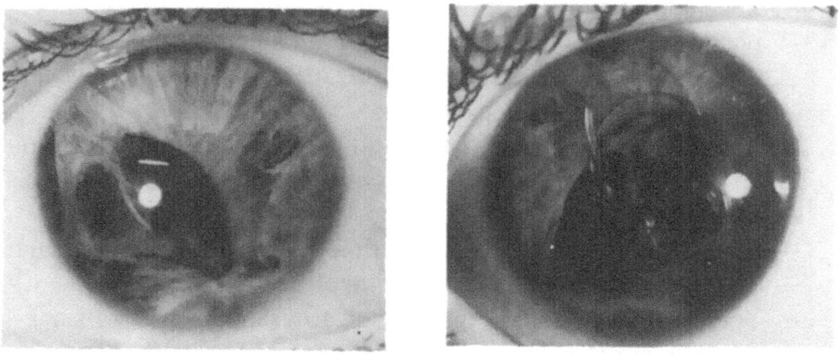

Fig. XI-11. — A case of secondary implantation of an iris clip lens. Note how the anterior synechiae have been dealt with. (Courtesy C.D. Binkhorst.)

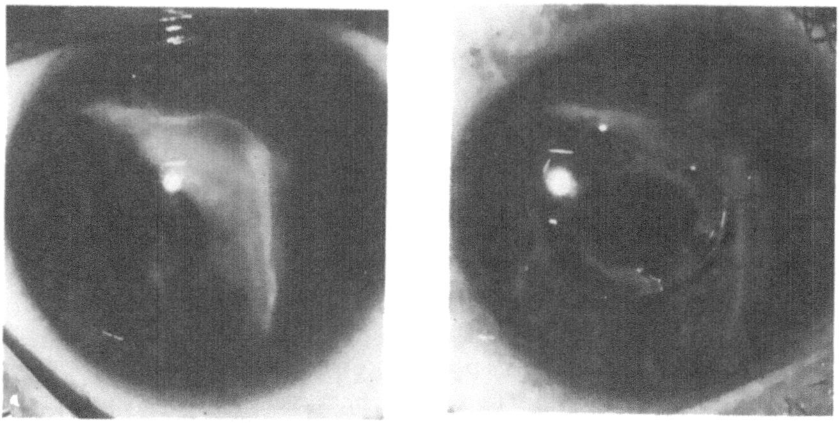

Fig. XI-12. — An apparently hopeless case provided with an iridocapsular lens with secondary implantation. (Courtesy C.D. Binkhorst.)

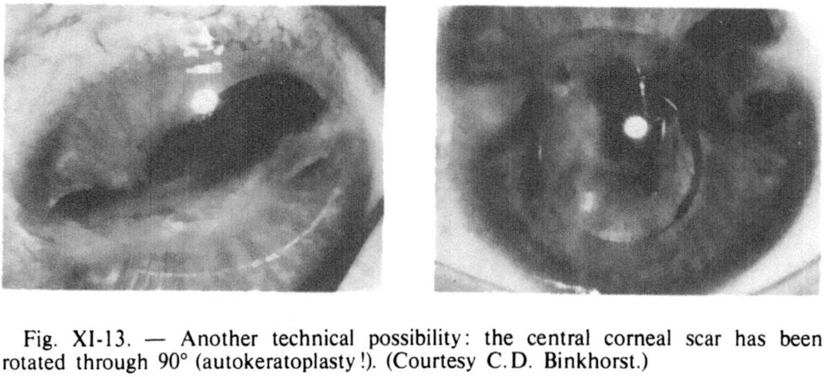

Fig. XI-13. — Another technical possibility: the central corneal scar has been rotated through 90° (autokeratoplasty!). (Courtesy C.D. Binkhorst.)

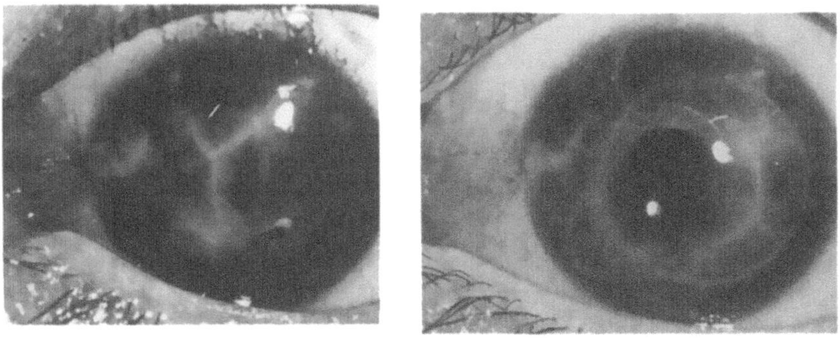

Fig. XI-14. — In this case of traumatic amiridia, the iridocapsular lens is held only by the lens capsule. Note also the rotating autokeratoplasty. (Courtesy C.D. Binkhorst.)

B. Reports by Other Surgeons

1. *A.T.M. Van Balen's Report on 37 Traumatic Cataracts in Children*

In 1974, A.T.M. Van Balen reported on the results of 37 traumatic cataracts in children treated at the Eye Clinic at Rotterdam by himself and other staff members. The series begins in September 1967, and the iridocapsular two-loop lens with metal loops was used. This report is of particular interest in two respects:

— It provides information on the problems encountered and results obtained by different surgeons using the same lens.
— It discusses the long-term results with 37 patients and confirms that lens implantation in children yields reproducible results if one adheres to Binkhorst's principles stated above.

In Van Balen's opinion, an artificial lens should always be considered when a child has a traumatic cataract because it offers the best chance for binocular rehabilitation. Some contraindications are: rupture of the posterior capsule by the trauma or during the operation because of the vitreous problems involved; extensive corneal scars that cause serious irregular astigmatism; large iris colobomata except when the lens can be secured by the methods Binkhorst has suggested.

Number and Age Distribution

Most of the patients had their accident between the ages of 4 and 10. Twenty-five patients could be implanted within the first few

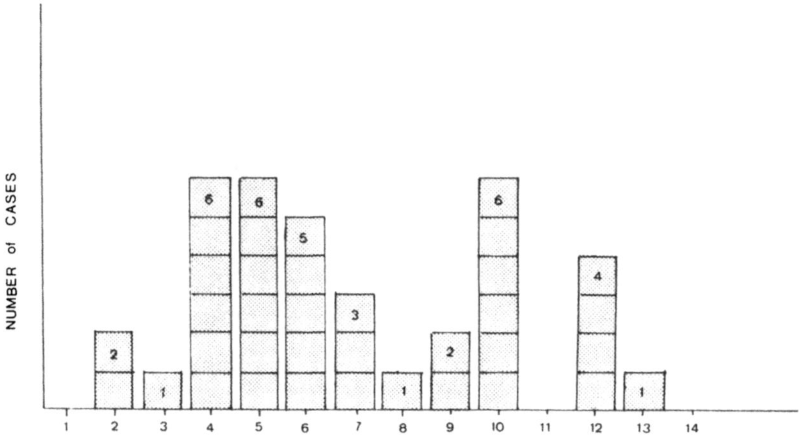

Fig. XI-15. — Age at injury of children with traumatic cataracts and supplied with intraocular lenses (A.T.M. Van Balen, 1975).

weeks after injury. Information is not available on the number of one-stage and two-stage procedures.

a. *Functional Results*

1) *Visual Acuity*

About 60% of the children regained visual acuity of 20/40 or better. Sixteen of them retained 20/25. However, two children with a postoperative visual acuity of 20/40 dropped to 20/200 because of amblyopia and retinal detachment.

TABLE XI-14. — *Corrected Visual Acuity of 37 eyes of Children with Traumatic Cataracts Treated with Intraocular Lenses (Van Balen, 1975)*

Corrected Visual Acuity	*Complete Series: 37 eyes* *Age at Injury: 2 years-13 years*
⩾20/40	22 eyes (59%)
⩾20/200	32 eyes (86%)
<20/200	5 eyes (14%)

Table XI-15 shows that the youngest group had the lowest visual acuity and that, from the age of 5 on, the results seem to stabilize.

TABLE IX-15. — *Corrected Visual Acuity of Three Groups according to Age at Time of Injury (Van Balen, 1975)*

Corrected Visual Acuity	*Group I 1-4 years 9*	*Group II 5-7 years 14*	*Group III ≥8 years 14*
≥20/40	2 (22%)	10 (71%)	9 (64%)
≥20/200	8 (89%)	11 (79%)	14 (100%)
<20/200	1 (11%)	3 (21%)	0 (0%)

2) *Binocular Vision*

Stereoscopic vision could be demonstrated in 27 patients, which means that 73% of the children obtained useful binocular vision. Van Balen noted that several cases with visual acuity of less than 20/40 had binocular vision or even stereoscopic vision. Van Balen, as does Binkhorst, stresses the importance of the correct selection of the power of the pseudophakos and strongly favors preoperative calculation of the lens power with ultrasonics. Also, in his opinion, a rather myopic correction is to be preferred.

b. *Implant Fixation and Postoperative Problems*

Van Balen contends that one should aim at firm capsular fixation, since iris support has proven to be insufficient for children, who have a long life expectancy. From the technical point of view, the implantation of an iridocapsular lens was not felt to be difficult, the problem being to remove sufficient lens material to get a clear posterior capsule while leaving sufficient lens material behind the iris for fixation of the loops.

Discisions had to be done in quite a few cases (60%) and in half of these more than once. Discision of the posterior capsule and after cataract membrane was not difficult in the presence of the pseudophakos. Indeed, inscision of the lens capsule even seemed to be facilitated because the loops of the pseudophakos apparently stretches it.

Uveal reactions were never a serious problem. Greyish white precipitates that sometimes patched the anterior and posterior surfaces of the lens during the postoperative course were considered to be related to the presence of after cataract. They disappeared after a few weeks.

Van Balen concluded that, although the iridocapsular lens with metal loops was the only lens then available that provided guarantees against material deterioration, lightweight lenses should be considered for the future. Like Binkhorst, Van Balen stressed the need to restrict this type of surgery to centers that are equipped to manage all the problems involved.

2. *D.A. Hiles's Report on 37 Traumatic Cataracts in Children*

The series of D. A. Hiles is significant in that it reflects the experience of one surgeon with different lens types. The follow-up, however, is less (maximum 36 months) than in Van Balen's series.

Number and Age Distribution

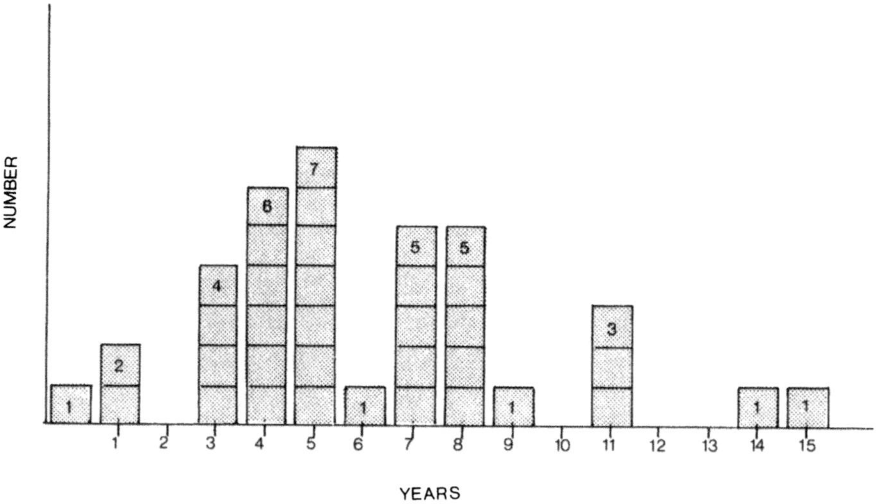

Fig. XI-16. — Age at injury of children with traumatic cataracts and supplied with intraocular lenses (D A. Hiles).

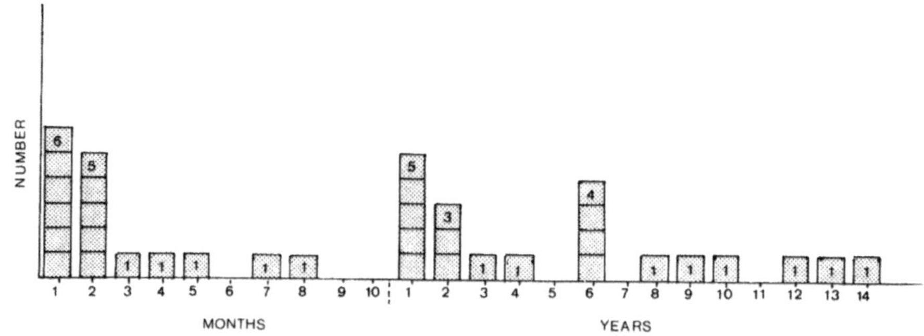

Fig. XI-17. — Injury-implant intervals (D.A. Hiles).

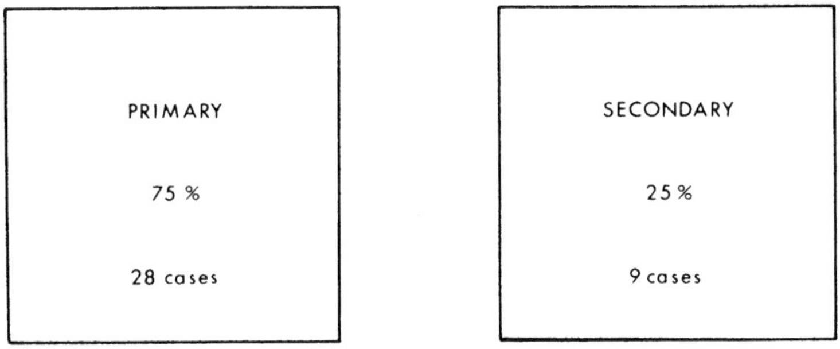

Fig. XI-18. — Distribution of primary and secondary procedures (D. A. Hiles).

a. *Functional Results*

1) *Visual Acuity*

Of the 37 pseudophakics, 21 (57%) demonstrated a corrected visual acuity of at least 20/40 and of these 10 attained at least 20/25 vision. Table XI-17 illustrates again that visual acuity increases with the age at the time of injury.

TABLE XI-16. — *Corrected Visual Acuity of 37 Pseudophakic Eyes, Hiles's Series*

Corrected Visual Acuity	*Complete series: 37 eyes* *Ages at injury: 6 months-15 years*
⩾20/40	21 (57%)
⩾20/200	28 (76%)
<20/200	6 (16%)
Unknown	3 (8%)

TABLE XI-17. — *Corrected Visual Acuity in Three Groups according to Age at Time of Injury, Hiles's Series*

Corrected Visual Acuity	*Group I* *1-4 years* *13 eyes*	*Group II* *5-7 years* *13 eyes*	*Group III* *8-15 years* *11 eyes*
⩾20/40	4 (13%)	8 (62%)	9 (82%)
⩾20/200	7 (54%)	11 (85%)	10 (81%)
<20/200	5 (38%)	1 (7.5%)	0
Unknown	1 (8%)	1 (7.5%)	1 (9%)

2) *Binocular Vision*

Twenty-six patients (70%) had no deviation in the primary position, 8 (22%) had exodeviation, and 3 (8%) had esodeviation. Fusion could be demonstrated in 17 cases (46%). In 14 cases (38%) fusion was not present and in 6 cases the binocular status was not recorded.

b. *Some Remarks on the Technique and Postoperative Problems*

The lenses used in this series were the Binkhorst iridocapsular lens, the Worst Medallion Lens, and the Worst Platina Lens. Hiles prefers the last two types because of the possibility of additional fixation. In his opinion, even though synechiae formation is likely to occur with children, extra fixation is still highly desirable.

Generally speaking, Hiles's approach is quite similar to that of Binkhorst, except for his more agressive attitude in the presence of vitreous loss, which Binkhorst considers to be a contraindication for lens implantation. When there is vitreous loss, Hiles applies standard vitreous management techniques: anterior chamber vitrectomy with mechanical vitrectors to clear the anterior chamber, the iris surface, and the incision before the surgery is completed.

It is also interesting to note that a lens glide was often found to be useful, especially when the anterior chamber collapsed.

Although Hiles did not give exact figures on the incidence of complications, some comments are in order.

Transient striated keratitis was common and was acribed to the inevitable contact between the lens and the endothelium before the anterior chamber could be restored. Again, this underlines the technical difficulties involved in lens implantation in chidren. Hiles notes that the striate keratitis always disappeared without clinical sequellae within 48 to 72 hours.

Postoperative iridocyclitis was also common and was generally associated with the preoperative condition created by the injury.

The routine treatment of both keratitis and iridocyclitis consisted of intravenous administration of dexamethasone upon completion of the operation, followed by daily administration of systemic prednisone (20 to 40 mg according to body weight) in decreasing doses for 8 to 10 days. Considering the moderate uveal reactions mentioned by

Binkhorst and Van Balen and observed by ourselves on many occasions, the need for such intensive and systemic corticosteroid treatment suggests, at least, that a reappraisal of the surgical procedure is in order.

3. *Hiles's Survey of Lens Implantation in Children, 1978*

At the request of the American Intra-Ocular Implant Society, D. A. Hiles compiled the results of lens implantation in children by surgeons in the United States.

One hundred forty-eight surgeons reported on 424 intraocular implants in children. Only 5 surgeons had implanted 11 or more lenses. Sufficient data were available on 296 implantations of which 166 were performed for traumatic cataract and 130 for infantile cataracts. Eight eyes were bilaterally implanted, the rest being unilateral cases. The value of the study is limited because the follow-up periods are not knwon, but certainly they did not exceed 3 years on the average so that various complications can still be expected to develop in the future. Nevertheless, the figures reported are significant in that they reflect what can be expected in the short-term when a number of surgeons using different lens styles enter this particular area of surgery.

a. *Traumatic Cataracts*

The distribution of primary and secondary procedures is given on Figure XI-19. Table XI-18 gives the different lens types used and their distribution.

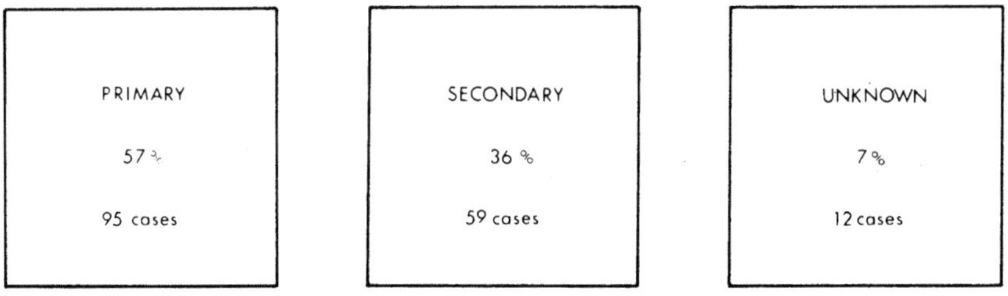
PRIMARY
57 %
95 cases
SECONDARY
36 %
59 cases
UNKNOWN
7 %
12 cases

Fig. XI-19. — Distribution of primary and secondary procedures, Hiles's survey (1978).

TABLE IX-18. — *Lens Types and Their Distribribution*

Lens Type	*Number of Traumatic Cataracts*
Medallion style	48 (29%)
Binkhorst 2-Loop	45 (27%)
Choyce style	31 (19%)
Others	27 (16%)
Binkhorst 4-Loop	13 (8%)
Unknown	2 (1%)
Total	166 (100%)

1) *Functional Results*

a) *Visual Acuity*

TABLE XI-19. — *Corrected Visual Acuity of 166 Pseudophakic Eyes, Hiles's Survey (1978)*

Corrected Visual Acuity	*Number of Eyes (Traumatic Cataracts)*
≥20/40	77 (46%)
≥20/200	115 (69%)
<20/200	20 (12%)
Unknownn	31 (19%)

TABLE XI-20. — *Corrected Visual Acuity in 4 Groups according to Age at the Time of Implantation, Hiles's Survey*

Corrected Visual Acuity	*Group I 1-4 years 26 eyes*	*Group II 5-8 years 45 eyes*	*Group III >8 years 63 eyes*	*Group IV Unknown 32 eyes*
≥20/40	6 (23%)	22 (49%)	37 (59%)	11
≥20/200	11 (42%)	35 (78%)	50 (79%)	17
<20/200	6 (23%)	3 (7%)	10 (16%)	4
Unknown	9 (35%)	7 (15%)	3 (5%)	11

Most of the 31 cases of unknown acuities were young or unresponsive children or patients lost for follow-up. As noted for the previous series discussed, the corrected visual acuity clearly increases with age at the time of implantation.

b) *Binocular Vision*

Some degree of binocular awareness or fusion was present in 81 cases (49%).

c) *Strabismic Deviation*

Squint was often reported to have been cured either spontaneously or after muscle surgery upon the implantation of an intraocular lens.

TABLE XI-21. — *Strabismic Deviation with Traumatic Cataracts before and after Lens Implantation*

	Before Implantation	*After Implantation*
Eso	18 cases	11 cases
Exo	30 cases	15 cases
Hyper	5 cases	None

2) *Complications*

TABLE XI-22. — *Distributions of Complications, Hiles's Survey*

Preoperative	121 (73%)
Peroperative	36 (22%)
Early Postoperative	66 (40%)
Late Postoperative	56 (34%)

a) *Preoperative Complications*

TABLE XI-23. — *Preoperative Complications, Hiles's Survey (1978)*

Complication	*Incidence*
Cornea: Corneal Scar	88 (53%)
Adherent Leucoma	28 (17%)
Iris: Traumatic Coloboma	40 (24%)
Iris Atrophy	26 (16%)
Atonic Pupil	16 (10%)
Iridodialysis	13 (8%)
Glaucoma	3 (2%)
Dislocated Lens	8 (5%)
Vitreous Opacities	7 (4%)
Macular Scars	11 (7%)
Optic Nerve Defects	1 (1%)
Others	4 (2%)

Table XI-23 shows that a large number of eyes presented preoperative pathologies, and some may have had several defects. These factors often adversely affected the final results.

b) *Peroperative Complications*

The two most significant peroperative problems were vitreous loss and rupture of the posterior capsule (Table XI-24). This group of surgeons, having had little experience, felt that these two conditions did not constitute contraindications for lens implantation. Peroperative hyphema and iris complications accounted for 4% of the complications. Globe collapse, a serious problem in 2% of the cases, seemed closely related to the size of the incision.

TABLE XI-24. — *Complications Occurring during the Lens Implantation, Hiles's Survey (1978)*

Complication	Incidence
Vitreous Loss	17 (10%)
Posterior Capsule Rupture	16 (10%)
Hyphema	7 (4%)
Iris Complications	6 (4%)
Globe Collapse	4 (2%)

c) *Early Postoperative Complications (within Two Weeks)*

The impressive amount of corneal involvement again shows that the insertion of an intraocular lens in a child's eye involves an additional trauma to the endothelium that may increase the danger of definitive decompensation of the cornea in the long run. The reported incidence of iridocyclitis (19%) seems acceptable if allowance is made for the proportion of one-stage procedures (57%), since one then has to deal more often with an irritable eye. Precise information is lacking about the 7 cases of early dislocation that occurred within 2 weeks of the operation.

TABLE XI-25. — *Early Postoperative Complications, Hiles's Survey*

Complications	*Incidence*
Cornea: Striate keratitis	34 (20%)
Corneal edema	30 (18%)
Iridocyclitis	32 (19%)
Vitritis	9 (5%)
Dislocated Lens	7 (4%)
Flat anterior chamber and wound dehiscence	4 (3%)
Pupillary block	2 (1%)
Iris prolapse	0
Endophtalmitis	0
Other	0

d) *Late Postoperative Complications*

As could be expected, about 50% of the posterior capsules became opaque and posterior capsulotomies were necessary in 43% of the cases. The rate of corneal endothelial dystrophy (4%) is low, considering the presence of pre-existing corneal pathology: 53% corneal scars and 17% adherent leucoma. In addition, there is the incidence of lens dislocation: 4% in the early postoperative period and 10% in the late postoperative period. Moreover, the incidence of flat anterior chambers was 3%. Although a child's cornea has an amazing capacity to recover, only the future wil tell how many of these corneas will ultimately decompensate. It all depends on the residual vitality of the endothelium.

TABLE XI-26. — *Late Postoperative Complications, Hiles's Survey (1978)*

Complications	*Incidence*
Endothelial corneal dystrophy	6 (4%)
Uveitis	10 (6%)
Precipitates on lens	16 (10%)
Iris atrophy	7 (4%)
Iris sphincter erosion	5 (3%)
Occluded pupil	6 (4%)
Glaucoma	4 (2%)
Dislocation	17 (10%)
Secondary membranes	80 (48%)
Retina: Cystoid macular edema	3 (2%)
Retinal detachment	5 (3%)
Optic atrophy	1 (0.6%)
Phthisis bulbi	2 (1%)
Enucleation	0
Lens removal	9 (5%)
Keratoplasty	5 (3%)

In addition to the 4% early dislocation incidence, a 10% late dislocation incidence was reported, either loop dislocation or total dislocation of unfixed implants. The Binkhorst 2-loop lens accounted for the largest part of the dislocations, although it was not used more often than the Medallion style lenses. Surprisingly, some of the Choyce style lenses, which were used less frequently, were also reported to have dislocated. Lens removal was necessary in 9 cases (5%): 4 of them because of corneal complications and 3 because of an additional trauma.

The other late complicatons—uveitis, retinal detachment, cystoid macular edema, glaucoma, and phthisis bulbi—are difficult to evaluate. The interaction between the preoperative condition, the operative trauma, and the aggression of the pseudophakos itself cannot be determined, particularly in eyes that have suffered a trauma and have been operated on by so many different surgeons.

Conclusions

In this heterogeneous group of traumatic cataracts in children treated by 148 different surgeons using at least 6 different lens models, nearly half of the children regained a visual acuity of at least 20/40 and half some degree of binocular vision. The exact rate of lens related complications is difficult to assess. Indeed, a fair amount of post-traumatic sequellae were present before the implantations, and complications may still develop in the years to come. It must be noted that some of the lenses are not well stabilized and that some of the corneas may ultimately decompensate.

b. *Infantile Cataracts*

The results of 130 cases of lens implantations used to treat infantile cataracts were also analyzed by Hiles. It is not clear, however, whether they all were congenital cataracts or if some had developed

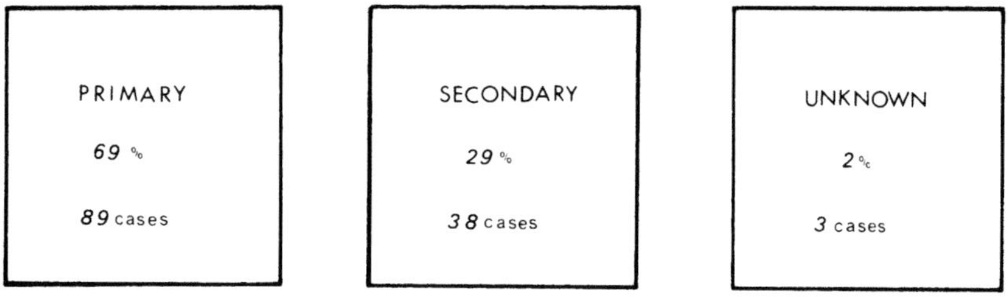

Fig. XI-20. — Division of primary and secondary procedures, Hiles's survey (1979).

TABLE XI-27. — *Lens Types and Distribution for Infantile Cataracts, Hiles's Survey (1978)*

Lens Type	*Number*
Medallion style	54 (42%)
Binkhorst 2-loop	35 (27%)
Others	20 (15%)
Choyce style	12 (9%)
Binkhorst 4-loop	9 (7%)
Total	130

in early childhood. Figure XI-20 gives the division of primary and secondary procedures, and Table XI-27 gives the distribution of lens styles.

1) *Functional Results*

a) *Visual Acuity*

It is noteworthy that only 23% of the cases yielded a visual acuity of 20/40 or better, and also that the youngest age group had the poorest visual performance. Hiles states that amblyopia was reported in 69% of the patients with infantile cataracts, whereas this incidence was only 33% for the group of traumatic cataract patients.

TABLE XI-28. — *Corrected Visual Acuity after Implantation for Infantile Cataracts. Hiles's Survey (1968)*

Corrected Visual Acuity	*Number*
⩾20/40	30 (23%)
⩾20/200	66 (51%)
<20/200	42 (32%)
Unknown	22 (17%)

TABLE XI-29. — *Corrected Visual Acuity of 4 Groups according to Age at Time of Implantation, Hiles's Survey (1978)*

Corrected Visual Acuity	*Group I 1-4 years 60 eyes*	*Group II 5-8 years 33 eyes*	*Group III >8 years 24 eyes*	*Group IV Unknown 13 eyes*
⩾20/40	4 (7%)	9 (27%)	14 (58%)	2 (15%)
⩾20/200	18 (30%)	20 (61%)	20 (83%)	6 (46%)
<20/200	15 (25%)	7 (21%)	3 (13%)	3 (23%)
Unknown	27 (45%)	6 (18%)	1 (4%)	4 (31%)

b) *Binocular Vision*

Some degree of binocular awareness or fusion was present in 31 cases (24%).

c) *Strabismic Deviation*

TABLE XI-30. — *Strabismic Deviation before and after Lens Implantation for Infantile Cataracts, Hiles's Survey (1978)*

	Before Implantation	*After Implantation*
Eso	45	26
Exo	21	22
Hyper	4	0

Esotropia was encountered more frequently among these patients than in the traumatic series.

2) *Complications*

TABLE XI-31.

Preoperative complications	32 (25%)
Peroperative complications	24 (18%)
Early postoperative complications	22 (17%)
Late postoperative complications	38 (19%)

a) *Preoperative Status*

TABLE XI-32. — *Preoperative Status of 130 Infantile Cataracts, Hiles's Survey (1978)*

	Number
Mircrophthalmia	7 (5%)
Cornea: Corneal scars	1 (<1%)
Adherent leucoma	4 (3%)
Iris: Congenital coloboma	6 (5%)
Atonic pupil	4 (3%)
Glaucoma	1 (<1%)
Persistent prim. vitreous	5 (4%)
Macular scars	1 (<1%)
Optic nerve defects	5 (4%)
Others	1 (<1%)

As in the traumatic series, the same eye may have had several defects that combined to prejudice the final results.

b) *Peroperative Complications*

TABLE XI-33. — *Peroperative Complications with Infantile Cataracts, Hiles's Survey (1978)*

Peroperative Complications	*Number*
Vitreous loss	13 (10%)
Posterior capsule rupture	7 (5%)
Hyphema	2 (2%)
Iris complications	2 (2%)
Globe collapse	1 (<1%)

Vitreous loss and rupture of the posterior capsule also were the commonest peroperative complications.

c) *Early Postoperative Complications*

TABLE XI-34. — *Early Postoperative Complications (Two Weeks after Surgery with Infantile Cataracts, Hiles's Survey (1978)*

Early Postoperative Complications	*Number*
Cornea: Striate keratitis	59 (45%)
Corneal edema	59 (45%)
Iridocyclitis	64 (49%)
Pupillary block	5 (4%)
Dislocation	4 (3%)
Flat anterior chamber	3 (2%)
Vitritis	1 (<1%)
Other	2 (2%)

The incidence of postoperative corneal problems and iridocyclitis is quite high. Since preoperative corneal pathology was virtually absent, this detrimental behavior of the cornea represents surgical trauma. The same observation may be made for the high incidence of postoperative iridocyclitis.

d) *Late Postoperative Complications*

TABLE XI-35. — *Late Complications with Infantile Cataracts, Hiles's Survey (1978)*

Late Postoperative Complications	*Number*
Endothelial Corneal Dystrophy	7 (5%)
Uveitis	6 (5%)
Precipitates on the lens	10 (8%)
Iris atrophy	2 (2%)
Iris sphincter erosion	5 (4%)
Occluded pupil	5 (4%)
Glaucoma	2 (2%)
Dislocation	4 (3%)
Secondary membranes	89 (68%)
Discisions	81 (62%)
Retina: Cystoid macular edema	0
Retinal detachment	0
Optic atrophy	0
Phthisis bulbi	0
Lens removal	2 (2%)
Ennucleation	2 (2%)

Since the average follow-up consists of only a few years, the value of these data is limited. In particular, the incidence of endothelial corneal dystrophy, iris atrophy, and lens dislocation may be expected to increase as time goes by.

Conclusion

In this group of patients with infantile cataracts, some 23% acquired a very useful corrected visual acuity of ⩾20/40 and half the group had ⩾20/200. Even without additional optical correction, the pseudophakic eye has a useful visual capacity that is superior to the rehabilitation offered by the classic optical correction for the aphakic eye.

Nevertheless, the incidence of post-operative problems was rather high. Many of these complications, which may constitue serious hazards to the ultimate fate of these eyes, would not have occurred if the surgeons had had more experience.

General Conclusions on Implantation in Children

Cataract removal and lens implantation in this particular age group always demands far more than usual surgical skill and judgment. Each case has to be considered separately and precise guidelines are difficult to lay down. The surgeon has to rely on his own experience and realize that the decisions he makes will have consequences for an entire lifetime.

In addition, the surgeon cannot deliver favorable results unless he can count on the active cooperation of all those who have a specific task to fulfill such as the parents, the nursing staff, the anesthesiologist, the orthoptist, and so on. The surgeon must also be able to make use of up-to-date equipment.

Insofar as these criteria are satisfied, a traumatic cataract in a child is certainly a positive indication for lens implantation. Indeed, the quality of binocular vision obtained is remarkable and longstanding.

The two most important problems that effect the final result are undoubtedly the pre-existing pathologies associated with the injury itself and the degree of amblyopia, particularly among the younger patients.

Regarding congenital cataracts, two important groups must be distinguished. There are unilateral cataracts, which are generally present at birth and for which lens implantation can offer no functional improvement at the present state of the art. But the situation is different for bilateral infantile cataracts for which the treatment of zonular cataracts is more promising. There is general agreement among the leading surgeons in this field, especially those in Europe, that lens implantation ought to be considered in these cases provided it is restricted to the eye with the poorest vision.

We are chary of drawing any definite conclusions as to the most suitable lens model, but since cataract surgery in these patients always has to be carried out extracapsularly, there is much to say for a lens that relies on capsular support. In the vast majority of the cases, such a lens makes additional suturing of the lens unnecessary, thus avoiding dangerous intraocular manipulations. Another point is the relatively small anterior eye segment in children, which is often still more restricted by the presence of traumatic synechiae. Thus, a lens with a small optical component is desirable, all the more since one has to take into account possible postoperative lens decentration because of traction due to shrinkage processes of the capsule and cortical remnants. Finally, the lens must allow good instrumental access to the retropupillary space in order to deal adequately with any secondary membrane formation or secondary posterior capsular opacities. The iridocapsular lens designed by Binkhorst meets these criteria.

At the present, the use of angle supported lenses seems less advisable. How long the scleral support can be maintained in these very young children is still controverted. Another problem with these lenses is that the anterior eye segment behaves unfavorably with a rigid pseudophakos when external pressure is applied. There have been occasional cases of hyphemata following contusion and also complaints of tenderness when the eye is rubbed. Finally, as the series cited above demonstrate, there is a frequent need for incision of secondary membranes in children, a procedure that is complicated by the presence of a large angle supported lens. The management of this problem may not be so difficult, however, with the angle supported lenses that have recently come on the market (Choyce Mark IX and Kelman lenses).

The extent to which posterior chamber lenses can be recommended for children has yet to be determined. Management of secondary membranes are even more difficult with these lenses than with the angle supported lenses, and the frequently encountered problem of early or late lens decentration because of capsular fibrosis can pose serious problems, especially with children.

Although, in our opinion, the biplanar, iridocapsular lens seems to be the lens of choice, there is still no ideal lens.

CHAPTER XII

LENS IMPLANTATION AND THE ENDOTHELIUM

Introduction

The inner face of the cornea is covered by a monocellular layer that separates it from the aqueous humor. The cells of this endothelium are flat and hexagonal (Fig. XII-1). At birth, the cornea has some 300,000 to 500,000 endothelial cells. The endothelium of a child or young adult has a cell density of about 1/2 that at birth because the surface area of the cornea increases and the cells spread out and grow. There is little morphological change between the ages of 15 and 50, but during the 60', the endothelial cells increase in size and develop irregular shapes (pleomorphism) (Laing et al., 1976, Kaufman, 1966).

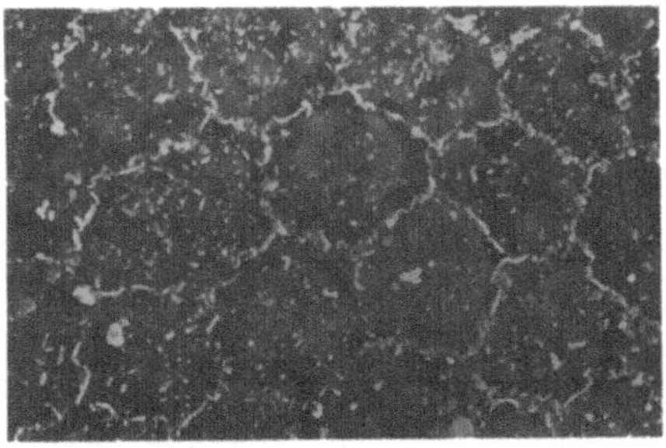

Fig. XII-1. — Scanning electron micrograph of human corneal endothelium. (Courtesy H. Van der Want.)

According to J. Capella (1972) and Kaufman et al. (1966), these changes probably are due to some cells enlarging to fill the gaps left by cells that die with age. Although regeneration of endothelial cells was thought to be possible, enough evidence has accumulated to allow the conclusion that human endothelial cells in adults probably never divide.

Together with the epithelium, the endothelium maintains the thickness and transparency of the cornea. Hydration of the cornea becomes abnormal if either the epithelium or the endothelium is damaged by trauma, inflammation or degenerative processes. The endothelium plays the major role in maintaining the constant thickness and hydration level of the cornea, since it is an active pumping mechanism that transfers fluid from the cornea to the aqeuous humor (Maurice, 1958). Since the endothelial cells are directly responsible for corneal transparency, this transparency may be compromised if large amounts of these cells are lost or damaged. As long as the number of cells suffice to cover the defect by spreading (the healing reserve), it is assumed that corneal decompensation will not occur (Bourne and Kaufman, 1976; Laing et al., 1976). At present, the critical number of endothelial cells needed to maintain corneal clarity is not known, but the critical factor is probably the fraction of the posterior corneal surface covered by normally functioning endothelial cells rather than the size and number of such cells. Forstot et al. (1977) have shown that corneal clarity can be maintained even with a cell count of only 380 cells per square millimeter.

In the history of lens implantation, decompensation of the cornea was the most dreaded complication, and it led to almost total abandonment of lens implant surgery in the late 1950's. The skepticism caused by the first generation of implants continues even today to tell against the diffusion of lens implantation.

At that time, the etiology of corneal dystrophy was a complex and puzzling problem since its clinical picture was very diverse. Indeed, the way in which endothelial corneal dystrophy developed led to a great deal of speculation as to its cause. Some corneas never cleared after surgery; others recovered temporarily but decompensated after a few weeks or months; some were clear for several years but ultimately deteriorated. Various mechanisms were incriminated: residual toxicity of the sterilizing agents, impurity of the materials used, allergic reactions to the plastic, and direct contact between the implant and the endothelium.

During the 1960's, a new generation of implants was developed that, after several years of trials, became the foundation for the modern lenses. The many changes in lens design and implantation technique of this period were essentially the result of the work done by C.D. Binkhorst and D.P. Choyce, who hoped to resolve the problem of corneal dystrophy by designing lenses that were situated as far as possible from the cornea without interfering with the other structures of the eye. After several years of clinical observation, Binkhorst adopted the posterior capsule for fixation, and Choyce chose refined angle fixation.

Among the early observations that led to the dramatic decrease of endothelial corneal dystrophy, the following are the most significant:

— Any form of traumatic surgery, which involved excessive intraocular manipulation, always leads to corneal problems.

— Even if the surgery is atraumatic, any contact—persistent or intermittent—between the lens and the endothelium always causes local or general endothelial damage.

— When there was pre-existing endotheliopathy of whatever origin, decompensation is more likely to occur.

— Postoperative endothelial corneal dystrophy is sometimes associated with other ocular pathology, such as chronic iridocyclitis or recurrent episodes of hypertension.

To a certain extent, these observations satisfactorily explained most cases of *early* corneal decompensation. More confusing, however, was *late* corneal dystrophy, especially in those eyes in which there was no contact between the lens and the endothelium. Binkhorst (1971) suggested that any intraocular surgical procedure causes a certain decline in corneal vitality (see Fig. XII-2a, XII-2b). Thus,

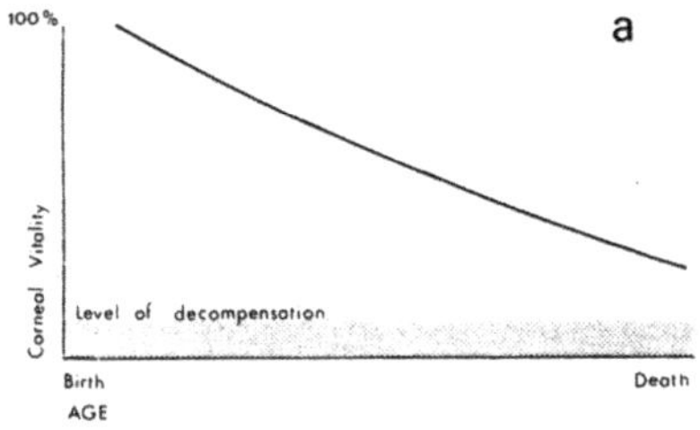

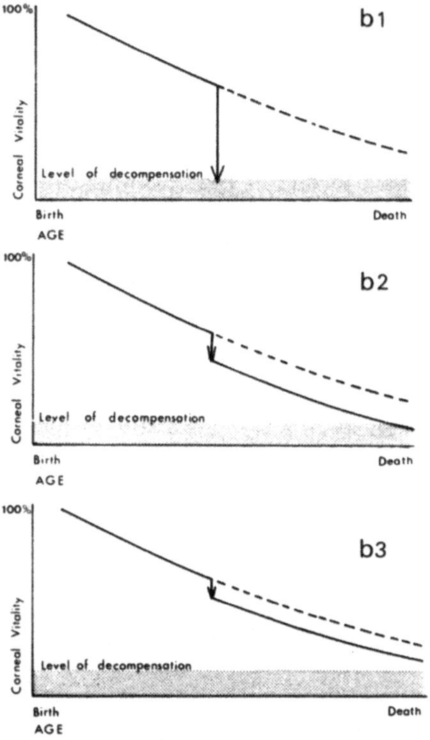

Fig. XII-2a. — Physiological decrease in corneal vitality relative to age. Corneal decompensation is unlikely to occur in the normal eye.

2b. — The influence of surgical trauma on corneal vitality.

1) Severe trauma will lead to immediate corneal decompensation.
2) Less severe trauma will lead to late decompensation.
3) Minor surgical trauma will not lead to late decompensation.

according to Binkhorst, after a marked endothelial trauma, physiological decrease in corneal vitality causes some eyes ultimate to decompensate.

In the sections that follow, we shall first examine how this surgical trauma is reflected in objective, measurable data obtained from pachometric studies conducted in the first few months after surgery and endothelial cell density studies. Then we shall consider in detail the peroperative and postoperative factors that can cause endothelial corneal dystrophy.

Finally, we shall discuss the incidence of endothelial corneal dystrophy as given in the series presented in the preceding chapters.

I. Postoperative Corneal Behavior as Evaluated by Pachometry and Specular Microscopy

A. Pachometric Studies

Miller and Dohlman (1970) and other investigators have suggested that measurements of corneal thickness be used to evaluate the relative aggressivity of different intraocular procedures. Indeed, pachometric recordings during the postoperative phase seem to be a good parameter for gauging the degree to which the endothelial function is affected: there seems to be a good correlation between the degree of hydration of the cornea and the dehydrating function and capacity of the endothelium (Harris and Nordquist, 1955) as well as between hydration of the corneal stroma and corneal thickness (Ytteborg and Dohlman, 1965). But there is no definite correlation between the tickness of the cornea and the presence of corneal edema (Norn, 1973).

Only a few reports are available on the evolution of corneal thickness during the first few months after intraocular lens surgery, they indicate that the cornea is slightly thicker after lens implantation than after cataract extraction without lens implantation.

After intracapsular cataract extraction without lens implantation, the data on Table XII-1 are noteworthy. The authors cited there observed that corneal swelling was marked during the first postoperative week but decreased to normal levels within 6 months unless there was previous endothelial disease.

W.J. Stark et al. (1977) found no significant difference between the evolution of postoperative central corneal thickness of 33 pseudophakics and that of 26 aphakics (see Fig. XII-3). Only patients who had

TABLE XII-1. — *Increase in Corneal Thickness after Classical Intracapsular Cataract Extraction Relative to Preoperative Thickness*

Source	*Number of patients*	*Average increase*	*Normalization*
M.S. Norn (1973)	114	15% (2nd day)	6 months
W.J. Wood and A.E. Maumenee (1975)	34	11.6% (4th day)	6 months
M. Tragakis et al. (1977)	55	16% (3rd day)	6 weeks

had an uneventful operation and no associated pathology were included in this study. The mean age of the implant patients was over 70 years old vs. 67 years old for the control group. Four-loop Iris Clip Binkhorst lenses were implanted after intracapsular cataract extraction and provided with a transiridectomy (9.0) suture.

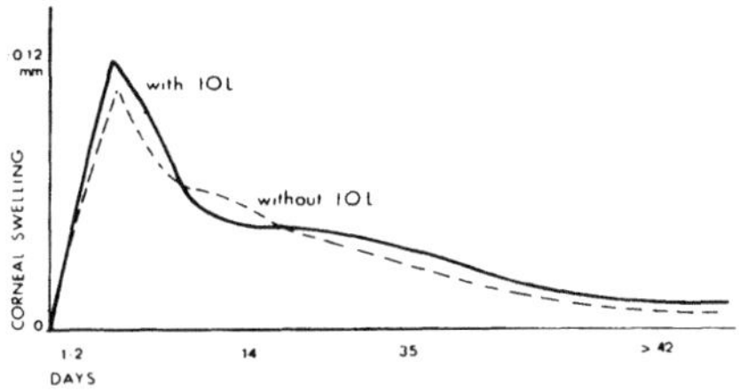

Fig. XII-3. — Corneal thickness changes after lens implantation surgery and after cataract surgery without lens implantation (Stark et al., 1977).

Although the corneas in the implant group showed more striate keratitis immediately after the operation, the corneal thickness in both groups increases about 0.12 mm on the first postoperative day. In 5 weeks, the corneal thickness had returned to the pre-operative level (Stark et al., 1977, p. 773).

Measuring corneal thickness 6 months after surgery, D.L. Praeger and H.A. Schneider (1977) found only a minor increase in corneal thickness after simple extracapsular cataract extraction and after phakoemulsification without lens implantation. Corneal swelling was more pronounced, however, after phakoemulsification combined with lens implantation. After intracapsular cataract extraction without lens implantation, corneal thickness was also above normal. The control group was a relatively young group of patients who did not undergo surgery (see Table XII-2).

Of the 31 eyes that had undergone phakoemulsification and lens implantation, only 2 registered a significant increase of corneal thickness (>0.057 mm) 6 months after the operation relative to the unoperated fellow eye (see Table XII-3).

TABLE XII-2. — *Mean Corneal Thickness at 6 Months after the Operation Various Surgical Procedures (Praeger and Schneider, 1977)*

Type of Procedure	*Number of Eyes*	*Mean Age of Patients (in years)*	*Corneal Thickness (in mm)*
None	38	45.5	0.453
Intracapsular cataract extraction	33	70	0.474
Phakoemulsification	77	64.9	0.467
Extracapsular cataract extraction	8	73	0.456
Phakoemulsification and lens implantation	31	72.5	0.480

TABLE XII-3. — *Corneal Thickness 6 Months after Phakoemulsification and Lens Implantation: Operated Versus the Unoperated Fellow Eye (Praeger and Schneider, 1977)*

	Number	*Corneal Thickness Mean ± Standard Error of the Mean (in mm)*	*Mean Age (in years)*
Unoperated eye	31	0.470±0.008	72.5
Operated eye	31	0.480±0.010	72.5
Difference		0.010±0.006	

Praeger and Schneider noted that corneal swelling was the most pronounced in the first few weeks after surgery, with the thickness increasing by 60% by the second and third postoperative day. After 8 weeks, the difference between the eyes was insignificant (see Fig. XII-4).

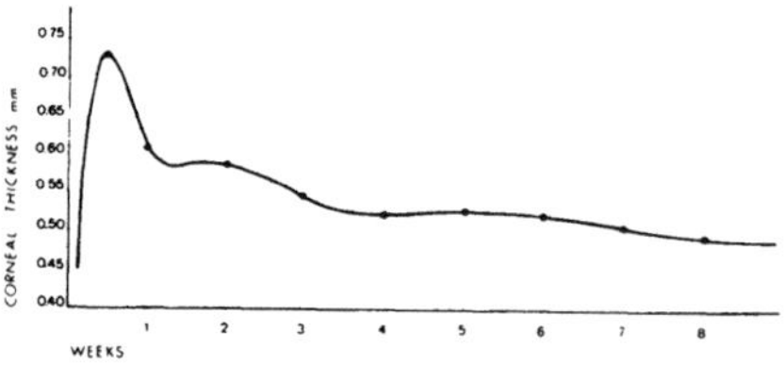

Fig. XII-4. — Corneal thickness measurements following intraocular lens implantations (Praeger and Schneider, 1977).

Similar observations were reported by Hung Cheng et al. (1977), who recorded the corneal thickness one day after the operation and again one month after for a group that had had simple cataract extractions and another group that had had cataract extractions and lens implantations (see Table XII-4).

Another study involving 100 eyes in which a lens was implanted after intracapsular cataract extraction confirms the findings of the authors cited above: corneal thickness after lens implantation was

TABLE XII-4 — *Mean Increase in Corneal Thickness at 5 Days and at 1 Month after Classical Intracapsular Cataract Extraction and Intracapsular Cataract Extraction with Lens Implantation (Cheng et al., 1977).*

Time of examination	*Intracapsular Cataract Extraction: Mean Increase in mm*	*Intracapsular Cataract Extraction and Lens Implantation: Mean Increase in mm*
After 5 days	0.0417 (N=23)	0.0750 (N=19)
After 1 month	0.0219 (N=17)	0.0145 (N=17)

found to be significantly increased during the first postoperative days but returned to normal after some weeks (Reshmi and Kondrot, 1976; see Tables XII-5 and XII-6).

TABLE XII-5. — *Changes in Corneal Thickness after Intracapsular Cataract Extraction and Lens Implantation in 100 Eyes (Resmi and Kondrot, 1978)*

	Average Corneal Thickness (in mm)	*Percent of Increase*
Preoperative	0.461	—
Postoperative		
3-5 days	0.555	+20.1%
30 days	≈0.461	not significant

TABLE XII-6. — *Percent of Patients Returning to Preoperative Thickness in Function of Elapsed Time (Reshmi and Kondrot, 1978, p. 1401)*

Postoperative Days	*% Patients*
3-10	38
11-15	50
16-20	71
21-30	94
40-60	100

All previous reports demonstrate that corneal swelling is more pronounced after cataract extraction followed by lens implantation than after cataract extraction alone, but in both instances recovery within 6 months is the rule. We may conclude that lens implantation of itself was responsible for these differences in corneal thickness as a result of disturbed endothelial functioning.

B. Studies with the Specular Microscope

The specular microscope is a biomicroscopic device for observation of the corneal endothelium in situ under large magnification. In his manual on slit-lamp biomicroscopy, Vogt noted in 1931 that the endothelium could be observed under large magnification by using th reflected light of a slit lamp. D.M. Maurice introduced the specular microscope in 1968, and the subsequent modifications by Laing, Sandstrom, and Leibowitz (1975) allowed photomicrography of the endothelium in vivo.

Fig. XII-5. — Specular micrographs of the corneal endothelium in vivo. Note the difference in cell density in the 2 pictures. (Courtesy C.D. Binkhorst and L. Loones.)

Usually, the area observed by the specular microscopes currently in use is very small and varies according to the kind of instrument being used. The size, shape, and number of cells filling a calibrated area can be established, and thus the number of cells per square millimeter can be calculated. Although there may be some differences between the central and the peripheral areas after profound cell loss, the central cornea does provide a measurable indication of the general endothelial cell population of the cornea (Blackwell, Gravenstein, and Kaufman, 1977).

According to the observations of Bourne and Kaufman (1976), the mean cell density in the central cornea as recorded in 40 normal eyes varies from more than 3000 cells per mm^2 for those under 20 years of age to an average of some 2500 cells per mm^2 for those 75 years old. There seems to be no correlation between cell density and corneal thickness (see Fig. XII-6).

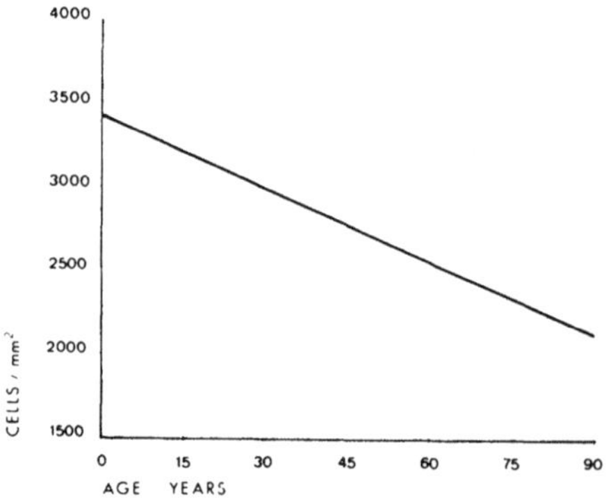

Fig. XII-6. — Endothelial cell density of 40 normal eyes vs. age (Bourne & Kaufman, 1976).

K.J. Hoffer (1978) found the average preoperative cell density of 600 normal cataract patients to be 2350 cells per mm^2 regardless of age. A more recent follow-up study with M. Kraff of 1600 eyes confirmed these findings and revealed no trend to higher density in younger patients relative to older patients. More information is required before definite conclusions can be drawn regarding cell densities and age.

At the present, the role to be attributed to specular microscopy in the field of lens implantation is not yet well defined. At least, it seems to be an interesting technique that allows objective comparison of pre- and postoperative data on the anatomical status of the endothelium in vivo. Studies indicate that the endothelium undoubtedly shows various degrees of decrease in cell density after surgery. Then, too, information on the preoperative status of the cornea may be able to indicate whether a particular surgical procedure is likely to precipitate definitive corneal decompensation. In the opinion of C.D. Binkhorst (1978), information provided by specular microscopy may be helpful in the future in deciding whether implantation should be undertaken in special cases, for example, in an already aphakic eye and in eyes that have suffered from uveitis, glaucoma, or an injury. Also the decision to perform simultaneous cataract extraction, lens implantation, and corneal grafting in an eye with known corneal diseases may well be largely influenced by specular microscopic findings.

The data reported below may be faulted since the investigators used different instruments and since the recordings were made at different times after the operation. Individual differences in the surgical approach may also have distorted the data to such an extent that no definite conclusions about the value of a particular technique or lens type may be made.

1. *Prospective Studies*

These studies are concerned with endothelial cell counts made by different authors before and after surgery.

a. *Cataract Extraction without Lens Implantation*

On the basis of the figures reported on Table XII-7, we may accept an endothelial cell loss of some 10% for uncomplicated intracapsular cataract extraction without lens implantation. But because the num-

TABLE XII-7. — *Cell Loss after Cataract Extraction without Lens Implantation*

Source	*Type of Surgery*	*Number of Patients*	*Average Cell Loss*
Bourne and Kaufman (1976)	ICCE and ECCE	16	−12%
Forstot et al. (1977)	ICCE	5	−8%
Hirst et al. (1977)	ICCE	26	−13%
Sugar et al. (1978)	ICCE	14	−8%
Galin et al. (1978)	ICCE and ECCE	20	−9.8%

ber of cases involved is rather small, more information is necessary for a definite conclusion. In addition, it would be well to have series giving the results after extracapsular cataract extraction with and without ultrasonic emulsification.

b. *Cataract Extraction with Lens Implantation*

TABLE XII-8. — *Cell Loss after Cataract Extraction with Lens Implantation*

Source	*Type of Surgery*	*Lens*	*Nr.*	*Average Cell Loss*	*Follow-Up*
Bourne and Kaufman (1976)	ECCE	Worst Medallion	5	−62.2%	Up to 15 weeks
Forstot et al. (1977)	ICCE	Binkhorst Worst	12	−35.7%	7-15 days
Hirst et al. (1977)	ICCE	Binkhorst	33	−14%	Avg. 69 days
			14	−21%	Avg. 109 days
Binkhorst et al. (1978)	ECCE	Binkhorst	41	−6.7%	Up to 6 months
Galin et al. (1978)	ICCE and ECCE	Binkhorst	85	−34%	N.A.
		Fyodorov Sputnik	44	−32.6%	N.A.
		Choyce Mk VIII	22	−21%	N.A.
Sugar et al. (1978)	ICCE	Binkhorst	56	−34.8%	
		Fyodorov Sputnik	32	−33.8%	Up to 6 months
		Choyce Mk VIII	5	−24.4%	
Kraff et al. (1979)	N.A.	Choyce Mk VIII	39	−18.6%	3 months
		Tennant	58	−12.4%	
Drews and Waltman (1978)	ICCE	Worst Medallion	11	−11.6%	N.A.
			15	−65.5%	

N.A. = Not available.

Table XII-8 gives the degree of cell loss in 472 eyes as from 7% to 65%. Interestingly, some authors indicated a significant decrease in cell density when the surgical procedure was complicated. For example, Forstot et al. reported and average of −28.6% cell loss in 10 uncomplicated cases, but they noted a cell loss of −57.6% in a case of postoperative sterile hypopion and a cell loss of −84.1% in a case of vitreous loss managed with sponge vitrectomy. These figures are comparable to those reported by Bourne and Kaufman (1976) who found cell loses ranging from −34% to −70% in 5 cases of which 2 were complicated by vitreous problems. Drews and Waltmann (1978) noted a 65% cell loss when the surgery was difficult, and less than 12% cell loss when it was easy.

2. *Retrospective Studies*

In these studies the cell density of pseudophakic eyes was compared to the cell density of the fellow eye, phakic or aphakic. Thus the eyes of the same patient were compared some time after surgery.

a. *Pseudophakic versus a Phakic Fellow Eye*

TABLE XII-9. — *Differences in Cell Density Between Pseudophakic Eyes and the Phakic Fellow Eye*

Source	*Type of Surgery*	*Lens*	*Nr.*	*Average difference in cell density*	*Follow-Up*
Forstot et al. (1977)	ICCE	Binkhorst 4-loop	21	−43.5%	1 week to 5 months
	ICCE	Copeland	5	−47.9%	3 to 7 years
	ICCE	Fyodorov I	1	−84.1%	2.5 years
	ECCE	Binkhorst 2-loop	9	−47.5%	7 months to 4 years
Sugar et al. (1978)	ICCE	Fyodorov Sputnik	59	−31.8%	
		Binkhorst 4-loop	44	−43.1%	2 weeks to 13 years
		Worst Medallion	7	−50.9%	
Sugar et al. (1978)	ICCE	Worst Medallion	83	−39.5%	1-19 months
		Circular loop	3		
Cozean et al. (1979)	ICCE	Choyce Mk VIII style	27	−22.5%	6-18 months
Kraff et al. (1978)	ICCE	Worst Medallion	80	−32.6%	—

Table XII-9 gives the average differences in cell density between pseudophakic and phakic eyes of the same patient.

Apart from the 22.5% difference reported by Cozean et al. (1979) the figures range from −32% to −50%. Significantly, Forstot et al. (1977) observed a −54.5% in a patient whose dislocated Binkhorst 4-loops lens had been repositioned with a conservative approach, and a −72.2% loss in another patient for whom a luxated lens had been surgically repositioned.

Noteworthy, too, is the conclusion reached by A. Sugar et al. (1978), who investigated decrease in cell density as a function of time (see Table XII-10). Since their data failed to demonstrate any significant influence of the passage of time, they suggested that most of the cell damage occurred at or near the time of surgery.

TABLE XII-10. — *Effect of Postoperative Duration on Cell Loss (Sugar et al., 1978)*

	Number	*Mean Postoperative Period*	*Cell Loss*
<1 year	67	4.1 months	36.2%
>1 year	49	27.8 months	37.3%

Further evidence demonstrating the influence of surgical trauma is provided by M.C. Kraff et al. (1978), who made clinical estimates of operative endothelial trauma at the time of surgery on a scale of 0 to 3+ (see Table XII-11). The mean decrease in endothelial cell density (relative to the unoperated eye) correlates directly with the increasing severity of the endothelial trauma.

TABLE XII-11. — *Mean Decreases in Endothelial Cell Density in Function of Endothelial Trauma (Kraff et al., 1978)*

Endothelial Trauma Ratings	*Mean % Decreases in Endothelial Cell Density*	*Number of Cases*
E.T. 0	−19%	33
E.T. 1+	−19%	13
E.T. 2+	−42%	16
E.T. 3+	−59%	

b. *Pseudophakic versus an Aphakic Fellow Eye*

Although the data given on Table XII-12 derives from a small number of cases, comparison of cell densities of eyes with a pseudo-

TABLE XII-12. — *Differences in Cell Density of Pseudophakic Eyes Relative to Aphakic Fellow Eyes*

Source	*Type of Surgery*	*Lens*	*Number*	*Average Difference in Cell Density*
Forstot et al. (1977)	ICCE	Copeland Binkhorst 4-loop	6 2	−41.4%
Hirst et al. (1977)	ICCE	Binkhorst 4-Loop	8	−17%
Sugar et al. (1978)	ICCE	Not available	35	−30.8%

phakos and fellow aphakic eyes indicates that the insertion of an intraocular lens accounts for significant decreases in cell density.

c. *Pseudophakic versus a Pseudophakic Fellow Eye*

C.D. Binkhorst (1978) made a retrospective study involving 23 patients with two intraocular lenses, one implanted after intracapsular cataract extraction and the other implanted after extracapsular cataract extraction. The cases were matched as well as possible: the average age was 71 years, the cataracts were all senile cataracts, the surgeries were all uneventful, and the follow-up periods were all relatively long (see Table XII-13). The average difference in cell density after intracapsular cataract extraction and implantation was a significant 50.8% less than after extracapsular cataract extraction and implantation.

TABLE XII-13. — *Average Cell Density after Intracapsular and Extracapsular Cataract Extraction and Lens Implantation in the Same Patient (Binkhorst, 1978)*

Procedure	*Intracapsular Binkhorst Lens*	*Extracapsular Binkhorst Lens*
Number	23	23
Follow-Up	Average 86.8 months	Average 85.7 months
Cell Density	Average 1064	Average 2166

Binkhorst explains this striking difference as follows:

— The lens is easier to insert after extracapsular extraction since the anterior chamber is easier to maintain.

— Additional manipulation for lens suturing procedures is not necessary after extracapsular extraction.
— There is the possibility of continuous cell loss after lens implantation with intracapsular extraction because of the Barrier Deprivation Syndrome (see pp. 250).
— There may be some toxic influence of the nylon loops in the intracapsular series.

Discussion

Although these studies are not really comparable, it may safely be concluded that lens implantation accounts for various degrees of cell loss, the amount of which depends on the individual surgeon, the method applied, and the lens implanted. As more investigators begin to use specular microscopy routinely, in a few years we should be able to conclude which method, which lens, and which surgeons maintain the highest endothelial cell densities. And since more and more devices are coming on the market that permit estimation of cell density simply and without the necessity of special skills, specular microscopy can also be a good way for each surgeon to evaluate his own performance.

Finally, these reports demonstrate that a surgeon, regardless of his interest in specular microscopy, must realize that he will sacrifice some 50% or more of the endothelial cell population if he persists in a lens implantation procedure when the peroperative conditions are unfavorable.

II. Endothelial Damage: Promoting Factors, Prevention and Treatment

A. Mechanical Damage

Mechanical damage can occur during and after surgery.

1. *Folding the Cornea*

Repeated folding of the cornea to allow access to the anterior chamber disturbs the normal corneal architecture as do traction folds during suturing. The cumulation of these traumas, especially in elderly people, results in prolonged corneal haze or marked striate keratitis or both.

M.S. Norn (1971) demonstrated that vital staining shows horizontal and slightly curved lines that indicate definite endothelial cell damage when the cornea is bent as is done in classic cataract extraction. The corneas he examined were previously normal.

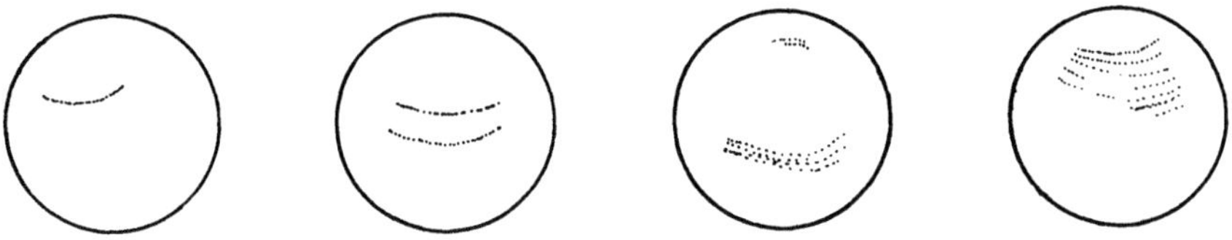

Fig. XII-7. — Vital staining patterns demonstrating definite endothelial cell damage as a result of manipulations during uncomplicated cataract extraction (Norn, 1971).

2. *Instrumental Touch*

Any instrument, whether it is used for incision, insertion, positioning, or steadying the implant, may injure Descemet's membrane at the inner edge of the incision. An instrument may also damage the endothelial layer when it is not kept in the proper posterior position. Such lesions can be revealed by vital staining of the cornea, both in vivo and in vitro (Norn, 1971; Völker-Dieben et al., 1979). Some implants require few instrumental manipulations while others require many delicate maneuvers in the anterior chambers for suturing procedures, closing safety devices, and so on. In this respect, lenses that require the minimum of intraocular manipulation are to be preferred.

3. *Damage by the Implant*

From the clinical observations of the pioneers in lens implantation, it was apparent that persistent or repeated contact between the endothelium and the lens parts results in localized and sometimes generalized corneal dystrophy. As we have already noted, these observations led to the development of new lens designs and better surgical techniques with the object of preventing corneal contact during and after surgery.

In the mid-seventies, J.L. Katz et al. (1977) demonstrated by scanning electron microscopy that contact between polymethylmethacrylate and the endothelium did indeed cause significant endothelial damage. This damage occurred almost instantaneously. Contact times ranging from 1 to 60 seconds resulted in cell losses of 20% to 35%. It appeared as though the cell membranes had been ripped off leaving the nuclei exposed. Moreover, this damage was independent of the kind of lens, the method of sterilization, and the wetness or dryness of the lens surface. It was apparently the result of the simple interaction of the methacrylate surface and the endothelial cells.

a. *Damage during Surgery*

Inadvertent contact between the lens and the endothelium is always possible, but is more likely to occur in a shallow anterior chamber. Even when the iris diaphragm is in a posterior position, unexpected forward displacement may occur if, for example, the anterior hyaloid ruptures or if air slips behind the lens while the lens is being positioned.

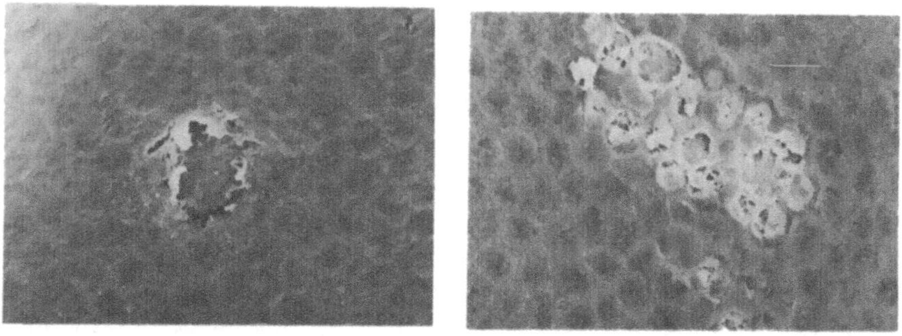

Fig. XII-8. — Scanning electron micrographs showing damage caused to a rabbit endothelium (left) after static touch and (right) after dynamic touch of a PMMA lens. (Courtesy Heyer Schulte.)

Prevention of endothelial damage by the implant requires accurate surgical judgment, precise technique, and proper management of adverse conditions. In this respect one should consider:

— Lens insertion using a formed chamber technique;
— The advantage offered by a lens glide; (see p. 131)
— Always maintaining a formed anterior chamber while suturing the incision;
— Aborting implantation when endothelial contact cannot be avoided.

Recently, the application of coating agents to the lens surface to neutralize the deleterious effect of polymethylmethacrylate on the endothelial cells has been investigated. So far, however, no definite conclusions can be made on the value and innocuousness of these agents in clinical practice.

According to P.U. Fechner (1977), a drop of a solution of 1% methylcellulose in Ringer's solution on the pseudophakos gives satisfactory results in preventing endothelial damage.

Good results in vitro were reported by Katz et al. (1977) with a 40% solution of polyvinyl pyrrolidone (PVP-K29-32) as a coating agent.

K. Scott et al. (1977) suggested using human albumin or the patient's own serum to coat implants prior to insertion. A comparative study with rabbits has shown that different coating agents make the methacrylate less agressive in varying degrees (see Table XII-14).

TABLE XII-14. — *Endothelial Cell Loss in Rabbits according to Coating Agents (n = 12 for each group)*
K. Scott et al. 1977

Coating agent	*Mean cell loss*
None	−43.33%
Saline	−34.17%
Plasma	−21.66%
TC 199	−20.83%
Albumin	−14.58%
Serum	−10.00%

Already in 1972, E.A. Balazs et al. reported on the use of hyaluronic acid for the replacement of vitreous and aqueous humor. In 1977, D. Miller et al. experimented with this product during intraocular lens implantation in rabbits. The Na-hyaluronate treated eyes had significantly less corneal edema and less iris engorgement and edema than did the control eyes.

In 1979, D. Miller and R. Stegmann reported their favorable results in a comparative study involving lens implantation in 40 human eyes. In 20 eyes, the anterior chamber was filled with a 1% Na-hyaluronate solution prior to pseudophakos implantation. The average cell loss was 17% versus 47% for the control group. No significant increase in intraocular pressure was observed in the eyes with the Na-hyaluronate. In the opinion of Miller and Stegman, this solution may also have some anti-inflammatory properties.

G.A. Payman and K. Zweig (1979) proposed that a 6% solution of bovine submaxillary mucin be used to coat the methacrylate surface. Experiments with animals failed to reveal any toxicity. Furthermore, uncoated lenses caused a 30.9% endothelial cell loss upon in vitro contact, while the coated lenses caused only a 4.3% loss.

Another possibility, which was investigated by L. Levy et al. (1979) in cat eyes, is interposition of a polymacon sheet (H.E.M.A.) between the anterior lens surface and the endothelium. These authors report that the polymacon shield reduces endothelial loss from 51% to 9%.

There is also the possibility of the lenses being made of different materials with other surface properties, for example, glass-silicon or H.E.M.A.

b. *Damage after Surgery*

Damage to the endothelium from some kinds of lenses is possible during the early postoperative period and even months or years later.

Shallow or Flat Anterior Chamber

When the clearance between the iris diaphragm and the posterior surface of the cornea is reduced for any reason, all lenses—except posterior chamber lenses—can come in contact with the endothelium. Obviously, the more volume occupied in the anterior chamber by the lens body, haptic parts, loops, struts, or clips, the more likely it is that contact will occur. And, just as obviously, contact is more apt to occur in a small anterior eye segment. When it does occur, it is a surgical emergency, and release must be achieved without delay.

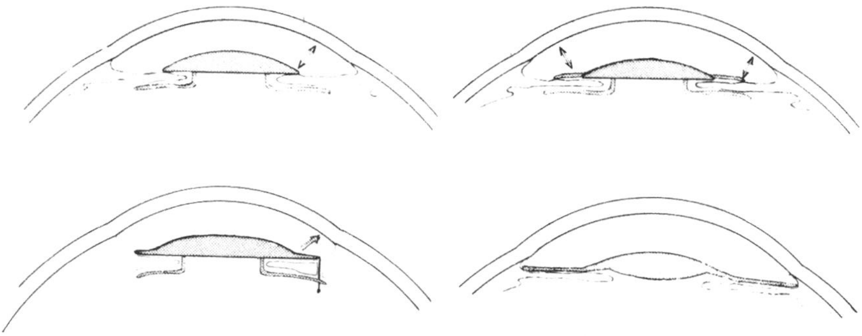

Fig. XII-9. — Various lens models and their location with respect to the endothelium.

In eyes with angle supported lenses, intermittent touching may occur should the eye be deformed by external pressure resulting, for example, from rubbing or compression during sleep.

Decentration

Whether decentration is caused by vitreous protrusion or incarceration, iris prolapse or atrophy, capsular fibrosis, or another mechanism, the main point is that here, too, the lens moves toward the cornea. Depending on the kind of lens, endothelial contact will occur more or less rapidly. This situation must be dealt with without delay by amputating the offending haptic parts, recentration of the lens, or even removing it if necessary.

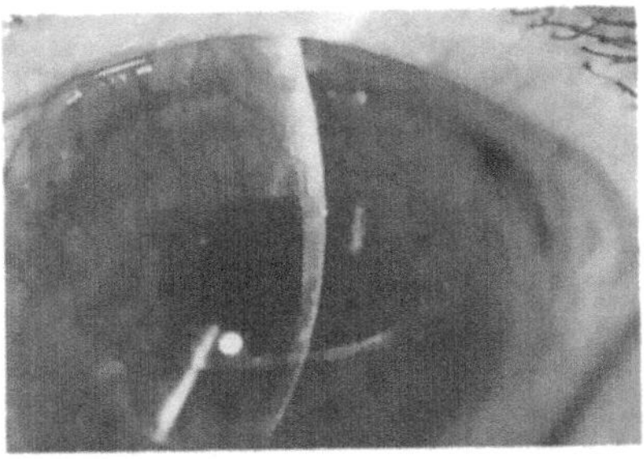

a

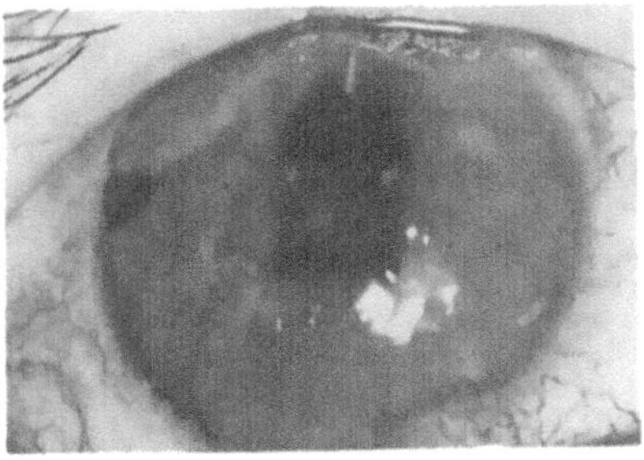

b

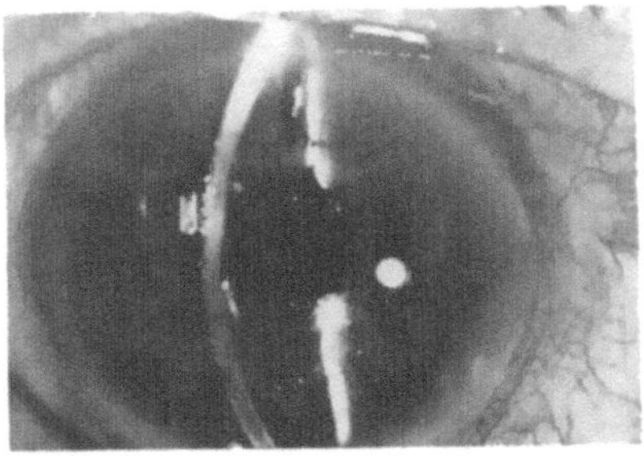

c

Fig. XII-10a. — Upwards decentration of an iris clip lens resulting from vitreous traction and causing localized endothelial corneal dystrophy.
b. — Upwards decentration of a platinum clip lens resulting from iris incarceration and causing localized endothelial corneal dystrophy.
c. — A platinum clip lens that is riding too high and causing localized endothelial corneal dystrophy. (Courtesy C. Kok van Alphen and H. Völker-Dieben.)

Lens Instability, Subluxation, Luxation

Due to the mobility and increasing laxness of the iris that occurs in time, most iris supported lenses after intracapsular cataract extraction show various degrees of instability (pseudophakodonesis). If certain conditions coincide—such as a small anterior eye segment, part of the implant extending toward the periphery, and the head being in a prone position—localized corneal dystrophy may develop where parts protrude from the lens, for example, lens loops, haptic rims, and clipping devices.

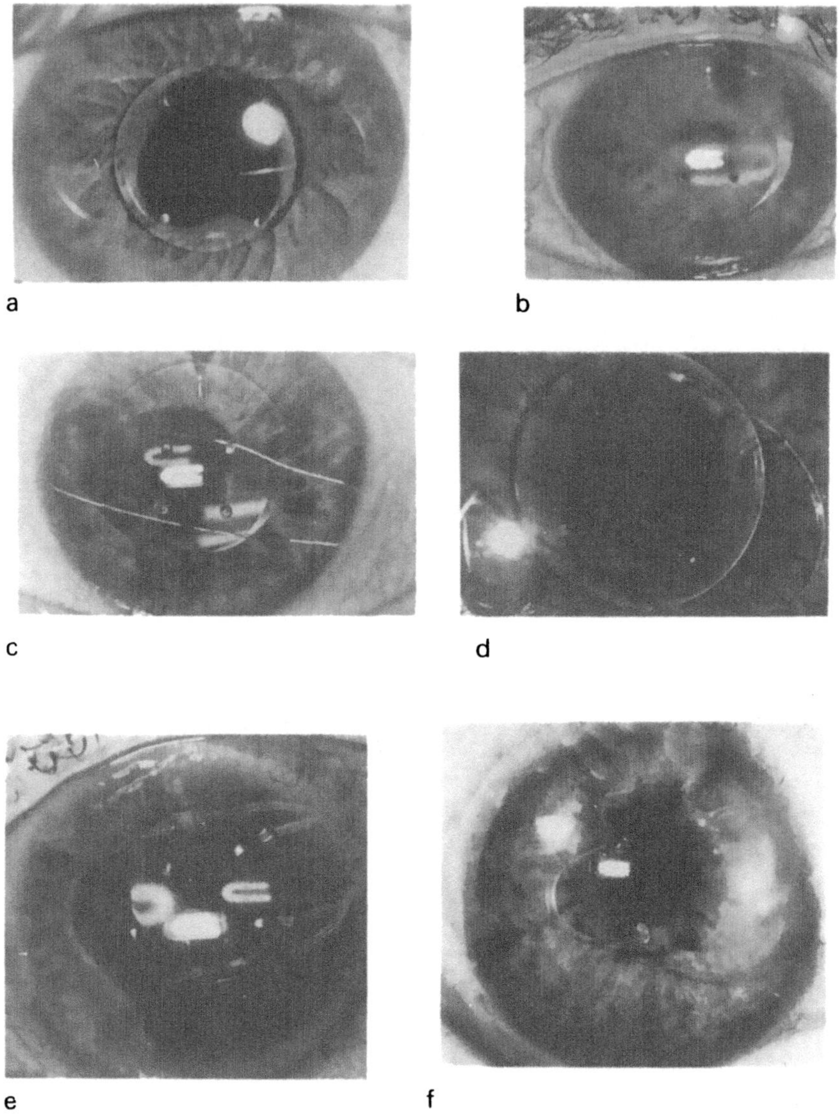

Fig. XII-11a. — Localized endothelial corneal dystrophy in an area overlying the tip of a loop of an iris clip lens caused by marked pseudophakodonesis.

b. — Forward tilting of a platinum clip lens causing endothelial corneal dystrophy.

c. — A Platinum Clip lens that had to be stabilized with a steel suture to release corneal contact.

d. — Iris clip lens from which an anterior loop was amputated to prevent incipient endothelial corneal dystrophy. (Courtesy C.D. Binkhorst.)

e. — Subluxated iris clip lens causing endothelial corneal endothelial dystrophy.

f. — Forward dislocation of a medallion lens causing endothelial corneal dystrophy. (Courtesy G. Baikoff.)

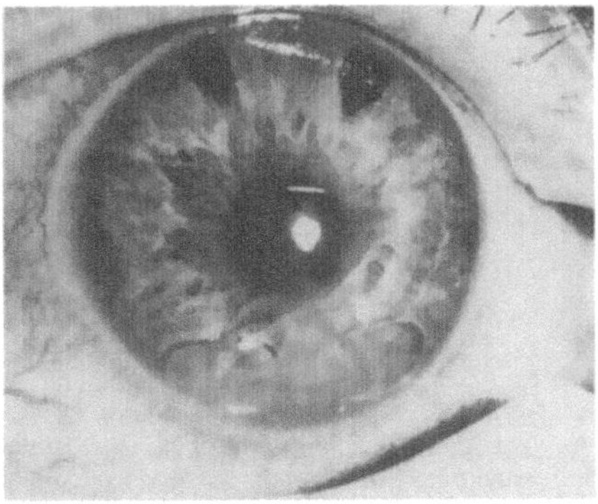

Fig. XII-11g. — Total dislocation of an iridocapsular lens with metal loops causing localized endothelial corneal dystrophy.

According to our surveys, the Sputnik and the Copeland lenses seem to be te most stable of the iris supported lenses used after intracapsular extraction. Subluxation and luxation will occur with any lens type, however, should the fixation mechanism fail, and corneal dystrophy may develop as a result of the ensuing endothelial damage caused by prolonged intermittent or persistent contact. The lens, therefore, has to be repositioned and measures taken to enhance fixation without delay. On occasion, the lens may have to be removed.

B. Other Factors

1. *Irrigating Solutions*

With the advent of extracapsular surgery in which large amounts of fluid are sometimes used, attention has been given to the possible influence of irrigating solutions on the endothelium.

On the basis of in vitro perfusions with both human and rabbit corneas, H. Edelhauser et al. (1976) compared the influence of various irrigating solutions on the endothelium. They concluded that a solution containing anorganic and organic constituents similar to those in the aqueous humor is to be preferred, and, in particular, the G.B.R. solution: Glutathione-Bicarbonate-Ringer (see Fig. XII-12 and Table XII-15). Although the osmolality and the pH of other solutions may be compatible with the endothelium, certain chemical constituents become necessary when the perfusion is prolonged: calcium is needed to maintain endothelial junctional complexes, glucose for aerobic metabolism, and glutathion for membrane protection (Kaye et al., 1968; McCarey, 1973; Mishima and Kudo, 1967).

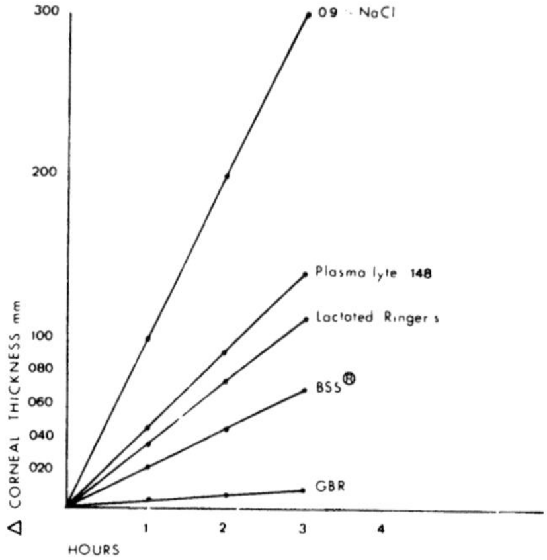

Fig. XII-12. — Changes in corneal thickness of rabbit corneas perfused with five different intraocular irrigating solutions (Edelhauser et al., 1976).

TABLE XII-15. — *Composition of Intraocular Irrigating Solutions in mM/l*

Chemical Constituent	*GBRS*	*BSS*	*LRS*	*P.L. 148*	*Saline*
NaCl	111.56	83.80	102.00	85.88	154.00
KCl	4.82	10.10	4.00	4.96	—
$CaCl_2$	1.04	4.32	3.00	—	—
$MgCl_26H_2O$	0.78	1.48	—	1.48	—
NaH_2PO_4	0.86	—	—	—	—
$NaHCO_3$	29.20	—	—	—	—
Glucose	5.01	—	—	—	—
Adenosine	0.50	—	—	—	—
Reduced Glutathione	0.30	—	—	—	—
Na Acetate	—	28.60	—	2.72	—
Na Citrate	—	5.78	—	—	—
Na Lactate	—	—	28.00	—	—
Na Gluconate	—	—	—	16.87	—
Osmolarity	306	270	277	299	308
pH	7.4	8.2	6.6	7.4	7.0

GBRS: Glutathione Bicarbonate Ringer Solution.
BSS: Balanced Salt Solution.
LRS: Lactated Ringer Solution.
P.L. 148: Plasma-Lyte 148.

Edelhauser and his colleagues propose the following guidelines: for low volume irrigation (as in routine cataract extraction in individuals with a normal corneal endothelium), any of the 5 solutions given on Table XII-15 would probably suffice; but in individuals with corneal endothelial decompensation (e.g., cornea guttata) or in individuals undergoing phakoemulsification, the solution that would cause the least harm to the endothelium would be the solution of choice, i.e., the G.B.R. solution.

Since the G.B.R. solution is not available commercially (it contains adenosine and reduced glutathione, which are labile when stored in solution for any prolonged period), other solutions were sought that would also protect the endothelium but would be easy to prepare or suitable for commercial distribution.

J. Christiansen et al. (1978) proposed solutions to be prepared in the operating room: Eighteen ml of commercial 5% dextrose in water and 20 ml of sodium bicarbonate solution (available in 50 ml ampules containing 50 ml Eq. of sodium bicarbonate) are injected aseptically into 1000 ml of Ringer's or lactated Ringer's solution.

D.R. Sanders et al. (1977) studied another solution, the Glucose-Phosphate-Ringer solution (G.P.R.), which contains all the essential electrolytes of G.B.R. except the labile elements (glutathion, adenosine, and bicarbonate). They substituted a stable phosphate buffer for the unstable bicarbonate buffer. The new G.P.R. solution seems to maintain corneal endothelial viability as well as does the G.B.R. solution.

J.K. McEnerney et al. (1978) investigated various electrolytic solutions and found that the T.C. Earle solution with glucose prolongs satisfactory endothelial vitality and preserves the endothelial function. These authors consider it to be one of the best commercially available solutions for intraocular irrigation.

TABLE XII-16. — *Composition of Solutions as Given by Sanders et al. (1977) and McEnerney et al. (1978) in gm/liter*

Chemical Composition	*GBR*	*GPR*	*T.C. Earle*
NaCl	6.521	8.143	6.800
Dextrose	0.901	0.404	1.000
KCl	0.359	0.410	0.400
$CaCl_2$	0.115	0.130	0.200
$MgCl_26H_2O$	0.159	0.180	0.000
$MgSO_4$	0.000	0.000	0.200
NaH_2PO_4	0.103	1.008	0.125
$NaH_2PO_4H_2O$	0.000	0.400	0.000
Sodium Gluconate	0.000	0.000	0.000
Sodium Acetate	0.000	0.000	0.000
NaH_2CO	2.454	0.000	2.200
Adenosine	0.134	0.000	0.000
Glutathione	0.092	0.000	0.000
Osmality	306	303	295
pH	7.40	7.20	7.45±0.05 [SE (n=6)]

2. *Mydriatics*

Intraocular epineprhine may be indicated to enlarge the size of the pupil. Hull et al. (1975) concluded on the basis of studies with laboratory animals that commercially available epinephrine 1:1000 with its sodium bisulfite preservative damaged the endothelial function and ultrastructure. They state that endothelial damage can be avoided, however, by diluting the commercially available epinephrine solution to 1:5000 or by mixing freshly prepared epinephrine bitartrate 1:1000 in a bicarbonate Ringer's solution without sodium bisulfite.

3. *Miotics*

According to J.L. Jay and M. MacDonald (1978), the following must be done to prevent endothelial corneal damage when pilocarpine is used. The pilocarpine should be prepared in a psysiological salt solution containing calcium. The osmolality should be near that of aqueous humor, approximately 300 m Os/liter, and no bacteriostatic perservatives should be added. These authors note that the low pH of pilocarpine solutions did not produce any adverse effects on cultured bovine corneal endothelia.

In the same experiments, 1% acetylcholine chloride in 5% manitol (Miochol) caused cell destruction, but it could not be determined if the toxic effect was caused by the active substance or by the hypertonicity of the preparation.

In another experiment, H. Völker Dieben et al. (1979) injected 2 ml of freshly prepared acetylcholine solution (1% in Ringer) into the anterior chambers of rabbit eyes. No endothelial cell damage could be demonstrated by vital staining of trephined corneal buttons.

4. *Antibiotics*

In vitro experiments with rabbit corneas by W.H. Coles (1975) showed that erythromycin and penicillin G. produced corneal thickness changes and morphological alterations when used in the ranges suggested for intracameral injections. Other antibiotics—bacitracin, chloramphenicol, oxacillin and cephalothin-produced dose-related and potentially harmful changes. Gentamycin, with and without preservatives (methylparaben and propylparaben), did not produce significant changes in corneal thickness.

Although Coles did draw some preliminary conclusions, he rightly argued that further investigations, both in vitro and in vivo, are necessary before guidelines can be drawn up regarding the intracameral use of antibiotics.

5. *Air*

Using air to separate the pseudophakos from the cornea has become routine, though there is some dispute as to whether this can damage the endothelial cells. Thus far, clinical observations have not revealed any detrimental effect, and M.A. Galin et al. (1979) reported that experiments with cats tended to confirm its innocuousness. However, both D.L. Van Horn et al. (1972) and H.M. Leibowitz and R.A. Laing (1974), using specular microscopy, observed various degrees of endothelial deterioration in rabbit eyes when the aqueous humor was replaced by air for 30 minutes. The morphological changes ranged from cytoplasmic abnormalities to cell explosion.

In any event, the benefits to be derived from the use of air in implant surgery outweigh the disadvantages observed in animal experiments. Of course, the air should not be left in the anterior chamber any longer than is strictly necessary.

6. *Iritis and Uveitis*

While it is clear from clinical observation that noticable alterations in transparency occur in the cornea in the presence of recurrent or severe uveitis, little is known about the underlying mechanisms. It is not even clear if inflammation causes a decrease in the cell density of the endothelium or if there is a decrease in vitality without the number of cells being affected.

Irreparable damage may be caused by antigen antibody complexes such as leucotoxins and lysozymes (Polack, 1977; Galin et al., 1979), and recurrent raises in intraocular pressure seem to be a contributing factor in some forms of uveitis (Setälä and Vannas, 1978; Vannas et al., 1977). In a study of the influence of unilateral iridocyclitis on cell density in 60 patients, K. Setälä (1979) found significant decreases in only 5 of the 7 patients who had "mutton-fat keratic precipitates". No significant differences in cell densities between the affected and the healthy eyes could be found in the remaining patients. Thirty-five of these patients had round, white keratic precipitates, and most of them had suffered from recurrent attacks of uveitis.

III. The Incidence of Endothelial Corneal Dystrophy

In assessing the performance of the modern refined lenses, the figures reported in the publications cited below are useful. They reflect the incidence of corneal pathology as observed by different surgeons using a single lens type. It must be noted that the reporting authors did not all use the same criteria: some mentioned endothelial corneal dystrophy only when the cornea was opaque, others only when the final visual acuity was less than 20/40, and others included pre-existing conditions and minor changes.

TABLE XII-17. — *Incidence of Endothelial Corneal Dystrophy according to Lens Type (Update Lens Models)*

Lens Type	*Number*	*Incidence of ECD*
Iris Clip Lens		
Schott (1977)	202	2.4%
Draeger (1977)	350	1.7%
Jaffe (1978)	698	0.6%
Kratz (1979)	332	0.9%
Medallion Lens		
Drews (1978)	300	0.7%
Kraff and Lieberman (1978)	500	0.5%
Copeland Lens		
Osher (1976)	100	1.0%
Snider and McReynolds (1977)	399	1.0%
Taylor et al. (1975)	196	1.0%
Sputnik Lens		
Fyodorov (1980)	2700	0.3%
Kwitko (1978)	100	1%
Galin (1978)	300	None
Iridocapsular Lens		
Binkhorst (1976)	500	1.4%
Rommel and Leonard	800	None
Kratz (1979)	308	2.3%
Platinum Clip Lens		
Sheets (1978)	757	1.5%
Pearce Lens		
Pearce (1979)	444	0.4%
Shearing Lens		
Kratz (1979)	756	None
Angle Supported Lens (Mark VIII)		
Choyce (Secondary) (1977)	1000	1.5%
Azar (1978)	800	None
Kratz (1979)	215	None

In view of the figures assembled on Table XII-17, one may conclude that these lenses give a rather low incidence of endothelial corneal dystrophy, all being under 2.5%. It may not be concluded, however, that this percentage will remain constant. "Clinically manifest" endothelial corneal dystrophy has been reported to develop as late as 8 years after implantation.

Indeed, all iris supported lenses that luxate or subluxate forward will increase the chances of endothelial corneal dystrophy, either as a direct result of the luxation or because of the intraocular manipulations involved in repositioning. Non-sutured iris clip lenses have a luxation rate of about 5%; sutured lenses luxate only when the suture fails, but subluxation is not infrequent; Copeland lenses that are not steadied by synechiae will luxate; iridocapsular lenses that are not fixated by synechiae or the posterior capsule will luxate, and particularly the metal looped lenses; and some platinum clip lenses will subluxate if they are not well fixed.

It may be that, in time, the Mark VIII lenses in Azar's and Kratz's series will turn out to have the same incidence of localized endothelial corneal dystrophy as did Choyce's series for which Pearce found a rate of 13.5%. As we have noted, Choyce himself considered this rate to be typical.

So far, endothelial dystrophy seems unlikely to develop at a high rate with posterior chamber lenses. Here too, however, those that are not well fixed may act like loose foreign bodies and come in contact with the endothelium as time goes on.

In many respects, the real situation is not reflected in the data given on Table XII-17. By including only data on the so-called refined original models, we have omitted the cases of corneal pathology that arose because tens of thousands of defective lenses were inserted in the United States.

We do not know the incidence of endothelial corneal dystrophy with metal looped lenses nor the incidence in U.G.H. cases. Also nearly nothing is available on the incidence of endothelial corneal dystrophy in the many thousands of cases operated on by non-publishing surgeons using refined lens models. We do know of several dozen eyes with bullous keratopathy, a condition frequently associated with cystoid macular edema and secondary glaucoma for which keratoplasty was necessary. (Kok van Alphen; Völker-Dieben; Winkelman; Otto; Van Ry, personal communications). The only valid conclusion that can be drawn seems to be that when qualified surgeons implant updated original lens models, one may expect a low incidence of clinically apparent corneal decompensation.

Summary and Conclusion

After three decades of lens implantation, the most important causal factors of endothelial corneal dystrophy seem to have been identified. Because the corneal endothelium is a good parameter for everything that occurs during and after the operation in the anterior chamber since it totalizes all adverse effects, our efforts in implant surgery must be directed to protecting this vital structure.

As we have shown in this chapter, there are many ways of avoiding iatrogenic endotheliopathy, and there are many or even more of precipitating it. In addition to atraumatic "instrumental surgery", irrigating solutions should be carefully selected and used in reasonable amounts. Until more is known about the effects of mydriatics, miotics, and antibiotics, the intraocular use of these agents should be considered with circumspection. Coating agents, in our opinion, are not imperative, since lens implantation is possible in most cases without endothelial contact.

Regarding the model of the lens, we can only state that the more the stability of the lens is assured, the less possibility there is of luxation or subluxation and subsequent deterioration of the cornea and, second, that the further the lens stays from the cornea, the less chance there is of endothelial corneal dystrophy occurring because of intermittent touch brought on by external causes.

Keratoplasty and Lensimplantation

Preventing contact between the pseudophakos and the endothelium is certainly one of the major problems in corneal grafting an eye that has an intraocular lens component in its anterior chamber.

In addition to the measures that must be taken to obtain a soft eye and to maintain a deep anterior chamber, the following measures must be considered:

— Using a coating agent to render the polymethylmethacrylate surface of the lens less aggressive.
— Covering the pseudophakos in situ while the first sutures are being placed through the graft by:
  - Using a lamellar membrane of Descemet's layer and the endothelium made from the patient's own corneal button, which is placed upside down on the pseudophakos (Drews, 1979).
  - Using a synthetic protective shield made, for example, of polymacon (HEMA) as suggested by Levy et al. (1979).
— Using retaining devices to keep the pseudophakos in the posterior position (see Fig. XII-13) as proposed by C.W. Simcoe.

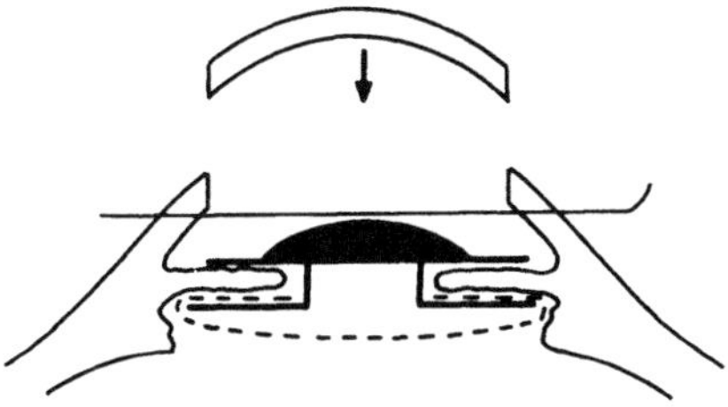

Fig. XII-13. — Retaining device to keep the pseudophakos in the posterior position.

— Using a larger corneal button from the donor eye, as Troutman (1976) has suggested.

The following situations arise:
— Penetrating keratoplasty, cataract extraction, and intraocular lens implantation (triple procedure);
— Penetrating keratoplasty and secondary lens implantation in aphakic patients with corneal disease;
— Penetrating keratoplasty for corneal disease in a pseudophakic eye.

A. **Triple Procedures**

A large variety of lens models have been used in the combined keratoplasty and implantation procedure: iris supported, iridocapsular supported, and capsular supported lenses.

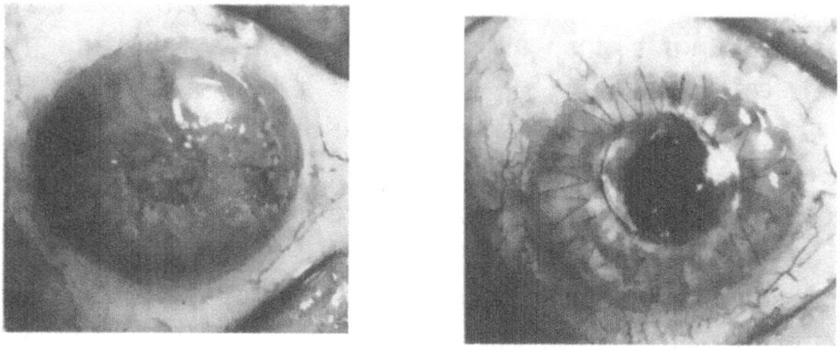

Fig. XII-14. — The "triple procedure". (Courtesy C.D. Binkhorst.)

Among them, the posterior chamber lenses seem to be of major interest since the iris diaphragm separates the graft from the implant both during and after the procedure.

Angle supported lenses raise practical problems in triple procedures. In contrast with the other lens types, a rigid anterior chamber lens cannot be introduced through the trephine opening.

In 1976, C.C. Kok van Alphen, A.J. Otto, and H.J.M. Völker-Dieben reported their results in 22 cases. In 15, the grafts retained good transparency, 4 regained reasonable transparence after mild rejection, and 3 grew opaque. After some 40 cases, these surgeons (personal communication, 1980) have come to the conclusion that triple procedures are to be restricted to non-inflammed cataractous eyes with Fuch's dystrophy, scrofulosis, etc.

Lee and Dohlman (1977) reported on 10 cases of penetrating keratoplasty, cataract removal, and artifical lens implantation with a follow up of 2 years. Graft failure occurred in 3 eyes. In 5 cases, visual acuity of ⩾20/40 was achieved. Sutured Medallion Lenses were inserted after intracapsular extraction. Lee and Dohlman noted that implantation during keratoplasty is much simpler than when it is done through a limbal wound since the large trepine opening (8 to 9 mm in diameter) allows easy access for the necessary manipulations.

J. Alpar (1978) reported on 18 cases of which 13 (72%) attained a visual acuity of ⩾20/40. The cataract extractions were about evenly divided between extracapsular and intracapsular. In the observation period, which ranged from 6 to 74 months (average: 21 months), 2 grafts were lost, 1 because of severe bleeding on the 3rd postoperative day and 1 because of a gradual shallowing of the anterior chamber with lens contact after 3 months.

D.M. Taylor et al. (1979) reported on 22 cases of which 12 (57%) attained a visual acuity of ≥20/40 and 17 (77%) had a clear graft. The maximum follow-up was 3½ years. The reasons for graft failure in 5 eyes included highly vascularized cornea of the recipient eye, faulty donor material, and chronic inflammation with secondary glaucoma. All the cataract extractions were intracapsular and, in the view of these authors, the presence of an intraocular lens during surgery prevented forward displacement of the vitreous and simplified graft suturing. Also after surgery, it reduced the possibility of graft failure from vitreous adhesions and diminished the incidence of retinal detachment.

J.D. Hunkeler and L.L. Hyde (1979) reported on 67 triple procedures. All the lens extractions but one were extracapsular. Iris sutured implants were used in 63 cases and 2-loop iridocapsular lenses in 4. The follow-up period ranged from 1 year to 5½ years (average: 2 years). Visual acuity ≥20/40 was attained in 72% of the cases. The graft remained clear in 64 eyes. These authors are of the opinion that the presence of the posterior capsule was one of the primary contributing factors for the low complication rate since it prevented vitreous interference during surgery and favored firm fixation of the pseudophakos later on.

B. Combined Procedures in Aphakia

Only a few surgeons have performed secondary implantation and simultaneous penetrating keratoplasty. We have data from 4 publications (Lee and Dohlman, 1977; Aquavella et al., 1977; Alpar, 1978; Taylor et al., 1979) giving the results of 40 cases. In most of the cases, keratoplasty was indicated because of Fuch's dystrophy or bullous keratopathy. Nearly all the cases involved intracapsular aphakia with a vitrectomy being performed at the time of the combined procedure. At the time of publication, 80% of the corneal grafts were clear. One out of 3 of these patients regained a visual acuity ≥20/40.

C. Keratoplasty in Pseudophakia

Various therapeutic measures are possible to prevent the advance of corneal edema in eyes containing a pseudophakos: amputation of the lens parts that touch the cornea such as loops, struts, the haptic rim, etc.; lens removal or exchange; and finally penetrating keratoplasty possibly combined with the previous measures. The incidence

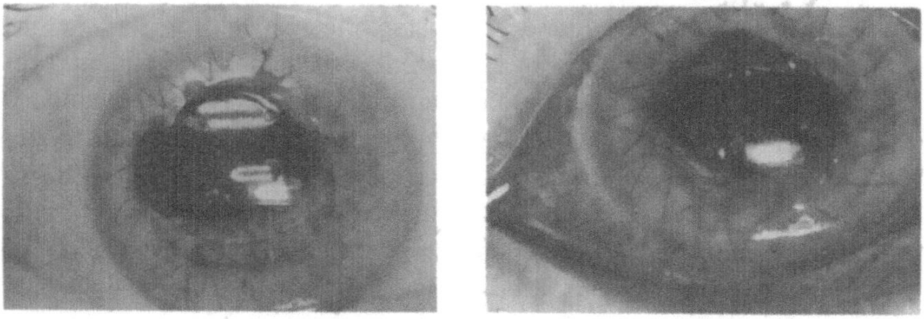

Fig. XII-15. — Perforating keratopolasty performed because of endothelial corneal dystrophy with a medallion lens. (Courtesy C.C. Kok van Alphen and H. Völker-Dieben.)

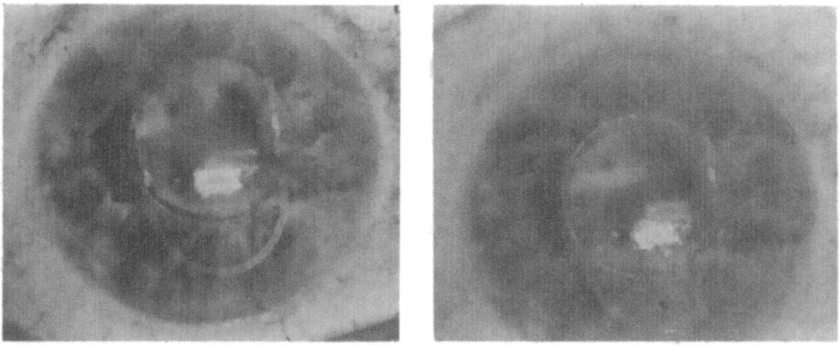

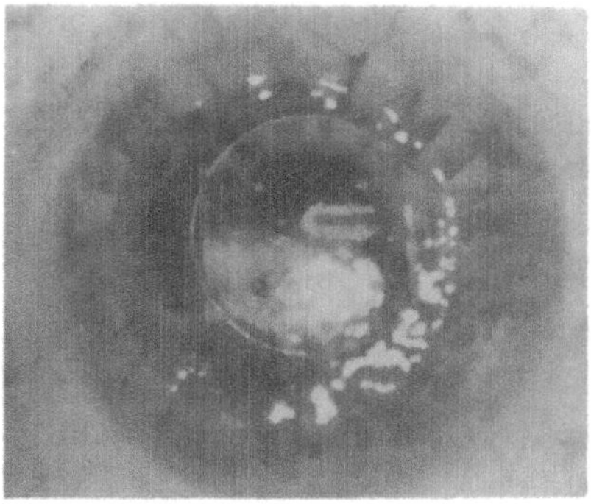

Fig. XII-16. — Progressive endothelial corneal dystrophy with an iris clip lens treated with perforating keratoplasty. (Courtesy C.C. Kok van Alphen and H. Völker-Dieben.)

of keratoplasty in pseudophakia is unknown, though the need for such procedures will undoubtedly increase as ever more surgeons enter the implant field. We have analyzed most of the reasons that promote endothelial corneal dystrophy elsewhere (cf. pp. 446).

Whether or not keratoplasty in pseudophakic eyes with corneal decompensation is rewarding depends on a number of factors. Indeed, concurrent pathological conditions such as glaucoma, uveitis, and diseases of the posterior pole and especially cystoid macular edema often seriously compromise the final result. C. Kok van Alphen and H. Völker-Dieben (1979), for example, have pointed out that when endothelial corneal dystrophy lasts more than 9 months, cystoid macular edema is very likely to be associated.

Conclusion

Keratoplasty in the presence of an intraocular lens has turned out to yield more favorable results than one could reasonably have expected. Predictions based on the incidence of complications after lens implantation and the rate of failure inherent in corneal grafting would certainly be bleak. However, the few dozen combined procedure cases that have been reported may yet, in view of the limited follow-up periods, develop problems with the lens, such as luxation, or with the graft.

In our opinion, the triple procedure should only be performed in very exceptional cases, but keratoplasty in an already pseudophakic eye should be performed whenever indicated, as it is often the only possibility left to improve the situation. Finally, keratoplasty and lens implantation in aphakic patients with corneal dystrophy should be considered with caution. Indeed, secondary lens implantation has its own specific limitations ad complications. To add the problems involved in grafting would seem to be difficult to justify.

CHAPTER XIII

LENS IMPLANTATION AND INFLAMMATORY RESPONSE AND GLAUCOMA

Introduction

According to our survey with regard to inflammatory reactions—uveitis, vitritis, endophthalmitis—and dysregulation of intraocular pressure, the eye responded favorably to lens implantation if the following conditions were fulfilled:

1. The eye was judiciously selected;
2. Adequately sterilized lenses with good "track records" were used;
3. The surgery was atraumatic and aseptic;
4. Adequate measures were taken to reduce postoperative inflammation and rises in intraocular pressure.

As illustrated by Table XIII-1, the uveitis incidence is acceptable. It must be noted, however, that higher doses of local or systemic corticosteroids were used than is usual after standard cataract extraction without lens implantation. As a rule, more pronounced uveal reactions were noticed in diabetic patients or in those that had a history of iritis or iridocyclitis. Although varying incidences of intraocular pressure dysregulation in the early postoperative period were recorded, the incidence of late glaucoma was insignificant.

I. Some Considerations on Postoperative Uveal Reaction

The common uveal reaction after cataract surgery is generally referred to as "surgical uveitis". The etiology of this reaction is complex since it is the result of the total of all the mechanical, chemical, and bacteriological agression that the uveal tissue suffers during surgery and the early postoperative phase.

Assuming that the influence of bacterial contamination on intraocular tissue is sufficiently well known, we shall limit our discussion here to some of the non-infectious factors that may account for early or late uveal reaction.

TABLE XIII-1. — *Statistical Survey of Complications*

	Number of Cases	*Iritis*	*Secondary Membranes*	*Glaucoma*		*Endophthalmitis*
				Early	*Persistent*	
Iris Clip Lens (ICCE)						
Scott (1977)	202	Rare	1%	1%	4.4%	N.A.
Draeger (1977)	350	Rare	N.A.	15%	1.7%	N.A.
Jaffe (1978)	698	Rare	1.9%	N.A.	N.A.	N.A.
Medallion Lens (ICCE)						
Drews (1978)	300	2%	1%	N.A.	0.7%	0.3%
Kraff and Lieberman (1978)	500	1%	N.A.	N.A.	N.A.	N.A.
Copeland Lens (ICCE)						
Osher (1976)	100	N.A.	2%	None	None	None
Snider and McReynolds (1977)	399	N.A.	N.A.	N.A.	0.5%	0.25%
Taylor et al. (1975)	196	9%	9%	N.A.	N.A.	N.A.
Sputnik Lens (ICCE)						
Fyodorov (1977)	2000	0.25%	3.4%	0.25%	None	N.A.
Galin (1978)	300	2%	1-11%	8%	None	N.A.
Kwitko (1978)	100	N.A.	1%	3%	0%	N.A.
Choyce Mark VIII						
Choyce (1976) (secondary implantation)	800	N.A.	N.A.	N.A.	N.A.	0.125%
Azar (1978)	800	2%	N.A.	3%	0.7%	None
Kratz (1979)	215	6.5%	N.A.	N.A.	N.A.	N.A.
Iridocapsular Lens (ECCE)						
Binkhorst (1976)	500	0.4%	*	N.A.	1.2%	N.A.
Rommel and Leonard	800	1.5%	*	1.8%	0.8%	None
Posterior Chamber Lenses (ECCE)						
Shearing Lens						
Kratz (1979)	756	3.3%	*	N.A.	0.4%	0.1%
Pearce Lens						
Pearce (1979)	444	2%	*	None	1.8%	None
Worst (1977)	1813	0.8% (vitritis 3.5%)	*	0.1%	N.A.	0.5%
Hirschman (1978)	1660	0.8%	*	1.1%	N.A.	0.2%
Shepard (1977)	500	2.4% (vitritis 4.6%)	2.6%	0.8%	1%	0%
Snider and McReynolds (1977)	500	N.A.	*	0.4%	N.A.	0.2%

N.A. = Not available.
* The distinction between secondary membrane and secondary opacification after extracapsular cataract extraction is rarely made in the literature and difficult to make in practice.

A sterile uveal reaction after lens implantation may be regarded as an irritative response to the implanted material. Historically, it does not seem that the material itself was the direct underlying cause for this, but rather the method of sterilization. Over the last three decades, enough clinical evidence has accumulated to confirm this. With the first implant lenses, the incidence of serious uveal reactions dramatically decreased with the introduction of the caustic soda method. Using this method as their standard procedure, manufacturers such as Rayner, Morcher, and Medical Workshop supplied thousands of lenses that were free from this problem. From the early fifties to the mid-seventies, reports of marked sterile uveal reactions are rare in the literature. But when manufacturers switched to other, supposedly superior, methods (γ-radiation and Ethylene oxyde sterilization) the problem of sterile uveal reactions reappeared

Another cause of postoperative sterile reactions may be incomplete removal of substances used in the manufacture of the lenses such as polishing and grinding agents (Binkhorst, 1957; Meltzer, 1980).

Another factor, which may precipitate unexpected uveal reaction, is the use of inappropriate materials in the manufacture of the lenses or the deterioration of that material during processing. Except for deterioration in the process of sterilization, the literature contains no reports of such cases over the last decade. However, as Yamanaka et al. (1979) and R. Drews (personal communication, 1979) have noted, manufacturers do not readily divulge the materials and products they use. This makes investigation difficult, if not impossible. There are very few ways of determining beforehand whether or not a given lens will be toxic. M. A. Galin et al. (1975) have suggested a tissue culture method: the lenses are placed in a culture of secondary rabbit kidney cells, which are observed daily. A less attractive method is implantation in animals. During the fifties, this was the only method available. Fedrizi (1955), De Poli and Ramagnoli (1955), King et al. (1957), and Lieb and Du Pont Guerry (1957) have published the results of their implantations of various plastic materials in rabbits, cats, dogs, monkeys, and other animals.

Finally, the irritative response of the uveal tissue to microtrauma must not be underrated as a cause of inflammatory reactions. Microtrauma is inevitable with any kind of intraocular surgery, and it is a particular concern for the implant surgeon because of the degree of it involved in lens implantation and because it may persist after surgery when the implant remains in close contact with the overlying

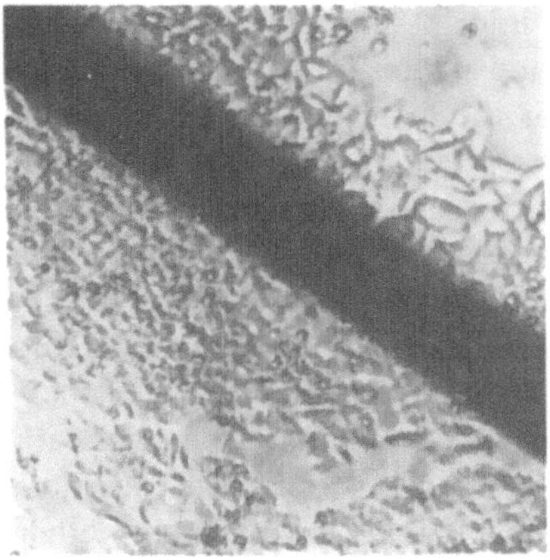

a

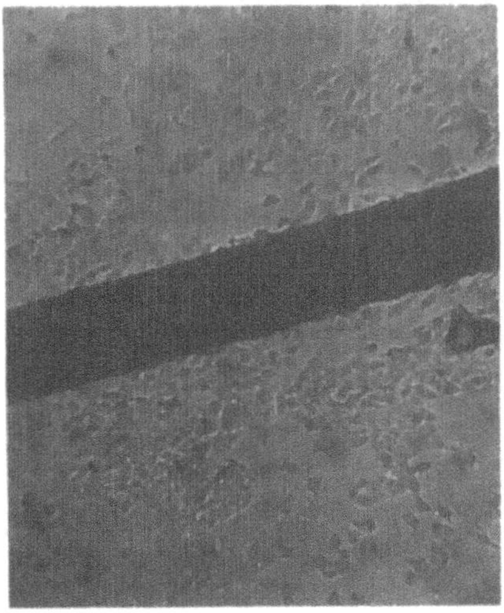

b

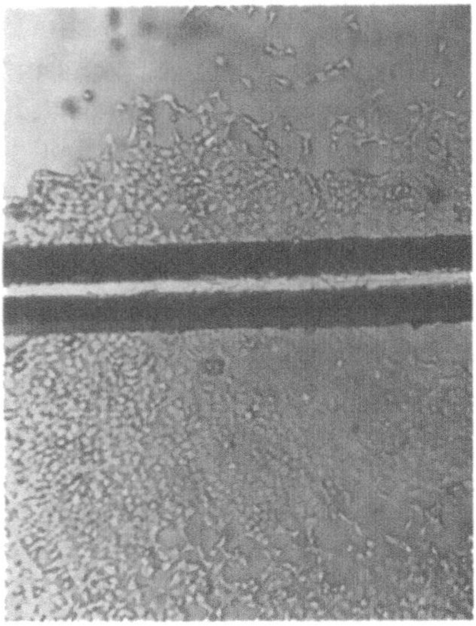

c

Fig. XIII-1a. — γ-sterilized polypropylene thread
b. — γ-sterilized nylon thread
c. — Platinum-iridium thread sterilized with the caustic soda method. The threads were placed in a medium containing secondary kidney cells. As shown in the photographs, the cellular density is unaffected by the presence of these materials. (Courtesy J. Verstraete.)

iris. Whether it is a matter of a mobile lens rubbing against the iris or a mobile iris rubbing against an immobile lens, the problem is essentially the same.

Both in laboratory animals and in human beings, paracentesis disrupts the blood-aqueous barrier, which is manifested by an increased degree of capillary permeability even for substances with high molecular weights. This vascular leakage or barrier breakdown of the iris vessels and the ciliary epithelium can be demonstrated by fluorescein angiography of the iris (Szaley et al., 1975; Kottow, 1978) or by measuring the concentration of protein in the aqueous humor.

Higher concentrations of protein after paracentesis have been shown to be present in the aqeuous humor of rabbits by Duke Elder already in 1931. In the early forties, Kronfeld et al. (1941) investigated this phenomenon in human beings, and Steiger et al. (1955) demonstrated that protein concentration rises to a maximum in human beings 30 to 45 minutes after parencentesis and returns to normal values after 48 hours.

The blood-aqueous barrier can also be broken down by other factors such as mechanical manipulation of the iris, chemical irritation, laser burn, scratching of the cornea, and blunt trauma of the anterior eye segment (Ambache, 1965; Cole and Unger, 1973; Bechetoile et al., 1978; Duke Elder, 1931; Davson and Guilliam, 1947).

The search for the chemical mediators that cause these profound disturbances in permeability has been intensive. Ambache (1955) and Ambache et al. (1965, 1966) isolated a substance from rabbit irides that has a potent smooth muscle contracting effect. Ambache named it "irin", and it was later identified to be a mixture of prostaglandins. These prostaglandins are fatty acids and are released into the eye as an irritative reaction to chemical or mechanical agression upon the iris tissue (among others, Cole and Unger, 1973; Janpol et al., 1975; Eakins, 1977).

The symptoms of this response include hyperemia of the conjunctiva, miosis, disruption of the blood-aqueous barrier, and transient increase in the intraocular pressure. According to Ambache et al. (1965), this response cannot be prevented by prior administration of either atropine or mepyramine, which indicates that it is not mediated by either acetylcholine or histamine. High concentrations of prostaglandins in the aqueous humor of human eyes has also been found in the presence of several types of uveitis (Whitelock et al., 1973; Masuda et al., 1973; Masuda et al., 1975).

The extent to which prostaglandins are stored in the undisturbed intraocular tissues is not known, but their release or synthesis in response to tissue damage is both rapid and massive. The conjunctiva and the iris of rabbits seem to be very active in prostaglandin production (Ambache, 1965).

The half-life of prostaglandins in the eye is extremely short, and they are rapidly removed by the ciliary processes and the posterior iris epithelium. Prostaglandins injected into the vitreous are removed rapidly and do not appear in the anterior chamber. This transport system is inhibited by probenecid and indomethacin, which allows prostaglandins to appear in the anterior chamber after vitreous injection (Bito, 1973).

Similarly, the ability to remove prostaglandins from the intraocular fluids in vivo was found to be severely inhibited during the course of inflammation and even several months after an episode of severe uveitis (Bito and Wallenstein, 1977). Certain drugs interfere with the availability of prostaglandins: aspirin, indomethacin, and the steroids were found to inhibit their synthesis at different stages. Polyfloretin phosphate, on the other hand, blocks their action.

Using the rise in total protein content in the aqueous humor as a parameter, Zimmerman et al. (1975) reported that the blood aqueous barrier stabilized after paracentesis for cataract extraction in patients pretreated with acetylsalicylic acid. According to Ferreira et al. (1971), Smith and Willis (1971), and Vane (1971), most of the aspirin-like drugs inhibit the initial stage of the synthetase reaction and thus block the formation of the whole series of compounds formed from the essential fatty acids and among them the prostaglandins. Indoxole is more potent than indomethacin in this respect, which is far more potent than aspirin (Podos and Becker, 1973; Bhattacherjee and Eakins, 1974).

In animals, the amount of systemic aspirin or indomethacin that is necessary to prevent the ocular irritative response after paracentesis or prostaglandin instillation is much higher than the human therapeutic dose (Podos and Becker, 1973; Bhattacherjee ad Eakins, 1974). And indomethacin administered systemically was reported to have no inhibitory effect in monkey eyes (Kass et al., 1975). It seems that it is very difficult for indomethacin to penetrate the eye from the circulatory system. Various investigators, however, have reported indomethacin to be effective when it is instilled (Hanna and Sharp, 1972; Conquet et al., 1975; Mishima and Masuda, 1977; Hung et al., 1977; Mochizuki et al., 1977; Myake 1978; Bechetoille et al., 1978).

Indeed repeated preoperative instillation of 0.5% indomethacin was found to suppress the irritative symptoms in the anterior ocular segment after cataract surgery and to cause the pupil to lose much of its tendency to constrict during surgery. Mishima and Masuda (1977) and Mochizuki et al. (1977) also noticed that preoperative instillation of indomethacin suppressed postoperative increase in corneal thickness. Since the effect of prostaglandins on the endothelium is still unknown, further investigation is necessary here.

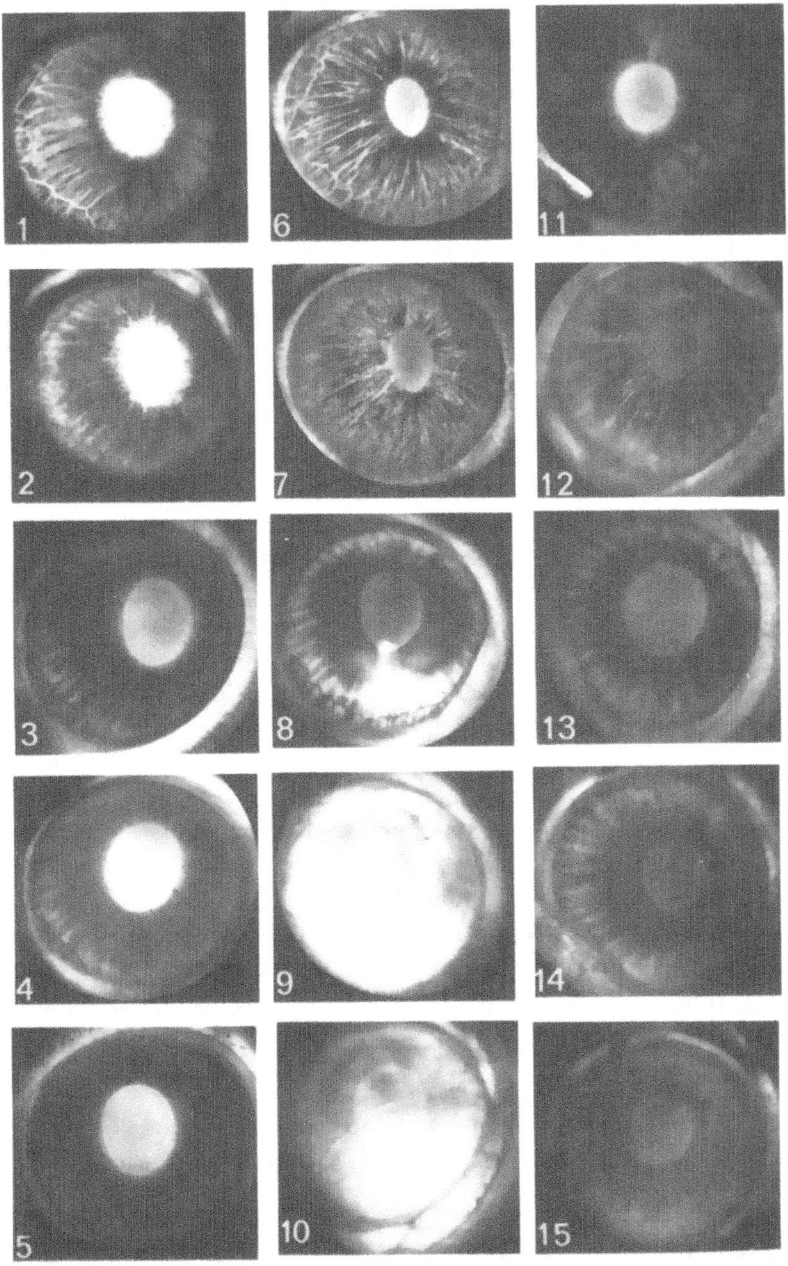

Fig. XIII-2. — Angiograms of normal anterior eye segments of rabbits (1, 2, 3, 4, 5) after blunt injury (6, 7, 8, 9, 10); after blunt injury and pretreatment with topical indomethacin (11, 12, 13, 14, 15). (Courtesy A. Bechetoille and J.J. Chananais.)

Unfortunately, indomethacin not only inhibits the synthesis of prostaglandins, but also suppresses dehydrogenase activity (Pace-Asciak and Cole, 1975) and thus the removal of prostaglandins from the eye by transport (Bito and Wallenstein, 1977). It is not impossible that this drug can intensify the effect of prostaglandins that are already released into the eye. There is evidence to suggest that it is reasonable to have a high concentration of indomethacin in the aqueous humor before any mechanical agression is begun, but that postoperative instillation probably is useless.

It may be concluded that, in addition to some not yet well defined chemical toxic substances, iris manipulation has to be included among the factors that promote postoperative, non-bacterial uveitis. Several investigators have demonstrated that mechanical trauma to the iris—stroking, rubbing, etc.—is responsible for an irritative response characterized by disruption of the blood-aqueous barrier, atropine-resistant miosis, hyperemia, elevation of intraocular pressure, and even various degrees of corneal swelling.

Prostaglandins seem to be one or the primary chemical mediators responsible for these symptoms.

The extreme sensitivity of the iris to trauma forces the implant surgeon to give close attention to what happens during the operation as well as to what can happen later on. There seems to be no reason to assume that a humoral mediator such as prostaglandin will not be released in a later stage when there is friction between the implanted lens and the iris. As we will have occasion to mention, some noteworthy forms of aseptic delayed uveal reactions have occured after the implantation of defective lenses.

In the future, the behavior of the iris of eyes containing implants will certainly be investigated thoroughly by means of iris angiography. It would be premature to draw any conclusions from this method at this time.

II. Uveal Behaviour and Intraocular Pressure Dysregulation during the Early Postoperative Period

A mild uveal tissue response classically characterized by the presence of some cells and flare is common.

Pigment cells or deposits can be seen in the anterior chamber located on the endothelium and the anterior hyaloid as in non-implant cataract surgery. In implant surgery, these cells also occur on both surfaces of the pseudophakos. C.D. Binkhorst has noted that, the amount of pigment loss may generally be correlated to the amount of trauma involved in the surgical procedure itself. Transillumination can detect some areas of pigment loss usually overlying the posterior haptics of the lens or near the sphincter.

When more severe tissue reaction occurs, in addition to an increase in cellular reaction and flare the classic fibrine cloud and even Descemet's precipitates may be seen. Both have a tendency to adhere to the implant material. Obviously, posterior synechiae may form during any uveal reaction. Depending on the lens type, these synechiae may adhere to the lens or the loops or to both.

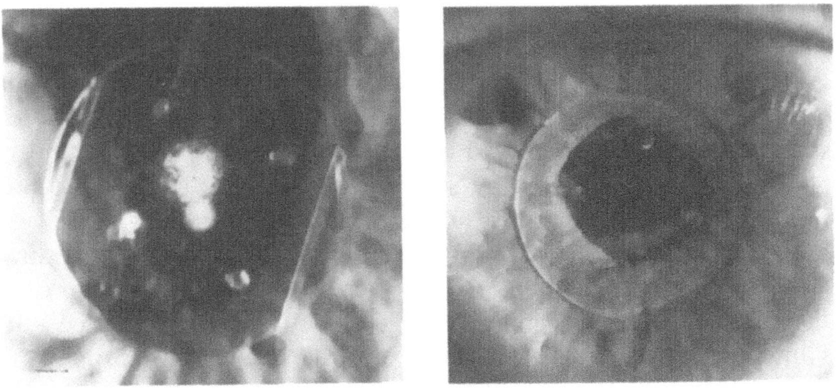

Fig. XIII-3. — Fatty precipitates and pigment deposits on the lens surfaces.

The formation of a cyclitic membrane, although infrequent, may be a matter of concern. Obviously associated with an uncommon degree of tissue reaction, it may develop at various times after surgery. This membrane can cover the anterior hyaloid face or the posterior capsule, and it may also adhere to the pseudophakos itself and especially to those parts located within the pupillary aperture.

Our survey indicated that the occurrence of hypopions is rather uncommon with the modern lens models. The few that we ourselves saw in our series were bacterial in origin and always reacted favorably to antibiotics. "Sterile hypopions", i.e. those not elicited by intraocular bacterial, fungal, or viral contamination, were rare until the late seventies. Galin et al. (1977) suggested the possibility of inadequate lens cleaning before sterilization in the cases he observed.

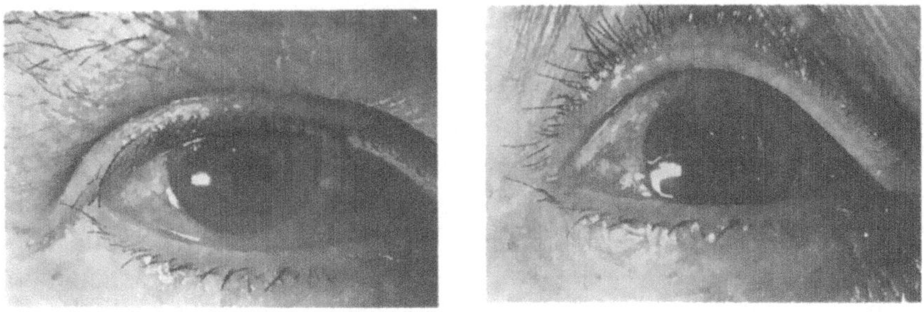

Fig. XIII-4. — Incipient bacterial endophthalmitis in a patient using high doses of corticosteroids and immuno-depressive drugs. The photographs were taken 1 week after surgery (left) and 2 weeks after surgery (right). The cyclitic deposit in the pupillary area disappeared completely, and the final visual acuity was 6/6. The patient died a year later because of generalized infection.

In the summer of 1976 in the U.S.A., 14 eyes implanted with lenses from a shipment of 388 γ-radiated Morcher lenses reacted vigorously with sterile hypopions. All of them responded well to steroid therapy and achieved good vision (Drews, 1978). Similar observations were reported by Schotz et al. (personal communication from C.D. Binkhorst). Other surgeons, however, including ourselves have implanted γ-radiated Morcher lenses without encountering any adverse reactions. Different reasons were suggested: degradation of the PMMA or the polypropylene or degradation of the balanced salt solution. W. Meltzer (1981) demonstrated the validity of the last hypothesis.

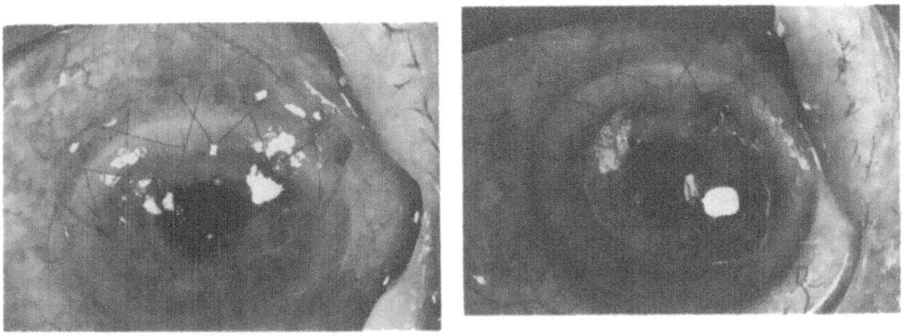

Fig. XIII-5. — Postoperative hypopion with γ-sterilized lens (left); the morning after intensive steroid therapy (right). (Courtesy J.J. Alpar.)

With the recent advent of ethylene oxide sterilization in the U.S.A., an unusually high incidence of postoperative hypopions has been noted, various reports placing it between 1% and 20%. These hypopions seem to be of non-infectious origin since they respond well to high doses of steroids. As a preventive measure, it is recommended that the ethylene oxide sterilized lenses be rinsed for a good half hour in saline (AIOIS Newsletter, 1978).

TABLE XIII-2. — *Incidence of Endophthalmitis*

Author	*Number of Operations*	*Incidence of Endophthalmitis*
Worst (1977)	1813	0.5%
Hirschman (1977)	1011	0.2%
Shepard (1977)	500	None
Drews (1978)	300	0.3%
Rommel and Leonard	1000	0.1%
Total	4624	±0.2%

Endophthalmitis is rare (see Table XIII-2), though a few outbreaks have been reported with lenses of U.S. origin. T.H. Pettit (1976) reported that 13 cases of fungal endophthalmitis (Paecilomyces lilacines) were observed in the United States in 1975. Eleven of these cases were caused by a contaminated lot of neutralizing solution ($NaHCO_3$). Seven of the cases ended up with enucleation, and, of the remaining 5, one had a visual acuity of 20/25, one had 20/200, two had light perception and one was phthisical with no light perception. T.H. Pettit noted that the delayed onset, which is typical for fungal endophthalmitis, was partly responsible for the surprisingly large number of cases from a single contamination source.

Another 8 cases of endophthalmitis caused by contaminated $NaHCO_3$ by Pseudomomas aerogenes were reported in the U.S.A. in the fall of 1976. The lenses had been shipped in the contaminated solution. Three eyes were functionally lost, but 5 were saved by means of intensive antimicrobial therapy (Poley, 1978).

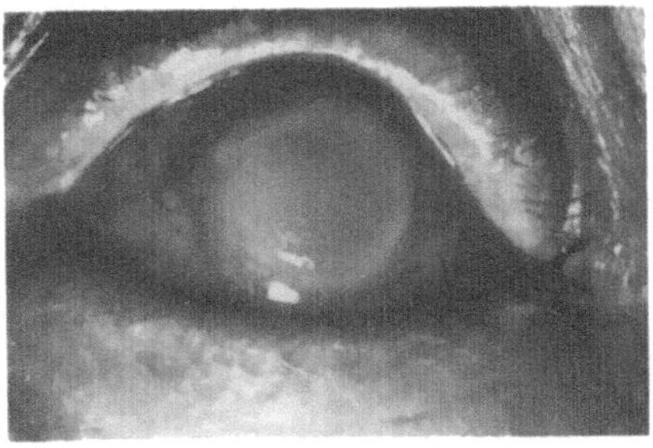

Fig. XIII-6. — Septic endophthalmitis. Photograph taken the second day after surgery. The anterior chamber was contaminated by *Klebsiella aerobacter*.

In most of the reported cases of early postoperative pressure dysregulation, the cause could be attributed to one of the following mechanisms:

1. Pupil block;
2. Steroid induced glaucoma;
3. Inflammatory reactions;
4. The use of α-chymotrypsin.

The incidence of early postoperative pressure dysregulation varies considerably depending on the surgical technique and the judgment of the surgeon. It is largely a matter of prevention: patients with borderline intraocular pressure should not be considered as routine candidates for implantation. In suspect cases, the outflow facility has to be assessed beforehand as well as possible sensitivity to corticosteroids.

In addition to performing adequate iridectomies, the use of anti-inflammatory agents is to be considered. J. Charleux (1978) has reported that systemic, preoperative administration of indomethacin has a beneficial influence. J. Pearce (personal communication, 1978) has had good results with non-steroidal drugs and particularly buviprofen. The routine administration of Diamox® in the early postoperative period, as C.D. Binkhorst recommends, is also indicated. We have obtained good results with the use of topical timolol 0.5% during the first few days after the operation.

1. *Iris Supported Lenses*

a. *Iris Clip, Medallion, Sputnik Lens*

The tissue reaction to the Iris Clip, Medallion, and Sputnik Lenses is low grade and easily controlled with topical corticosteroids.

Usually, any slight synechia formation can be controlled by judicious administration of mydriatics. Small synechiae are harmless with an Iris Clip or a Medallion Lens. And, to a certain extent, synechiae between the pupil margin and the anterior hyaloid or the lens supports may be advantageous since they stabilize the lens and prevent luxation. Asymmetric synechiae formation with a Sputnik Lens is undesirable because decentration of the lens may cause the subluxation of, for example, an anterior strut.

The consequences of a more pronounced uveal reaction that is characterized by extensive synechia formation is of more concern. They may lead to seclusion of the pupil and eventual pupillary block

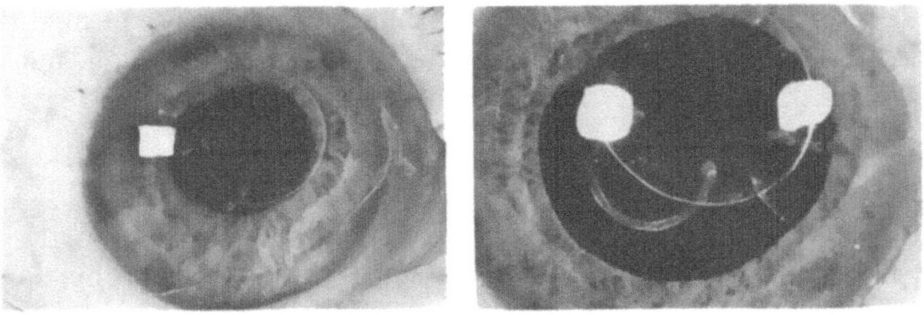

Fig. XIII-7. — Asymmetric posterior synechia formation with Sputnik lens leading to subluxation of the anterior strut (at 5 o'clock) without further complications. (Courtesy J.J. Alpar).

if the peripheral colobomas are not functioning. In exceptional cases, such a reaction results in membrane formation involving the iris border and the anterior vitreous face, which requires secondary procedures.

Although pupillary block in the hands of a skillful surgeon is infrequent, it may constitute a major problem for the inexperienced implant surgeon. The bulging iris makes the anterior chamber shallower increasing the risk of the lens touching the cornea, which is always to be considered an emergency. When the anterior chamber is shallow, of course, other causes such as wound leak or ciliary block should not be overlooked.

b. *Copeland Lens*

Unlike the other models, iris reactions after the insertion of a Copeland Lens is more pronounced in the early and late postoperative period. As we have had occasion to note, this reaction is caused by the special one-plane design of the lens that leads to extensive contact between the 4 flat haptic supports and the adjacent iris tissue. Consequently, physiological changes in the pupil width are prevented, and the facility of aqueous flow through the pupillary aperture is slightly diminished. Synechia formation between the iris and the lens is frequently reported to occur in the immediate postoperative period. Due to the special anatomical location of the lens in the pupillary area, the synechia may involve the anterior hyaloid, which lies in close contact to the surface of the pseudophakos. If adequate measures are taken, however, it seems that the consequences of the early uveal reaction to this lens type can be substantially lessened. Routine peroperative subtenonal or parabulbar injection of corticosteroids is recommended. Judicious use of mydriatics also seems to be strongly indicated to prevent seclusion, pupillary block, and early membrane formation (Blumenthal et al., 1977).

2. *Iridocapsular Supported Lenses*

B. Drews summarized in 1976 some of the current opinions against extracapsular lenses as follows (Boyd, 1978): "In the presence of too much cortical material left after surgery one may expect problems with uveitis that the cortex induces; furthermore if a secondary procedure is required to evacuate excessive cortical material in the pupillary aperture, this is to be done mostly under general anesthesia, because one cannot well anesthetize an inflammed eye with local anesthesia."

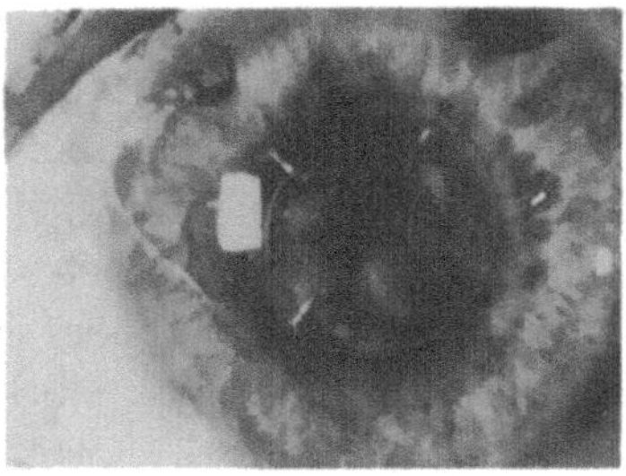

Fig. XIII-8. — Cortical remnants left after surgery. Photograph taken 10 days after implantation.

Thus as late as 1976 extracapsular surgery was thought to be associated with problems of uveitis if cortical material remained in the eye.

This opinion is in marked contrast to the clinical findings of C. D. Binkhorst, the followers of his school, and all the surgeons using extracapsular techniques. They all reported low uveal reactions after planned and well-conducted extracapsular cataract extraction.

Usually, a mild cellular reaction and flare occurs during the first few days. Our own observations indicate that pericorneal injection is mostly absent and that neither photophobia nor pain occur. Pigment deposits can be observed on the lens surface or Descemet's membrane or both. Within a week, the corticosteroid drops can be reduced to a dose of 3 times daily and eventually stopped. The postoperative administration of miotics that is routine for the Binkhorst-type of iridocapsular lens causes the pupil to be miotic for the first postoperative day. Weak mydriatics are judiciously applied thereafter to mobilize the pupil.

In the case of a more pronounced inflammatory response, which in our experience is rare, the tendency to posterior synechia formation is aggravated. White, fatty precipitates sticking to the lens surface can also be noted. In these cases, more aggressive pupil dilation and anti-inflammatory treatment is mandatory. The white, fatty precipitates and the slight tendency to synechia formation are the only things that seem to be related to what is commonly called the phacotoxic reaction after extracapsular cataract extraction. The use of corticosteroids has probably reduced this complication to a rarity.

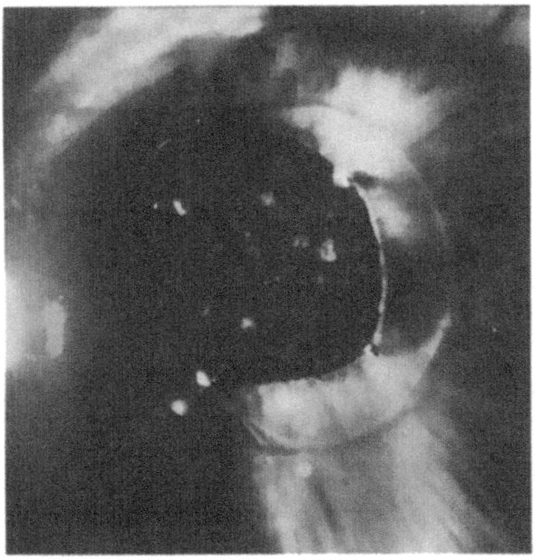

Fig. XIII-9. — White fatty precipitates on the lens surface. (Courtesy A.T.M. Van Balen).

Early formation of a secondary membrane overlying the posterior capsule usually starts when fibrin production occurs. Clinically, it appears as if the fibrin sticks to the posterior capsule, sometimes involving the posterior loop attachments and the pupillary margin. This is probably a major component in early opacification of the posterior membrane. Mostly, if adequate management is promptly instituted, the condition can be reversed in a few days.

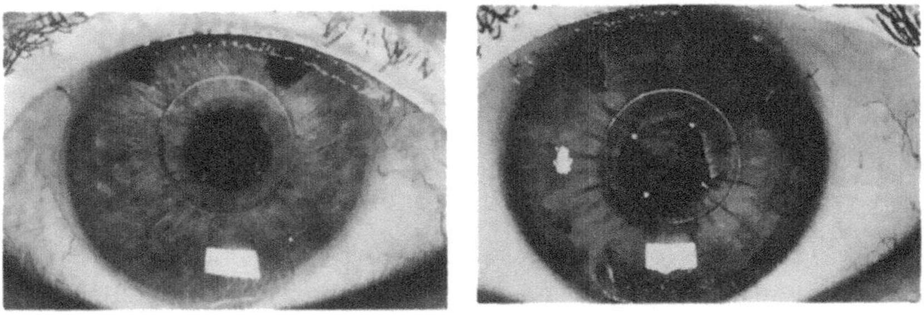

Fig. XIII-10. — Examples of fibrine deposition on the posterior capsule.

It has been noted (cf. Chapter XI) that the inflammatory reaction pattern in children after the insertion of iridocapsular lens is basically the same as that in adults. Our own experience with a few dozen cases confirms the observations of C.D. Binkhorst and A.T.M. Van Balen.

The posterior chamber lenses designed by J.L. Pearce and by S. Shearing are reported to give only low-grade early postoperative reactions. The possibility of early postoperative pupil dilation probably contributes to the low-grade uveal response.

3. *Angle Supported Lenses*

The precise incidence of early postoperative uveitis with anterior chamber lenses is difficult to determine. D.P. Choyce did not report the incidence of iritis in his series of 800 Choyce Mark VIII lens implantations. We do know that 11 Mark VIII lenses of the first 500 Choyce implanted had to be removed because of intractable iritis (Choyce, 1975). R.F. Azar (1978) reported a 2% incidence, and R.P. Kratz (1979), who also used the original Rayner Mark VIII lenses, reported and incidence of more than 6%.

Because of the specific anatomical location of the Mark VIII lens, early postoperative iritis can be complicated by pupillary block. The clinical picture more or less depends on the degree of iris edema and the residual possibility of aqueous passage. When the latter is prevented because of inadequately functioning iris colobomas, the edematous iris touching the overlying lens first shows iris bulge and very soon the pupillary block will develop since the pupillary aperture is plugged by the lens itself.

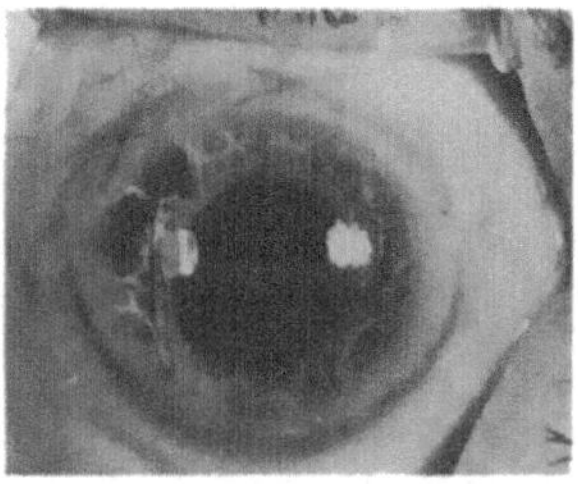

Fig. XIII-11. — Additional iridectomies performed because of pupil block glaucoma with a Choyce Mark VIII lens. (Courtesy J.J. Alpar.)

J.L. Tenant (1976) suggest the following treatment:

1. Aggressive control of the iritis to eliminate the iris edema as quickly as possible.

2. Vigorous dilation of the pupil beyond the border of the lens.
3. If the pupil block cannot be reversed medically, surgery is indicated (making an additional peripheral iris aperture).

As already mentioned in the chapter on anterior chamber lenses, the more recently developed lenses (Tennant, Choyce Mark IX) have a more anteriorly placed optic. Since this increases the clearance between the iris and the pseudophakos with respect to that of the Mark VIII lens, it is expected that early postoperative reactions will be of less concern.

Oval pupils or eliptically distorted pupils in the meridian of insertion have little or no harmful effects on the eye. These conditions are reported by various authors (Choyce, 1977; Tennant, 1976; Kratz, 1978), though its incidence is unknown. Reviewing 300 cases, M. Kraff (1979) reported gonioscopic evidence of peripheral iris incarceration (iris tuck) in some 28% of the cases.

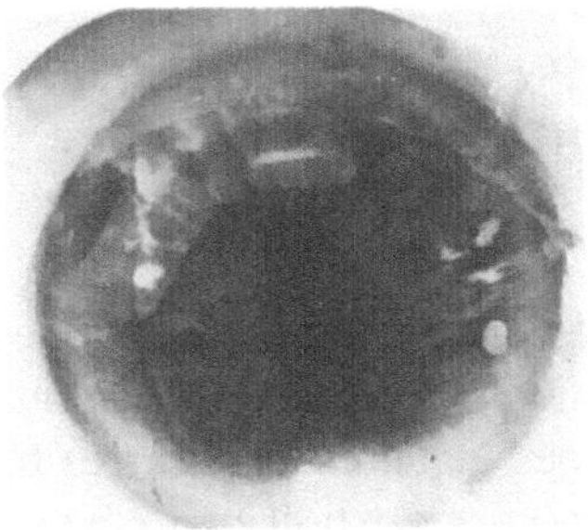

Fig. XIII-12. — Oval pupil with Choyce Mark VIII lens. (Courtesy J.J. Alpar.)

During lens insertion, irido- or cyclodialysis may occur due to the improper placement of the distal feet. J.L. Tenant (1976) notes that the disinsertion of the iris root may result in a hemorrhage into the vitreous and the anterior chamber.

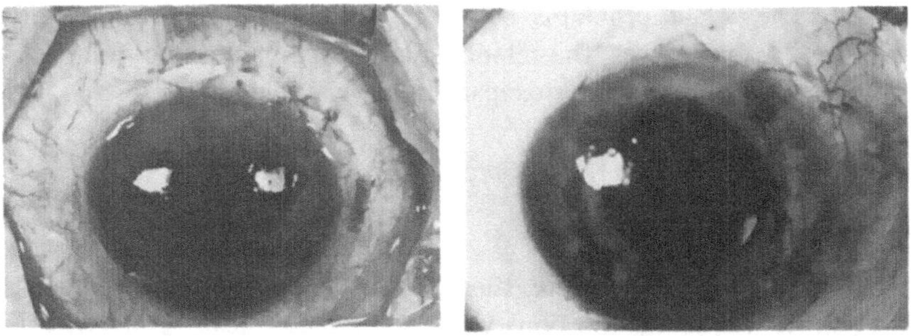

Fig. XIII-13. — Left: Hemorrhage on the 4th postoperative day with a Choyce Mark VIII lens (Rayner).
Right: Secondary glaucoma that led to corneal decompensation. (Courtesy J.J. Alpar.)

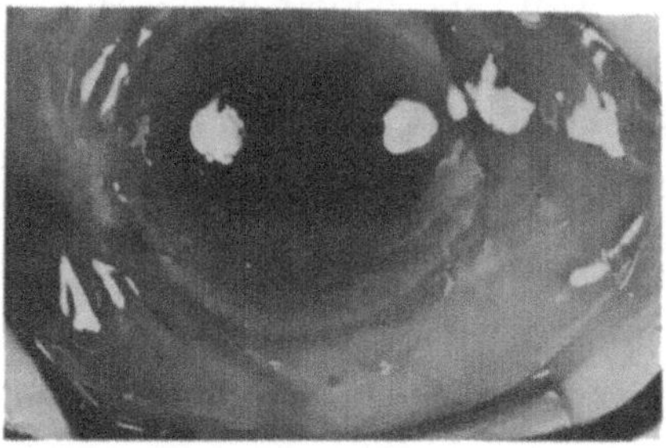

Fig. XIII-14. — Postoperative hemorrhage at a foot of a Choyce Mark VIII lens (Rayner). Ten days after the operation, the entire anterior chamber was filled with blood, and irrigation-aspiration was necessary. (Courtesy J.J. Alpar.)

R.P. Kratz (1979) reported a 6.4% incidence of postoperative hyphema. He does not attribute this to too long or poorly finished lenses, but rather to minimal trauma to the trabecular meshwork: hyphema occurred in 4.7% at the time of insertion and 1.4% in the late postoperative period.

III. Uveal Behaviour and Intraocular Pressure Dysregulation during the Late Postoperative Period

A. Late Uveal Behaviour

When good lenses with a proven track record are implanted under optimal conditions, late uveal inflammatory responses or serious damage to the iris structure is rare. Nor does glaucoma appear to be a problem. Major complications have occurred, however, when improperly designed lenses were used or when there were errors in the implantation procedure. Particular problems occurred when metal-looped iris supported lenses were implanted after intracapsular cataract extraction and also with the defective anterior chamber lenses. These late problems could be attributed to mechanical iris damage. In some cases, the relationship between a chronic inflammatory reaction and cystoid macular edema was obvious.

1. *Iris Supported Lenses*

a. *Chronic Uveal Reactions*

According to the literature, there is satisfactory long-term evidence to indicate that uveal reactions were never a significant problem with Iris Clip Lenses, Sputnik Lenses, or Medallion Lenses.

Occasionally, secondary membrane formation impairing vision was reported, even after uneventful intracapsular extraction. Jaffe suggests that fibrous metaplasia resulting from adhesions between the anterior surface of the vitreous and the iris may be the cause. The cellular source of this metaplasia is uncertain, though it may come from the pigment epithelium of the iris (Jaffe, 1978). J. Pearce and T. Ghosh (1977) ascribed consensation on the vitreous face to prolonged postoperative uveitis. C.D. Binkhorst has observed that continuous use of miotics could promote retrolenticular membrane formation, and M.A. Galin (1978) reported that discontinuing miotics dramatically reduces the incidence of membrane formation (cf. Table XIII-3).

TABLE XIII-3. — *Percentage of Membrane Formation with Fyodorov Lenses (Galin, 1978)*

Year	*Postoperative Treatment*	*Percentage of Cases*
1969	Miotics	8
1970	Miotics	11
1971	Miotics	10
1972	No miotics	4
1973	No miotics	2
1974-76	Mydriasis	1

The low incidence of needling required for secondary membranes illustrates the sporadic occurrence of late uveal reactions. In a series of 692 cases of Iris Clip Lens implantations after intracapsular extraction performed by C.D. Binkhorst, Nordlohne (1975) reported an incidence of needling of 1.3%, with the average interval between surgery and the secondary procedure being 411 dyas. N.S. Jaffe (1978) reported that 2% of 559 Iris Clip Lens implants after intracapsular extraction required needling or a transparsplana vitrectomy. Pearce and Ghosh (1977) reported 4 cases of needling necessary out of 537 implants (0.7%),and J. Worst (1977) found 13 cases of secondary membrane formation in 1519 primary lens implantations (0.8%). About one-third of the latter were Iris Clip Lenses and the remaining were Medallion Lenses. Fyodorov (1977) reported and incidence of 3.4% for 2000 Sputnik Lens implants.

Secondary membrane formation is more frequent with a Copeland Lens, both with regard to the higher degree of uveal reactions observed in the early postoperative period as well as to chronic inflammatory reactions later on. The clinical findings of the few authors who have reported on the matter, however, are divergent:

Kulvin (1975): retrolenticular membrane formation:

15% (694 ICCE)

Taylor (1978): retrolenticular membrane formation: 9% (196 ICCE)
Osher (1976): retrolenticular membrane formation: 2% (100 ICCE).

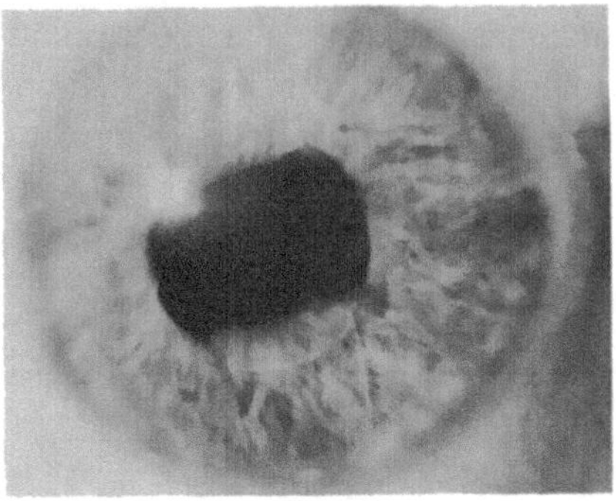

Fig. XIII-15. — Secondary membrane formation with Copeland lens.

As we have already noted, the Copeland Lens violates one of the essential lens design requirements: no part of the lens should be in constant friction with one of the delicate structures of the eye. When the iris tissue that is woven between the solid haptics of this lens is not completely immobilized by synechiae, friction is inevitable over a considerable surface.

The question of whether mydriatics can prevent late membrane formation is controversial. T.N. Hamdi (1976) does not routinely dilate the pupil, whereas Osher (1976) and Blumenthal (1977) argue that pupil dilation has advantages.

D. Praeger (personal communication, 1978) and T. Hamdi (1976) have noted that uveal reactions, both early and late, were always less pronounced when the Copeland Lens was inserted after extracapsular cataract extraction.

b. *Late Atrophic Changes*

A well-designed lens will cause only minimal damage to the iris. Localized areas of pigment loss may be seen by means of a slit lamp and retroillumination. These zones generally overlie the contact areas between the iris and the posterior loop tips. According to C.D. Binkhorst, pigment loss immediately after surgery suggests traumatic insertion or individual predisposition; later on, it is the result of friction. Continuous friction of the lens components is aggravated by the instability of the iris membrane in the aphakic eye after intracapsular extraction.

According to J. Alpar's (1979) clinical observation, progressive iris pigment loss is not a purely mechnical phenomenon, but rather a phenomenon with both mechanical and chemical factors, and it is both a cause and an effect of inflammatory changes.

Late damage to the pupillary margin from pressure atrophy is a common finding if the observation time is long enough. It generally begins at those points where the sphincter touches the posterior loop attachments. Data on the incidence of this phenomenon are lacking, but C.D. Binkhorst has observed that most of the eyes with Iris Clip lenses for more than 10 years show this defect. Occasionally, progressive atrophy of the sphincter muscle and adjacent iris tissue develops, which can lead to lens instability and luxation.

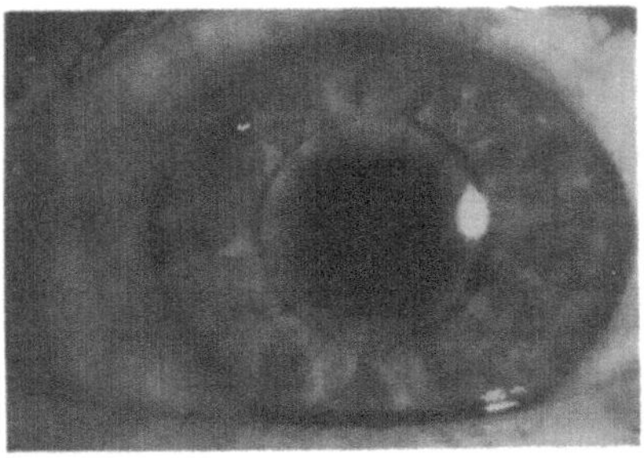

Fig. XIII-16.

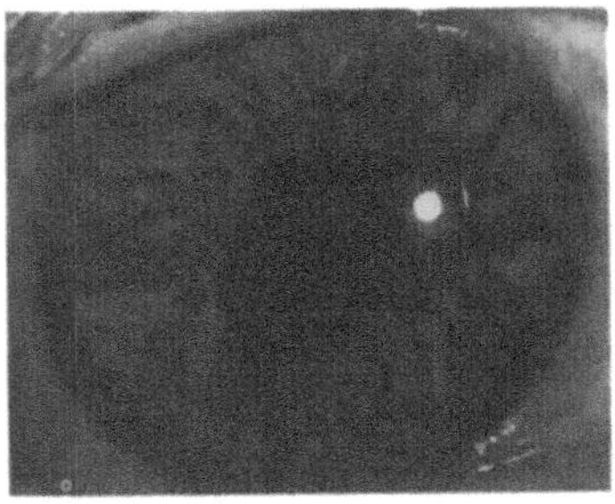

Fig. XIII-18.

Fig. XIII-17.

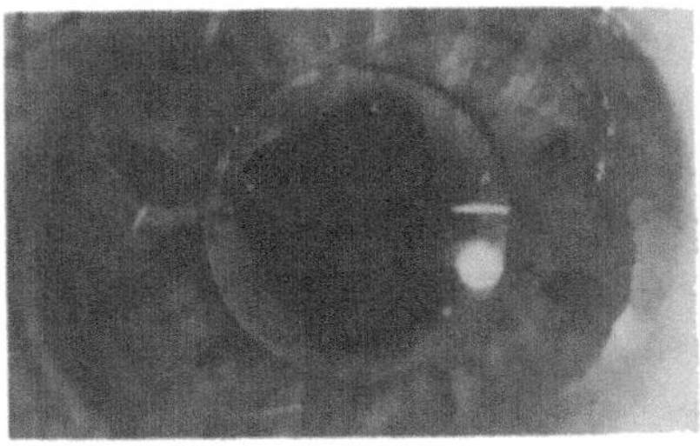

Fig. XIII-19.

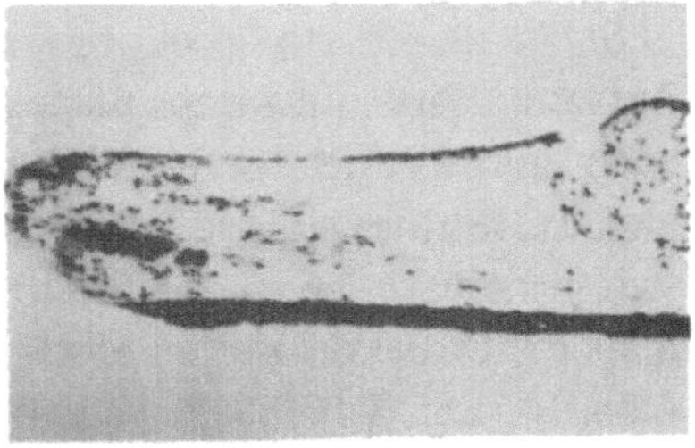

Fig. XIII-16. — Mild sphincter erosion with an iris clip lens.

Fig. XIII-17. — Marked sphincter erosion with an iris clip lens.

Fig. XIII-18. – Extreme sphincter damage with an iris clip lens after ten years.

Fig. XIII-19. — Atrophy of pupillary margin caused by iris clip lens. The sphincter muscle has almost disappeared. (H.-E., ×76; Neg. PA 26730). (Manchot, 1974, p. 866).

Posterior synechiae prevent excessive bouncing of the pupillary margin against the posterior loop attachments, but stable fixation by spontaneous synechiae formation is not very predictable. C.D. Binkhorst has tried various methods of promoting posterior synichae formation but without success. Although myotics prevent pupil mobility—especially the long-acting agents such as carbachol and physostigmin—they do not prevent local atrophy.

Iris sutures have not caused any adverse tissue reactions. If there are any, they remain well below the level that can be detected by present clinical investigative methods. From a mechanical point of view, the traction exerted on the iris by a loose suture holding a lens weighing a few milligrams in aqueous may be considered negligible. But there is still a question whether stainless steel sutures (Worst technique) will not erode through the iris stroma as time goes on.

It may be concluded that various degrees of sphincter and even iris atrophy are inherent in the use of lightweight lenses that rely on the pupil for support. Since the iris has a normal tendency to become more or less atrophic with age even without an implant, the long-term fate of an eye containing an iris supported lens is dubious. Therefore, iris supported lenses should only be given to candidates with suitable irides and relative short life expectancies.

c. *Problems with Metal-Looped Iris Supported Lenses*

The guidelines put out by C.D. Binkhorst resticted the use of metal-looped lenses to those cases in which capsular fixation was likely to occur. Nevertheless, a number of manufacturers in the U.S.A. started to produce metal-looped lenses intended to be implanted after intracapsular cataract extraction. The introduction of such devices after the possibilities and limits of iris fixation had been already fully evaluated remains surprising. In retrospect, there were two principal reasons for this: the fear of eventual breakdown of the loop material and the ease with which metal can be handled during manufacture, which allowed the massive demand to be met.

The incidence of complications with these heavy lenses after intracapsular extraction is not known. From the survey conducted by K.J. Hoffer (1978) we know that here were several thousand metal-looped lenses implanted after intracapsular extraction up to March 1977—at least 6000 metal-looped Medallion-style lenses (U.S. origin) and 2000 Binkhorst-style lenses (U.S. made). Hoffer also reported that 3000 metal-looped Platina-style lenses had been implanted, but the exact number of those implanted after intracapsular extraction is not known. The large circular-loop lens, which was specifically intended for use after intracapsular extraction was implanted in 2442 cases. According to another source (Drews, 1978), one U.S. firm alone produced 44,000 metal-looped lenses, 33,000 of which were implanted after intracapsular cataract extraction.

Using these rather heavy metal-looped lenses after intracapsular surgery was simply asking for problems involving not only the anterior segment but also the entire eye. Indeed, the adverse conditions to which the eye was being exposed could not be worse:

— The introduction of a sometimes bulky implant with rigid loops over the bare vitreous was very demanding and often resulted in peroperative damage to the pigment layer of the iris and rupture of the anterior hyaloid face.

— Major postoperative problems started after a few months. The amount of eye damage varied depending on the type of lens, the specific weight of the lens, its momentum, the diameter of the metal wire used for the construction of the loops, the finish, and the presence or absence of posterior synechiae.

The combination of a mobile iris rubbing over a metal device constituted a continual source of uveal irritation and destruction. In some eyes, entire iris sectors were eroded away, sometimes accompanied by hyphemas. The chronic inflammatory status of other eyes was striking. This condition was frequently associated with episodes of secondary glaucoma and/or corneal haze, along with vitritis (Baikoff, 1975; Worst, personal communication, 1977) and cystoid macular edema (Shepard, 1978, reported an incidence of 39%). Because of gravity, nearly all these lenses from which the loop attachment gradually eroded the iris tisue (cheese wiring) sagged to the 6 o'clock position. Frequently, loose lenses dislocated either into the anterior

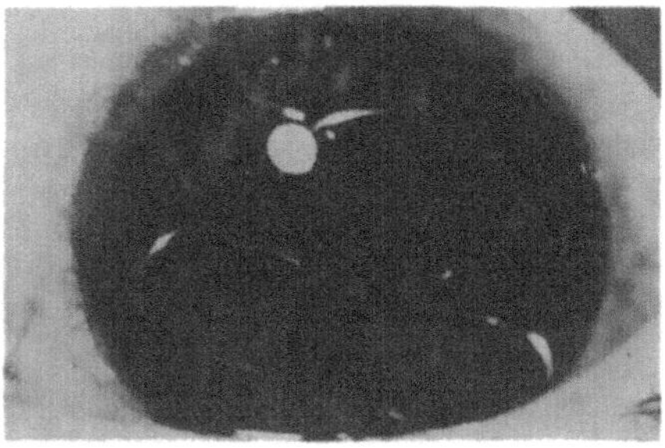

Fig. XIII-20. — A Fyodorov-style lens with metal loops cutting through the lower iris sector. (Courtesy J.J. Alpar.)

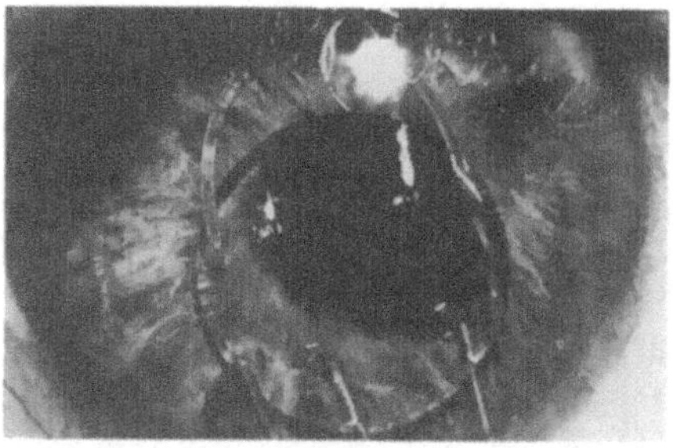

Fig. XIII-21. — An iris clip lens with metal posterior loops showing anterior dislocation after having eroded the sphincter margin. (Courtesy J.J. Alpar.)

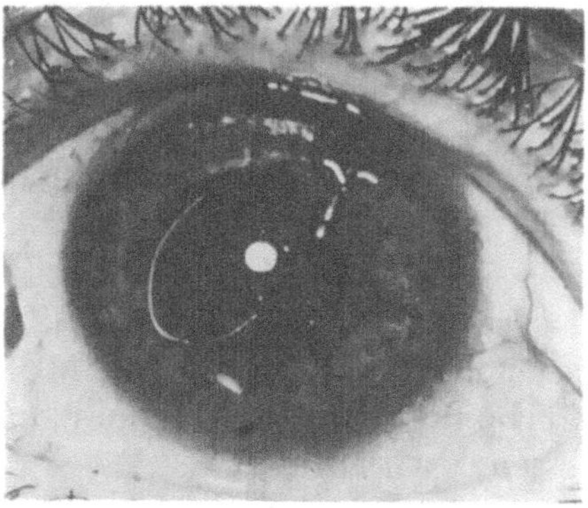

Fig. XIII-22. — Large circular loop lens showing recurrent dislocation. (Courtesy J.J. Alpar.)

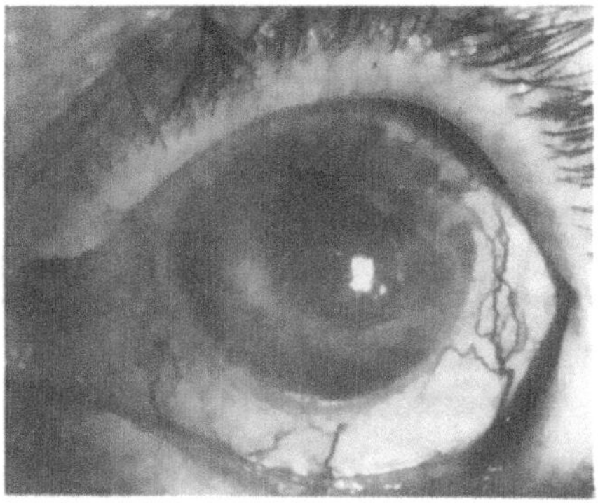

Fig. XIII-23. — Total corneal dystrophy, the ultimate complication in some patients who received iris supported lenses with metal loops. Because these eyes also often have chronic cystoid macular edema, corneal grafting does not always yield good vision. (Courtesy R. Drews.)

chamber or into the vitreous. Never in the history of implant surgery had the deleterious influence of iridodonesis and pseudophakodonesis been so striking.

Depending on the stage of the damage, the following rescue operations were more or less successful:

— Instillation of long-acting myotics;

— Binkhorst-McCannel iris suture through one or more loops;

— Transscleral fixation thread (Strampelli Principle);
— Lens removal or exchange.

The ultimate fate of the many thousands of eyes containing lenses that predictably would never yield good results is still obscure. We may well presume that many of these eyes were definitely lost.

2. *Iridocapsular Supported Lenses*

So far, late iris atrophy or chronic uveitis with lightweight, well-fixed two-loop iridocapsular lenses without metal loops seem to be minimal. But the first of these lenses came only in use in 1976.

In some cases, however, delayed formation of pigment precipitates on the lens accompanied by minor inflammatory signs has been observed. The incidence of this condition among our patients was 1%, and it generally responded favorably to topical corticosteroids. While the etiology of this phenomenon is still a matter of speculation, we have the impression that it indicates a "sick eye" or a "sick patient" as it occurs mostly in patients, for example, who have retina pigmentosa or a cataract of unknown origin or who are alcoholic.

a. *Chronic Uveal Reactions with Metal-Looped Lenses*

Loose metal-looped lenses implanted after extracapsular cataract extraction caused chronic uveitis, secondary glaucoma, and cystoid macular edema only when the loops were improperly finished. The exact incidence of these complications is unknown. In our cases, which were followed for 2 to 8 years, chronic inflammation never occurred.

b. *Late Atrophic Changes with Metal-Looped Lenses*

With a stable metal-looped lens well fixed by capsular adhesions late erosion of the pupillary margin may occur where the mobile pupil margin meets the posterior loop attachments (bouncing effect). The thickness of the posterior loop attachment seems to play a role: there is some clinical evidence that pressure atrophy is more pronounced with loop material with a thickness of 0.1 mm than with material with a thickness of 0.2 mm (cheese wiring effect).

This type of localized atrophy of the pupillary margin is innocuous. Indeed, the capsular fixated lenses do no rely on the pupil for fixation or proper centration.

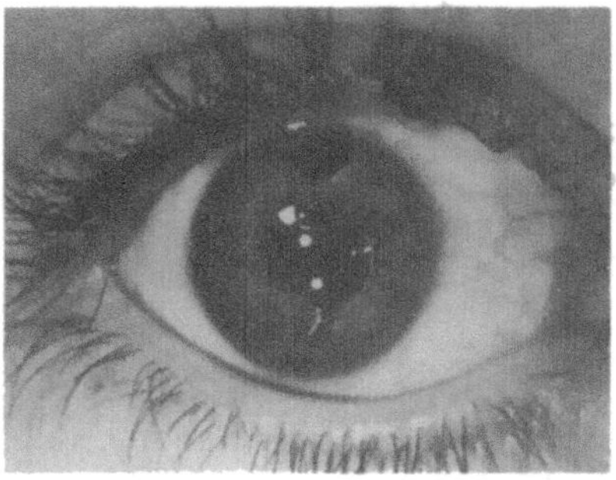

Fig. XIII-24.

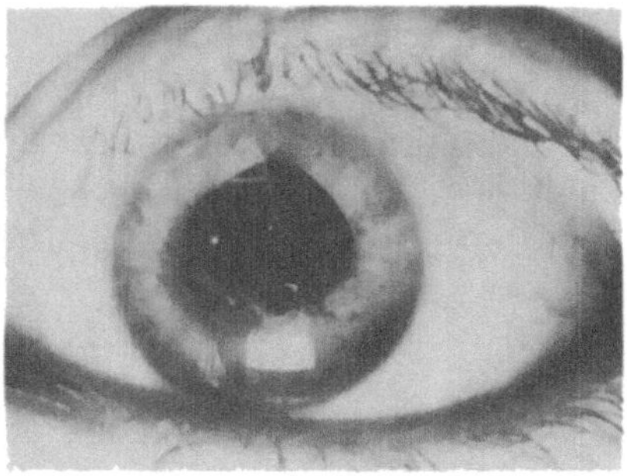

Fig. XIII-25.

Fig. XIII-24. — Mild iris erosion below in an area overlying a lens loop that was not inserted properly between the 2 capsular loops.

Fig. XIII-25. — Marked iris sphincter atrophy because of the chafing effect of the metal loop on the pupillary border. This case has been followed for 6 years, and no irritation has occurred in the eye.

More pronounced damage to the iris was observed when only one of the loops of the metal looped lens was properly placed in the capsular cleft. The other loop, generally the upper one, would then sometimes occupy a more forward position and interfere with normal iris activity. After years or even months of this continuous rubbing of the iris over the lens loop, local atrophy developed and the iris sector disappeared completely without any sign of inflammatory reactions. The exact incidence of this type of pathology is unknown. In our patients, it occurred in less than 0.5% of the cases.

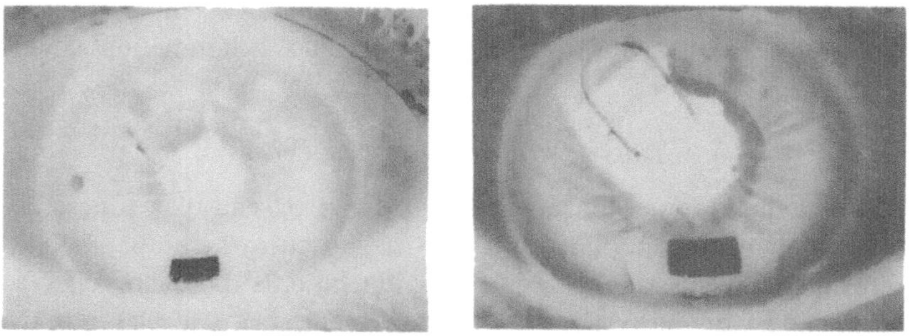

Fig. XIII-26. — Photographs taken 1 year (left) and 2 years (right) after implantation. The upper metal loop is not embedded in the cortical remnants and has eroded. The lens has been in place for 5 years with no other side effects.

A third category of iris damage from metal looped lenses occurred when neither capsular fixation nor any other type of firm iris fixation was achieved. In these eyes, a combination of both of the patholog-

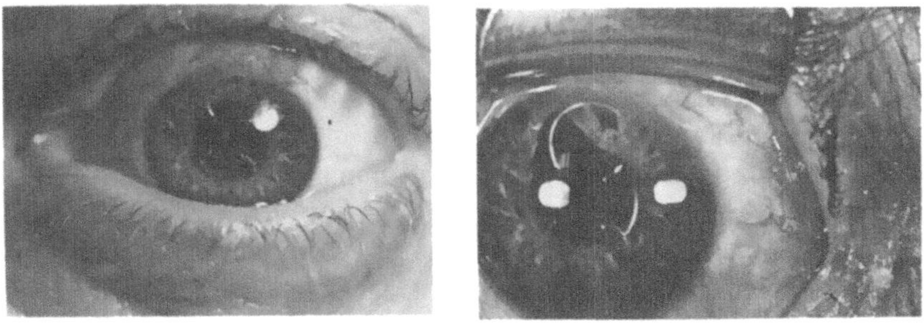

Fig. XIII-27. — Photographs taken 1 year (left) and 3 years (right) after implantation of an iridocapsular lens, the upper loop of which was not placed between the capsular flaps. (Courtesy of J.J. Alpar.)

ical conditions described above developed: cheese wiring of the sphincter and continuing iris atrophy. Initially, the metal loop attachments started to erode the inferior pupillary border. Gravity then caused progressive cheese wiring of the adjacent iris sector. Finally, if the situation was not cured, the heavy lens sagged more and more through the iris.

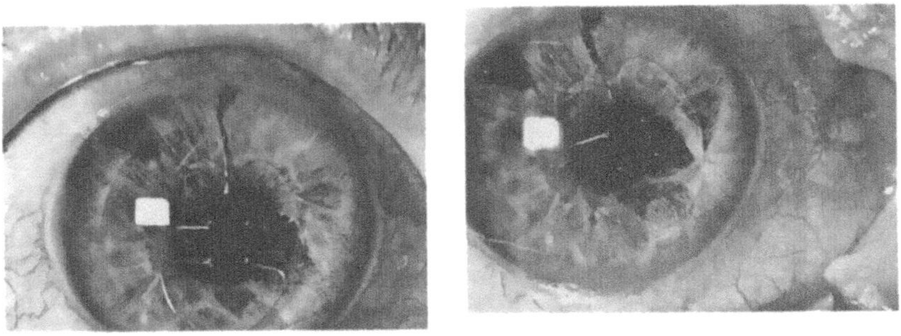

Fig. XIII-28. — A small incision lens with metal loops from which the inferior loop dislocated after having eroded the pupillary margin. (Courtesy J.J. Alpar.)

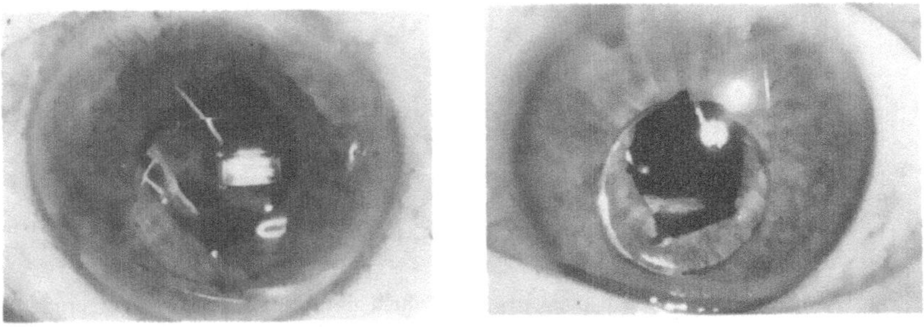

Fig. XIII-29. — Gravity-caused progressive downward decentration of a loose iridocapsular lens with platinum-iridium loops.

Similar conditions developed in eyes containing platinum style lenses with metal loops and in other heavy lenses that rely partially or totally on transiridectomy support (Householder, 1977). When these heavy lenses were not properly fixed by iridocapsular adhesions, iris atrophy started both at the pupillary margin and at the iridectomy site. In all cases, the chafing effect of the metal loop was more pronounced when the loop material was poorly finished.

Various therapeutic measures have been devised to rescue eyes containing loose, metal-looped iridocapsular lenses.

— Placing a Binkhorst-McCannel suture through the iris or through both the iris and the posterior capsule;
— Embedding one or more of the loops in a capsular pocket by means of a secondary procedure;
— Steadying the lens by reversing the optic portion through an opening in the poster capsule (the collar button principle);
— Using a transscleral fixation thread (the Strampelli fixating principle);
— Removing the lens or exchanging it for a Shearing posterior chamber lens or an angle supported lens.

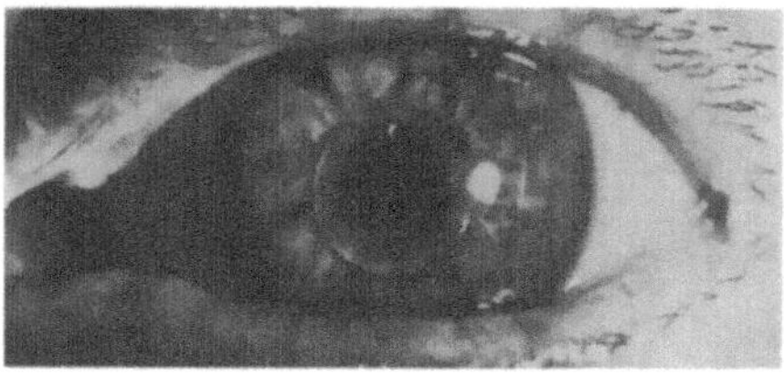

Fig. XIII-30. — Iridocapsular lens steadied with a Binkhorst-McCannel suture.

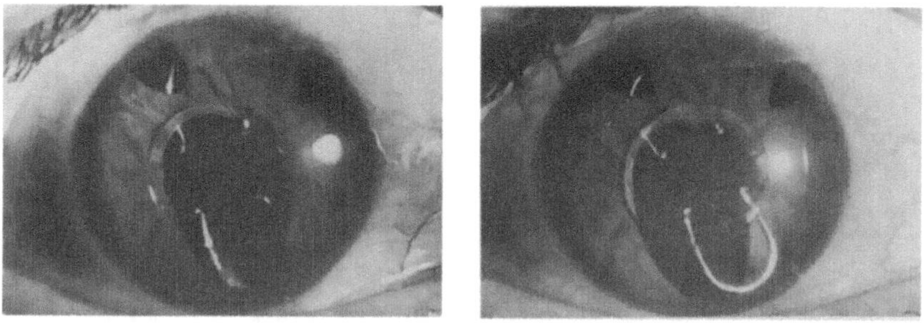

Fig. XIII-31. — An iridocapsular lens from which the inferior loop was not properly positioned between the capsular flaps. After complete anterior dislocation (left), the lens was stabilized by making a pocket in the inferior cortical remnants into which the loop was introduced (right). (Courtesy C.D. Binkhorst and L. Loones.)

3. *Angle Supported Lenses*

a. *Chronic Uveal reactions*

With a well-manufactured anterior chamber lens, late inflammatory uveal responses and uveal damage are of minor concern provided these two conditions are fulfilled:

— The lens has to fit exactly, being neither too long nor too short.

— The lens must be fitted into the scleral ring and remain immobile and parallel to, but clear of, the iris diaphragm.

When the lens is too long, D.P. Choyce (personal communication, 1977) has observed that late and mild uveitis are significant and that complaints of more than usual pain and tendernesss are common. He also noted the occasional occurence of dialysis of the iris root or disinsertion of the cillary body. This situation may be accompanied by hyphemas and even massive hemorrhages.

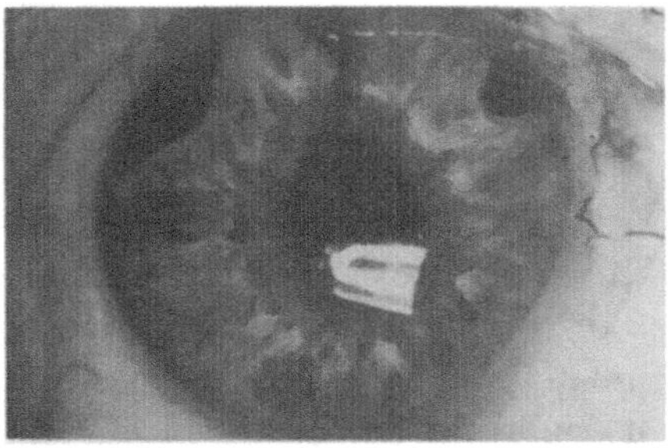

Fig. XIII-32. — Iridodialysis caused by a Choyce lens (since removed). (Courtesy M. Kraff.)

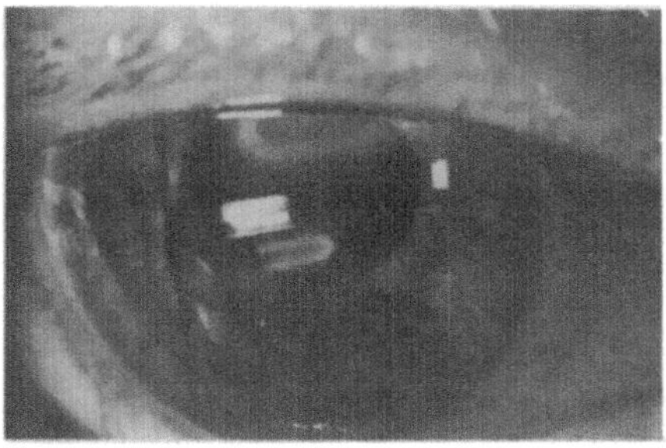

Fig. XIII-33. — Clot on a Choyce lens after resorption of the blood. (Courtesy M. Kraff.)

When the lens is too short, persistent, low-grade iritis may occur. To a certain extent, this reaction can be advantageous since it may stabilize the lens by promoting the development of peripheral localized synechiae. Some surgeons (Shepard, personal communication,

1978) rely on this secondary fixation mechanism and administer strong miotics (Diflupyl) to promote some uveal reaction.

When the lens is improperly positioned, for example, when a foot penetrates a peripheral coloboma, the ciliary body is indented, as has been shown by gonioscopy. This may also be a source of irritation and pain.

b. *Late Atrophic Changes*

When intimate continuous or intermittent contact occurs between the anterior iris surface and a lens, localized contact atrophy will develop as time goes by. Marked late iris atrophy is apt to occur with younger patients so lenses with colored haptics are recommended for them.

A relatively narrow anterior chamber and a lens that is too long can be contributory factors for this condition along with, of course, poor surgical judgment and bad positioning.

To our knowledge, there have been no reports of serious sequellae to contact atrophy.

c. *The U.G.H. Syndrome*

We have discussed the U.G.H. syndrome (uveitis-glaucoma-hyphema) in detail in Chapter VIII. Enough evidence has accumulated to conclude that the outbreak of complications characterized by serious uveal damage and inflammatory reactions was caused by improperly manufactured lenses. It could not be confirmed that the deterioration of the material itself released toxic elements. In the same way as the explosive demand for iris supported lenses was met by industry by turning out lenses that were far from innocuous, the same sad experience was repeated with anterior chamber lenses. Several U.S. manufacturers began to mass produce these lenses with techniques that differed significantly from the original, tedious process. Instead of cutting them from a solid sheet of perspex, these "Choyce style" lenses were produced by injection molding, which accelerated the production process. Many of these lenses were poorly finsished: sharp edges and tips and rough irregularities were common. Some of the lens feet curled (warpage), a defect that could sometimes be spotted even before implantation.

These manufacturing flaws caused a mechanical type of uveal involvement that led to complications that Ellingson (1977) called the U.G.H. Syndrome. This syndrome was the result of interaction between the fixed implant and the mobile iris. Iridodonesis was also a factor, and Kratz, among others, noted that the U.G.H. syndrome was less pronounced after extracapsular than after intracapsular extraction. Although a great deal has been published on this problem, the exact incidence is unknown.

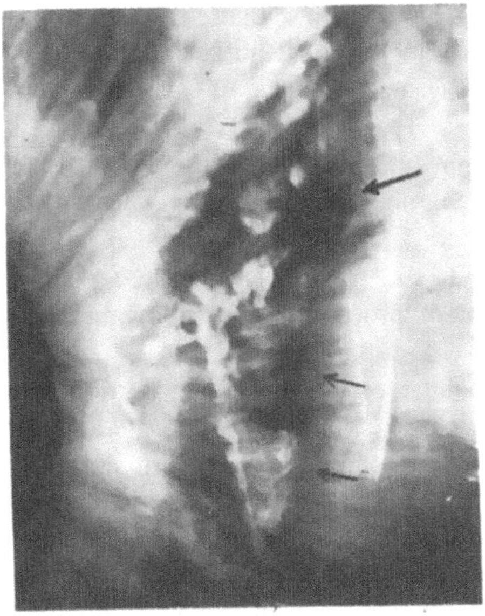

Fig. XIII-34. — The rough edges of this injection molded Choyce lens has badly chewed into the iris as the pupil dilates and constricts. The chronic iritis and the erosion of the iris surface has reached vessels, and recurrent hyphema has developed. The UGH syndrom was completed in this patient by secondary glaucoma. Such a lens must be removed early, or cystoid macular edema and corneal dystrophy will often follow. (Courtesy R. Drews.)

B. Late Intraocular Pressure Dysregulation

After lens implantation, persistent or late intraocular pressure dysregulation seems to be rare, provided, of course, that the surgical procedure was well-conducted, safe lenses were implanted, and the eye was carefully selected. Indeed, our investigation indicates that the vast majority of persistent or late glaucoma cases were associated with, for example, preoperative borderline intraocular pressure and that they decompensated because of defects in the surgical procedure, chronic inflammatory reactions, or prolonged use of corticosteroids. The therapeutic measures include vigorous control of any form of uveitis, systemic use of Diamox®, topical administration of timolol, judicious application of mydriatics or miotics, and, possibly, replacement of corticosteroids by preparations that have less effect on the intraocular pressure.

When postoperative intraocular pressure gets out of medical control, it has to be normalized by means of filtering procedures. This is a very serious problem since the most feared complication in an eye containing an intraocular implant is peroperative and early postoperative loss or even shallowness of the anterior chamber. Endothelial contact is unlikely to occur with only a few lens types, for example, the posterior chamber lenses and, to a lesser degree, the angle supported and Copeland lenses. At the present, guarded sclerotomies (trabeculotomy, trabeculectomy, cautery under the scleral flap, etc.) are preferable since they offer the best chance of maintaining a formed anterior chamber (Drews, 1978). Simcoe (1979) suggests retaining devices during glaucoma surgery when lenses with parts that protrude into the anterior chamber are involved. The use of viscuous agents has been suggested.

When there is a possibility that the intraocular pressure will be adversely influenced by the implant procedure, the following solutions may be considered:

— Surgical control of the intraocular pressure and lens insertion at a later stage. The filtering procedure should be performed in an area where it will not interfere with the subsequent implantation, e.g., the superior nasal quadrant. Techniques such as iridencleisis that would lead to an eccentric pupil are to be avoided.

— Combined cataract extraction, lens implantation, and a filtering procedure that offers the best chance for an uneventful outcome with posterior chamber lenses. There have been too few case reports, however, to assess the benefits of this combined procedure.

Finally, lens implantation is not contraindicated of itself with controlled narrow-angle glaucoma. A great deal depends on the underlying mechanisms. It is favorable when there is evidence that the removal of the cataractous lens will deepen the anterior chamber.

IV. Lens Implantation after Glaucoma Surgery

In cataractuous eyes that have successful glaucoma surgery, the additional step of lens implantation does not seem to precipitate intraocular pressure disregulation provided that the postoperative inflammatory reaction is minimal or adequately controlled. Neither the lens type nor the technique (intracapsular vs. extracapsular) seem to exercise a significant influence.

Since angle supported lenses do not rely on the pupil for centration, their insertion after iridencleisis was found to be advantageous by Choyce. It is important that the pupillary aperture coincide with the optic center of the lens, which sometimes requires that a sphincterotomy be performed in the 6 o'clock direction. Obviously, too, the angle must be free enough from peripheral anterior synechiae to allow correct and atraumatic placement of the lens.

Lenses that have to have their optics centered by the pupil require special techniques. In the late sixties, J. Worst began reconstruction of the pupil when iris colobomas pre-existed. These techniques allow adequate centration of iris supported and iridocapsular supported lenses as well.

These same "iridoplasty" techniques can be used when the pupil is rigid, for example, after prolonged use of miotics when a sphincterotomy is required to allow for cataract extraction and lens implantation.

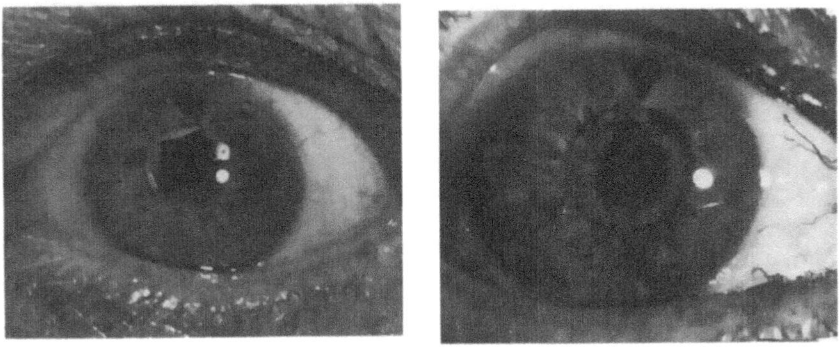

Fig. XIII-35. — Iris clip lens after intracapsular cataract extraction and iridocapsular lens after extracapsular cataract extraction in cases previously operated on for glaucoma. (Courtesy C.D. Binkhorst.)

The incision site for cataract removal and lens insertion is optional but it should not involve the filtering area. A corneal section just below he inferior limit of the filtering bleb, a temporal approach, or an inferior incision are all possibilities.

C.D. Binkhorst (1979) has presented the results and conclusions of 33 prepupillary lens implantations in eyes with open-angle glaucoma that had undergone various filtering procedures.

Intracapsular extraction was performed in the first 7 cases, and extracapsular in the rest. The follow-up periods ranged from 1 to 7 years with an average of 3 years.

In all but 2 cases, the intraocular pressure was within the normal limits without any medication. One case was controlled medically, the other required repeated glaucoma surgery. In 18 eyes, the anterior chamber depth was measured and found to be similar to that of non-glaucomatous pseudophakic eyes, i.e. 2.7 mm from the endothelium to the anterior lens vertex. No cases of endothelial corneal dystrophy were observed.

The technique preferred by Binkhorst is a pre-bleb, pure corneal incision and extracapsular extraction. The pre-bleb incision facilitates reconstructive iris surgery when it is necessary.

As could be observed, the temporary presence of lens material in the anterior chamber did not adversely affect the intraocular pressure provided enough reserve outflow capacity exists.

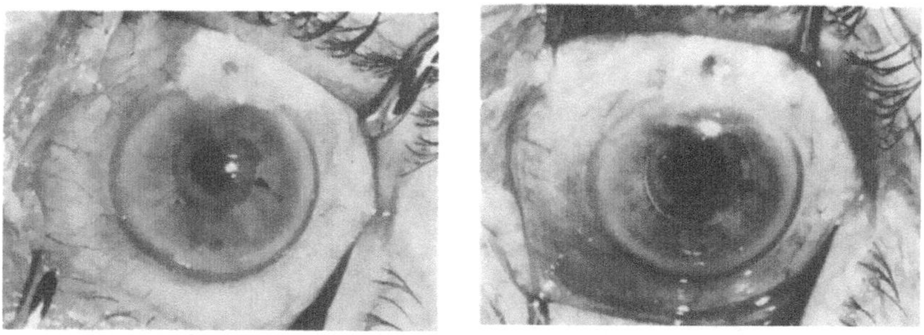

Fig. XIII-36. — Eye with large filtering bleb (left) and same case after intracapsular cataract extraction and implantation of an iris clip lens (right). (Courtesy C.D. Binkhorst.)

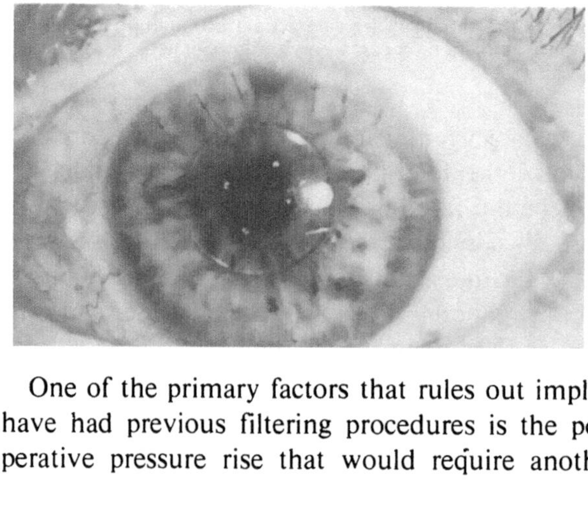

Fig. XIII-37. — Example of corneal incision as proposed by C.D. Binkhorst.

One of the primary factors that rules out implantation in eyes that have had previous filtering procedures is the possibility of a postoperative pressure rise that would require another glaucoma proce-

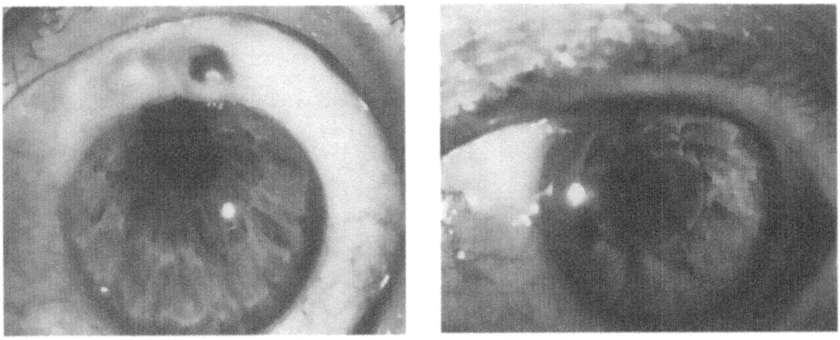

Fig. XIII-38. — Eye with iridencleisis and typical updrawn pupil (left) in which an iridocapsular lens was inserted after extracapsular cataract extraction and pupil reconstruction. (Courtesy C.D. Binkhorst.)

dure, thus increasing the chance of endothelial contact. Therefore, cases with borderline intraocular pressure values and even those with normal tension but poor outflow capacity should be rejected.

J. Alpar (1979) reported on the results obtained in 27 cases. In twenty of them (74%) there was no persistent intraocular pressure disregulation, but medical therapy had to be instituted in the remaining 7.

Conclusion

As we noted in the introduction, uveal reactions and chronic pressure dysregulation after lens implantation are infrequent if certain conditions are fulfilled. Nevertheless, certain lens models are apt to cause local atrophic changes in the iris.

We also stress that cataractous eyes that were previously operated on for glaucoma also come under consideration for lens implantation.

CHAPTER XIV

LENS IMPLANTATION AND CYSTOID MACULAR EDEMA

I. Introduction

A. The Clinical Picture

The Irvine-Gass Syndrome, commonly referred to in the literature as aphakic cystoid macular edema, is a microcystic edema of the macular region, sometimes accompanied by an edema of the papilla, that can occur after cataract extraction, even when uneventful. The interval ranges from a few days to several years, with the peak incidence being between the first and the third month after surgery. S.R. Irvine (1953) first drew attention to this syndrome and studied the associated modifications of the vitreous, and J.D. Gass and E.W. Norton (1966) described the biomicroscopic and angiographic characteristics.

The typical clinical picture is that of a patient who undergoes an uneventful cataract extraction and regains good visual acuity but who suddenly starts to complain of an irritable eye or photophobia, generally associated with a drop in central visual acuity. The decrease in visual acuity may be restricted to one or more lines, but more pronounced drops have been reported (Gass and Norton, 1969). The use of a stenopeic aperture does not improve central vision. Associated visual disturbances such as micropsia, macropsia, metamorphopsia, and erythropsia are common.

Further clinical examination may reveal a rupture of the anterior hyaloid, which occurs in some 30% to 40% of the cases, with or without vitreous adherences to the wound (Bonnet, 1972; Coscas, 1972). Posterior vitreous detachment seems rather common (Gass and Norton, 1966; Tolentino and Schepens, 1965; Iliff, 1966).

Alteration of the retrovitreal cavity in front of the macular region is frequently observed, along with the presence of flare, cellular debris and degenerated fibrillar material (Tolentino and Schepens, 1965; Gass and Norton, 1966). Vitreous-macular adhesions do not seem to be specifically associated with macular edema.

Ophthalmoscopic findings generally are restricted to modifications of the foveal reflex, which suggest some edema of the macular region. Occasionally, moderate papilledema can be observed (11-19%), and also small peripapillar hemorrhages. When adequate biomicroscopic examination of the posterior pole is feasible, characteristic foveal cysts with a honeycomb appearance complete the clinical picture.

The diagnosis is confirmed with fluorescein angiography. Gass and Norton (1966, p. 654) describe the characteristic pattern as follows:

> Leakage of dye usually appears initially within the retina in the perifoveal area in an irregular circular or wreathlike pattern, and progresses both centrally and peripherally at a variable rate. As the dye converges on the foveal area, a remarkable and diagnostic geometric dark stellate figure develops centrally on the background of fluorescein staining (Fig. XIV-1). The accumulation of intraretinal fluorescein lies deep to the larger paramacular vessels, which stand out as dark lines against the background of pooled flourescein. The time required for the development of the characteristic macular pattern of staining is variable. In most it is well developed in 5 to 15 min whereas in others it becomes evident only after 30 min or longer... Leakage of dye into the optic nerve and surrounding retina occurs in those patients with papilledema. This is most apparent approximately 10 to 15 min after injection of the dye.

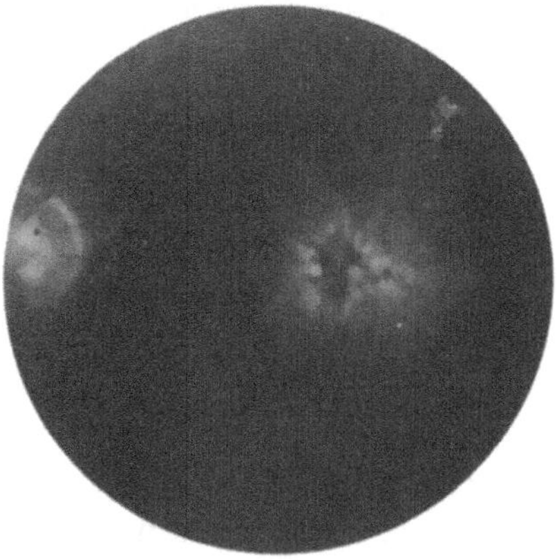

Fig. XIV-1. — Angiographic pattern of cystoid macular edema.

In the most positive cases, the iris also hyperfluorescence (Kottow and Hendrickson, 1975). There seems to be no correlation with the depth of visual loss and the amount of staining present. Resolution of staining, however, usually parallels visual improvement (Gass and Norton, 1966).

B. Evolution and Prognosis

The evolution of the syndrome varies. In most instances, aphakic macular edema is transient and thus spontaneous resolution with visual improvement may be expected. Of the 64 eyes followed by Gass and Norton (1969), half were cleared within 6 months and 72% in 3 years (see Table XIV-1), all with a visual acuity ⩾20/40. In most of the cases, the macula regained a normal appearance, with only a few showing cystic degeneration, cellophane wrinkling of the inner retina, or pigment mottling. When macular edema persists, partial or full-thickness macular holes may develop that, in the opinion of Gass and Norton, probably preclude regaining good central visual acuity.

TABLE XIV-1. — *Evolution of Cystoid Macular Edema in Aphakics (Gass and Norton, 1969)*

Resolution time	*Number*	*Percent*
6 months	32/64	50%
6-12 months	6/64	6.6%
12-36 months	10/64	15.6%
Total	46/64	72%

Following 33 eyes that presented aphakic macular edema 6 weeks after surgery, R.A. Hitchings (1977) found that the edema had resolved 2 years later in all but 4 cases. And in these 4 cases, visual acuity had improved in spite of persistent edema in the macular region.

The factors that cause aphakic macular edema to persist are still obscure. The prognosis seems to be poorer when the following conditions are present:

— An extended free interval between cataract extraction and the onset of fhe clinical picture (Bonnet, 1972).

— Vitreous incarceration in the wound (vitreous strands and peaked pupil). Gass and Norton (1969) noted that the average time required for the macular edema to clear in eyes without vitreous incarceration was 25 weeks, but with vitreous incarceration 65 weeks was required.

— A prolonged period of macular edema (Bonnet, 1975).

— Associated chronic ocular inflammation (Norton et al., 1975; Martin et al., 1977; Deutman and Van Balen, 1976; Irvine, 1976).

Other factors that may contribute, though apparently to a lesser degree, are cardiovascular diseases, systemic hypertension (Gass and Norton, 1969), and continuous topical adrenergic therapy (Kolker and Becker, 1968; Gass and Norton, 1969). The presence of optic disc edema also seems less favorable (Bonnet, 1975).

C. **Pathogenesis**

Three theories have been advanced to explain the pathogenesis of cystoid acular edema:

1. *Traction Theory*

Traction by the vitreous on the retina was first suggested by S.R. Irvine (1953) as an underlying cause. Other authors have also suggested the influence of vitreous traction on the macular region (Tolentino and Schepens, 1965; Reese et al., 1967).

2. *Vascular Theory*

Gass and Norton (1969) noted that patients with cardiovascular diseases, hypertension, or diabetes had a higher incidence of aphakic cystoid macular edema, which suggests the involvement of a vascular component. Added weight is given to this hypothesis by the precipitation or aggravation of macular edema by topical adrenergic therapy, which seems to have adverse effects on the capillary bed of the macular region (Kolker and Becker, 1968; Gass and Norton, 1966).

3. *Inflammatory Theory*

J.D. Gass and E.W. Norton (1966) were among the first to suggest that inflammation and increased vascular permeability may combine to cause cystoid macular edema. Associated inflammatory changes—cyclitis, vitritis, and retinal phlebitis—have been noted in cases submitted to histopathological examination (Michels et al., 1971; Norton et al., 1975).

Since no one theory seems to be conclusive, one may reasonably assume that the etiology is multifactorial. Increased abnormal permeability of the capillaries in the posterior pole seems to be a crucial and universal factor. Since increased vascular permeability is not ruled out by vitreo-retinal traction, vascular imbalance, or inflammatory reactions, all these theories still hold.

Attempts to identify the common biochemical component leading to abnormal capillary permeability have yet to meet with success. In recent years, it has often been suggested that prostaglandins acts as a humoral mediator responsible for a temporary disruption of the blood-aqueous barrier (Cole and Unger, 1973; Eaking, 1977; Mochizuki et al., 1977; Mishima and Masuda, 1977; Miyake et al., 1978). It would be premature, however, to conclude that the problem of the pathogenesis of cystoid macular edema has been solved.

D. **Treatment**

Since aphakic cystoid macular edema is known to heal spontaneously in a high percentage of the cases, it is difficult to assess the effect of treatment. C. Iliff (1966) suggested that vitreous adherences to the wound be released surgically. Corticosteroids have been administered topically and systemically with and without success, and photocoagulation of leaking points in the posterior pole has been considered. D.R. Jacobson and A. Dellaporta (1974) have concluded that no medical or surgical treatment has been demonstrated to improve the rate of natural and spontaneous resolution of cystoid macular edema after cataract extraction.

Various preventive measures, however, can be taken. During surgery, it seems imperative that vitreous loss be prevented and that vitreous-wound adherences be released. Postoperatively, adequate control of inflammatory reactions also seems to be an important factor. Various authors advise caution in using adrenergic eye drops after intracapsular cataract extraction because they can precipitate cystoid macular edema (Kolker and Becker, 1968; Maumenee, 1976). Finally, assuming that cystoid macular edema is primarily caused by a disruption of the blood-aqueous barrier that may be triggered by the release of biochemical components such as prostaglandin, presurgical treatment with the so-called prostaglandin-synthetase inhibitors may have advantages. Some of the drugs were administered topically and others systemically (Neufeld et al., 1972; Cole and Unger, 1973; Eakins, 1977; Bechetoille et al., 1978).

The role of non-steroidal anti-inflammatory drugs in cataract surgery in humans is now being studied. Preliminary reports suggest that the release of prostaglandin caused by the surgical trauma, the hypothetical disruption of the blood-aqueous barrier, and the occurrence of cystoid macular edema are related. According to M. Myake (1978), the incidence and severity of cystoid macular edema in eyes treated topically with indomethacin before and after surgery was less than in the untreated fellow eye, as demonstrated by fluorescein angiography. Similarly, R.M. Klein et al. (1979) found that postoperative oral administration of indomethacin caused a statistically significant decrease in the incidence of aphakic cystoid macular edema as shown by fluorescein angiography.

II. Incidence of Cystoid Macular Edema without Lens Implantation

A. Clinical Cystoid Macular Edema (C.C.M.E.)

It is generally recognized that clinical macular edema is not frequently encountered among the complications that occur after cataract operations. Irvine (1953) reported a 2% incidence of the Irvine Syndrome in a group of 891 aphakics after intracapsular extraction; R.B. Welch and J.C. Cooper (1958) reported that 1.25% of 1600 aphakics had edema of the posterior pole; F.I. Tolentino and C.L. Schepens (1965) reported a 1.7% rate for 1000 aphakics; J.D.M. Gass and E.W. Norton (1966) noted an incidence greater than 2%; D. Easty et al. (1977) reported cystoid macular edema present in 2% of 200 aphakics after intracapsular extraction; and M. Bonnet et al. (1975) reported a 2% incidence of clinical cystoid macular edema.

An incidence of clinical cystoid macular edema of some 2% may be taken as normal after intracapsular cataract extraction. The literature cites this figure as being widely accepted (Duke-Elder, 1969; Fasanella, 1960; Theodore, 1962; Coscas, 1972)..

As A. Lefrançois (1976) noted, the incidence of clinical cystoid macular edema may increase from 2% to about 10% when the cataract extraction encounters complications, but precise figures in this regard do not seem to be available in the literature.

The advent of intentional extracapsular cataract extraction raises the question of whether the presence of the intact posterior capsule influences the onset of clinical cystoid macular edema. As yet, there is no clear answer to this question. Certainly, the incidence is low when the posterior capsule is intact and it increases when the capsule has been ruptured at surgery, which may involve vitreous loss, or opened later, which may cause a certain degree of vitreous disturbance.

J. Little found an incidence of 1% clinical cystoid macular edema when the posterior capsule was intact, and an incidence of 3% to 4% when it had been opened or removed.

R. Kratz (1978) reported an incidence of 0.5% when the posterior capsule was intact, 4.8% when it had been incised at surgery, and 4.2% when it had been opened later on.

C. Kelman (3000 cases) and D. Praeger (1500 cases), as cited by Berrocal (1977), reported rates of 1% and 1.5% respectively, when the capsule was intact and 5% and 6% respectively when the posterior capsule was ruptured.

B. Angiographic Cystoid Macular Edema (A.C.M.E.)

When fluorescein angiography is routinely used after cataract extraction to assess the status of the posterior pole, the angiographic pattern typical for cystoid macular edema occurs far more frequently than the classic clinical picture. A.R. Irvine et al. (1971) reported an incidence of 40% angiographic cystoid macular edema (ACME) 4 to 16 weeks after uneventful cataract extraction; R.A. Hitchings (1975) reported a 50.6% rate 6 to 7 weeks after surgery; M. Bonnet et al. (1975) a rate of 18%; Yoshioka and Kawashima (1971, as cited in Hitchings, 1977) reported 60%; M.S. Jaffe (1978), for a series of 113 eyes after intracapsular extraction, reported incidences of 15% at 4 months after surgery, 14.8% at 8 months, and 9.6% at 16-24 months. R.M. Klein and L. Jannuzzzi (1976) reported an incidence of less than 5% for the first week after surgery but 50% after 4 to 6 weeks. W. Fung, (as cited by Norton and Johnson, 1977), reporting on 30 phakoemulsification cases after 4 months, gave incidences of 5.5% (1/19) when the posterior capsule was intact, and 54% (6/11) when it was ruptured. Finally, Kensaku Miyake (1978) reported 50% after uneventful intracapsular extraction at 5 weeks.

Therefore, we may conclude that the incidence of angiographic cystoid macular edema in aphakia peaks around the 6th postoperative week and may involve as many as half the cases.

III. Incidence of Cystoid Macular Edema with Lens Implantation

A. Clinical Cystoid Macular Edema (C.C.M.E.)

Various authors using different techniques and lens models report incidences of clinical cystoid macular edéma ranging from 0.45% to

8.4% (see Table XIV-2). The wide difference in incidence can be partially attributed to the varying criteria applied: Jaffe and Hirshman, for example, only counted those cases in which the final visual acuity was less than 20/40, and others, like Galin, excluded all cases in which the surgical procedure was not uneventful.

TABLE XIV-2. — *Incidence of Clinical Cystoid Macular Edema with a Pseudophakos*

Lens	*Source*	*Number*	*Incidence*
Iris supported lenses after ICCE			
Iris Clip	K. Schott (1977)	202	4.4%
	J. Draeger (1977)	350	3.4%
	M.S. Jaffe (1978)	698	1.5%
Medallion	Kraff-Lieberman (1978)	500	3.6%
	Drews (1978)	300	2%
Copeland	Osher (1976)	100	3%
	Snider and McReynolds (1977)	399	4.2%
Sputnik	Galin (1978)	300	3%
Iridocapsular lenses after ECCE			
	Binkhorst (1976)	500	1.2%
	Rommel and Leonard	800	1.4%
	Kratz (1979)	320	4.7%
Posterior chamber lenses			
Pearce	Pearce (1979)	444	0.45%
Shearing	Kratz (1979)	756	2.1%
Angle supported lenses			
Mark VIII	Choyce (1977)	1000	6%
	Azar (1978)	800	2.5%
	Kratz (1979)	215	8.4%
Combined Results			
	Hirschman (1970)	1660	2.5%
	Worst (1977) ICCE	1519	4.1%
	ECCE	199	1%
	Shepard (1977)	500	15.4%
	Snider and McReynolds (197)	500	7.4%

Although this heterogeneous material comprising some 11,000 cases does not permit any precise conclusions on the incidence of clinical cystoid macular edema with pseudophakia, we do note that there are few series in which the incidence is equal to or less than 2%.

Much higher incidences have been occasionally reported. D. Shepard (1978) reported a 38% incidence of clinical cystoid macular edema in 60 cases with iris supported lenses with metal loops after intracapsular extraction and 12% for 440 cases with iris supported lenses with supramid loops. L.M. Loewenthal (1978) reported an incidence of 22.2% with 4-loop lenses with titanium loops after intracapsular cataract extraction and 4% with Supramid® and Prolene® loops.

Cystoid macular edema was also frequently associated with the U.G.H. syndrome. The actual incidence is unknown.

Noteworthy are the differences in incidence reported for intracapsular and extracapsular cataract extraction and for intact or non-intact posterior capsules.

— J. Worst (1977), for a series of implants of various lens styles, reported incidences of clinical cystoid macular edema of 4.1% for 1519 intracapsular cases but only 1% for 199 extracapsular cases.

— O. Kline (1978) found a 16% incidence with Copeland lenses implanted after intracapsular extraction but none after extracapsular extraction. Equally striking are the figures he cites for the 4-loop Binkhorst lens: 11% after intracapsular extraction and none after extracapsular.

— J.W. Maida and J.H. Sheets (1978) reviewing 1000 lens implantations reported an incidence of 11% clinical cystoid macular edema after extracapsular extraction when the posterior capsule was not intact but only 1% when the posterior capsule was intact.

— In contrast to the above findings L. Moses (1979), in a series of various lens styles implanted after phakoemulsification, found a 1.4% incidence of clinical cystoid macular edema in 501 cases with open posterior capsules and the same incidence in 573 cases with intact posterior capsules.

B. Angiographic Cystoid Macular Edema (A.C.M.E.)

1. *Retrospective Study by R.L. Winslow et al. (1978)*

The results of a retrospective study conducted by R.L. Winslow et al. (1978) are given on Table XIV-3. All the patients underwent fluorescein angiographic examinations at about 5 months after lens implantation. The authors noted that the average incidence of angiographic cystoid macular edema for aphakic patients at this time is around 15%. Thus, considering only those cases with an intact

TABLE XIV-3. — *Incidence of Angiographic Cystoid Macular Edema ±5 Months after Implantation in Fuction of the Procedure and the Status of the Posterior Capsule and the Vitreous (Winslow et al., 1978, p. 190)*

Procedure	*Status of the Posterior Capsule or the Vitreous*	*Number*	*ACME*	
			Number	*Percent*
Phakoemulsification	Intact posterior capsule	120	13	11%
	Ruptured posterior capsule	25	10	40%
	Vitrectomy	23	10	43%
	Discision	14	8	57%
Extracapsular	Intact posterior capsule	5	0	0
Intracapsular	No vitreous loss	45	4	9%
	Vitreous loss	10	7	70%
	Vitrectomy	5	2	40%
Secondary Implantation	No vitreous loss	3	0	0
	Total:	250	54	22% Avg:

posterior capsule after extracapsular extraction and those without vitreous loss after intracapsular extraction, the average 10% incidence (17/173) compares favorably. But when vitreous loss occurred or when the posterior capsule did not remain intact, the incidence increased to an average of 48% (37/77).

2. *Preliminary Comparative Study by N.S. Jaffe et al. (1978)*

The incidence of angiographic cystoid macular edema was reported by N.S. Jaffe et al. (1978) for 303 patients aged 67 or older for the periods of 4-8 and 16-25 months after lens implantation. Binkhorst 4-loop lenses were implanted after intracapsular cataract extraction, and Binkhorst 4- or 2-loop lenses after extracapsular cataract extraction. The intracapsular pseudophakic series includes cases with peroperative vitreous loss; the extracapsular pseudophakic eyes all had

TABLE XIV-4. — *Incidence of Angiographic Cystoid Macular Edema after Intraocular Lens Implantation and after Intracapsular Cataract Extraction without Lens Implantation (Control Group) in 771 Angiograms (303 eyes) (Jaffe, 1978)*

	Postoperative time in months	*Total Number of Cases*	*ACME*	
			Number	*Percent*
All implants	4	190	27	14.2%
	8	158	16	10.1%
	16-24	138	18	13.0%
Controls	4	113	17	15.0%
	8	89	13	14.8%
	16-24	83	8	9.6%

TABLE XIV-5. — *Incidence of Angiographic Cystoid Macular Edema after Intraocular Lens Implantation in 486 Angiograms (190 Eyes) (Jaffe, 1978, p. 157)*

Procedure	*Postoperative time in months*	*Total Number of Cases*	*ACME*	
			Number	*Percent*
Intracapsular	4	145	24	16.6%
	8	113	14	12.4%
	16-24	109	17	15.6%
Extracapsular	4	45	3	6.7%
	8	45	2	4.4%
	16-24	29	1	3.4%

intact posterior capsules. All the surgery was performed by the same surgical team. Some cases were dropped from the study because of patient refusal to undergo further angiography, death, severe illness, onset of other fundus disease, or poor quality of the angiograms.

Jaffe et al. concluded that, in this particular series, there was a comparable incidence of angiographic cystoid macular edema at the two testing periods for the routine intracapsular cases and the total group of pseudophakic cases. Extracapsular cases with Binkhorst lenses and intact posterior capsules appeared to have a significantly lower incidence of angiographic cystoid macular edema than either the cases of routine cataract extraction or of Binkhorst lens implants after intracapsular extraction. Jaffe noted, however, that the group of extracapsular implant cases was too small to justify definite conclusions.

3. *Preliminary Study of ACME and the Status of the Posterior Capsule by R.L. Winslow et al. (1978)*

In the study by R.L. Winslow et al. (1978) on the incidence of angiographic cystoid macular edema in pseudophakia as a function of the status of the posterior capsule, all the cases underwent extracapsular cataract extraction, some by means of phakoemulsification. Most of the implanted lenses were platinum clip lenses (N = 59). As shown on Table XIV-6, the incidence declined from 44% at 6 weeks to 20% at one year. Of the 16 patients with persistent angiographic cystoid madular edema, 8 had a visual acuity ⩾20/40 and 8 a visual acuity ⩾20/60. Macular edema alone accounted for the poor visual acuity in 6 of these cases, macular edema associated with corneal edema accounted for it in one, and macular edema associated with atrophic macular degeneration in the other.

TABLE XIV-6. — *Evolution of the Incidence of ACME in Pseudophakia over 12 Months (Winslow et al., 1978)*

Number of Eyes	*6 Weeks*	*6 Months*	*12 Moths*
79 100%	35 44%	23 29%	16 20%

To evaluate the influence of the status of the posterior capsule on angiographic cystoid macular edema, Winslow and his colleagues recorded that status at the time of surgery and during the postoperative examinations. They discovered that the integrity of the posterior capsule made little difference in the incidence at 6 weeks, but significant differences did apear at 6 and 12 months: when the capsule was intact, the incidence progressively declined. However, as these authors stressed, the causes of capsule rupture varied and they could had significantly different effects on the persistance of the edema. The effects of a deliberate capsulotomy, an unplanned posterior capsule rupture, at surgery, vitreous loss, and a vitrectomy differ in degree and influence on the behavior of the eye. Since the reasons why the capsules were open were not given, no conclusions are possible as to the influence of each procedure on the occurrence of persistent angiographic cystoid macular edema.

TABLE XIV-7. — *Influence of the Posterior Capsule Status on the Incidence of ACME (Winslow et al., 1978)*

	Intact Posterior Capsule (45)		*Open Posterior Capsule (34)*	
	Number	*Percent*	*Number*	*Percent*
6 weeks	20	44%	15	44%
6 months	8	18%	15	44%
12 months	3	7%	13	38%

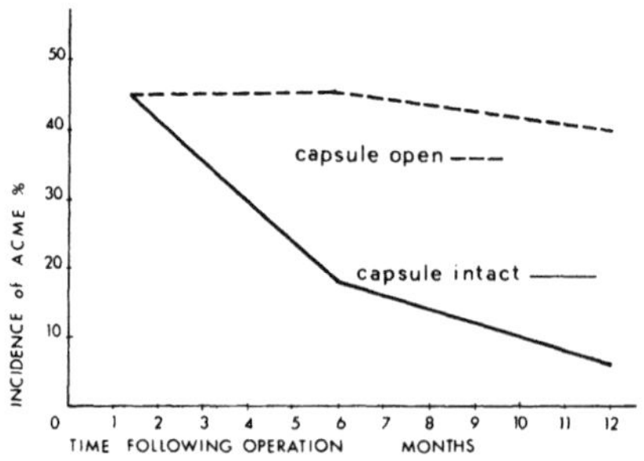

Fig. XIV-2. — Incidence of angiographic cystoid macular edema with respect to time after operation and intact posterior capsule versus open posterior capsule. An open posterior capsule can result from a deliberate capsulotomy, capsule rupture, vitreous loss, or a vitrectomy (Winslow et al., 1978).

We can only say that, in view of the studies cited above, the lowest incidence of angiographic cystoid macular edema occurs when the posterior capsule is intact, regardless of the type of implant used.

IV. Discussion and Conclusions

We must realize that we are concerned here with a complication that only occurs in 2% of ordinary cataract operations, and then more than half of them heal without any treatment. The etiology is multifactoral in ordinary aphakia, with the common denominator being an abnormal permeability of the capillaries of the macular region.

The chemical releasers that trigger this breakdown of the blood-aqueous barrier have not yet all been identified. It has been determined that pre-treatment with substances that inhibit prostaglandin synthesis causes a decline in abnormal vascular premeability, but the studies on the matter are far from sufficient.

Regarding implant surgery, some basic questions must be considered.

A. Is the incidence of cystoid macular edema the same in aphakia as in pseudophakia?

— After intracapsular cataract extraction, the incidence of cystoid macular edema with a lens implant is the same as that with plain aphakia only in a few series. Most often it is somewhat higher.

— After extracapsular cataract extraction and lens implantation, the incidence of both angiographic and clinical cystoid macular edema is lower or at least comparable to the incidence in plain aphakia. The incidence increases when the posterior capsule is not intact.

— As reported above, very high incidences of clinical cystoid macular edema were observed when defective lenses were implanted after intracapsular cataract extraction. It is well to point out that what is involved here are several thousand eyes. If we estimate the average incidence in these cases at between 20% and 30% and we know that, for example, one U.S. firm alone has produced some 44,000 metal looped lenses (Drews, personal communication, 1978) of which 75% were implanted after intracapsular cataract extraction, then, for this one single manufacturer, between 6,600 and 10,000 cases are involved.

B. How is the occasional higher incidence after lens implantation to be explained?

This problem can be partially resolved in the light of information from the history of lens implantation. Indeed, there was always more cystoid macular edema in series in which there was more chronic uveitis. The early Copeland lens series had high incidences of both cystoid macular edema and uveitis. This clear association was repeated when the defective iris supported and defective angle supported lenses came on the scene. Although sufficient statistical data is lacking, on can perceive a clear difference in the cystoid macular edema incidence when defective lenses were used after intracapsular extraction and when they were used after extracapsular extraction (Kratz, 1978; Worst, personal communication, 1978). In the latter case, the incidence was lower. Another clinical observation is that cystoid macular edema was frequently found to occur in eyes suffering from endothelial corneal dystrophy after lens implantation. Nordlohne (1975) has pointed out that these two conditions occurred together in the same eye oftener than the normal distribution would lead one to expect. N.S. Jaffe (1978) made the same observation. Kok van Alphen and Völker-Dieben (1979) found a high incidence of cystoid macular edema in several cases of endothelial corneal dystrophy after lens implantation. They also reported that cystoid macular edema was always associated with endothelial corneal dystrophy that lasted over 9 months. So far the etiological correlations between these two conditions has not been clarified.

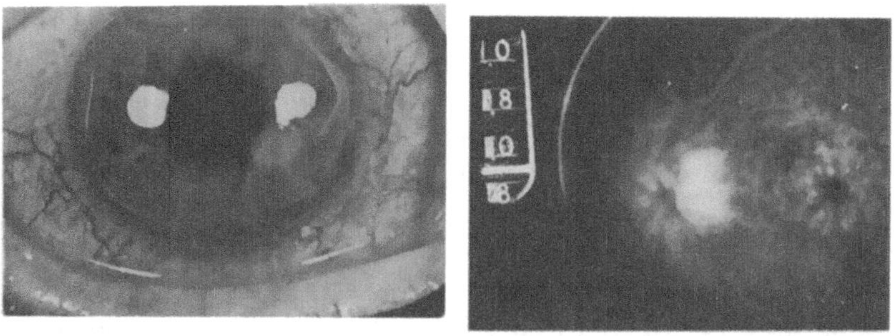

Fig. XIV-3. — A Copeland lens after intracapsular cataract extraction. Chronic uveitis has developed showing clinical and angiographic evidence of persistent cystoid macular edema. (Courtesy J.J. Alpar.)

Another factor is vitreous loss, but, as we have pointed out, the results in this regard are not consistent, and it is yet to be shown if a good quality implant after adequately managed vitreous loss significantly influences the incidence of cystoid macular edema.

C. Does pseudophakic cystoid macular edema have the same characteristics as ordinary cystoid macular edema and what are the therapeutic consequences?

The data we have from our own series, those of Binkhorst, and some others, in which few cases of clinical cystoid macular edema occurred, seem to indicate that pseudophakic cystoid macular edema acts like the normal variety and that the lens has no influence on its natural evolution. From these series, no therapeutic conclusions can be drawn.

In contrast, there are numerous examples cited in the literature in which the implant itself was responsible for a malignant form of cystoid macular edema that did not respond to any therapy until the implant was finally removed. These lenses were defective.

Between these two extremes, there are the cases whose characteristics are difficult to catalogue and of which there is no ready therapy. These are the cases with a concurrence of many factors that sometimes spontaneously evolve favorably and sometimes not.

When one is certain that the lens causes chonic irritation, the appropriate measures must be taken: secondary fixation of a loose lens, amputation of loops that come in contact with the cornea, or lens removal. But if there is no mechanical irritation and if the lens type has a good track record, one can do little more than what is prescribed for ordinary aphakia.

Since it is clear that the incidence of cystoid macular edema can be decreased by eliminating contributory factors, the question for implant surgery is and remains one of prevention. This includes avoiding defective lenses, and, in general, vitreous involvement and chronic inflammation. Whether or not the administation of prostaglandin synthetase inhibitors will prove to be beneficial is still controverted.

Finaly, as to the question of whether extracapsular cataract extraction reduces the incidence of clinical and angiogaphic cystoid macular edema in implant surgery has yet to be satisfactorally dealt with. In favor of extracapsular extraction, we may submit the following.

A well-conducted extracapsular extraction precludes vitreous loss which is recognized as a contributing factor. Furthermore, the presence of the posterior capsule inhibits iridodonesis and pseudophakodonesis, and this, according to Binkhorst, diminished irritation of the eye (see p. 250 on the barrier deprivation syndrome).

In 1974, J. Worst suggested that the compartimentation constituted by an intact posterior capsule would prevent penetration of aqueous biotoxic complexes (ABC factors) into the posterior eye segment. In Worst's opinion, when the posterior capsule is open or absent, the penetration of aqueous and its biotoxic factors via Cloquet's canal damages the macular region and leads to cystoid macular edema provided that some specific anatomical changes in the vitreous structure in front of the premacular region have occurred.

Although these hypotheses of Binkhorst and Worst come very close to the every day reality, in that cystoid macular edema is less frequent in extracapsular aphakia with the posterior capsule intact, it will probably be several years before microbiological research will succeed in satisfactorily explaining theory and practice.

CHAPTER XV

LENS IMPLANTATION AND RETINAL DETACHMENT

Introduction

In the general population, the incidence of retinal detachment seems to be about one in ten thousand. Among aphakics, however, this incidence varies from 0.5% to about 3%, an increase by a factor of 300, which confirms the irrefutable influence of cataract extraction. A survey of the literature indicates that the incidence among pseudophakics seems to be of the same order.

I. Data on Aphakic Retinal Detachment without Lens Implantation

A. Incidence

As shown on Table XV-1, the incidence of aphakic retinal detachment varies from 0.5% to 3.4%, the generally accepted mean being some 2% (Theodore, 1962; Fasanella, 1960, Urrets-Zavelia, 1968; Duke Elder, 1967). According to Duke Elder (1967), the incidence of aphakic retinal detachment after uneventful surgery is the same for intracapsular and extracapsular cataract extraction.

TABLE XV-1. — *Incidence of Retinal Detachment among Aphakics*

Source	*Number*	*Aphakic Retinal Detachment*
Shaplad (1934)	1281	2.2%
Knapp (1936)	500	1.2%
Beach and Adams (1938)	100	2%
Berens and Bogart (1938)	1001	2%
Hughes and Owens (1947)	2086	0.5% to 3.4%
Nonenmacher (1951)	2818	0.93%
Polychronakos (1962)	1000	1.2%
Witmer (Balkoff, 1976)	1150	2.3%
Charamis (Baikoff, 1976)	6594	1.85%
Pasinoand Satori (Baikoff, 1976)	1592	2.76%
François et al. (1917)	910	2.74%
Total	19032	

B. Time Interval between Cataract Extraction and Retinal Detachment

In view of the figures given on Table XV-2, it may be concluded that about 40% of the aphakic retinal detachments occur within a year after cataract surgery.

TABLE XV-2. — *Interval between Cataract Extraction and Retinal Detachment*

Source	*Number of Cases*	*Interval*		
		≤*6 months*	≤*1 year*	>*1 year*
Ravault (1977)	226	30%	40%	60%
Menezo (1977)	109	—	45%	55%
Norton (1964)	119	38%	—	—
Schepens (1951)		—	40%	60%
Malbran and Dodds (1964)	81	—	33%	67%
Guillaumat et al. (1972)	111	23%	43%	57%
Morax and Pouliquin (1963)	32	—	63%	27%
François et al. (1977)	86	30%.	38%	62%

C. Age

Because of the tendency in unilateral cases to lower the age limit for lens implantation, data on ages may be significant. Unfortunately, most of the available information does not distinguish cases of high myopia, traumatic cataracts, and congenital cataracts, thus making conclusions difficult.

Ravault (1977) reviewed 226 cases of retinal detachment and found that the majority of the patients were over 60. Table XV-3 gives the distribution reported by Menezo (1977), Norton (1964), and Guillaumat (1972). Approximately 40% of the patients were under the age of 60 but congenital, traumatic, and myopic cases are common in this group.

TABLE XV-3. — *Age Distribution of 341 Cases of Retinal Detachment (Menezo, 1977; Norton, 1964; Guillaumat, 1972)*

Age	*Menezo*	*Norton*	*Guillaumat*
<60	47	64	39
≥60	52	75	64
Total	99	139	108

D. Factors Contributing to Aphakic Retinal Detachment

1. *Preoperative Conditions*

The following preoperative factors may contribute to aphakic retinal detachment:

— Myopic and other degenerative changes on the periphery of the retina, which are usally referred to as lattice or palisade degeneration (Schepens, 1952; Straatsma, 1977; Byer, 1965).

— Chronic inflammatory processes in the region of the ora serrata. Schepens (1951) suggested that this might be an underlying cause of retinal weakness, but this does not seem to be widely accepted (Malbran and Dodds, 1963; Urrets- Zavalia, 1968).

— Blunt or perforating trauma.

— A history of retinal detachment in either eye, even though ophthalmoscopic evidence of retinal pathology may not be present in the eye for which cataract surgery is planned. Maumemee (1957) and Shafer (1964) reported frequencies of retinal detachment ranging up to 25% if there had been prior retinal detachment in either eye.

2. *Peroperative Factors*

The single most important factor contributing to aphakic retinal detachment is undoubtedly operative vitreous loss. Baurmann (1929) reported 16 cases (1.6%) of aphakic retinal detachment in 931 cases of uneventful surgery and 10 cases (10%) of retinal detachment in 99 cases in which there had been vitreous loss during surgery. Hughes and Owen (1945) reported a retinal detachment incidence of 0.9% among 1720 aphakics who were operated on without vitreous loss and incidences of 5.7% in 141 cases with moderate vitreous loss and 10.9% in 46 cases with severe vitreous loss. L. Guillaumat and H. Massin (1972) also reported that vitreous loss had occurred in 40% of 111 aphakic retinal detachment cases. Ravault and Marion (1977), however, found vitreous loss associated with only 17.2% of 226 aphakic retinal detachment cases.

According to some authors (Schepens, 1951; Malbran and Dodds, 1964), one has to distinguish between the loss of the more fluid vitreous of elderly patients and the loss of solid vitreous of younger patients. In particular, massive retraction developing after the loss of solid vitreous seems to compromise seriously the final result.

It may be assumed that these problems will be solved with the advent of advanced vitrectomy techniques. Indeed, after an adequately conducted vitrectomy, the anterior eye segment looks definitely better: the pupil is round and there are no vitreous strands extending to the wound. Unfortunately, as Norton (1977) noted, there are no large matched series comparing the incidence of aphakic retinal detachment in eyes in which vitreous loss was managed with vitrectomy procedures and the incidence when it was not.

3. *Postoperative Factors*

a. *Endophthalmodonesis*

As postulated by Hilding (1954, cited by Urrets-Zavalia, 1968), the increased mobility of the vitreous body after intracapsular cataract extraction could contribute to the development of retinal detachment since traction at the sites of vitreoretinal adherences necessarily increases.

b. *Late Rupture of the Anterior Vitreous Face*

The question of whether the disruption of the anterior hyaloid face after intracapsular cataract extraction constitutes a contributing factor for aphakic retinal detachment does not seem to have throughtly investigated. Harrington (1952) and Kirsh and Steinman (1954, cited by Urrets-Zavalia, 1968) attributed a certain degree of influence to this phenomenon if late dehiscence of the anterior hyaloid face was followed by massive vitreous prolapse into the anterior chamber.

c. *Vitreous Hemorrhage*

Schepens (1951) considers that the danger of retinal detachment is increased when a sizable vitreous hemorrhage occurs because of the greater tendency for vitreous retraction. Malbran and Dodds (1964) reported 7 cases of early vitreous hemorrhage that soon were complicated by retinal detachment.

d. *Inflammation in the Regio of the Ora Serrata Retinae*

As Schepens (1951) has noted, inflammation in the ora serrata retinae, in addition to being a possible precipitating factor, may worsen the prognosis because of the increased possibility of vitreous retraction. Malbran and Dodds (1964) also attribute an important role to the recurrence of pars planitis.

E. Aphakic Retinal Detachment after Extracapsular Cataract Extraction (Phakoemulsification)

Although it may be argued that there have been major improvements in the technique of intracapsular cataract extraction over the last decade, E.W. Norton and J.C. Johnson (1977) contend that no convincing evidence has been presented to justify the position that cyro-extraction, zonulolysis, or round pupil extraction have lowered the incidence of aphakic retinal detachment.

With the reintroduction of extracapsular cataract surgery, it has been suggested that the incidence of aphakic retinal detachment has decreased. The data we have compiled do not entirely confirm this, unless the cases complicated with vitreous loss are excluded.

C.P. Wilkinson et al. (1978) reviewed a consecutive series of 1500 extracapsular cataract extractions with phakoemulsification of which 94.7% had had posterior capsulotomies or capsulectomies. The follow-up periods ranged from less than 1 month to more than 3 years, but 58% of the periods were less than 1 year. For the entire series, the incidence of retinal detachment was 3.6%. Vitreous loss occurred in 4.2% of the cases, and these cases had a 14% retinal detachment rate.

W.G. Everett et al. (1977) reported an incidence of 1.7% of retinal detachment for 1107 aphakics after phakoemulsification. Patients with congenital or traumatic cataracts as well as those with a history of retinal detachment were excluded from the series. The follow-up period was at least 15 months. Of the 19 cases of retinal detachment, the posterior capsule was intact in 12 and ruptured in 7.

D.M. Shaffer (1974) reported a retinal detachment incidence of 0.97% for 1450 aphakics after phakoemulsification.

R. Kratz (1976) reported a 1.2% incidence of retinal detachment for 1400 cases of phakoemulsification with a 2 year follow-up. Relative to the status of the posterior capsule and the vitreous, Kratz noted the following retinal detachment rates:

- Intact posterior capsule: 0.5%
- Posterior capsulotomy at surgery: 1.6%
- Posterior capsulotomy after surgery: 1.4%
- Vitreous loss at surgery: 7%

J. Little (Emery, 1976), who performed 2900 phakoemulsifications reported a 1% incidence of retinal detachment among those patients followed for at least 1 year. The maximum follow-up was 3 years. The incidence was 0.5% when the posterior capsule was intact, 2.5% when the capsule had been opened or removed, and 6.7% when vitreous loss had occurred.

These data do not indicate that phako emulsification has eliminated aphakic retinal detachment or reduced it to a rare complication. Further, according to Jungschaffer and Fritch (1977), the location, number, and character of tears seem to be quite similar to those that occur after intracapsular procedures. In the patients they observed:

— The average tear size was 1 mm, with horseshoe type tears predominating;
— The average number of tears was 2 per patient;
— Most of the tears were located near the equator and in the superior half of the retina;
— Reattachment rates also seemed similar.

Of the 78 eyes for which retinopexy had been performed by Jungschaffer and Fritch, the posterior capsule was intact in 10 and not intact in 60.

The same conclusions as to the characteristics of retinal detachment after phakoemulsification were reached by C.P. Wilkinson (1979), who reviewed 100 such cases. He also noted that the characteristics of retinal breaks and the configuration of the detachments were similar to those that occurred after intracapsular cataract extraction, and that the reattachment rates also compared favorably.

II. Aphakic Retinal Detachment with Lens Implantation

A. Incidence

As shown on Table XV-4, the incidence of retinal detachment with pseudophakia ranges from 0.5% to 3.6%, which is very close to the incidence for aphakic patients without a lens implantation.

B. Characteristics

On the basis of the literature, pseudophakic retinal detachment shares most of the characteristics of simple aphakic retinal detachment.

TABLE XV-4. — *Incidence of Retinal Detachment after Intraocular Lens Implantation by Lens Type and Reporting Surgeon*

Lens Type	*Source*	*Number*	*Retinal Detachment*
Iris Clip	Schott (1977)	202	2.0%
	Draeger (1977)	350	2.3%
	Jaffe (1978)	698	0.5%
	Kratz (1979)	332	1.2
Medallion	Drews (1978)	300	2.0%
	Kraff (1978)	500	1.4%
Copeland	Osher (1976)	100	1.0%
	Snider and McReynolds (1977)	399	1.0%
	Taylor et al. (1975)	196	0.5%
Sputnik	Fyodorov (1980)	2700	1.7%
	Galin (1978)	300	2.0%
Iridocapsular	Binkhorst (1976)	500	1.0%
	Rommel and Leonard	800	1.2%
	Kratz (1979)	308	1.2%
Shearing	Kratz (1979)	756	1.3%
Pearce	Pearce (1979)	444	None
Choyce Mark VIII	Choyce (1976) (secondary implantation)	800	1.5%
	Azar (1978)	800	None
	Kratz (1979)	215	3.1%
Various Lens Models			
	J. Worst (1977)	1813	2.0%
	Hirschmann (1978)	1660	2.1%
	Shepard (1977)	500	3.6%
	Snider (1977)	500	1.0%

O.H. Jungschaffer (1977) concluded on the basis of 43 cases that retinal detachment in the presence of an intraocular lens implant has the same characteristics as simple aphakic detachment. He noted that the retinal breaks varied from a pinpoint horseshoe tear at the ora to a giant tear. There were 51 tears in all in 39 eyes. The large horseshoe tears were near the equator, and the smaller tears between the equator and the ora and at the ora. No differences in shape, size, location, or number of tears were noted between the intracapsular cases and the extracapsular cases.

Discussing 22 cases, G.P. Johnston et al. (1977) also mention the similarity of the location and shape of the retinal breaks. In addition, they were impressed with the unusual degree of anterior segment and vitreous inflammatory reactions in 4 of these 22 cases.

A. Norton (1978) found no difference between implanted and non-implanted retinal detachment in 61 cases (31 intracapsular and 30 extracapsular) except for visibility problems.

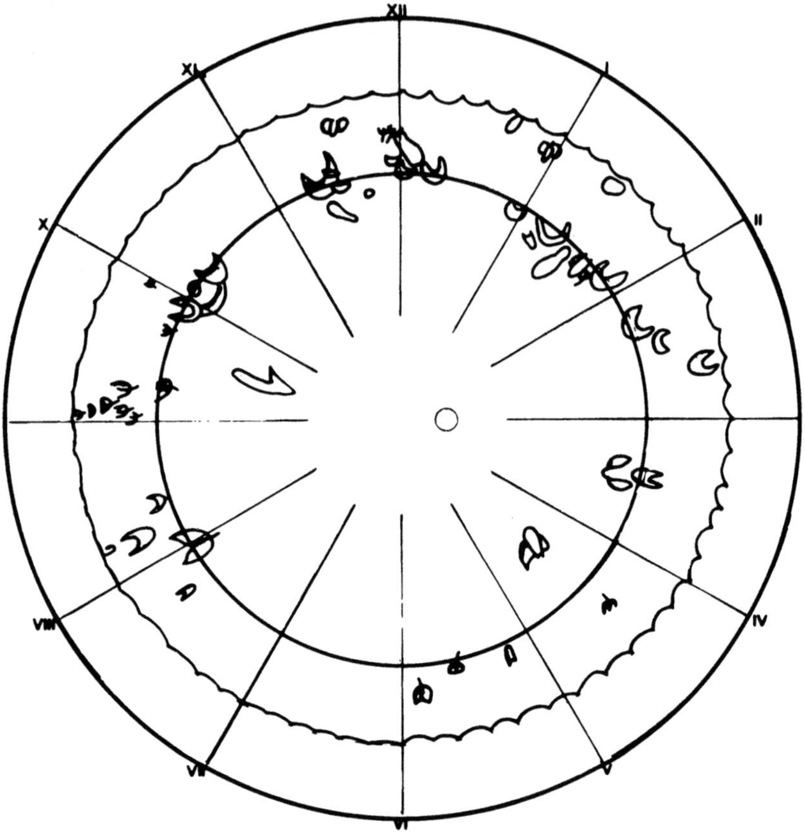

Fig. XV-1. — Location of breaks in 39 cases of retinal detachment (Jungschaffer 1977, p. 1203.)

H.F. Spalter 1980, investigating 15 cases, found no difference from routine aphakic detachment in the location or type of the breaks.

D.A.E. Mertens et al. (1979), having treated 37 cases of pseudophakic retinal detachment, remarked that the type of detachment was quite similar to that in ordinary aphakia. The breaks were mostly of the horseshoe type.

W.B. Snyder et al. (1979) compared 30 cases of pseudophakic retinal detachment with a matched group of 30 cases of aphakic retinal detachment: both groups had a similar distribution of retinal breaks by meridians, and the majority of the retinal defects were located in the temporal region. There was an important difference, however, in the distribution of equatorial and oral holes: 53% of the holes in the pseudophakic group were oral as opposed to only 34% in the aphakic group.

C. **Problems Related to Pseudophakic Retinal Detachment**

All retinal surgeons would agree that perhaps the most important factor in successful reattachment of the retina is visual access, both for preoperative identification and for peroperative location of the defects.

Depending on the type of lens and the technique used, visibility ranges from excellent to poor and is even sometimes impossible. Special procedures are sometimes indicated to improve visual access.

1. *Visualization of the Retina*

The following may interfere with good visualization of the peripheral retina:

— Corneal opacities or corneal dystrophy;
— Blood or cellular debris in the anterior chamber;
— Reflections or light scatter from loop attachments, metal loops in particular give bright reflections;
— Precipitates on the pseudophakos such as pigment dots, blood, and fibrine;
— Posterior synechiae on the pupil border, the lens body or loops, the posterior capsule, the vitreous membrane, etc. that preclude adequate pupil dilation;
— Cortical lens remnants in the pupillary area or on the periphery;
— Opacities of the posterior capsule: stress lines, capsular fibroses, Elshnig pearls, etc.;
— Opacities of the vitreous.

The problems revealed in one multicenter study dealing with 252 pseudophakic retinal detachments are illustrative. Mackenzie Freeman (1979) reported that retinal breaks were not seen in 18% of the cases, and that prominent lens precipitates resulting from iridocyclitis were present in 16%. In 38% of te eyes, pupil dilation was poor because of synechiae formation, and in 10%, excessive lens remnants (extracapsular extraction) interfered with good visual access.

In order to evaluate the potential of funduscopy in pseudophakic eyes, D.E. Dikerson (1977) examined 75 cases without dilating the pupil and without any special selection. Fifty-four of the lenses had been implanted after intracapsular extraction and 21 after phakoemulsificaton. Table XV-5 gives the breakdown of the lens styles, and Table XV-6 gives the retinal areas observed. Dikerson emphasized that not all the eyes had perfectly clear media and that not all the patiens were fully cooperative.

TABLE XV-5. — *Lenses Used in the Dikerson Fundoscopy Study*

Lens style	*Intracapsular Extraction*	*Phakoemulsificaion*
Medallion sutured	34	9
Fyodorov Type I	17	4
Medallion Platina	3	2
Iridocapsular	—	4

TABLE XV-6. — *Retinal Areas Observed in Dikerson Fundoscopy Study*

	Intracapsular Extraction	*Phakoemulsification*
Equator seen	100%	100%
Ora serrata seen	90%	85%
Without depression	20%	5%
With depression	70%	80%
Superior half of ora		
Without depression	53%	9%

In Dikerson's opinion, the examination of the peripheral fundus of an eye containing an implanted lens is not impossible, provided there is a minimal pupil opening allowing indirect binocular ophthalmoscopy. In the eyes he examined the lens types kept the pupil from constricting smaller than 2 mm square, which provided a diagonal distance of approximately 2.8 mm. This distance was found to be sufficient for peripheral fundus examination using the small pupil indirect ophthalmoscope.

D.A.E. Mertens et al. (1979) stated that the Panfunduskop of Schlegel was a very valuable tool and permitted detection of most retinal breaks situated anterior to or on the equator.

Adequate examination for pseudophakic retinal detachment frequently requires an extraordinary amount of time. O.H. Jungschaffer (1977) reported that observation times were increased by 50% after intracapsular extraction and lens implantation and by 100% after extracapsular extraction and lens implantation. Occasionally, several sessions totaling 6-10 hours were necessary.

Therefore, eyes with clear media and pupils that can be well dilated without interfering with lens stability are optimal for retinal examination and, should retinal detachment occur, for subsequent surgery.

TABLE XV-7. — *Retinal Visualization Factors*

Type of Lens	*Reflections and Scatter*	*Pupil Dilation*	*Visibility*
Angle supported	−	++	++
Posterior chamber	−	++	+
Iris supported			
Iris clip without iris sut.	+	−	+
with iris sut.	+	+	++
Copeland	−	+/−	+
Medallion with iris sut.	+	+	++
Sputnik	+	+/−	+
Iridocapsular			
Two-loop Binkhorst	+	+	+/−
Platinum clip	+	+	+/−

++ = very good
\+ = good
+/− = fair
− = poor.

As shown on Table XV-7, good visibility may be expected when angle supported lenses are implanted after intracapsular extraction. With iris supported lenses, pupil dilation may be limited by the presence of posterior synechiae to the lens. But if full dilation is achieved, subluxation and even luxation is to be feared with some models. Although eyes containing iridocapsular lenses may be fully dilated without disturbing lens stability, dilation is often limited in practice by posterior synechiae. For posterior chamber lenses, the visual pathway generally is not really affected in spite of the extracapsular extraction. Most surgeons, however, perform a large posterior capsulotomy at the time of implantation when using these lenses.

2. *Measures to Improve Visual Access*

In difficult situations visualization of the peripheral retina can be improved by taking certain measures, some of which are harmless but others of which involve surgical intervention bearing some risk. The following progression of procedures is based on the assumption that the surgeon should be as unaggressive as possible (Norton, 1978):

Intracapsular	*Extracapsular*
Mydriasis	Mydriasis
Photocoagulation	Photocoagulation
Synechiolysis	Synechiolysis
Iridectomy	Iridectomy
Membranotomy	Capsulotomy
VISC procedures	VISC procedures

Mydriasis: As we have mentioned, uncontrolled pupil dilation with an iris supported lens may cause subluxation or luxation of the lens. Moreover, pupil deformation caused by scleral indentation during the examination of the peripheral parts of the retina can increase the danger of implant dislocation.

Photocoagulation: The elimination of pigmented obstructions in the pupilary area by photocoagulation cannot yet be recommended. Although investigations with animals and in vitro experiments seem to indicate that photocoagulation with an implant lens is harmless, there are not enough clinical data available for this procedure to be used in human eyes (Norton, 1978; Poole and Galin, 1977).

Synechiolysis and Additional Iridectomies: These are the first to be considered among the surgical procedures. Obviously, they may result in instability of the implant or inadvertent luxation. A. Norton (1978) suggested that lens stability be carefully checked beforehand and that the consequences of procedures such as removing a sector of the iris be evaluated. The Francescetti hook has been found to be very useful for sector iridectomies because it

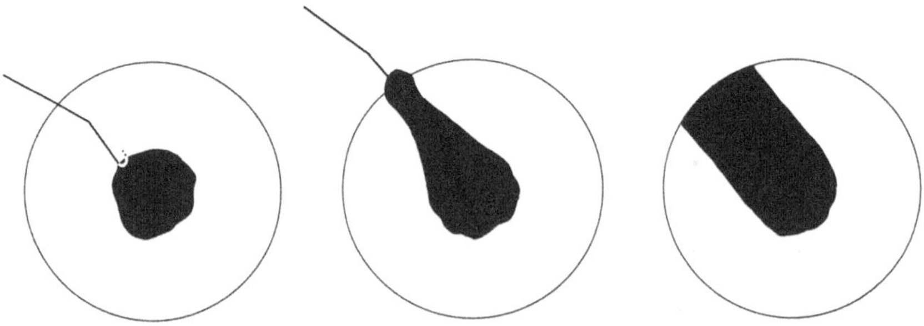

Fig. XV-2. — Francescetti method for performing a sector iridectomy.

requires only a minimal opening of the anterior chamber. Francescetti's method can also be repeared in different quadrants.

Membranotomy — Capsulotomy: Most secondary membranes in the pupilary aperture can be managed with small and simple instruments. Any discission needle or sharp microhook that can be introduced through a small incision is of value.

Vitreous Suction and Cutting (VISC) Procedures: G. Girard (1974) was one of the first to show European implant surgeons how membranes could be removed from behind the implant through the pars plana by using vitreous suction and cutting devices. Although VISC procedures are not to be embarked upon lightly, it seems, in the view of some, that trans-pars plana vitrectomy may be useful in dealing with thick secondary membranes, especially if there is extensive involvement of the iris, with or without opacification of the anterior vitreous (Eichenbaum, 1977; Jaffe, 1978; Deutman, 1978).

D. Results in Pseudophakic Retinal Detachment

Only a few documented series of pseudophakic retinal detachment have come to our attention.

Otto Jungshaffer (1977)

43 cases: 2 eyes were not operated on because of atrophia bulbi in the one and because of extreme cloudiness of the media in the other.
41 eyes were operated on:
— 4 remained detached
— 37 reattached
— Visual results: 22 = 20/40
4 = 20/100
3 = 20/200
8 = 3/200 – 10/200

The follow-up period after the retinal surgery ranged from 3 months to 7 years. The case of poor visual acuity shared no common denominator, nor dit there appear to be a direct relationship with the intraocular lens.

C.P. Johnston et al. (1977)

22 cases: 3 eyes were inoperable because of serious inflammatory reactions and massive vitreous retraction.

19 were operated on. One case failed because of a pre-existing moderately severe iridocyclitis, which increased after retinal surgery and ultimately developed into massive vitreous retraction. Eighteen cases reattached.

The visual results were disappointing with only 6 patients attaining visual acuity equal to or better than 20/40. Four of the fellow eyes of the 22 also had retinal breaks. The lens types used were:

Worst Medallion	14
Copeland	4
Iris Clip	3
Binkhorst 2-Loop	1

D.D. Shepard (1978)

18 cases: 3 eyes were not operated on and 1 case was found to be irreparable.

Visual resuls: 6 achieved useful vision of ≥20/50.

Types of lenses used after intracapsular extraction:

Medallion with supramid loops	8
Fydorov I with supramid loops	6
Platina with supramid loop	2
Medallion with metal loop	1
Platina with metal loop	1

H.F. Spalter (1980)

15 cases: All 15 were operated on.

3 failures: In none of these was the tear found. In two cases, there was persistent inflammation of the anterior chamber and the vitreous body accompanied by chronic ciliary injection and vitreous fibrosis.

12 successes.

Poor visualization was not a significant problem in any of these 15 cases.

W.B. Snyder et al. (1979)

30 cases: Complete anatomic reattachment was achieved in 29 cases, the 1 failure being due a massive preretinal proliferation.

The final visual acuity of 25 eyes did not differ statistically from the visal acuity attained in a matched group of apakic retinal detachment without lens implantation. However, significantly poorer visual acuity was found in 5 eyes that had marked anterior segment inflammation prior to the scleral buckling procedures.

D.A.E. Mertens, et al. (1979)

37 cases: Anatomic reattachment after 1 operation: 29
Anatomic reattachment after 2 operations: 3
Total: 32 (89%)

The reasons for failure in 5 eyes were massive preretinal proliferation (4 cases) and abandonment after 3 interventions because of advanced age.

Ten cases achieved visual acuity of ⩾20/40 and 26 cases ⩾20/200.

H. MacKenzie-Freeman (1979): Multicenter Study

252 cases: The rate of successful anatomic reattachment was found to be 5% less than that of aphakic retinal detachment patients without lens implantation. The overall visual results were also not as good as those achieved with retinal detachment in simple aphakia.

E. Remarks on the Presence of a Pseudophakos during the Treatment of Retinal Detachment

The reports cited above indicate that the methods used for reattachment with a pseudophakos were similar to those used for normal aphakia: scleral buckling and encircling procedures combined with diathermy, cryocoagulation, and photocoagulation.

As was to expected, some lenses subluxated or luxated after pupil dilation, scleral depression, or intravitreal gas insufflation. The angle supported and capsular supported lenses were the most stable. As A. Krieger (1978) commented, rigid angle supported lenses require special attention since scleral indentation or encircling procedures may cause a slight displacement of one of the haptic feet. R. Kratz (1979) remarked that patients with rigid angle supported lenses complained of pain upon scleral depression, thus making examination of the peripheral fundus difficult.

Occasionally, contact occurred between the implant and the corneal endothelium either because intravitreal gas insufflation drove the lens forward or because the anterior chamber became more shallow afterwards, for example, when extensive choroidal detachment developed following scleral buckling.

As a number of authors have observed, the prognosis of some of the interventions was prejudiced for two reasons:

— poorer visual access;
— the presence of chronic inflammation.

III. Summary and Conclusions

Our survey indicates that the incidence of pseudophakic retinal detachment is comparable to that of aphakic retinal detachment and is even lower in some series. Careful case selection and avoidance of lens implantation when conditions were unfavorable probably played a significant role in this. More statistical data is needed to determine whether the presence of the posterior lens capsule significantly influences the incidence of retinal detachment.

According to most retinal surgeons the characteristics of pseudophakic retinal detachment are similar the those of aphakic retinal detachment.

The anatomical and functional resuls of the reattachment procedures are good, provided that visual access to the retinal periphery is possible and that no chronic inflammatory reaction is present.

The presence of an intraocular lens may constitute an additional complication in the diagnosis and treatment of retinal detachment, so the insertion of a pseudophakos in an eye prone to retinal detachment should not be undertaken lightly. This implies, among other things, thorough examination, if possible, of the peripheral retina of both eyes if there are any doubts. Implantation is contraindicated if any retinal breaks are or were present in either eye. Nor should implantation be performed if there is latice degeneration in either eye, and special attention should be given to a patient having a family history of retinal detachment. Lens implantation in the presenile group should be regarded cautiously because of the frequent associaton of vitreoretinal degeneration (Mertens e tal. 1979). Because of the high incidence of retinal detachment with high myopia, one should also proceed cautiously if the patient has an axial myopia exceeding 6 or 7 diopters.

Whether or not prophylactic treatment can be an adequate safeguard is still controverted.

Since peroperative loss of formed vitreous is known to be a precipitating factor, lens implantation in these cases is not recommended unless more statistical evidence is found that demonstrates that well-conducted vitrectomy procedures significantly reduce the incidence of aphakic retinal detachment.

Because chronic uveitis was found to prejudice the final visual result, lens implantation should be avoided in patients with a history of chronic uveitis, and any form of inflammatory reaction after lens insertion should be dealt with aggressively.

Once a patient is provided with an intraocular lens, prompt attention should be paid to the slightest subjective complaints that may indicate incipient retinal detachment such as the occurrence of black spots, showers, or light flashes. And since visual fields are normalized with a pseudophakos, repeated evaluation of the visual field in these cases is mandatory.

CHAPTER XVI

GUIDELINES

Introduction

Lens models and implant techniques are constantly changing, so the guidelines we offer here must be considered tentative. These guidelines are based on our study of the literature and our own experience. Our position is that before deciding to implant a pseudophakos, the parameters presented on Figure XVI-1 must be taken into consideration. We shall discuss them in turn.

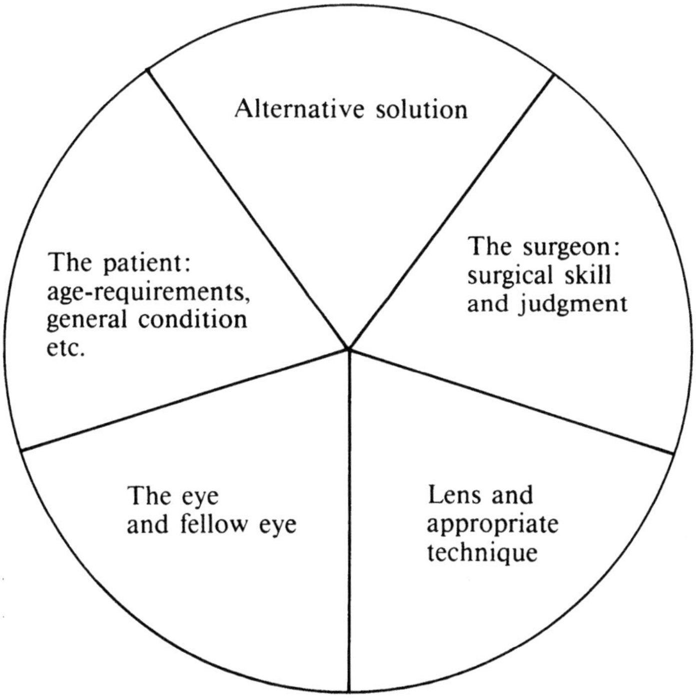

Fig. XVI-1. — Factors involved in the decision to implant a lens.

I. Alternative Solutions

While lens implantation offers a new dimension in the optical correction of aphakia, the possibilities provided by the other methods must not be overlooked. Much is being done to improve the quality and long-term tolerance of contact lenses. Indeed, it is not at all out of the question that continuous-wear contacts will be able to offer in the future substantial guarantees for the long-term revalidation of the aphakic patient. The problem of aniseikonia, especially for the unilateral cataractous patient, however, still remains a limiting factor. Spectacle correction methods are also undergoing continuous improvement.

According to R.C. Welsh (1979), the temporal fields of the larger, nonlenticular aspheric lenses having 4 to 6 diopters of peripheral power drop equal 65° with a range of 56° to 74°. In addition, the newer designs of aphakic spectacle frames that have a 6 to 8 mm vertex distance can significantly decrease magnification (Dabezics Ir., 1979).

II. Surgical Skill and Judgment

The surgeon himself is one of the primary factors that influence the final result. Implant surgery, as J. Worst commented, has its own rights and cannot be considered merely an adjunct to cataract removal. Perfect cataract surgery is necessary and the implant techniques must be mastered, the latter being, perhaps fortunately, in constant evolution. It is, therefore, advisable for the neophyte implant surgeon to limit himself to low-risk cases and not to modify any of the steps in the technique on his own initiative.

III. The Patient

A. Age

The calendar age of the patient is not as important as the life expectancy. Indeed, both the integrity of the materials and the period in which the pseudophakos must remain solidly fixed in the eye must at least exceed the patient's life expectancy. Most of the materials we use have only a limited clinical history: polymethylmethacrylate seems to be time proven; supramid or nylon has its own limitations; and polypropylene, although reported to be innocuous in other human tissues, has only a 3-year track record in intraocular surgery. With regard to lens stability, none of the lens models have gone more than 15 years without being substantially modified. Lens implantation in younger age groups is still, therefore, a matter of some controversy.

The lenses that relied on pure iris support have not withstood the test of time. The angle-supported lenses (Choyce Mark VIII), although stable, did have problems that were important enough to require design changes. The iridocapsular supported lenses with metal loops also had to be modified, even though they were stable in the vast majority of the cases.

From this, one may not conclude that most of the eyes containing the Mark VIII or metal looped iridocapsular lenses could be expected to develop problems that would put the eye in jeopardy. We ourselves have examined many eyes containing metal-looped lenses implanted by C.D. Binkhorst in the rate sixties that are still behaving extremely well. We have also seen eyes with angle supported lenses placed by D.P. Choyce that were holding up well after 20 years.

B. The Patient's Requirements

1. *Restoration of Binocular Vision*

Lens implantation can restore binocular vision, so patients with unilateral cataract or unilateral aphakia are considered as good candidates.

2. *Professional and Environmental Requirements*

Pilots, drivers, and other professions as well as people who have to be in dusty, windy, or chemical-laden environments (farmers, divers, firemen) cannot wear contact lenses. Diseases of the outer eye, such as blepharitis, and conjunctivitis sicca, also make the wearing of contact lenses almost impossible.

3. *Some Mental and Physical Conditions*

Parkinsonism, rheumatoid diseases, palsy, cerebral syndromes, and mental conditions such as severe oligophrenia and senile dementia make the classic corrective methods less desirable.

4. *Unilateral Aphakia*

The already unilateral aphakic patient with a contact lens may profit from having the second eye implanted. Indeed, the implanted eye is highly appreciated in order to execute the manipulations necessary with a contact lens. However, as we noted in Chapter IV on optics, some special problems may arise with regard to binocular vision.

5. *The One-Eyed Patient*

Since lens implantation involves additional risk during surgery and the postoperative course, there seem to be few arguments in favor of supplying a one-eyed patient with an implant lens. In any event, the experienced surgeon will have to weigh very carefully the possible benefits and the attendant dangers.

6. *Bilateral Lens Implantation*

Bilateal implantation may be considered with patients with senile cataracts. Since much can be learned from the behavior of the first eye, it is prudent to perform the implantation in the second eye only after a reasonable delay: 6 months to a year. Bilateral implantation places the surgeon in a very delicate situation since abortion of the procedure in the second eye can mean a great disappointment for both the patient and the surgeon. And new problems arise in managing a situation in which the patient has an implant in one eye and the other eye is rendered aphakic. Therefore, the implantation in the second eye should not be undertaken lightly and certainly should be avoided by the neophyte.

In presenile groups, for example those patients between 50 and 60 years of age, the problem is more complex. In such cases, the delay between the two interventions should be significantly extended, up to 5 years if need be. This delay will be sufficient to assess the behavior of the operated eye and to rule out any pathology that was not manifest before surgery and particularly any pathology of the posterior eye segment, vitreitis, retinal breaks, and retinal detachment. If there is any doubt about the opportuneness of lens implantation in the second eye, one should consider regular intracapsular or planned extracapsular cataract extraction, the latter technique offering the possibility of secondary implantation.

When the patient is under 50 and has bilateral cataracts, which sometimes occurs on a familial or predispositional basis, lens implantation is not indicated. One alternative solution would be to perform planned extracapsular extraction in both eyes, which makes secondary lens implantation possible at a later stage.

7. *General Conditions as Restrictive Factors*

Malignant forms of diabetes can lead to additional eye pathology such as rubeosis iridis and retinopathy. When rubeosis iridis develops, some lens types may provoke recurrent hyphemas (anterior chamber and iris supported lenses). The pseudophakos may also hamper visual access to the posterior eye segment. Mild forms of senile diabetes that are easily controlled by oral hypoglycemic agents or by diet alone are not contraindications.

Some general conditions make the eye more prone to infection. Decreased immunity can be idiopathic or acquired by the use of immunodepressants, high dosages of corticosteroids, or cytostatic drugs.

The use of anticoagulants is not a real restriction, so long as their administration is discontinued temporarily as is done for cataract surgery without lens implantation. Since both iris supported and angle supported lenses can cause late intraocular hemorrhaging, only capsular supported lenses should be considered when anticoagulants are being used.

C. **Racial Factors**

Up till now, little is known about whether race is a factor in the complications that arise in lens implantation. It is not impossible that the pigmented irides of the negroid race could contribute to secondary glaucoma or be prone to loss of pigment by friction with some lens models.

IV. The Eye

Some eyes are more and some are less suitable for lens implantation. For example, eyes that manifest slight uveal reactions before lens implantation may remain irritable thereafter, regardless of the type of lens used; eyes with borderline intraocular pressures may decompensate definitely; and eyes with poor endothelial vitality may suffer corneal breakdown upon lens implantation.

Since many of these problems can be predicted beforehand, the correct implant policy consists of recognizing that some eyes are high-risk cases and others not. The eyes that come into consideration for lens implantation can be divided into four categories:

— The low-risk group is the largest and is constituted by the regular, non-complicated senile cataractous eyes having healthy corneas, normal intraocular pressure with good outflow capacity, and normal anterior eye segments. If there is an increased danger of retinal detachment, implantation should not be performed. Senile macular degeneration is not considered a contraindication. Indeed, having a full field of vision is much apprecated by patients with this condition.

— The second group of eyes are less routine and thus less frequent but lens implantation in them gives acceptable results. This group includes senile cataractous eyes that have, for example, iriscolobomas, small anterior eye segments, or simple anterior or posterior synechiae. In addition to demanding more experience on the part of the surgeon, some of these cases require that an appropriate lens type be selected.

— The third group, which also occurs less frequently, consists of eyes of adults that manifest more pronounced anatomical or functional disturbances, for example, eyes that have been subjected to filtering procedures, eyes with corneas that are prone to decompensation, already aphakic eyes, and eyes with mutilated anterior segments.

— The last category consists of traumatic cases in younger people and possible some cases of congenital cataracts. The anterior segments of these eyes tend to collapse during surgery, which demands adequate technical measures to prevent immediate or late damage to vital eye structures. Favorable results have been reported for lens implantation in children with traumatic cataracts and for unilateral implantation in eyes wih congenital, zonular cataracts. However, the more complex the condition, the more surgical skill and judgment are required to manage the problems involved.

Independently of the skill of the surgeon and the lens type used, some eyes are not suitable for implantation. There is general agreement that the following conditions constitue contraindications:

— Congenital unilateral total cataract;

— Congenital cataract as a consequence of rubella;

— Microphthalmos or an extremely shallow anterior eye segment not due to a swollen cataract;
— Cataract associated with chronic uveitis (anterior or posterior);
— A severely injured eye in which long-term fixation cannot be assured;
— High myopia.

The following are disputable or relative contraindications:

— Eyes with an increased risk of retinal detachment possibly, but not necessarily, because of traumatic or degenerative causes;
— Eyes that require optimal visualization of the posterior eye segment for diagnostic or therapeutic purposes, generally for vascular diseases of the retina such as Coats' Disease, Eales' Disease, or mild diabetic retinopathy;
— Eyes with conditions about which too little is known to be able to predict how they will react to lens implantation. In this group we would include eyes with retina pigmentosa, iris atrophy, heterochromia of the iris, or a unilateral cataract in a patient with pronounced bilateral myopia.

Finally, some peroperative situations may constitute a relative or absolute contraindication such as eyes with serious peroperative problems that may compromise the final result such as peroperative absence of the anterior chamber, hemorrhaging, and substantial vitreous loss;

V. The Lens and the Appropriate Techniques

The choice of an intraocular lens is always a compromise. Some are easy to insert but offer few guarantees for their long-term behavior in the eye. Others demand a far more difficult surgical technique but their long-term performance is better. The question of whether lens implantation is better combined with intracapsular cataract extraction or extracapsular cataract extraction is still controverted. Our survey indicated that the eyes that were implanted after properly conducted extracapsular extraction fared better than those implanted after intracapsular extraction, regardless of the lens model used and even if they were defective. Often, too, the presence of posterior capsule was felt to be an advantage in that it improved the conditions for lens implantation. When intracapsular extraction and implantation were restricted to elderly patients and when peroperative conditions were favorable, most eyes did welll.

A. Lens Types after Intracapsular Cataract Extraction

1. *Angle Supported Lenses*

Angle supported lenses are best in a rather large and deep anterior eye segment. If properly wedged in the scleral spur, they are stable and lie far from the endothelium and free of the iris. Because of their special fixating principle, they can be used even in the presence of large iris colobomas. Colored haptics can be obtained on request (the Choyce Mark VIII lens). Among the technical disadvantages of the rigid angle supported lenses, one of the most significant is the exacting technique demanded that requires the selection of the exact length and the correct placement of all the haptic tips.

The lens models that may be used in a primary procedure after intracapsular extraction—Choyce Mark IX, Tennant, Azar, and Kelman—have only limited follow-up periods to date.

2. *Iris Supported Lenses*

The iris supported lenses, such as the Iris Clip, the Medallion and the Sputnik Lenses, give acceptable results in those eyes in which good iris support can be expected. The iris diaphragm should be non-atrophic, and the pupil rather narrow. Among the disadvantages are the technical difficulties in suturing the lens to the iris and the possibility of subluxation. And since the natural tendency of the iris stroma is to thin out in time, these lenses should be restricted to patients having a short life expectancy (5 to 10 years).

The Copeland Lens, although claimed to be technically one of the easiest to insert, seems to yield to high an incidence of uveal reactions and cystoid macular edema for it to be recommended after intracapsular extraction.

B. Lens Types after Extracapsular Cataract Extraction

1. *Angle Supported Lenses*

The angle supported lenses—Choyce Mark IX, Tennant, Azar, and Kelman Lenses—will probably perform well because the posterior capsule stabilizes the vitreous, iridodonesis is markedly reduced, and intermittent or constant iris/lens friction is largely prevented, which in turn gives less mechanical iris involvement. In the long term, however, it is still conjectural how the surrounding structures of the chamber angle will support these lenses. Because of its flexibility, we expect the non rigid angle supported lenses to be slightly superior to the other, rigid models.

2. *Iris Supported Lenses*

All the iris supported lenses—Iris Clip, Medallion, Copeland, and Sputnik Lenses—can be implanted after extracapsular extraction. The results obtained with these lens types after planned extracapsular extraction are favorably influenced by the presence of the posterior capsule. Indeed, after ECCE, the mobility of the iris diaphragm is considerably decreased, which results in less pseudophakodonesis and less agression to the uveal tissue. The Copeland lens is also reported to perform better when the posterior capsule is present. (T. Hamdi and D. Praeger, personal communication, and D. Praeger, 1979).

3. The Iridocapsular Lens and the Platinum Clip Lens

The lens capsule is an avascular and insensitive membrane that can provide stable support to a pseudophakos. Additional stabilization by the iris is not essential. The iridocapsular lenses fulfill the two main criteria of a successful intraocular lens: stability and non-interference in the delicate surrounding eye structures. The limiting factors are the exacting technique required, the development of late but innocuous atrophic changes at the pupil margin, and the occasional occurrence of lens decentration.

4. *Posterior Chamber Lenses* (Pearce, Shearing, Anis, etc.)

Because no long-term follow-up data are availabe, we cannot yet recommend posterior chamber lenses for patients with a long life expectancy, although the advantages are significant. More clinical data have to be accumulated.

Conclusion

Bearing all these considerations in mind, the final decision in each particular case must be arrived at after weighing the risks and benefits before and during the operation.

POSTWORD

After three decades of continuous refinement, lens implantation has developed to a point where it can yield very positive results. The failures that have occurred can be laid at the door of bad judgment and inexperience, rather than of any unforeseen reaction of the human organism. Such failures, we hope, will constitute permanent object lessons for the future.

It is difficult to be very categorical about the choice of lens model and technique, for, indeed, several techniques and models are quite satisfactory. Neverthelesss, all the models and all the techniques are undergoing constant change, which can be very frustrating for the neophyte surgeon.

It is precisely for this reason that lens implantation can be called a "method art" that can only be practiced with success by surgeons who are willing to devote themselves particularly to this procedure, who are willing and able to follow its evolution closely, and who have the opportunity to apply it regularly.

These last three decades of evolution of lens implantation have opened up vast new areas of research for the non-inplant surgeon, too. These areas range from the study of materials, optical performance, and sterilization problems to the more profound investigation of the biological response of the eye to the entire implantaion event.

All these areas are providing continual impetus for research that extends well beyond the specific concerns of the ophthalmologist.

No one can say whether or not lens implantation is the ultimate answer for the optimal rehabilitation of aphakic patients. It may be, for example, that replacement of the content of the cristallin by a highly refractive material will turn out to be a reliable technique, and keratorefractive surgery is not beyond the realm of possibility.

It is a matter of regret that the cost and complexicity of implant surgery and the pressure of time upon the available medical manpower restricts its large scale application in the non-industrialized countries, where cataracts are a major endemic problem.

Although intraocular lens implantation certainly constitutes a major step forward in the history of medicine, the final judgment of its utility for the human race will have to be rendered by the future.

INDEX

BIBLIOGRAPHY

ALLEN, A. and N.S. JAFFE: Cystoid macular edema: A preliminary study. *Trans. Am. Ac. Ophthal. & Otol.* 81: 133-134, 1976.

ALPAR, J.J.: Guidelines for indications of intraocular lens implantation and selection of the proper lens. *Ophthal. Surg.* 6: 31-46, 1975.

ALPAR, J.J.: Removal of an artificial lens. *Am. Intraoc. Impl. Soc. J.* 2: 29, 1976.

ALPAR, J.J.: A new technique to suture the Binkhorst two-loop and four-loop and Fyodorov lenses. *Cont. & Intraoc. Lens Med. J.* 3: (1) 37-46, 1977.

ALPAR, J.J.: A suggestion for handling intraocular lenses. *Am. Intraoc. Impl. Soc. J.* 3: 45, 1975.; *Cont. & Intraoc. Lens Med. J.* 3:: 71, 1977.

ALPAR, J.J.: A simple and safe suture for fixation of intraocular lenses. *Ophthal. Surg.* 8: 95-104, 1977.

ALPAR, J.J.: The significance and handling of anterior segment hemorrhages in artificial lens-implantation surgery. *An. Ophthal.* 9: 901-907, 1977.

ALPAR, J.J.: Iatrogenic hemorrhages of the anterior segment in artificial lens implantation surgery. *Am. Intraoc. Impl. Soc. J.* 3: 94-117, 1977.

ALPAR, J.J.: Progressive iris pigment loss following cataract operation: Part I. *Cont. & Intraoc. Lens. Med. J.* 4(4): 70-86, 1978.

ALPAR, J.J.: Intraocular lens implantation in a desert environment. *Cont. & Intraoc. Lens. Med. J.* 4(1): 46-53, 1978.

ALPAR, J.J.: Keratoplasty with primary and secondary lens implantation. *Ophth. Surg.* 9(5): 58-66, 1978.

ALPAR, J.J.: Progressive iris pigment loss following cataract operation: Part II. *Cont. & Intraoc. Lens. Med. J.* 5(1): 102-110, 1979.

ALPAR, J.J.: Progressive iris pigment loss following cataract operation: Part III. *Cont. & Intraoc. Lens. Med. J.* 5(2): 81-91, 1979.

ALPAR, J.J.: Intraocular lens implantation into eyes with pre-existing filtering blebs. *Cont. & Intraoc. Lens. Med. J.* 5(1): 111-117, 1979.

ALPAR, J.J.: Cataract extraction and lens implantation in eyes with pre-existing filtering blebs. *Am. Intraoc. Impl. Soc. J.* 1: 33-44, 1979.

ALPAR, J.J.: A comparative study of different intraocular lenses. *Cont. & Intraoc. Lens Med. J.* 6(2): 171-184, 1980.

AMBACHE, N.: Irin, a smooth-muscle-contracting substance present in rabbit iris. *J. Physiol.* 129: 65, 1955.

AMBACHE, N.: Properties of irin, a physiological constituent of the rabbit's iris. *J. Physiol.* (London) 135: 114, 1957.

AMBACHE, N.: Further studies on the preparation, purification and nature of irin. *J. Physiol.* (London) 135: 114, 1959.

AMBACHE, N., L. KAVANAGH and J.M.C. WHITING: Effects of mechanical stimulation on rabbits eyes: release of active substances in anterior chamber perfusates. *J. Physiol.* (London) 176: 378-408, 1965.

ANDERSON, D.R.: Phacoemulsification. *Audio J. Review in Ophthal.* 2: 2, 1976.

ANDERSON, D.R.: Specular microscopy of corneal endothelium. *Audio J. Review in Ophthal.* 3(5): 1977.

ANIS, A.Y.: The Anis Posterior Chamber Lens. *Cont. & Intraoc. Lens. Med. J.* 6(3): 286-290, 1980.

ANOCH, J.M.: Physiology of monocular aphakia. *Trans. Am. Ac. Ophthal. & Otol.* 86: 391-398, 1979.

APOLLONIO, A.: La mia lente acrilica da camera anteriore con piede fistolizzante. *Atti Soc. Oftalm. Lombarda.* 9: 59-61, 1954.

APOLLONIO, A.: Lenti acriliche fisse in camera anteriore. *Boll. Ocul.* 35: 314-318, 1956.

APOLLONIO, A.: Lenti acriliche endobulbari. *G. Ital. Oftal.* 13: 200-205, 1960.

AQUAVELLA, J.V., E.L. SHAW and G.N. RAO: Intraocular lens implantation combined with penetrating keratoplasty. *Ophthal. Surg.* 8(3): 113-116, 1977.

AQUAVELLA, J.V.: Intracapsular cataract extraction with intraocular lens implantation. *Cont. & Intraoc. Lens. Med. J.* 4(4): 89-94, 1978.

AQUAVELLA, J.V. and G.N. RAO: The extended-wear contact lens vs. the intraocular lens: a comparison of risks. *Trans. Am. Ac. Ophthal. & Otol.* 86: 662-666, 1979.

ARNOTT, E.J.: Kelman phaco-emulsification, results and complications. *Trans. Ophthal. Soc. U.K.* 97: 60-63, 1977.

ARON-ROSA, D., J.J. ARON, M. GRIESEMANN and R. THYSEL: Use of the neodymium-YAG laser to open the posterior capsule after lensimplant surgery. *Am. Intraoc. Impl. Soc. J.* 6: 352-354, 1980.

ASCHER, K.W.: Prosthetophakia two hundred years ago. *Am. J. Ophthal.* 59: 445, 1965.

ASHTON, N. and D.P. CHOYCE: Pathological examination of a human eye containing an anterior chamber acrylic implant. *Brit. J. Ophthal.* 43: 577-583, 1959.

ASHTON, N. and J. BOBERG-ANS: Pathology of an aphakic eye containing an anterior chamber implant. *Brit. J. Ophthal.* 45: 543-549, 1961.

AZAR, R.F.: Intraocular lens implantation vs. conventional cataract surgery. *Cont. & Intraoc. Lens. Med. J.* 2(3): 72-80, 1976.

AZAR, R.F.: Complications of anterior chamber implants. *Cont. & Intraoc. Lens. Med. J.* 4(1): 30-33, 1978.

AZAR, R.F. The Azar anterior chamber tripod lens. *Communication Am. Intraoc. Soc. meeting. L.A.* March, 1978.

BAIKOFF, G.: Aphakie unilatérale de l'adulte et cristallin artificiel. Thesis, 1975: Université de Nantes, France.

BAILEY, P.F.: A new instrument for transiridectomy clip closure. *Am. Intraoc. Impl. Soc. J.* 4: 351-352, 1979.

BARASCH, K.R. and S. POLER: A glass intraocular lens. *Am. J. Ophthal.* 88: 556-559, 1979.

BARON, A.: Tolérance de l'œil à la matière plastique. Prothèses optiques cornéenne. Prothèses optiques cristalliniennes. *Bull. Soc. Ophtal.* 53: 982-988, 1953.

BARON, A.: Prothèses cornéennes et cirstalliniennes en matière plastique. *Bull. et Mémoires Soc. Franc. Ophtal.* 67: 386-390, 1954.

BARON, A.: Discussion of the paper by J. Barraquer and N. Bailbé (1957). *Bulletin et Mém. Soc. franç. Ophtalmol.* 70: 247-248, 1957.

BARRAQUER, J. and N. BAILBE: Ensenanzas deducidas de nuestra estadistica operatoria en casos de substitucion del cristalino cataratoso por el lente de Ridley, *Estudios e Informaciones Oftalmologicas.* Instituto Barraquer, Barcelona 5: 13, 1953.

BARRAQUER, J.: Nuestro primer caso de inclusion de lente plastico de Strampelli en la camara anterior. *Communicacion al XXXII Cong. de la Soc. Oftal. H.A.*, Madrid, October, 1954.

BARRAQUER, J.: Lentilles plastiques dans la chambre antérieure. Indications. Technique. Expérience personnelle sur cent cas. *Bull. soc. Belge Ophtal.* 114: 503-516, 1956.

BARRAQUER, J.: Use of plastic lenses in anterior chamber: indications-technique-personal resuls. *Trans. Ophthal. Soc. U.K.* 75: 537, 1956.

BARRAQUER, J. and N. BAILBE: Incidents, accidents et complications possibles au cours de l'inclusion de lentilles plastiques dans la chambre antérieure. Expérience personnelle basée sur les 132 premiers cas. *Bull. et Mém. Soc. franç. Ophtalm.* 70: 233-251, 1957.

BARRAQUER, J. and N. BAILBE: Lentilles plastiques dans la chambre antérieure. Facteurs essentiels pour obtenir de bons résultats. (Lentes plasticos de camara anterior, Estudios e Informaciones Oftalmologicas-Instituto Barraquer, Barcelona, Agosto, 1954). *Acta concil. ophthal. Belgica.* 11: 1709-1711, 1958.

BARRAQUER, J.: Anterior chamber plastic lenses: Results of and conclusions from five years' experience. *Trans. Ophthal. Soc. U.K., Session 1959.* 79: 393-424, 1960.

BARRAQUER, J.: Complicaciones de la inclusion segun los diversos tipos de lentes. *Ann. Inst. Barraquer.* III-4: 588-592, 1962.

BARRON, G.J.: Correction of induced astigmatism after cataract surgery with introduction of an intraocular lens. *Ophthal. Surg.* 8(3): 110-112, 1977.

BARHOLOMEW, R.S., C.I. PHILLIPS and C.G.F. MUNTON: Vicryl (Polyglactin 910) in cataract surgery: A controlled trial. *Brit. J. Ophthal.* 60: 536-538, 1976.
BAURMANN, 1929, cited by DUKE ELDER and DOBREE (1967).
BEACH, S.J. and Mc. ADAMS, W.R.: Intracapsular extraction of cataract in the average practice. *Arch. Ophthalmol.* 15: 95-100, 1936.
BEAUCHAMP, J.O., H.M. CLAYMAN and N.S. JAFFE: Transiridectomy suture for the Binkhorst iris-clip implant. *Am. J. Ophthal.* 82: 795-796, 1976.
BEALE, Jr. J.P.: Closed eye technique of intracapsular cataract extraction with intraocular lens implantation. *Ann. Ophthal.* 11: 801-811, 1979.
BEARLE, J.F. and J. THOMSITT: Anaesthesia for cataract surgery. *Trans. Ophthal. Soc. U.K.* 97: 109-111, 1977.
BECHETOILLE, A. and H. SARAUX: Biometrie oculaire ultra sonique. *Ann. oculist. Franç.* 203(2): 131-149, 1970.
BECHETOILLE, A., J.L. CHABANAIS, G. JALLET and H. SARAUX: Contusion et perméabilité de la barrière hémato-aqueuse à la fluorescéine. *J. Fr. Ophth.* 1, 2: 139-143, 1978.
BECKER, B. and R.N. SCHAFFER: Diagnosis and therapy of glaucomas. 4th ed. by A.E. Kolker and J. Hetherington. St. Louis 1976.
BECKER, S.C.: Personal experience with intraocular lens implants. *Cont. & Intraoc. Lens. Med. J.* 1: 8-11, 1975.
BECKER, S.C.: The prevention of complications associated with lens implantation surgery. *Cont. & Intraoc. Lens. Med. J.* 2: 3-7, 1976.
BECKSTEIN, E.H.: The importation of intraocular lenses under the medical device act. *Am. Intraoc. Impl. Soc. J.* 2: 125-126, 1977.
BEGUNOVA, G.B.: Determination of the resolving power of intraocular lenses. *Vest. Oftal.* 2: 62-66, 1974.
BEIDNER, B., L. ROTHKOFF and M. BLUMENTHAL: The effect of acetazolamide on early increased intraocular pressure after cataract extraction. *Am. J. Ophthal.* 83: 565-568, 1977.
BENJAMIN, S.N. and O.R. SHERMAN: Comparison of intracapsular and extracapsular cataract extraction with and without intraocular lens implantation. *Am. Intraoc. Impl. Soc. J.* 3-4: 202-203, 1977.
BENOLKEN, R.M., J.M. EMERY and D.J. LANDIS: Temperature profiles in the anterior chamber during phaco-emulsification. *Invest. Ophthal.* 13, 1974.
BERENS, C. and D. BOGART: Certain postoperative complications of cataract operations, with especial reference to a study of 1004 operations. *Am. J. Surg.* 42: 39-61, 1938.
BERROCAL, J.A.R.: Incidence of cystoid macular edema after different cataract operations. *Mod. Probl. Ophthal.* 18: 518-520, 1977.
BETSCH, A.: Über die menschliche Refractionskurve. *Klin. Mbl. Augenheilk.* 82: 365-379, 1929.
BETTMAN, Jr., J.W. and J.W. BETTMAN Sr.: One-day hospitalization for extracapsular cataract surgery without phacoemulsification. *Ophthal. Surg.* 8(4): 81-84, 1977.
BETTMAN, J.W. and J.W. BETTMAN, Jr.: The extracapsular cataract extraction without phacoemulsification. *Trans. Am. Ac. Ophthal. & Otol.* 85: 41-45, 1978.
BETTMAN, J.W.: Medicolegal hazards of intraocular lens implanting. *Am. J. Ophthal.* 86: 496-500, 1978.
BHATTACHERJEE, P. and H.E. EAKINS: Inhibition of the prostaglandin synthetase systems in ocular tissues by indomethacin. *Br. J. Pharmacol.* 50: 227-230, 1974.
BHATTACHERJEE, P. and B.R. HAMMOND: Inhibition of increased permeability of the blood-aqueous barrier by non-steroidal anti-inflammatory compounds as demonstrated by fluorescein angiography. *Exp. Eye Res.* 21: 499-505, 1975.
BIEDNER, B., L. ROTHKOFF, T. MONOS and M. BLUMENTHAL: Two special indications for intraocular lens implantation. *Brit. J. Ophthal.* 62: 468-469, 1978.
BIERLAAGH, J.J.M., A. VAN DER WEE, A. KATS, P.A.M. LEONARD and C.D. BINKHORST: Technique and perspectives of lens implants (pseudophakia). In: *Proceedings of the Second Congress of Orthoptics.* Amsterdam, Excerpta Medica Foundation, pp. 194-202, 1972. *Int. Congr. Series,* Nr. 245, 1971.
BIESHEUVEL, K. and A.T.M. VAN BALEN: Ervaringen met implantatie van artificiële lenzen. *Ned. T. Geneesk.* 114-489, 1970.

BIESHEUVEL, K. and A.T.M. VAN BALEN: Experience with the implantation of artificial lenses. *Ophthalmologica*, Basel, 163: 2-7, 1971.
BIETTI, G.B.: Discussion al trabajo de Baron, *S.F.O.*, 1955; *Acta Ophtal.*, Fasc. 1, 1954.
BIETTI, G.B.: The present state of the use of plastics in eye surgery. *Acta Ophthal.* (Kopenhagen) 33: 337-370, 1955.
BIGAR, F., R. SCHIMMELPFENNING and R. GIESELER: Routine evaluation of endothelium in human donor corneas. *Albrecht v. Graefes Arch. Klin. Exp. Ophth.* 200: 195-200, 1976.
BIGAR, F., R. WITMER and A. THAER: Die Spiegelmikroskopie des Hornhautendothels. *Klin. Mbl. Augenheilk.* 173: 691, 1978.
BINDER, S.: Corneal endothelial damage. *Am. J. Ophthal.* 82(1): 48-54, 1976.
BINKHORST, C.D.: De prognose van de aangeboren en in de eerste levensjaren ontstane staar. *Ned. T. Geneesk.* 87: 343-350, 1943.
BINKHORST, C.D. and F.P. FLU: Sterilization of intra-ocular acrylic lens protheses with ultra-violet rays. *Brit. J. Ophthal.* 40: 665-668, 1956.
BINKHORST, C.D.: Intra-oculaire lensprothese volgens Ridley. Resultaten bij 12 patiënten. *Ned. T. Geneesk.* 100: 3522-3528, 1956.
BINKHORST, C.D.: Ridley's intraocular lens prothesis. The postoperative reaction. Results obtained in 12 cases. *Ophthalmologica* (Basel) 133: 384-392, 1957.
BINKHORST, C.D.: De implantatie van kunststoflenzen in het oog. Een nieuwe fixatiemethode: de pupillens of iris-cliplens. *Ned. T. Geneesk.* 103: 1289-1294, 1959.
BINKHORST, C.D.: Iris-supported artificial pseudophakia. A new development in intraocular artificial lens surgery (iris clip lens). *Trans. Ophthal. Soc. U.K.* 79: 569-584, 1959.
BINKHORST, C.D.: Über die Endgültige Verträglichkeit künstlicher Augenlinsen bei der Aphakie und deren Verbesserung Mittels Fixation der Linse in der Pupille ("Pupillar-Linse" oder "Iris-Clip Linse"). *Klin. Mbl. Augenheilk.* 134: 536-543, 1959.
BINKHORST, C.D.: Ervaringen van de implantatie van verschillende typen lens-prothesen bij enkelzijdige afakie: de pupil-lens of iris-cliplens een nieuwe fixatiemethode. *Ned. T. Geneesk.* 104: 754-755, 1960.
BINKHORST, C.D.: Results of implantation of intraocular lenses in unilateral aphakia with special references to the pupillary or iris clip lens: A new method of fixation. *Am. J. Ophthal.* 49: 703-710, 1960.
BINKHORST, C.D.: Indikation und Implantationstechnik der "Pupillarlinse" oder "Iris-Clip-Linse" bei der Aphakie. *Klin. Mbl. Augenheilk.* 136: 35-43, 1960.
BINKHORST, C.D.: Experience with implantation of various types of lens protheses in unilateral aphakia: The pupillary lens or iris clip lens. A new method of fixation. *Ophthalmologica* (Basel) 139: 500-503, 1960.
BINKHORST, C.D.: The pupillary lens (iris clip lens). An artificial lens for aphakia completely supported by the iris. *Ophthalmologica* (Basel) 141: 479-480, 1960.
BINKHORST, C.D.: Iris clip lens, een door de iris gefixeerde artificiële lens bij afakie. *Ned. T. Geneesk.* 105: 1118-1119, 1961.
BINKHORST, C.D.: Aktive und rationelle Behandlung des Altersstars mit der 'iseikonischen' Pupillarlinse (Iris-Klipp-Linse). *Ber. 64. Zus. dtsch. ophthal. Ges. Heidelberg* 1961: 486-488, 1962.
BINKHORST, C.D.: Lensimplantatie. *Ned. T. Geneesk.* 106: 908-912, 1962.
BINKHORST, C.D.: Use of the pupillary lens (iris clip lens) in aphakia. Our experience based on the first fifty implantations. *Brit. J. Ophthal.* 46: 343-356, 1962.
BINKHORST, C.D.: Artificial pseudophakia. Long-term results obtained with the pupillary lens (iris clip lens) in the first twenty cases of unilateral aphakia. *Brit. J. Ophthal.* 46: 496-502, 1962.
BINKHORST, C.D.: The pupillary lens (iris clip lens). A third method of intraocular artificial lenses in aphakia. *An. Inst. Barraquer*, III-4: 562-569, 1962.
BINKHORST, C.D. and M.H.M.A. GOBIN: Oogletsels met lenstroebeling bij jonge kinderen. *Ned. T. Geneesk.* 108: 978-985, 1964.
BINKHORST, C.D. and M.H.M.A. GOBIN: Injuries to the eye with lens opacity in young children. *Ophthalmologica* (Basel) 148: 169-183, 1964.
BINKHORST, C.D., B.C. CARDON, R.G. VAN DAMME and H. HOMMERS: The pupillary lens. A substitute for the caractous crystalline lens. *Med. Radiogr. Photogr.* 42: 16-23, 1966.

BINKHORST, C.D.: Iris-clip and irido-capsular lens implants (pseudophakoi). Personal techniques of pseudophakia. *Brit. J. Ophthal.* 51: 767-771, 1967.
BINKHORST, C.D.: Lens implants (pseudophakoi) classified according to method of fixation. *Brit. J. Ophthal.* 51: 772-774, 1967.
BINKHORST, C.D.: Eigene Verfahren der Pseudophakie. Iris-clip-Pseudophako und iridokapsulärer Pseudophakos. *Klin. Mbl. Augenheilk.* 151: 21-28, 1967.
BINKHORST, C.D. and M.H.M.A. GOBIN: Pseudophakia after lens injury in children. *Ophthalmologica* (Basel) 154: 81-87, 1967.
BINKHORST, C.D. and P.A.M. LEONARD: Results in 208 iris-clip pseudophakos implantations. *Am. J. Ophthal.* 64: 947-956, 1967.
BINKHORST, C.D.: The fixation of pseudophakoi. Perspect. Ophthal. 1: 191-194. *Excerpta Med. Found.* Amsterdam, 1968.
BINKHORST, C.D. and P.A.M. LEONARD: Implantation of the iris clip pseudophakos. Results in the first 208 cases. *Perspect. Ophthal.* 1: 195-214, 1968. *Excerpta Med. Found.* Amsterdam, 1968.
BINKHORST, C.D.: De bevestiging van pseudophakoi. *Ned. T. Geneesk.* 113: 2258-2259, 1969.
BINKHORST, C.D., M.H.M.A. GOBIN and P.A.M. Leonard: Posttraumatic pseudophakia in children. In: J. François. *Occupational and medicative hazards in ophthalmology*, pp. 284-291. Karger, Basel, 1969.
BINKHORST, C.D., M.H.M.A. GOBIN and P.A.M. LEONARD: Posttraumatic pseudophakia in children. *Proc. Centennial Symp. Manhattan Eye, Ear and Throat Hosp.* pp. 72-86, ed. A.I. Turtz. Mosby, St. Louis, 1969.
BINKHORST, C.D., M.H.M.A. GOBIN and P.A.M. LEONARD: Posttraumatic artificial lensimplants (pseudophakoi) in children. *Brit. J. Ophthal.* 53: 518-529, 1969.
BINKHORST, C.D. and M.H.M.A. GOBIN: Treatment of congenital and juvenile cataract with intraocular lens implants (pseudophakoi). *Brit. J. Ophthal.* 54: 759-765, 1970.
BINKHORST, C.D.: The attachment of pseudophakoi. *Ophthalmologica* (Basel) 162: 205-207, 1971.
BINKHORST, C.D. and M.H.M.A. GOBIN: Congenital cataract en lensimplantatie. *Ned. T. Geneesk.* 115: 822-823, 1971.
BINKHORST, C.D.: Letter to the editor. *Am. J. Ophthal.* 70: 311, 1970.
BINKHORST, C.D.: The attachment of pseudophaki. *Ophthalmologica.* (Bazel) 162: 205-207, 1971.
BINKHORST, C.D.: Power of the prepupillary pseudophakos. *Brit. J. Ophthal.* 56: 332-337, 1972.
BINKHORST, C.D.: Praxis und Theorie der 'Iris Klipp Linse' und der 'Irido-Kapsular Linse'. *Sitzungsber. 125. Vers. Ver. Rhein.-Westfäl. Augenärzte Bonn.* Grafischer Betr. Zimmerman, Balve/Sauerland, 1972.
BINKHORST, C.D.: Perspektiven der Iris-Klipp-Linse und der Irido-Kapsularlinse. *Klin. Mbl. Augenheilk.* 161: 477-481, 1972.
BINKHORST, C.D.: Power of the prepupillary pseudophakos. *Brit. J. Ophthal.* 56: 332-337, 1972.
BINKHORST, C.D.: Perspektiven der Iris-Klipp-Linse und der Iridokapsularlinse. *Klin. Mbl. Augenheilk.* 161: 447-481, 1972.
BINKHORST, C.D., M.H.M.A. GOBIN: Congenital cataract and lens implantation. *Ophthalmologica* (Basel), 164: 392-397, 1972.
BINKHORST, C.D., A. KATS and P.A.M. LEONARD: Extracapsular pseudophakia. Results in 100 two-loops iridocapsular lens implantations. *Am. J. Ophthal.* 73: 625-636, 1972.
BINKHORST, C.D.: The iridocapsular (two-loop) lens and the iris clip (four loop) lens in pseudophakia. *Trans. Am. Ac. Ophthal. & Otol.* 77: 589-617, 1973.
BINKHORST, C.D.: Lens Implants. In: Sorsby, A. (ed.): *Modern Trends in Ophthalmology.* London, Butterworths, 5; 154-163, 1973.
BINKHORST, C.D.: Dioptric value of artificial eye lenses. *Klin. Mbl. Augenheilk.* 162(3): 354-361, March, 1973.
BINKHORST, C.D.: Some thoughts on the fixation of the intraocular lenses. *First International Symposium on Artificial Lens Implantation.* Utrecht, April 1974. Edited by A.T.M. Van Balen, The Netherlands, 1975, Junk Publishers, pp. 99-128.

BINKHORST, C.D. and H.D.S. ONG: Heutige Technik der intra- und extrakapsulären Linsenextraction mit Einpflanzung einer künstlicher Linse. *Augenärtzliche Fortbildung.* 2(3): 1974.

BINKHORST, C.D.: Evaluation of intraocular lens fixation in pseudophakia. *Am. J. Ophthal.* 80: 184-191, 1975.

BINKHORST, C.D.: Interview. *Highlights of ophthal.* pp. 244-345, 1975-76.

BINKHORST, C.D.: Pseudophakia—Why extracapsular surgery? *Am. Intraoc. Impl. Soc. J.* 2: 4, 1976.

BINKHORST, C.D., A. KATS, T.T. TJAN and L.H. LOONES: Retinal accidents in pseudophakia: intracapsular versus extracapsular surgery. *Am. Intraoc. Impl. Soc. J.* 2: 24, 1976.

BINKHORST, C.D., A. KATS, T.T. TJAN and L.H. LOONES: Retinal accidents in pseudophakia: intracapsular vs. extracapsular surgery. Symposium: Intraocular Lenses. *Trans. Am. Ac. Ophthal. & Otol.* 81: 120-127, 1976.

BINKHORST, C.D. and L.H. LOONES: Intraocular Lens Power. Symposium: Intraocular Lenses. *Trans. Am. Ac. Ophthal. & Otol.* 81: 70-79, 1976.

BINKHORST, C.D.: Twenty years experience with Pseudophakia. Some Thoughts on the fixation of intraocular lenses. *Cont. & Intraoc. Lens Med. J.* 1(1-2): 115-120, 1975.

BINKHORST, C.D.: Pseudophakia, intracapsular or extracapsular technique? *Documenta Ophthalmol.* Proceedings Series - Oct. 1975. The Hague. Junk Publishers, pp. 251-263, 1976.

BINKHORST, C.D.: Intraocular lens power. *Trans. Am. Ac. Ophthal. & Otol.* 81: 70-79, 1976.

BINKHORST, C.D.: Five hundred planned extracapsular extractions with irido-capsular and iris clip lens implantation, in senile cataract. *Ophthal. Surg.* 8(3): 37-44, 1977.

BINKHORST, C.D. and W.A. MANSCHOT: The mechanism of capsular fixation of intraocular lenses in the human eye. *Am. Intraoc. Impl. Soc. J.* 2: 110-112, 1977.

BINKHORST, C.D., L.H. LOONES and P. NYGAARD: The clinical specular microscope. *Am. Intraoc. Impl. Soc. J.* 3-4: 184-192, 1977.

BINKHORST, C.D., P. NYGAARD and L.H. LOONES: Specular microscope of the corneal endothelium and lens implant surgery. *Am. J. Ophthal.* 5: 597-605, 1978.

BINKHORST, C.D., B, GREAVES, A. KATS and A.K. BERMINGHAM: Lens injury in children treated with irido-capsular supported intraocular lenses. *Am. Intraoc. Impl. Soc. J.* 2: 34-49, 1978.

BINKHORST, C.D., P. NYGAARD and L.H. LOONES: Corneal endothelium and lens implant. *Am. J. Ophthal.* 85: 597-605, 1978.

BINKHORST, C.D., L.H. LOONES and P. NYGAARD: Die Bedeutung der Spiegelmikroskopie und -graphie des Hornhautendothels für die Einpflanzung künstlicher Augenlinsen-Beschreibung einer Tiefkammertechnik für Einpflanzung. In: *Kunststoff implantate in der Ophthalmologie Red.* W. Jaeger, Ed., J.F. Bergmann Verlag, Munich, pp. 93-103, 1978.

BINKHORST, C.D. and C. HUBER: Cataract extraction and intraocular lens implantation after fistulizing glaucoma surgery. *Am. Intraoc. Impl. Soc. J.* 7(2): 133-139, 1981.

BINKHORST, R.D.: A weightless iseikonic intraocular lens. *Am. J. Ophthal.* 58(1):73-78, 1964.

BINKHORST, R.D.: The optical design of intraocular lens implants. *Ophthal. Surg.* 6(3): 17-31, 1975.

BINKHORST, R.D.: Intraocular lens power calculation manual. A complete guide to the author's TI-59 Programs. R.D. Binkhorst, New York (s.d.).

BINKHORST, R.D.: Pitfalls in the determination of intraocular lens power without ultrasound. *Ophth. Surg.* 7(3): 69-82, 1976.

BINKHORST, R.D.: The cuse of excessive astigmatism with intraocular lens implants. *Trans. Am. Ac. Ophthal. & Otol.* 86: 672-675, 1979.

BINKHORST, R.D.: Intraocular lens power determination. In: *Pseudophakia, Current Trends and Concepts.* Ed. by M.L. Kwitko and D.L. Praeger. Williams & Wilkins, Baltimore-London, 1980, pp. 53-66.

BITO, L.Z. and E.V. SALVADOR: Intraocular fluid dynamics III. The site and mechanism of prostaglandin transfer across the blood intraocular fluid barriers. *Exp. Eye Res.* 14: 233, 1972.

BITO, L.Z.: Concentration accumulation of prostaglandins by the iris-ciliary in vitro and facilitated removal of prostaglandin E_1 from intraocular fluids in vivo. *Exp. Eye Res.* 14: 175, 1972.
BITO, L.Z.: Absorptive transport of prostaglandins from intraocular fluids to blood. *Exp. Eye Res.* 16: 299, 1973.
BITO, L.Z.: The effects of experimental uveitis on anterior uveal prostaglandin transport and aqueous humor composition. *Invest. Ophthal.* 13: 959, 1974.
BITO, L.Z. and M.C. WALLENSTEIN: Transport of prostaglandine across the bloodbrain and blood-aqueous barriers and the physiological significance of these absorptive transport processes. *Exp. Eye Res. Suppl.* 229-243, 1977.
BITO, L.Z., E.V. SALVADOR and L. PETRINOVIC: Intraocular fluid dynamics. IV. Intraocular sites of solute utilization and transport as revealed by studies on aphakic eyes. *Exp. Eye Res.* 26: 47-55, 1978.
BLACKWELL, W.L., N. GRAVENSTEIN and H.E. KAUFMAN: Comparison of central corneal endothelial cell numbers with peripheral areas. *Am. J. Ophthal.* 84: 473-476, 1977.
BLAKER, J.W.: Quality control of intraocular lens optics. *Am. Intraoc. Impl. Soc. J.* 2: 128-129, 1977.
BLANKSMA, L.J. and J.V. SIERTSEMA: Changes in the structure of intraocular nylon. *Doc. Ophthalmologica.* 44(1): 223-229, 1977.
BLAYDES, J.E.: Cataract wound closure with polyglactin 910 following insertion of a 4-loop Binkhorst lens: Preliminary report. *Am. Intraoc. Impl. Soc. J.* 4: 225-226, 1978.
BLUMENTHAL, M.: Iris plane pseudophakic (Copeland lens): Prevention or synechiae formation. *Ophth. Surg.* ((3): 105-109, 1977.
BOBERG-ANS, J.: Experience with twelve cases of intraocular anterior chamber implants for aphakia. Two new models of lenses are described. *Brit. J. Ophthal.* 45: 37-43, 1961.
BOBERG-ANS, J.: Pathology of an aphakic eye, containing an anterior chamber implant. *An. Inst. Barraquer.* 111-4: 585-589, 1962.
BOBERG-ANS, J.: Complications from intraocular lenses in aphakia. In: *Complications after cataract surgery*, ed. F.H. Theodore, Little, Brown & Co.: Boston, pp. 443-448, 1964.
BOBERG-ANS, J.: Complications from intraocular lenses in aphakia. *Int. Ophthal. Clin.* 5/1: 107-122, 1965.
BOBERG-ANS, J.: Reconstructive surgery in the anterior chamber. *Ophthalmologica* (Basel). Addit. ad 158: 279-283, 1969.
BOBERG-ANS, J.: Reconstructive surgery in the anterior chamber. *Acta Ophthal.* (Kopenhagen) 47: 489-497, 1969.
BOBERG-ANS, J.: Management of anterior synechia: Iris disruption, traumatic cataract and lens remnants, vitreous adhesions. *Adv. Ophthal.* 27: 148-149, 1972.
BOBERG-ANS, J.: Differences and similarities in a series of cases bilateral intraocular lenses and evaluation of the results. *Brit. J. Ophthal.* 61: 622-627, 1977.
BOBERG-ANS, J.: 22 Jahre Erfahrungen mit Intraokularen Linsen. *Klin. Mbl.* 171: 303-316, 1977.
BOEDER, P.: Aniseikonia: theorical aspect. *Acta XVI, Conc. Ophthal.* 2: 720-726, 1950.
BOEDER, P.: Spectacle correction of aphakia. *Arch. Ophthal.* (Chicago) 68: 870-874, 1962.
BÖGER, R.: Erfahrungen mit Vorkammerlinsen. *Klin. Mbl. Augenheilk.* 139: 583-586, 1961.
BONNET, R., J.P. GERHRAD and M. MASSIN: Les verres de contact. *Bull. Soc. Ophtal. Fr.* Rapport annuel, 1966.
BONNET, M.: Le syndrome d'Irvine-Gass. *Arch. Ophthal.* (Paris) 32: 705-720, 801-814, 1972.
BONNET, M., J.D. GRANGE and C. PINGAULT: Fréquence de l'œdème maculaire après extraction de la cataracte. *An. Ocul.* 208: 217-220, 1975; *Bull. Soc. Ophtal. Fr.* 2: 231-233, 1975.
BONNET, M.: Les facteurs de pronostic du syndrome d'Irvine-Gass. *An. Ocul.* 208: 275-278, 1975.
BORUCHOFF, S.A.: Degradation of "non-absorbable" sutures. *Ophthal. Surg.* 8: 42-43, 1977.

BOURNE, W.M. and H.E. KAUFMAN: Cataract extraction and the corneal endothelium. *Am. J. Ophthal.* 82: 44-47, 1976.

BOURNE, W.M. and H.E. KAUFMAN: Endothelial damage associated with intraocular lenses. *Am. J. Ophthal.* 81: 482-485, 1976.

BOURNE, W.M. and H.E. KAUFMAN: Specular microscopy in human corneal endothelium in vivo. *Am. J. Ophthal.* 81: 319-323, 1976.

BOURNE, W.M., R.F. BRUBAKER and W.M. O'FALLON: Use of air to decrease endothelial loss during intraocular lens implantation. *Arch. Ophthal.* 97: 1473-1475, 1979.

BOYD, B., A.E. MAUMENEE & Co.: Discussion: Prevention of aphakic retinal detachment. Current Concepts in cataract surg. St. Louis: C.V. Mosby Co., 1974.

BOYD, B.F.: Intraocular lenses vs. around-the clock soft contact lenses in aphakics. Highlights of Ophthal. 111(3): 1-6, 1974.

BOYD, B.F.: What are the new trends and different orientations in the field of intraocular lenses? *Highlights of Ophthal. Monthly Letter.* 4(2): 1-5, 1976.

BOYD, B.F.: Dr Jaffe's final results on his perfectly matched series. *Highlights of Ophthal., Monthly Letter.* 5(4): 1977.

BOYD, B.F.: Long term wear contact Lenses: A reality. *Highlights of Ophthal. Monthly Letter.* 5(15): 1-7, 1977.

BOYD, B.F.: What are the new trends in intraocular lenses? What new problems have developed? *Highlights of Ophthal., Monthly Letter.* 5(1): 1-5, 1977.

BOYD, B.F.: The changing scene of lens implant surgery (Part I). *Highlights Ophthal., Monthly Letter,* 6(14): 1-5, 1978.

BOYD, B.F.: The changing scene of lens implant surgery. Part II. *Highlights of Ophthal., Monthly Letter.* 6(15): 1-5, 1978.

BOYD, B.F.: What are the newest developments in ophthalmic sutures and needles. *Highlights of Ophthal., Monthly Letter.* 6(2): 1-4, 1978.

BOYD, B.F.: The treatment of traumatic cataract in childhood with lens implantation. *Highlights of Ophthal., Monthly Letter.* 6(7), 1978.

BOYD, B.F.: Why the new, strong tendency toward a posterior chamber intraocular lens? *Highlights of Ophthal., Monthly Letter.* 7(11): 1-3, 1979.

BRAS, J.F.: Review of Binkhorst intraocular lenses. *Brit. J. Ophthal.* 61: 631-633, 1977.

BRENNER, L.: Patient-acceptance of macular edema with intraocular lenses. In: *Current concepts in cataract surgery,* pp. 219-220 St. Louis, C.V. Mosby, 1976.

BRESNICK, G.H.: Eyes containing anterior chamber acrylic implants. Pathological complications. *Arch. Ophthal.* 82: 726-737, 1969.

BRINKMAN, C.J.J. and R.M. BROEKHUYSE: Cell mediated immunity in relation to cataract and cataract surgery. *Brit. J. Ophthal.* 63: 301-305, 1979.

BRODRICK, J.D.: The cornea and intraocular lenses. *Am. Intraoc. Impl. Soc. J.* 4(2): 30-33, 1978.

BRODSTEIN, R.S.: Letter to the editor, *Am. Intraoc. Impl. Soc. J.* 4(1): 64-65, 1978.

BRONNER, A. and C. HEYDACKER: La correction optique de l'aphaque. *Conférences d'optique médicale: Lab. H. Faure* 11: 1-27, 1970.

BROWN, S.I. and J.M. McLEAN: Peripheral corneal edema after cataract extraction a new clinical entity. *Trans. Am. Ac. Ophthal. & Otol.* 79: 465-468, 1969.

BROWN, S.I.: Peripheral corneal edema after cataract extraction. *Am. J. Ophthal.* 70: 326-328, 1970.

BROWN, R.M. and J.M. ENOCH: Combined rules of thumb in aniseikonic prescriptions. *Am. J. Ophthal.* 69: 118-126, 1970.

BROWN, C.A.: Intraocular lenses in retrospect. *Proc. R. Soc. Med.* 63: 310, 1970.

BROWN, C.A.: Anterior chamber implants with the Ridley tripod lens. *Proc. Roy. Soc. Med.* 69: 908-911, 1976.

BROWN, H.F.: A review of 21 cases of the Medallion circular loop metal clip lens. *Am. Intraoc. Impl. Soc. J.* 3-4: 182-183, 1977.

BROWN, H.F.: A report on the Medallion Circular loop lens. *Cont. & Intraoc. Lens Med. J.* 4(1): 41-42, 1978.

BUCCI, M.G.: Changes in weight of the rabbit vitreous by oral administration of glycerin. *Boll. Ocul.* 42: 569-577, 1963.

BURIAN H.M.: Optics: Fusion in unilateral aphakia. *Trans. Am. Ac. Ophthal. & Otol.* 66: 1962.

BUXTON, J.N., C.F., BARER, M.S. JAFFE and F.A. MANOPOLI: Clinical evaluation of the Kelman anterior intraocular lens. *Am. Intraoc. Impl. Soc. J.* 4: 216-218, 1978.
BUXTON, J.N. and M.S. JAFFE: Combined keratoplasty, cataract extraction and intraocular lens implantation. *Am. Intraoc. Impl. Soc. J.* 3: 110, 1978.
BYER, N.E.: Clinical study of lattice degeneration of the retina. *Trans. Am. Ac. Ophthal. & Otol.* 69: 1064-1082, 1965.
BYRON, H.M.: Intraocular implant surgery for beginner. *Cont. & Intraoc. Lens Med. J.* 3(2): 66-70, 1977.
BYRON, H.M.: Malpractice aspects of implant surgery. *Cont. & Intraoc. Lens Med. J.* 3(3): 41-47, 1977.
BYRON, H.M.: Anterior segment complications of implant surgery. *Trans. Am. Ac. Ophthal. & Otol.* 86: 621-624, 1979.
BYRON, H.M.: Case report on long term implant tolerance. *Am. Intraoc. Impl. Soc. J.* 5(1): 46-48, 1979.

CAPELLA, J.A.: Regeneration of endothelium in diseased and injured corneas. *Am. J. Ophthal.* 74: 810-817, 1972.
CASTLEMAN, L.D.: Pseudophakia anterior surface membrane. *Am. Intraoc. Impl. Soc. Newsletter.* 1: 48, September 1975.
CASTLEMAN, L.D.: Initial results with the Choyce Mark VIII lens. *Cont. & Intraoc. Lens Med. J.* 4(1): 34-40, 1978.
CATCHPOLE, B.N.: *Lancet.* I: 531 (letter) 1958.
CAUDELL, P.M.: The first twelve years of intraocular lens construction. *An. Inst. Barraquer.* 11-4: 531-542, 1962.
CHAPIRO, A.: Reductions induced by Ionizing Radiations. In: *Encyclopedia of Polymer Science and Technology.* 11: 702-760, 1962.
CHENG, H. and G.D. STURROCK, B. RUBENSTEIN and C. BULPITT: Corneal oedema and enthelial cell loss after iris-clip lens implantation. *Trans. Ophthal. Soc. U.K.* 97: 91-94, 1977.
CHENG, H.: Corneal edema: Iris-clip lens implantation and simple intracapsular extraction compared. *Ophthal. Surg.* 8(3): 64-69, 1977.
CHOWDHURY, A.M. and J.F. BRAS: Posterior dislocation of an intraocular lens implant and its removal. *Brit. J. Ophthal.* 61: 327-328, 1977.
CHOYCE, D.P.: Correction of uni-ocular aphakia by means of anterior chamber acrylic implants. *Trans. Ophthal. Soc. U.K.* 78: 459-470, 1958.
CHOYCE, D.P.: Correction of uni-ocular aphakia by means of anterior chamber acrylic implants. *Acta Concil. Ophthal. Belgica* (Brussels) II: 1705-1708, 1958.
CHOYCE, D.P.: Corrections of uni-ocular aphakia by means of all-acrylic anterior chamber implants. Review of 100 cases. *Brit. Med. J.* 3: 609-612, 1959.
CHOYCE, D.P.: The correction of uniocular aphakia by means of all-acrylic anterior chamber implants. *Am. J. Ophthal.* 49: 417-439, 1960.
CHOYCE, D.P.: The uses of acrylic anterior chamber implants illustrated by cases shown. *Proc. Royal Soc. Med.* 54: 849-856, 1961.
CHOYCE, D.P.: All-acrylic anterior-chamber implants in ophthalmic surgery. *Lancet.* II: 165-171, 1961.
CHOYCE, D.P.: All-acrylic anterior chamber implants. New developments and uses. *Arch. Ophthal.* 66: 188-200, 1961.
CHOYCE, D.P.: Anterior-chamber implants with built-in stenopaeic aperture. *Lancet.* II: 1233-1234, 1961.
CHOYCE, D.P.: A Galilean telescope uwing an anterior chamber inplant as eyepiece. *Lancet.* I: 794-796, 1963.
CHOYCE, D.P.: *Intra-ocular lenses and implants.* 211 pages, London, H.K. Lewis, 1964.
CHOYCE, D.P.: Mark VI, VII & VIII fixed-length all-acrylic Strampelli Choyce anterior chamber implants. *J. Soc. Science Med.*, Lisbon, 128: 665, 1964.
CHOYCE, D.P.: The Mark VI, Mark VII and Mark VIII Choyce anterior chamber implants. *Proc. Royal Soc. Med.* 58: 729-731, 1965.
CHOYCE, D.P.: Intraocular lenses and implants. *E.E.N.T. Digest 28*, 83-90, 1966.
CHOYCE, D.P.: Intra-cameral and intra-corneal implants. A decade of personal experience. *Trans. Ophthal. Soc. U.K.* 86: 507-525, 1966.

CHOYCE, D.P.: The present status of intra-cameral and intra-corneal implants. *Canad. J. Ophth.* 3: 295-311, 1968.
CHOYCE, D.P. and G.H. BRESNICK: Eyes containing anterior chamber acrylic implants. Correspondence. *Arch. Ophthal.* 84: 703-704, 1970.
CHOYCE, D.P.: Intra-ocular implants. Nursing Times 28th May and 4th June. St. Albans, Fisher, Knight & Co. Ltd. 1970.
CHOYCE, D.P.: Long-term tolerance of Choyce Mk. 1 and Mk. VIII anterior chamber implants. *Proc. Royal Soc. Med.* 63: 310-313, 1970.
CHOYCE, D.P.: History of Intraocular Implants. *An. Ophthal.* 5(10): 1113-20, 1973.
CHOYCE, D.P.: Intracameral lenses and implants. In: *Cataract and Abnormalities of the Lens*, ed. by J.G. Bellows, Grune & Stratton, inc. pp. 412-419, 1975.
CHOYCE, D.P.: The latest facts and figures on anterior chamber lens implant. *Cont. and Intraoc. Lens Med. J.* 2(4): 60-62, 1976.
CHOYCE, D.P.: The Choyce Mk. VIII anterior chamber implant secondary or primary insertion. *Cont. & Intraoc. Lens Med. J.* 2(4): 56-58, 1976.
CHOYCE, D.P.: Interview. *Highlights Ophthal.* pp. 244-345, 1975-1976.
CHOYCE, D.P.: The theoretical ideal for an artificial lens implant to correct aphakia. *Trans. Ophth. Soc.* U.K. 97: 94-95, 1977.
CHOYCE, D.P.: The Choyce Mk. VIII anterior chamber implant: Primary and secondary implantation compared. *Ophthal. Surg.* 8(3): 49-53, 1977.
CHOYCE, D.P.: Restoration of binocular vision. *Ophthal. Surg.* 8(3): 102-104, 1977.
CHOYCE, D.P.: New eyes for old? *Spectrum International.* Vol. XX(3): 41-46, 1978.
CHOYCE, D.P.: Complications of the A.C. implants of the early 1950's and the U.G.H. or Ellingson syndrome of the late 1970's. *Am. Intraoc. Impl. Soc. J.*, 2: 22-29, 1978.
CHOYCE, D.P.: The evaluation of the anterior chamber up to, and including the Choyce Mark IX. *Trans. Am. Ac. Ophthal. & Otol.* 86(2): 197-206, 1979.
CHOYCE, D.P.: The Choyce Mark VIII and Mark IX anterior chamber implants. *Am. Intraoc. Impl. Soc. J.* 3: 217-221, 1979.
CHRISTIANSEN, J.M., C.R. KOLLARITS, H. FUKUI, M.L. FISHMAN, R.G. MICHELS and I. MIKUNI: Intraocular irrigating solutions and lens clarity. *Am. J. Ophthal.* 82: 594-597, 1976.
CHRISTMAN, E.H.: Correction of aniseikonia in monocular aphakia. *Arch. Ophthal.* (Chicago), 85: 148-149, 1971.
CLAYMAN, H.M., N.S. JAFFE, D.S. LIGHT and D.M. EICHENBAUM: Lens implantation surgery in the second eye. *Ophthal. Surg.* 8(3): 45-48, 1977.
CLAYMAN, H.M., N.S., JAFFE and D.S. LIGHT: Lens implantation and diabetes mellitus. *Am. J. Ophthal.* 88: 990-999, 1979.
CLAYMAN, H.M., N.S. JAFFE, S. LIGHT and D.M. EICHENBAUM: Lens implantation, miosis and glaucoma. *Am. J. Ophthal.* 87: 121-123, 1979.
CLEASBY, G.B.: The uses of vitreous surgery instruments in lens implant problems. *Am. Intraoc. Impl. Soc. J.* 4(3): 88-89, 1978.
CLEVENGER, C.E.: Clinical prediction versus ultrasound measurement of IOL power. *Am. Intraoc. Impl. Soc. J.* 4(4): 222-224, 1978.
COGAN, D.G.: A new method for studying endothelial regeneration: Biomicroscopic observations on normal and vitamin C deficient animals. *Ophthalmologica* (Basel) 118: 440-443, 1949.
COHAN, B.E., A.C. PEARCH and S. SCHWARTS: Broken nylon iris fixation sutures. *Am. J. Ophthal.* 88: 982-989, 1979.
COLE, D.F. and W.G. UNGER: Prostaglandins as Mediators for the responses of the eye to trauma. *Exp. Eye Res.* 17: 357-368, 1973.
COLEMAN, D.J.: Ophthalmic biometry using ultrasound. *International Ophthalmology Clinics.* 9(3): 667-683, 1969.
COLENBRANDER, M.C.: Plastic voorkamerlenzen in de oogheelkunde. *Ned. T. Geneesk.* 106: 278, 1962.
COLENBRANDER, M.C.: Calculation of the power of an iris clip lens for distent vision. *Brit. J. Ophthal.* 57: 735-740, 1973.
COLES, W.H.: Effect of antibiotics on the in vitro rabbit corneal endothelium. *Invest. Ophthal.* 14(3): 246-249, 1975.
CONQUET, P., B. PLAZONNET and J.C. LE DOUAREC: Arachidonic acid—induced elevation of intraocular pressure and anti-inflammatory agents. *Invest. Ophthal.* 14: 772-775, 1975.

COPPER, A.C.: *An introduction to clinical orbitotonometry.* Thesis, Leiden, 1948.
CORBOY, J.M.: Choyce lens warp testing: Effect of temperature and pressure changes. *Am. Intraoc. Impl. Soc. J.* 3: 111-112, 1978.
CORBOY, J.M.: Traumatic loss of an anterior chamber lens. *Am. Intraoc. Impl. Soc. J.* 5(1): 54-56, 1979.
COSCAS, G. and G. HALIMI: La correction optique des aphaques. *Arch. Ophtal* (Paris), 26: 295-308, 1966.
COSCAS, G.: Maculopathies Œdémateuses. *Bull. des Sociétés d'ophtalmologie de France. Rapport annual Soc. d'ophtal. de Paris.* Special issue, 1972.
COZEAN, C.H. and S.R. WALTMAN: Endothelial cell loss with the Choyce anterior chamber lens. *Am. Intraoc. Impl. Soc. J.* 1: 13-14, 1979.

DABEZIES, O.H., Jr.: Defects of vision through aphakic spectacle lenses. *Trans. Am. Acad. Ophthal. & Otol.* 86: 352-387, 1979.
DALLAS, N.L.: Five-year trial of the Binkhorst iris-clip lens in aphakia. *Trans. Ophthal. Soc. U.K.* 90: 725-732, 1970.
DALLAS, N.L.: The history of intraocular lenses. *Cont. & Intraoc. Lens Med. J.* 2(3): 68-70, 1976.
DALLAS, N.L.: The safer operation for iris-clip lens implants. *Trans. Ophthal. Soc. U.K.* 97: 82-83, 1977.
DANNHEIM, H.: Vorderkammerlinse mit elastischen Halteschlingen. *Ber. Dtsch. Ophthal. Ges. Heidelberg* 60: 267-268, 1956.
DANNHEIM, H.: Types of anterior chamber lenses with elastic loops. *An. Inst. Barraquer.* III-4: 570-572, 1962.
DANNHEIM, H. JR. In: Abstract of meeting French Implant Soc. Cannes, May 2.5.1979. *Newsletter Internat. Intraocular Implant Club*, Sept. 1979 nr. 9.
DARIN, J.J.: Survey on secondary lens implantation. *Am. Intraoc. Impl. Soc. Newsletter.* 1: 32-36, sept. 1975.
DARIN, J.J.: Survey of secondary lens implantation. *Am. Jntraoc. Jmpl. Soc. J.* 1: 31-33, 1977.
DAVIDSON, B., B.P. KRATZ, T.B. MAZZOCCO and W.F. MALONEY: An evaluation of the Honan intraocular pressure reducer. *Am. Intraocular Impl. Soc. J.* 3: 237, 1979.
De HAVEN, C.R.: Letter to the editor. *Am. Intraoc. Impl. Soc. J.* 4: 67, 1978.
DELMARCELLE, Y. and J. LUYCKS-BACUS: Biométrie du segment antérieur dans la cataracte sénile. *Acta Ophthalmologica.* 49: 454-466, 1971.
DELMARCELLE, Y., J. FRANÇOIS, F. GOES, J. COLLIGNON-BRACH, J. LUYCKX-BACUS and H. VERBRAEKEN: Biometrie Oculaire Clinique. *Bull. Soc. Belge d'Ophtal.* 172.1, 1976.
DE POLI, A. and M.A. ROMAGNOLI: Experimental research on acrylic lenses in the anterior chamber and the tissue tollerance for plastic materials. *Atti. Soc. Oftal. Lombarda.* 10: 143-150, 1955.
DE ROETH, A.: Ridley's cataract operation. *Am. J. Ophthal.* 36: 1568-1570, 1953.
DETHMERS, H.W.: Management of some complications of the Medallion circular loop lens. *Am. Intraoc. Impl. Soc. J.* 1: 36-38, 1978.
DETTINGER, G.B. and W.F. BOWERS: Tissue response to Orlon and Dacron sutures. *Surgery.* 42: 325-335, 1957.
DEUTMAN, A.F. and A.T.M. VAN BALEN: Macular oedema after intraocular lens implantation. *Ophthalmologica* (Basel). 173: 196-199, 1976.
DEUTMAN, A.F., W.F. TREFFERS and P.J.M. CUJPERS: Die Netzhaut nach extrakapsulären Linsen. In: *Kunststoffimplantate in der Ophthalmologie.* W. Jaeger, Ed., J.F. Bergmann Verlag Munich, pp. 93-103, 1978.
DE VOE, A.G.: Monocular aphakia and intraocular lenses (editorial). *Arch. Ophthal.* 72: 152-153, 1964.
DICKERSON, D.E.: Peripheral fundus examination in the pseudophakic eye. *Am. Intraoc. Impl. Soc. J.* 3(1): 34-35, 1977.
DIDDIE, K.R. and R.E. SMITH: Intraocular gas injection in the pseudophakic patient. *Am. J. Ophthal.* 89: 659-661, 1980.
DODEN, W. and H. SCHMITT: Veränderungen an Kunststoff-Fäden nach langer Verweildauer im Hornhautgewebe. *Klin. Mbl. Augenheilk.* 164: 155-159, 1974.

DODEN, W. and H. SCHMITT: Mikroskopische Befunde an unbenutzten bestrahlten und unbestrahlten Kunststoff-Fäden. *Klin. Mbl. Augenheilk.* 167: 291-294, 1975.
DOHLMAN, C.H. and H.M. FREEMAN: Recent advances in the use of alloplastic materials in ocular surgery. *Docum. Ophthal.* 25: 1-20, 1968.
DOHLMAN, C.H.: Report of 2nd Meeting of Intra-Ocular Implant Club in Budapest. *Arch. Ophthal.* 88: 693, 1972.
DOLLFUS, M.A. and I. BORSOTTI: Étude expérimentale de la tolérance intra-oculaire des aciers et alliages inoxydables industriels. *Soc. Ophth. Paris.* 5: 188-194, 1938.
DRAEGER, J.: Some methodical aspects of the implantation of Binkhorst lenses. *Ophthal.* 5: 35-37, 1976.
DRAEGER, J.: Probleme der Indikationsstellung der Nachbehandlung und der Komplikationen bei Kunststofflinsenimplantation. *Manuscript read before the German Ophth. Soc. Meeting, Heidelberg, Sept. 1977.*
DRAEGER, J.: Surgical Technique: Intracapsular Symposium: Intraocular Lens. *Trans. Am. Ac. Ophthal. & Otol.* 81: 97-101, 1977.
DRAEGER, J., A. KOUDELKA and P. MODZANOWSKI: Erfahrungen mit der Implantation von Vorderkammerlinsen. *Klin. Mbl. Augenheilk.* 172: 295-305, 1978.
DRAEGER, J.: Probleme der Indikationsstellung der Nachbehandlung und der Komplikationen bei Kunststofflinsenimplantation. In: *Kunststoffimplantate in der Ophthalmologie.* W. Jaeger, Ed., J.F. Bergmann Verlag, Munich, pp. 116-121, 1978.
DREWS, R.C.: Use of millipore filters. *Am. J. Ophthal.* 50: 159-160, 1960.
DREWS, R.C.: Clean Eye Surgery. *Current Concepts in Cataract Surgery.* Ed. J.M. Emery & D. Paton, St. Louis: C.V. Mosby Co., pp. 33-36, 1976.
DREWS, R.C.: Clean eye surgery. *Revista Brasileira de Oftalmologica.* 35(2): 13-18, 1976.
DREWS, R.C.: A lens implant holder. *Trans. Am. Ac. Ophthal. & Otol.* 81: 912-913, 1976.
DREWS, R.C.: The management of patients with intraocular lenses. Guidelines for those who do not perform this operation. *Trans. Ophthal. Soc. U.K.* 97: 78-81, 1977.
DREWS, R.C.: Refractive error for intraocular lens of known power program for Hewlett Packard 25/25 c computers. *Am. Intraoc. Impl. Soc. J.* 2: 109, 1977.
DREWS, R.C.: The moving fluid field in ophthalmic surgery. *Arch. Ophthal.* 95: 669, 1977.
DREWS, R.C.: A practical approach to lens implant power. *Am. Intraoc. Impl. Soc. J.* 3-4, 170-176, 1977.
DREWS, R.C.: A new needle for iris sutures—especially for the Medallion intraocular lens. *Ophthal. Surg.* 8(5): 100, 1977.
DREWS, R.C.: Calculation of intraocular power: A program for the Hewlett Packard 97 calculator. *Am. Intraoc. Impl. Soc. J.* 3-4: 209-212, 1977.
DREWS, R.C.: Programs for the HP-25/C calculators for lens implant power. *Am. Intraoc. Impl. Soc. J.* 1: 48-49, 1977.
DREWS, R.C.: Management of subluxated intraocular lenses. *Cont. & Intraoc. Lens Med. J.* 3(3): 36-40, 1977.
DREWS, R.C.: Lens implantation: premises and promises. *Palestra oftalmologica panamericana.* 1(2): 16-39, 1977.
DREWS, R.C.: Polypropylene. *Am. Intraoc. Impl. Soc. J.* 4(4): 209, 1978.
DREWS, R.C.: Penetrating keratoplasty combined with intraocular lens implantation in aphakia. XXII Concilium Ophthalmologicum Kyoto, 1978, Acta Pars II, p. 1406, *Excerpta Medica*, Amsterdam-Oxford, 1979.
DREWS, R.C.: Inflammatory response, endophthalmitis, corneal dystrophy, glaucoma, retinal detachment, dislocation, refractive error, lens removal and enucleation. *Trans. Am. Ac. Ophthal. & Otol.* 85: 164-175, 1978.
DREWS, R.C., M.E. SMITH and O. OKUN: Scanning electron microscopy of intraocular lenses. *Trans. Am. Ac. Ophthal. & Otol.* 85, 1978.
DREWS, R.C. and S.R. WALTMAN: Endothelial cell loss in intraocular lens placement. *Am. Intraoc. Impl. Soc. J.* 2: 14-16, 1978.
DREWS, R.C.: The management of patients with intraocular lenses. Guidelines for those who do not perform this operation. *Ophthal. Surg.* 10(2): 56-64, 1979.
DREWS, R.C.: New trends on intraocular lenses. *Highlights of Ophthal. B.F. Boyd.* 15: 252, 1978-1979.

DREWS, R.C.: A pigtail suture guide. *Trans. Am. Ac. Ophthal. & Otol.* 86: 851, 1979.
DUBOIS-POULSEN, A.: L'inadaptation de l'aphakie. *Année thérapeutique et clinique en Ophthalmologie.* 17: 231-234, 1966.
DUDRANGE, R.: *Prothèses optiques oculaires. Théorie optique.* Vol. I, Éditions Labor. de Recherches optiques, 49 Blvd. de Courcelles, Paris 1955.
DUFFNER, L.R., W.K. WALLACE and W.R. STILES: The Miami cooperative community study on the Copeland intraocular lens. *Am. J. Ophthal.* 82: 590-593, 1976.
DUFFNER, L.R.: The Miami Pseudophakos Study—A suggested community study protocol. *Trans. Am. Ac. Ophth. & Otol.* 81: 128-131, 1976.
DUKE ELDER, P.M. and W.S. DUKE ELDER: The vascular responses of the eye. *Proc. Roy. Soc.*, London (B), 109-79, 1931.
DUKE-ELDER, S. and K.C. WYBAR: *System of Ophthalmology* vol. II 93-94, 1961.
DUKE ELDER, W.S.: *The Foundation of Ophthalmology. System of Ophthalmology.* Vol. VII, Ed. by Henry Kimpton, London, 1962.
DUKE ELDER, W.S. and J.H. DOBREE: *Diseases of the Retina. System of Ophthalmology.* Vol. X, Ed. by Henry Kimpton, London, 1967.
DUKE ELDER, W.S.: *Ophthalmic Optics and refraction. System of Ophthalmology.* Vol. V, Ed. by Henry Kimpton, London, 1970.
DULANEY, D. and W.F. MALONEY: Technique for closed-chamber insertion of trans-iridectomy prolene clip lens. *Am. Intraoc. Impl. Soc. J.* 4(2): 8-10, 1978.
DULANEY, D.: I.O.L.'s and iris erosion. *Am. Intraoc. Impl. Soc. J.* 4(4): 208, 1978. (Letters to the editor).
DULANEY, D.: A double guide technique to ensure capsular fixation. *Am. Intraoc. Impl. Soc. J.* 5(2): 156, 1979.
DUMAS, J. and L. SCHEPENS: Chorioretinal lesions predisposing to retinal breaks. *Am. J. Ophthal.* 61: 620, 1966.
DU PONT GUERRY, III: Present status of the anterior chamber lens. *Am. J. Ophthal.* 50: 250-258, 1960.
DUNN, M.J.: Factors influencing the specification of intraocular lens dioptric power. *Am. Intraoc. Impl. Soc. J.* 2: 130-133, 1977.
DUNN, M.J.: The resolving power of intraocular lens implants. *Am. Intraoc. Impl. Soc. J.* 4(2): 126-129, 1978.
DUNN, M.J.: A method for correlating spectacle and intraocular lens prescriptions. *Am. Intraoc. Impl. Soc. J.* 4(2): 18-21, 1978.
DYER, J.A. and K.A. OGLE: Correction of unilateral aphakia with contact lenses. *Am. J. Ophthal.* 50: 11-17, 1960.

EAKINS, K.E.: Prostaglandin and non-prostaglandin mediated breakdown of the blood-aqueous barrier. *Exp. Eye Res.* Suppl. 483-498, 1977.
EASTY, D., N. DALLAS and R. O'MALLEY: Aphakic macular oedema following prosthetic lens implantation. *Brit. J. Ophthal.* 61: 321-326, 1977.
EDELHAUSER, H.F., D.L. VAN HORN, R.O. SCHULTZ and R.A. HYNDIUK: Comparative toxicity of intraocular irrigating solutions on the corneal endothelium. *Am. J. Ophthal.* 81(4): 473-481, 1976.
EDELHAUSER, H.F., R. CONNERING and D.L. VAN HORN: Intraocular irrigating solutions. *Arch. Ophthal.* 96: 516, 1978.
EHRICH, W.: Plexiglas (P.M.M.A.) in der Vorderkammer. *Klin. Mbl. Augenheilk.* 168: 493, 1976.
EICHENBAUM, D.M.: Pars plana vitrectomy for complications of intraocular lens implantation. *Ophthal. Surg.* 8(3): 127-128, 1977.
EICHENBAUM, D.M., N.S. JAFFE, H.M. CLAYMAN and D.S. LIGHT: Pars plana vitrectomy as a primary treatment for acute bacterial endophthalmitis. *Am. J. Ophthal.* 86: 167-171, 1978.
ELLINGSON, F.T.: Complications with the Choyce Mark VIII anterior chamber lens implant (uveitis-glaucoma-hyphema). *Am. Intraoc. Impl. Soc. J.* 3-4: 199-201, 1977.
ELLINGSON, F.T.: Importance of inspecting Choyce Mark VIII lenses. *Am. Intraoc. Impl. Soc. J.* 2: 118, 1977.
ELLINGSON, F.T.: The uveitis-glaucoma-hyphema syndrome associated with the mark VIII anterior chamber lens implant. *Am. Intraoc. Impl. Soc. J.* 2: 50-53, 1978.

EIFRIG, D.E.: Intracapsular plastic lens-loop fixation in the rabbit. *Arch. Ophthal.* 94: 1167, 1976.

ELLIOTT, J. and J.D. MORRISON: Anaesthesia for ophthalmic surgery. In: *Anaesthesia for Eye, Ear, Nose and Throat Surgery.* Ed. by W.F.K. Morrow and J.D. Morrison, Churchill Livingstone, pp. 112-127, 1975, Edinburgh.

EMERY, J.M., D.J. LANDIS and R.M. BENOLKEN: The phacoemulsifier: an evaluation of performance safety margins. *Curr. Concepts in Cataract Surgery: Selected Proceedings of Third Biennial Cataract Surgical Congress.* Ed. by J.M. and D. Paton St. Louis, C.V. Mosby Co., pp. 208-222, 1974.

EMERY, J.M. and D. PATON: Phacoemulsification: A survey of 2875 cases. *Current Concepts in Cataract Surgery: Selected Proceedings of Third Biennial Cataract Surgical Congress.* St. Louis, C.V. Mosby Co., 1974, pp. 222-224.

EMERY, J.M. and D. PATON: *Current Concepts in Cataract Surgery: Selected Proceedings of the Third Biennial Cataract Surgery Congress.* St. Louis, C.V. Mosby Co., 1974.

EMERY, J.M. and D. PATON: *Current Concepts in Cataract Surgery: Selected Proceedings of the fourth Biennial Cataract Surgery Congress.* St. Louis, C.V. Mosby Co., 1976.

EMERY, M., K.A. WILHELMUS and S. ROSENBERG: Complications of phacoemulsification. *Trans. Am. Ac. Ophthal. & Otol.* 85: 141-150, 1978.

EMMRICH, K.: Vorderkammerlinsen aus Silikatglas. *Klin. Mbl. Augenheilk.* 132: 254-256, 1958.

ENOCH, J.M.: Physiology of monocular aphakia. *Trans. Am. Ac. Ophthal. & Otol.* 86: 391-398, 1979.

EPSTEIN, D.L.: Cystoid macular edema occuring 13 years after cataract extraction. *Am. J. Ophthal.* 83: 501-503, 1977.

EPSTEIN, E.: The Ridley lens implant. *Brit. J. Ophthal.* 41: 368-376, 1957.

EPSTEIN, E.: Modified Ridley lenses. *Brit. J. Ophthal.* 43: 29-33, 1959.

EPSTEIN, E.: Experience with modified Ridley lenses and others. *An. Inst. Barraquer.* 3(4): 555-561, 1962.

EPSTEIN, L.J. and W.J. GEERAETS: On the determination of the power of a lens implant. *Am. Intraoc. Impl. Soc. J.* 3: 87, 1977.

ERLICH, D.R. and R.H. KEATES: The use of an aspheric spectacle (Varilux-2) for implant patients. *Cont. & Intraoc. Lens Med. J.* 2: 75-76, 1979.

ESTERBROOK, M., P.G. TUFFNELL and J.C. HILL: Bacterial decontamination of polymethylmethacrylate in opthalmology. *Canad. J. Ophthal.* 4: 247-257, 1969.

EVERETT, W.G., G. HURITE and M. SORR: Retinal detachment following cataract extraction by phacoemulsification. *Mod. Probl. Ophthal.* 18: 503-507, 1977.

FAHMY, J.A., S. MØLLER and M. WEIS: Bacterial flora in relation to cataract extraction. *Acta Ophthalmologica.* 54: 271-280, 1976.

FASANELLA, R.M.: *Modern advances in cataract surgery.* Philadelphia, J.B. Lip, 1953.

FASANELLA, R.M.: *Prevention et traitement des complications de la chirurgie oculaire.* Paris, Masson et Co., 1960.

FAULBORN, J. and G. MACKENSON: Spätkomplikationen bei Vorderkammerlinsen. *Klin. Mbl. Augenheilk.* 169: 774, 1976.

FAULBORN, J., B.P. CONWAY and R. MACHEMER: Surgical complications of pars plana vitreous surgery. *Trans. Am. Ac. Ophthal & Otol.* 85, 1978.

FAULKNER, G.D.: Letter. in: Consultation section. Ed. by D.D. Shepard. *Am. Intraoc. Impl. Soc. J.* 5: 359, 1979.

FECHNER, P.U.: Methylcellulose in lens implantation. *Am. Intraoc. Impl. Soc. J.* 3(3-4): 180-181, 1977.

FECHNER, P.U.: Laser-coagulation of ruptured fixation suture after lens-implantation. *Am. Intraoc. Impl. Soc. J.* 2: 54, 1978.

FECHNER, P.U.: Erfahrungen mit der Implantation einer künstlicher Augenlinsen. *Klin. Mbl. Augenheilk.* 1722: 852-862, 1978.

FECHNER, P.U.: Methylcellulose als Gleitsubstanz für die Implantation künstlicher Augenlinsen. *Klin. Mbl. Augenheilk.* 174: 136, 1979.

FECHNER, P.U.: Tadini, the man who invented the artificial lens. *Am. Intraoc. Impl. Soc. J.* 5(1): 22-23, 1979.

FECHNER, P.U., M.U. FECHNER and H. REIS: Der Okulist Tadini zur Geschichte der Künstlichen Augenlinsen *Klin. Mbl. Augenheilk.* 176: 1003-1011, 1980.

FECHNER, P.U.: *Intraocularlinsen: Grundlagen und Operationslehre. Bücherei des Augenarztes.* Heft 82, F. Enke Verlag, Stuttgart, 1980.
FEDRIZZI, G.: Tolerance of the acrylic lens of the Strampelli type in the aphakic rabbit eye. *Atti, Soc. Oftal. Lombarda.* 10: 339-343, 1955.
FERREIRA, S.H., S. MONCADA and J.R. VANE: Indomethacin and aspirin abolish prostaglandin release from the spleen. *Nature, New Biol.* 231: 237-239, 1971.
FINE, M.: Keratoplasty for bullous keratoplasty with intraocular lens. *Am. Intraoc. Impl. Soc. J.* 4(2): 12-13, 1978.
FINK, A.I., D.B. GOLDBERG and H.L. GOULD: Canula modification of the Fink-Weinstein Syringe. *Cont. & Intraoc. Lens Med. J.* 5(2): 45-47, 1979.
FLIERINGA, H.J.: Procedure to prevent vitreous loss. *Am. J. Ophthal.* 36: 1618-1619, 1953.
FLOCKS, M.F., C.S. LITTWIN and L.E. ZIMMERMAN: Phacolytic Glaucoma. *Archives of Ophthal.* 4: 37-45, 1955.
FORGIE, R.E., J. MORTIMER and B.H. LORIMER: Clinical evaluation of an inexpensive ultrasound oculometer for ocular biometry. *Am. J. Ophthal.* 87: 292, 1979.
FORSTOT, S.L., W.L. BLACKWELL, N.S. JAFFE and H.E. KAUFMAN: The effect of intraocular lens implantation on the corneal endothelium. *Trans. Am. Ac. Ophthal. & Otol.* 83: 195-212, 1977.
FRANÇOIS, J., M. GDAL-ON, T. TAKEUCHI and V. VICTORIA-TRONCOSO: Ocular hypotension and massage of the eyeball. *Annals of Ophthal.* 5: 645-662, 1973.
FRANÇOIS, J.: Fortschritt und Rückschritt in der Kataraktchirurgie. *Klin. Mbl. Augenheilk.* 166: 745-751, 1975.
FRANÇOIS, J., H. VERBRAEKEN and I. STRANSKI: Aphakic retinal detachment. *Ophthalmologica*, Basel. 175: 181-184, 1977.
FRANÇOIS, J. and H. VERBRAEKEN: Complications in 1000 consecutive intracapsular cataract extractions. *Ophthalmologica.* Basel. 180: 121-128, 1980.
FRANÇOIS, J., and H. VERBRAEKEN: Complications dans mille extractions intracapsulaire consécutives de cataracte. *Bull. Soc. Belge.* Vol. 187-II, 59-70, 1980.
FREEMAN, H.M., J.G. DOBBIE, M.W. FRIEDMAN, G.P. JOHNSTON, O.H. JUNGSCHAFFER, A.R. McPHERSON, D.H. NICHOLSON, H.F. SPALTER, C.P. WILKINSON and S. TASMAN: Pseudophakic retinal detachment. *Mod. Probl. Ophthal.* 20: 345-353, 1979.
FREEMAN, H.M.: Discussion of presentation by Dr. Williams Snyder, et al. *Ophthal.* (AAOO) 86: 239-241, 1979.
FREY, T., D. FRIENDLY and D. WYATT: Re-evaluation of monocular cataracts in children. *Am. J. Ophthal.* 76: 381-388, 1973.
FRIEDMAN, M.W.: The treatment of 4 cases of retinal detachment following insertion of an intraocular lens. *Mod. Probl. Ophthal.* 18: 494-495, 1977.
FUNG, W.E.: Phacoemulsification. *Trans. Am. Ac. Ophthal. & Otol.* 85: 46-51, 1978.
FYODOROV, S.N.: On preliminary results of implantation into eye of artificial lens made out of Soviet plastic masses. *Oftal. Z.* 17: 19-24, 1962.
FYODOROV, S.N.: Application of intraocular pupillary lenses for aphakia correction. *Vestn. Oftal.* 78: 76-83, 1965.
FYODOROV, S.N.: Methods employed to fix intraocular lenses. *Vestn. Oftal.* 82: 38-43, 1969.
FYODOROV, S.N.: Combined implantations of the intraocular iris clip lens in posttraumatic lens opacifications and secondary cataracts. *Ophthalmologica* (Basel). *Addit. ad* 158: 301-302, 1969.
FYODOROV, S.: N.: Implantation of iris-clip-lenses with single stage removal of the crystalline lens through basal coloboma of the iris. *Vestn. Oftal.* 82: 58-61, 1969.
FYODOROV, S.N. and E.V. EGOROVA: Auto-alloplastic model of the anterior chamber intraocular lens. *Vestn. Oftal.* 2: 33-38, 1972.
FYODOROV, S.N.: Modern concepts of intraocular lenses. *Rep. Moscow Inst. Med. Stomatol.* 41-47, 1973.
FYODOROV, S.N. and E.V.EGOROVA: Surgery in traumatic cataract with the use of intraocular correction. *Vestn. Oftal.* 2: 22-26, 1974.
FYODOROV, S.N., M.A. GALIN and A. LINKSZ: Calculation of the optical power of intraocular lenses. *Invest. Ophthal.* 14(8): 625-628, 1975.

FYODOROV, S.N.: Long-term results of 2000 operations of implantation of Fyodorov intraocular lenses performed in the Soviet Union. *Am. Intraoc. Impl. Soc. J.* 2: 101, 1977.

FYODOROV, S.N.: 3000 cases of Sputnik-style lens implantation. *Am. Intraoc. Impl. Soc. J.* 1: 37-39, 1980.

GALAND, A.: L'Abord des cataractes secondaires par la pars plana du corps ciliaire. *Bull. Soc. Belge d'Ophtal.* 186: 87-96, 1979.

GALIN, M.A., R.D. BINKHORST and M.L. KWITKO: Ocular dehydration. *Am. J. Ophthal.* 66(2): 233-235, 1968.

GALIN, M.A.: Intraocular lens implants. *Am. J. Ophthal.* 65: 932, 1968.

GALIN, M.A., E. CHOWCHUVECH and A. GALIN: Tissue culture methods for testing the toxicity of ocular plastic materials. *Am. J. Ophthal.* 79(4): 665-669, 1975.

GALIN, M.A.: Optical and mechanical consideration of intraocular lenses. *Am. Intraoc. Impl. Soc. J.* 2(1): 22-23, 1976.

GALIN, M.A., E. CHOWCHUVECH and L. TURKISH: Uveitis and intraocular lenses. *Trans. Ophthal. Soc. U.K.* 96: 166-167, 1976.

GALIN, M.A., L. TURKISH and E. CHOWCHUVECH: Detection, removal and effect of unpolymerized methylmethacrylate in intraocular lenses. *Am. J. Ophthal.* 84: 153-159, 1977.

GALIN, M.A., S.A. OBSTBAUM, V. BONIUK, A. GALIN and D. SILVERSTONE: Iris-supported lens implantation vs. simple cataract extraction. An analysis of data. *Trans. Ophthal. Soc. U.K.* 97: 74-77, 1977.

GALIN, M.A.: Fyodorov Sputnik lens implant. in: '*Pseudophakos*', C.V. Mosby C°, p. 206-207, 1978.

GALIN, M.A., E.C. FETHEROLF, L.K. LIN and S.A. OBSTBAUM: Surgery and the endothelium. *Abstract of communication,* Am. Intraoc. Impl. Soc. Meeting, Los Angeles, March, 1978.

GALIN, M.A., E. FETHEROLF, L. LIN and A. SUGAR: Experimental cataract surgery: part I. *Ophthalmology.* 86: 213-218, 1979.

GALIN, M.A., E. FETHEROLF, L. LIN and D.L. VAN HORN: Experimental cataract surgery. Electron microscopy: part II. *Ophthalmology.* 86: 608-620, 1979.

GALIN, M.A., T.A. POOLE and S.A. OBSTBAUM: Retinal detachment in pseudophakia. *Am. J. Ophthal.* 88: 49-51, 1979.

GALIN, M.A., L.L. LIN, E. FETHEROLF S.A. OBSTBAUM and A. SUGAR: Time analysis of corneal endothelial cell density after cataract extraction. *Am. J. Ophthal.* 88: 93-96, 1979.

GALIN, M.A. and L. TURKISH: Sodium hydroxide sterilization of intraocular lenses. *Am. J. Ophthal.* 88: 560-564, 1979.

GALIN, M.A.: Studies of intraocular lens sterilization: The effect of NaOH on B. Subtilis spores. *Am. Intraoc. Lens Impl. J.* 1: 18-20, 1980.

GARTNER, S.: Optic Neuritis and macular edema after cataract surgery. In : *Complications after Cataract Surgery.* Ed. by F. Theodore. Boston, Little Brown and Co., 321-327, 1965.

GASS, J.D.M. and E.W.D. NORTON: Cystoid macular edema and papilloedema following cataract extraction. *Arch. Ophthal.* 76: 646-661, 1966.

GASS, J.D.M. and E.W.D. NORTON: Follow-up study of cystoid macular edema after cataract extraction. *Trans. Am. Ac. Ophthal. & Otol.* 73: 665-681, 1969.

GASS, J.D.M.: Lamellar Macular hole. A complication of cystoid macular edema after cataract extraction. *Arch. Ophthal.* 94: 793-800, 1976.

GASSET, A.R., L. LOBO and W. HOUDE: Permanent wear of soft contact lenses in aphakic eyes. *Am. J. Ophthal.* 83: 115-120, 1977.

GASTEIGER, H.: Beitrag zur Frage der Implantation von Vorderkammerlinsen. *Klin. Mbl. Augenheilk.* 132: 609-617, 1958.

GENTRY, J.H.: Results of 100 implants over two years. *Am. Intraoc. Impl. Soc. J.* 2: 119, 1977.

GERNET, H.: Ultraschall biometrie des Auges. *Klin. Mbl. Augenheilk.* 151: 853, 1967.

GERNET, H. and E. OLBRICH: L'excès de la courbe de réfraction de l'œil humain et ses causes. *Bull. de la Soc. Belg. d'Ophtal.* 149: 424-432, 1968.

GERNET, H.: Oculometriedaten bei Augengesunden. *Ber. 70. Zus. Dtsch. Ophth. Ges.* 598-599, 1969.
GERNET, H., H. OSTHOLT and H. WERNER: Neue klinische Grundlagen zur Binkhorst-Linseneinpflanzung bei Altersstar. *Klin. Mbl. Augenheilk.* 159: 135-136, 1971.
GERNET, H., H. OSTHOLT and H. WERNER: L'évaluation pré-opératoire des cristallins artificiels intra-oculaires. *Bull. Mém. Soc. Fr. Ophtal.* 84: 537-546, 1971.
GERNET, H. and H. OSTHOLT: Augenseitige Optik. Ein neues Gebiet der Klinischen Okulometrie. *Ophthalmologica* (Basel), 166: 120-143, 1973.
GILLS, J.P.: Intraocular lens in perspective. *Cont. & Intraoc. Lens Med. J.* 1(3): 39-47, 1975.
GILLS, J.P.: Suture fixation of iridocapsular lenses. *Cont. & Intraoc. Lens Med. J.* 2(2): 17, 1976.
GILLS, J.P.: Extracapsular cataract extraction with intraocular lens insertion by Gills'technique. *Abstract of the Am. Intraoc. Impl. Soc. Meeting L.A. March 1978.*
GILS, J.P.: Power of I.O.L. *Am. Intraoc. Impl. Soc. J.* 4(4): 163-164, 1978.
GILLS, J.P. and T.L. LOYD: Extracapsular cataract extraction with intraocular lens insertion. *Am. Intraoc. Impl. Soc. J.* 1: 9-12, 1979.
GILLS, J.P.: Constant mild compression of the eye to procedure hypotension. *Am. Intraoc. Impl. Soc. J.* 1: 52-53, 1979.
GILLS, J.P. and J.Mc.H. NIELSEN: Removal of wire-loop intraocular lenses and the insertion of Choyce lenses—tertiary lenses. *Cont. & Intraoc. Lens Med. J.* 2: 77-80, 1979.
GILLS, J.P.: Delivery of the lens nucleus in extracapsular surgery. *Cont. & Intraoc. Lens Med. J.* 1: 46-47, 1980.
GILLS, J.P.: Minimizing postoperative refractive error. *Cont. & Intraoc. Lens Med. J.* 1: 56-59, 1980.
GILLS, J.P.: Triple Procedures. *Cont. & Intraoc. Lens Med. J.* 1: 51-52, 1980.
GILLS, J.P.: Discissions with extracapsular cataract extraction. *Cont. & Intraoc. Lens Med. J.* 1: 48-50, 1980.
GILLS, J.P.: Preparations for surgery: Anaesthesia and ocular compression. *Cont. & Intraoc. Lens Med. J.* 1: 42-45, 1980.
GINSBERG, S.F.: The intraocular lens implant and cataract surgery. *Cont. Lens J.* 9: 21-28, 1976.
GIOVINCO, J. and D.L. THOMAS: A preliminary report of fifty consecutive cases of Choyce Mark VIII implantations. *Cont. & Intraoc. Lens Med. J.* 3(1): 54-59, 1977.
GIRARD, L.J., B. FRIEDMAN, C.D. MOORE, R.I. BLAU, C.D. BINKHORST and M.H. GOBIN: Intraocular implants and contact lenses. *Archives of Ophthal.* 68: 762-775, 1962.
GIRARD, L.J.: A scleral expander for prevention of scleral collapse during intraocular surgery. *Annals of Ophthal.* 5: 223-240, 1973.
GIRARD, L.J.: Cataract extraction by ultrasonic aspiration, vitrectomy by ultrasonic aspiration. In: *Current Concepts in Cataract Surgery.* Ed. J.M. Emery & D. Paton, St. Louis, C.V. Mosby Co., 109-111, 1976.
GIRARD, L.J.: Management of the peaked pupil and vitreous adherence to the wound. In: *Current Concepts in Cataract Surgery.* Ed. J.M. Emery & D. Paton, St. Louis, C.V. Mosby Co., 1976.
GIRARD, L.J.: Cystoid macular edema. In: *Current Concepts in Cataract Surgery.* Ed. J.M. Emery & D. Paton, St. Louis, C.V. Mosby Co., 1976.
GIRARD, L.J.: Ultrasonic fragment for Retroimplant Membranes and pupillary block. *Ophthal. Surg.* 8(3): 130-133, 1977.
GIRARD, L.J.: Phacoprothesis in unusual cases. *Am. Intraoc. Impl. Soc. J.* 3(1): 28-30, 1977.
GOLDBERG, M.F.: Hazards of mannitol. *Arch. Ophthal.* 69: 687, 1963.
GOULD, H.L.: Keratoplasty and intraocular lenses. *Am. Intraoc. Impl. Soc. J.* 1: 42-44, 1980.
GOULD, H.L.: Extracapsular cataract extraction and pseudophakia. *Cont. & Intraoc. Lens Med. J.* 1(3): 49-53, 1975.
GOULD, H.L.: Astigmatism and cataract surgery. In: *Current Concepts in Cataract Surgery.* Ed. by J.M. Emery and D. Paton, St. Louis, C.V. Mosby Co., 1974.
GOWAN, Mc. B.L.: Letter to the editor. *Am. Intraoc. Impl. Soc. J.* 4: 66-67, 1978.

GRABNER, G., G. ZEHETBAUER, H. BETTELHEIM and W. DORDA: Immediate changes in Protein-Concentration in aqueous humor induced by intracapsular lens extraction in human eyes. *Graefes Arch. Klin. Ophthal.* 210: 275-289, 1979.

GUERRY, D.: Present status of the anterior chamber lens. *Am. J. Ophthal.* 50: 250-258, 1960.

GUERRY, D. and W.J. GEERAETS: Complications of anterior chamber lenses. *Am. J. Ophthal.* 54: 229-292, 1962.

GUILLAUMAT, L., M. MASSIN, D. LEVY and H.P. THERON: Expérience clinique du décollement de rétine postaphakie. Analyse de 111 cas traités aux Quinze-Vingts. *An. Ocul.* 205: 1281-1305, 1972.

GUILLAUME, F. and M. RINGOT: Utilisation de la Neuroleptanalgésie dans la chirurgie de la cataracte. *Clinique Ophthal.* 4: 93-98, 1976.

GUILLAUME, F.: Neuroleptanalgésie avec association de diazépam (Valium) dans les interventions pour cataracte. *Ann. Anesth. Franç.* 10(2): 243-245, 1969.

GUTMAN, H., R.M. SINSKEY and W. CAIN, Jr.: A comparison of lidocaine and etidocaine in retrobulbar anaesthesia for cataract surgery. *Am. Intraoc. Impl. Soc. J.* 2: 120-122, 1979.

HAGER, G.: Das Blickfeld Gesichtsfeld und Umblickfeld von Brillenträgern sowie von Patienten mit kornealen Haftschalen und Patienten mit intraocular Korrektur. *Klin. Mbl. Augenheilk.* 139: 317-338, 1961.

HAGLER, W.S.: Aphakia and retinal detachment. In: *Current Concepts in Cataract Surgery.* Ed. J.M. Emery, D. Paton, St. Louis, C.V. Mosby Co., 333-336, 1976.

HAMDAN, Y.M.: The intraocular acrylic implants. *Bull. Ophthal. Soc. Egypt.* 51: 349-355, 1958.

HAMDI, T.: Aphakia treated by a flexibly supported anterior chamber lens. *Trans. Am. Ac. Ophthal. & Otol.* 68: 35-39, 1964.

HAMDI, T.: The Copeland intraocular lens: Five to ten years later. *Trans. Am. Ac. Ophthal. & Otol.* 86: 984-996, 1979.

HANNA, C.H. and H.C. KEATES: Indomethacin in ocular inflammation in rabbits. *Arch. Ophthal.* 77: 554, 1967.

HANNA, C.H. and J.D. SHARP: Ocular absorption of indomethacin by the rabbit. *Arch. Ophthal.* 88: 196-198, 1972.

HARDENBERGH, F.E.: Secondary intraocular lens implantation. *Ophthal. Surg.* 8(3): 70-81, 1977.

HARDENBERGH, F.E.: Techniques in secondary intraocular lens implantation. *Cont. & Intraoc. Lens Med. J.* 4(2): 65-69, 1978.

HARNISH, J.P. and G. LÖSCHAU: Rasterelektronenmikroskopische Untersuchungen an Kunststoff-Fäden. *Klin. Mbl. Augenheilk.* 166: 131-136, 1975.

HARRIS, J.E. and L.T. NORDQUIST: The hydratations of the cornea: I. *Am. J. Ophthal.* 40: 100-111, 1955.

HARRIS, W.S., B.C. TAYLOR and R.L. WINSLOW: Cystoid macular edema following intraocular lens implantation. *Ophthal. Surg.* 8(3): 134-137, 1977.

HARRIS, W.S.: A study of posterior chamber intraocular lenses and an introduction of a new posterior chamber intraocular lens. *Acta Pars II*, Kyoto 1978, Excerpta Medica, p. 1397, 1979.

HARRIS, W.S.: Current status of posterior chamber lens implantation. *Cont. & Intraoc. Lens Med. J.* 5(3): 67-69, 1979.

HARRIS, W.S.: Cystoid Macular Edema in Extracapsular and Intracapsular Aphakia and Pseudophakia. In: *Pseudophakia, Current Trends and Concepts.* Ed. by M.L. Kwitko and D.L. Praeger, Baltimore/London: Williams & Wilkins, pp. 367-373, 1980.

HARRISON, J.H. and R.H. ADLER: Nylon as a vascular prosthesis in experimental animals with tensile strength studies. *Surg. Gynecol. Obstet.* 103: 613-617, 1956.

HARRISON, S.W. and B.G. PRATER: Trauma and the anterior chamber lens. *Cont. & Intraoc. Lens Med. J.* 4(3): 100-102, 1978.

HARRY, J.: Newsletter of the *Internat. Intraocular Implant Club.* Nr. 5, p. 1, July 1977.

HARTSTEIN, J.: The hard contact lens versus the intraocular lens. *Cont. & Intraoc. Lens Med. J.* 1(3): 28-29, 1975.

HARTSTEIN, J.: The techniques of intraocular lens implantation: The advantages, disadvantages and indications. *Cont. & Intraoc. Med. J.* 1(3): 30-33. 1975.

HAVENER, W.H.: Osmotic agents. In: *Ocular Pharmacology.* 3rd ed., St. Louis, C.V. Mosby Co., pp. 429-452, 1974.
HAVENER, W.H.: Secretory inhibitors. In: *Ocular Pharmacology.* 3rd ed., St. Louis, C,V. Mosby Co., pp. 464-485, 1974.
HAWKINS, W.R.: Irvine-Gass syndrome. In: *Current Concepts in Cataract Surgery.* Ed. by J.A. Emery & D. Paton, St. Louis, C.V. Mosby Co., pp. 300-302, 1974.
HAWKINS, W.R.: Aphakic macular edema. In: *Current Concepts in Cataract Surgery.* Ed. by J.A. Emery and D. Paton, St. Louis, C.V. Mosby Co., pp. 339-342, 1974.
HAYAND, S.: 3 cases of anterior chamber lens implant. *Acta Soc. Ophthal. Jap.* 64: 2043-2048, 1960.
HAYAND, S.: Acrylic lens implant and its limitations. *J. Jap. Cont. Lens Soc.* 13(10): 87-90, 1971.
HAYAND, S., K. TAKAHASHI and K. SUZUKI: Intraocular implant: Medallion lens. *Folio Ophthal. Jap.* 26: 63-67, 1975.
HEDBYS, B.O. and S. MISHIMA: The thickness-hydration relationship of the cornea. *Exptl. Eye Res.* 5: 221-228, 1966.
HESLIN, K.B.: Is "white-to-white" right? *Am. Intraoc. Impl. Soc. J.* 1: 50-51, 1979.
HIGHMAN, V.N.: Stereopsis and aniseikonia in uniocular aphakia. *Brit. J. Ophthal.* 61: 30-33, 1977.
HILDRETH, H.: Digital ocular compression proceeding cataract surgery. *Am. J. Ophthal.* 51: 1237-1239, 1961.
HILES, D.A.: Intraocular lens implantation in children. *An. of Ophthal.* 9: 789-797, 1976.
HILES, D.A.: The need for intraocular lens implantation in children. *Ophthal. Surg.* 8(3): 162-169, 1977.
HILES, D.A.: AIOIS survey of intraocular lenses in children—1978. *Am. Intraoc. Impl. Soc. J.* 4: 166-172, 1978.
HILES, D.A., A.W. BIGLAN and E.C. FETHEROLF: Central corneal endothelial cell counts in children. *Am. Intraoc. Impl. Soc. J.* 4: 292-300, 1979.
HILES, D.A.: Peripheral iris erosions associated with pediatric intraocular lens implants. *Am. Intraoc. Impl. Soc. J.* 3: 210-212, 1979.
HILES, D.A. and B.A. WATSON: Complications of implant surgery in children. *Am. Intraoc. Impl. Soc. J.* 1: 24-32, 1979.
HILES, D.A.: Pseudophakia in children. In: *Pseudophakia, Current Trends and Concepts.* Ed. by M.L. Kwitko and D.L. Praeger. Baltimore/London: Williams & Wilkins 1980, pp. 93-114.
HIRSCHMAN, H.: Intraocular iris-clip-lens. *Am. J. Ophthal.* 68: 1113, 1969.
HIRSCHMAN, H.: *Communication* Internat. Impl. Soc. Meeting, Budapest, April 1972.
HIRSCHMAN, H.: Advantages and disadvantages of the types of intraocular lens available. *Trans. Am. Ac. Ophthal. & Otol.* 81: 89-92, 1976.
HIRSCHMAN, H.: Intraocular lens implantation: Faster, more complete, rehabilitation of the cataract patient. *Journal of the Am. Geriatrics Soc.* 25(1): 35-38, 1977.
HIRSCHMAN, H.: Various lenstypes. Results. in '*Pseudophakos*' Ed. by C.V. Mosby C°, St. Louis 1978 pp. 208-215.
HIRSCHMAN, H.: Complications with the four-loop lens of Binkhorst (the irisclip lens). *Trans. Am. Ac. Ophthal. & Otol.* 86: 655-658, 1979.
HIRST, L.W., R.C. SNIP, W.J. STARK and E. MAUMENEE: Quantitative corneal endothelial evaluation in intraocular lens implantation and cataract surgery. *Am. J. Ophthal.* 84: 775, 1977.
HIRTHE, C.H.: Ergebnisse mit künstlichen Vorderkammerlinsen. *Klin. Mbl. Augenheilk.* 153: 527-530, 1968.
HITCHINGS, R.A. and I.H. CHISHOLM: Incidence of aphakic macular oedema. *Brit. J. Ophthal.* 59: 444, 1975.
HITCHINGS, R.A.: Aphakic macular oedema: a two-year follow-up study. *Brit. J. Ophthal.* 61: 628-630, 1977.
HOBBS, B.C. and G.S. WILSON: *The disinfectant activity of caustic soda.* J. Hygiene (Canterburry). 42: 436, 1942 (cited by F. Ridley, 1957).
HOFFER, K.: Accidental suture engagement by posterior loop while inserting a Medallion lens. An easy method of correction. *Am. Intraoc. Impl. Soc. Newltr.* 1: 42-43, 1975.

HOFFER, K.J.: Selection of lens power for implantation in infants and children. *Am. Intraoc. Impl. Soc. J. Newsltr.* 1: 49, Sept. 1975.
HOFFER, K.J.: Preliminary report of independent testing of intraocular lenses. *Am. Intraoc. Impl. Soc. J.* 3-4: 206-208, 1977.
HOFFER, K.J. and D.R. ALLEN: A simple lens power calculation program for the HP-67 and HP-97 calculators. *Am. Intraoc. Impl. Soc. J.* 4: 197-199, 1978.
HOFFER, K.J.: Survey on the use of intraocular lenses. *Trans. Am. Ac. Ophthal. & Otol.* 85: 400-407, 1978.
HOFFER, K.J. and G. PHILLIPPI: A cell membrane theory of endothelial repair and vertical cell loss after cataract surgery. *Am. Intraoc. Impl. Soc. J.* 1: 18-25, 1978.
HOFFER, K.J.: Phacoemulsification and ultrasound. *Am. Intraoc. Impl. Soc. J.* 4(4): 209, 1978.
HOFFER, K.J.: Clinical importance of preoperative endothelial cell counts. *Newsltr. Medical Optics Center,* April 1979.
HOFFER, K.J., T.V. SCOTT and R.W. DION: X-ray technique for discovering metal loops of intraocular lenses. *Am. Intraoc. Impl. Soc. J.* 1: 58-59, 1979.
HOFFER, K.J.: Vertical endothelial cell disparity. *Am. J. Ophthal.* 87: 344, 1979.
HOFFER, K.J.: Intraocular lens in the ciliary sulcus. *Am. J. Ophthal.* 92: 268-272, 1981.
HOFMANN, H.: Erfahrungen mit Vorderkammerlinsen. Vereins Reinisch-Westfälischer Augenärtze. 125: 50-53, 1972. *Klin. Mbl. Augenheilk.* 161: 481, 1972.
HOLYK, P.R. and D.E. EIFRIG: Effects of monomeric methylmethacrylate on ocular tissues. *Am. J. Ophthal.* 88: 385-395, 1979.
HONAN, P.R.: Some observations on the use of a pneumatic eye softener for intraocular surgery. *Cont. & Intraoc. Lens Med. J.* 3: 78-80, 1979.
HONEGGER, H.: Quantitative Untersuchungen über die Hornhautendothelregeneration in vivo. *Graefes Arch. Klin. Ophthal.* 165: 31-42, 1962.
HOUSEHOLDER, J.A.: Preliminary report of the survey on the use of metal looped lenses in intracapsular surgery. *Am. Intraoc. Impl. Soc. J.* 1: 50-52, 1977.
HOVLAND, K.R.: Vitreous findings in fellow eyes of aphakic retinal detachment. *Am. J. Ophthal.* 86: 350-353, 1978.
HUANG, K., G.A. PEYMAN, J. McGETRICK and JANEVICIUS: Indomethacin inhibitor of prostaglandin mediated inflammation following intraocular surgery. *Invest. Ophthal.* 16: 760-762, 1977.
HUBER, C.: Indikation und Resultate der extrakapsulären Linsenimplantation beim Patientengut von Dr. C.D. Binkhorst im Jahre 1967. *Klin. Mbl. Augenheilk.* 174: 876-881, 1979.
HUBER, C. and C.D. BINKHORST: Iseikonic lensimplantation in anisometropia. *Am. Intraoc. Impl. Soc. J.* 3: 194-202, 1979.
HUBERMAN, J.P.: Capsulectomy for planned extracapsular cataract extraction with lens implantation. *Cont. & Intraoc. Lens Med. J.* 3(4): 45-46, 1977.
HUBERMAN, J.P.: Management of secondary membranes in extracapsular cataract surgery with lens implantation. *Cont. & Intraoc. Lens Med. J.* 4(1): 43-45, 1978.
HUGES, W.F. and W.C. OWENS: Extraction of senile cataract. A statistical comparison of various techniques and the importance of preoperative survey. *Am. J. Ophthal.* 28: 40-49, 1945.
HULL, D.S., M.T. CHEMMOTTI, H.F. EDELHAUSER, D.L. VAN HORN and R.A. HYNDIUK: Effect of epinephrine on the corneal endothelium. *Am. J. Ophthal.* 79(2): 245-250, 1975.
HULL, D.S.: Use of IOL with retinitis pigmentosa. *Am. Intraoc. Impl. Soc. J.* 4(4): 208, 1978.
HUNKELER, J.D. and L.L. HYDE: The triple procedure: combined penetrating keratoplasty, cataract extraction and lens implantation. *Am. Intraoc. Impl. Soc. J.* 3: 222-224, 1979.
HYDE, L.L.: Corneal astigmatism after cataract extraction. In: *Astigmatism and cataract wounds: Current Concepts in Cataract Surgery.* Ed. by J.M. Emery and D. Paton, St. Louis: C.V. Mosby Co., 1974.

ILLIF, C.E.: A surgical soft eye by posterior sclerotomy. *Am. J. Ophthal.* 61: 276-277, 1966.

IRVINE, S.R. and A.R. IRVINE, Jr: Lens-induced uveitis and glaucoma: Part I, Endophthalmitis phaco-anaphylactica. *Am. J. Ophthal.* 35: 177-186, 1952.
IRVINE, S.R. and A.R. IRVINE, Jr.: Lens-induced uveitis and glaucoma: Part II, The "phacotoxic" reaction. *Am. J. Ophthal.* 35: 370-375, 1952.
IRVINE, S.R. and A.R. IRVINE, Jr.: Lens-induced uveitis and glaucoma. Part III, "phacogenetic glaucoma" lens induced glaucoma, mature or hypermature cataract; open iridocorneal angle. *Am. J. Ophthal.* 35: 489-499, 1952.
IRVINE, S.R.: A newly defined vitreous syndrome following cataract surgery. *Am. J. Ophthal.* 36(5): 599-619, 1953.
IRVINE, A.R., R. BRESKY, B.M. CROWDER and S.M. KULVIN: Macular edema after cataract extraction. *Ann. Ophthal.* 3: 1234-1243, 1971.
IRVINE, A.R.: Cystoid maculopathy (review). *Survey ophthal.* 21: 1-17, 1976.
IRVINE, A.R., R.P. KRATZ and J.J. O'DONNELL: Endothelial damage with phacoemulsification and intraocular lens implantation. *Arch. Ophthal.* 96: 1023-1026, 1978.

JACOBSON, D.R. and A. DELLAPORTA: Natural history of cystoid macular edema after cataract extraction. *Am. J. Ophthal.* 77: 445-447, 1974.
JAFFE, N.S. and D.S. LIGHT: Oral glycerin in cataract surgery. *Archives Ophthal.* 73: 516-518, 1965.
JAFFE, N.S.: Cystoid Macular Edema (Irvine's Syndrome). In: *Complications of Cataract surgery.* St. Louis: C.V. Mosby Co., 210-222, 1972.
JAFFE, N.S.: Current status of intraocular lenses. *Eye, Ear, Nose, Throat Mon.* 51: 290-296, 1972.
JAFFE, N.S.: The lens. Annual review. *Arch. Ophthal.* 87: 453-486, 1972.
JAFFE, N.S.: *Cataract surgery and its complications.* St. Louis: C.V. Mosby Co., 1972-1976.
JAFFE, N.S.: The lens: Annual review. *Arch. Ophthal.* 90: 136-171, 1973.
JAFFE, N.S.: The iris-plane (Copeland) pseudophakos. *Arch. of Ophthal.* 94: 420-424, 1976.
JAFFE, N.S.: Indications and contraindications. Symposium: Intraocular Lenses. *Trans. Am. Ac. Ophthal. & Otol.* 81: 94-96, 1976.
JAFFE, N.S.: Suggested guidelines for intraocular lens implant surgery. *Arch. Ophthal.* 94: 214-216, 1976.
JAFFE, N.S. and L.R. DUFFNER: The iris-plane (Copeland) pseudophakos. *Arch. Ophthal.* 94: 420-424, 1976.
JAFFE, N.S.: Postoperative complications early and late. Symposium: Intraocular Lenses. *Trans. Am. Ac. Ophthal. & Otol.* 81: 118-119, 1976.
JAFFE, N.S.: Interview. *Highlights Ophthal.* pp. 244-345, 1975-1976.
JAFFE, N.S.: The molecular basis of intraocular implant lens materials. *Am. Intraoc. Impl. Soc. J.* 2: 9, 1976.
JAFFE, N.S.: Initiation of the Implant Surgeon. *Cont. & Intraoc. Lens Med. J.* 3(2): 55-57, 1977.
JAFFE, N.S., H.M. CLAYMAN and D.M. EICHENBAUM: Communication by D. Eichenbaum, Implant Symposium, April 1977, Israel.
JAFFE, N.S.: Controversity in intraocular lens implant surgery. In: *Controversity in Ophthalmology.* W.S. Saunders Co., pp. 254-268, 1977, Philadelphia.
JAFFE, N.S.: Results of intraocular lens implant surgery. Implants vs. routine cataract extraction. *Am. J. Ophthal.* 85(1): 13-24, 1978.
JAFFE, N.S., M.A. GALIN, H. HIRSCHMAN and H.N. CLAYMAN: *Pseudophakos,* St. Louis: C.V. Mosby Co., 1978.
JAFFE, N.S.: Intraocular lenses: Secondary membranes, cystoid macular edema. *Trans. Am. Ac. Ophthal. & Otol.* 85: 157-163, 1978.
JAFFE, N.S., D.M. EICHENBAUM, H.M. CLAYMAN and D.S. LIGHT: A comparison of 500 Binkhorst implants with 500 routine intra-capsular cataract extractions. *Am. J. Ophthal.* 85: 24, 1978.
JAFFE, N.S.: Intraocular lenses. Current status. *Trans. Am. Ac. Ophthal. & Otol.* 85: 52-58, 1978.
JAFFE, N.S., D.M. EICHENBAUM, H.M. CLAYMAN and D.S. LIGHT: Dislocation of Binkhorst four-loop lens implant. *Trans. Am. Ac. Ophthal. & Otol.* 86: 207-211, 1979.

JAFFE, N.S.: Symposium: Contact lens and spectable lens. Correction of aphakia. Introduction. *Trans. Am. Ac. Ophthal. & Otol.* 86: 345-346, 1979.
JAFFE, N.S.: The changing scene of intraocular implant lens surgery. *Am. J. Ophthal.* 88: 819-828, 1979.
JAFFE, N.S., H.M. CLAYMAN, M.S. JAFFE, D.S. LIGHT: The results of lensimplantation in eyes with operative loss of vitreous. *Am. Intraoc. Impl. Soc. J.* 6: 243-245, 1980.
JAGGER, W.S. and K.W. JACOBI: An analysis of pseudophakodonesis and iridodonesis. *Am. Intraoc. Impl. Soc. J.* 3: 203-206, 1979.
JAMPOL, L.M., A.H. NEUFELD and L.M. SEARS: Pathways for the response of the eye to injury. *Invest. Ophthal.* 14: 184-189, 1975.
JANSSON, F. and E. KOCK: Determination of the velocity of ultrasound in the human lens and vitreous. *Acta Ophthal.* 40: 420-433, 1962.
JARDINE, P. and J.H. SANDFORD-SMITH: Fedorov iris-supported intra-ocular acrylic lens. *Brit. J. Ophthal.* 58: 718-724, 1974.
JAY, J.L. and M. McDONALD: Effect of intraocular miotics on cultured bovine corneal endothelium. *Brit. J. Ophthal.* 62: 815-820, 1978.
JEWETT, E.P.: A report on eighteen implant cases with recalled lenses. *Am. Intraoc. Impl. Soc. J.* 4(4): 227-228, 1978.
JOHNSTON, G.P., E. OKUN, I. BONUIK, N. ARRIBAS and R. ESCOFFERY: Pseudophakic retinal detachment. *Mod. Prob. Ophthal.* 18: 499-602, 1977.
JONKERS, G.H.: Intra-ocular acrylic lenses: a case report. *Ophthalmologica* (Basel). 126: 55-57, 1953.
JUNGE, J.: Cystoid macular edema associated with PVP coating of an intraocular lens. *Am. Intraoc. Impl. Soc. J.* 1: 28-29, 1980.
JUNGSCHAFFER, O.: Iris Clip lens and retinal detachment. Examination and surgery of three eyes. *Arch. Ophthal.* 88: 594-595, 1972.
JUNGSCHAFFER, O.: Intraocular lenses and retinal detachment. *Mod. Probl. Ophthal.* 18: 4896-4898, 1977.
JUNGSCHAFFER, O. and C.D. FRITCH: Phacoemulsification and retinal detachment. *Mod. Probl. Ophthal.* 18: 508-510, 1977.
JUNGSCHAFFER, O.: Retinal detachment after intraocular lens. *Arch. Ophthal.* 95/7: 1203-1204, 1977.

KAHN, W.J.: Cellular precipitates on IOL's. *Am. Intraoc. Impl. Soc. J.* 4(4): 214, 1978.
KALVIN, N.H.: Surgical treatment for aphakic fibrous downgrowth associated with persistent cystoid macular edema. *Current Concepts in Cararact Surgery.* Ed. by J.M. Emery & D. Paton, St. Louis: C.V. Mosby Co., 1974.
KANTER, Y.C.: A suggestion for handling intraocular lenses sterilized by Ridley method. *Cont. & Intraoc. Lens Med. J.* 4(4): 87-88, 1978.
KASNER, D.: Cited by J.L. Tennant in "*A lens for all seasons*" 1976.
KASS, M.A., A.H. NEUFELD and M.L. SEARS: Systemic aspirin and indomethacin do not prevent the response of the monkey eye to trauma. *Invest. Ophthal.* 14: 604-6, 1975.
KATZ, J.L., H.E. KAUFMAN, E.P. GOLDBERG and J.W. SHEETS: Prevention of endothelial damage from intraocular lens insertion. *Trans. Am. Ac. Ophthal. & Otol.* 83: 204-212, 1977.
KAUFMAN, H.E., A. CAPELLA and J.E. ROBBINS: The human corneal endothelium. *Am. J. Ophthal.* 67(5): 835-841, 1966.
KAUFMAN, H.E.: Human corneal endothelium: New insights. *Invest. Ophthal.* 15(1): 2-3, 1976.
KAUFMAN, H.E. and J. KATZ: Endothelial damage from intraocular lens insertion. *Invest. Ophth.* 15: 996-1000, 1976.
KAYE, G.I. and S. MISHIMA: Studies on the cornea. Effects of perfusion with a Ca^{++} free medium on the corneal endothelium. *Invest. Ophthal.* 7: 53, 1968.
KEATES, R.H.: The place of intraocular lenses in ophthalmic training programs. *Cont. & Intraoc. Lens Med. J.* 1(4): 4-6, 1975.
KEATES, R.H. and D.R. EHRLICH: "Lenses of chance" complications of anterior chamber implants. *Trans. Am. Ac. Ophthal. & Otol.* 85: 408-414, 1978.

KEATES, R.H. and S.B. LICHTENSTEIN: Surgical complications of choyce-type implants. *Trans. Am. Ac. Ophthal. & Otol.* 86: 625-631, 1979.
KELMAN. C.D.: Phaco-emulsification and aspiration. *Am. J. Ophthal.* 75: 764-768, 1973.
KELMAN, C.D.: Summary of personal experience. *Trans. Am. Ac. Ophthal. & Otol.* 78: 22-27, 1974.
KELMAN, C.D.: *Communication* Implant Society Meeting Cannes May 1979.
KENYON, K.R., D.L. VAN HORN and H.F. EDELHAUSER: Endothelial degeneration and posterior collagenous proliferation in aphakic bullous keratopathy. *Am. J. Ophthal.* 85: 329-336, 1978.
KERN, R.: Erste Erfahrungen mit der Einpflanzung von Vorderkammerlinzen. (Iris-clip-linsen nach Binkhorst). *Ophthalmologica* (Basel). 170: 165-171, 1975.
KERN, R.: Weitere Erfahrungen mit der Vorderkammerlinse. *Ophthalmologica* (Basel). 172: 149-154, 1976.
KERN, R.: Möglichkeiten zur Korrektur der Aphakie unter besonderer Berücksichtigung der Linsenimplantation. *Ophthalmologica* S.O.Z. 1: 5-9, 1977.
KERN, R.: Iridocapsular lenses versus iris-clip lenses: Comparison of the results and complicatons of 100 of each. *Ophthal. Surgery.* 8(3): 82-88, 1977.
KERN, R.: Komplicationen und ihre Vermeidung vor, während und nach Implantation von intraokulären Linsen. *Klin. Mbl. Augenheilk.* 172: 426-430, 1978.
KESSLER, J.: Experiments in refilling the lens. *Arch. Ophthal.* 71: 412-417, 1964.
KING, J.H., Jr.: Acrylic lenses in the anterior chamber. *Arch. Ophthal.* 58: 392-395, 1957.
KIRK, S., R.W. BURDE and S.R. WALTMAN: Minimizing corneal endothelial damage due to intraocular lens contact. *Invest. Ophthal.* 16(11): 1053-1056, 1977.
KIRSCH, R.E. and W. STEINMAN: Digital pressure, an important safeguard in cataract surgery. *Arch. Ophthal.* 54: 697-703, 1955.
KIRSCH, R.E.: Further studies on the use of digital pressure in cataract surgery. *Arch. Ophthal.* 58: 641-646, 1957.
KIRSCH, R.E.: Intraocular lenses: The conservative approach. In: *Controversity in ophthalmology.* W.B. Saunders Co., pp. 269-278, 1977.
KIRSCH, R.E.: Intraocular lenses: The conservative approach. In: *Controversity in ophthalmology.* W.B. Saunders Co., pp. 269-278, 1977.
KLEIN, R.M. and L. YANNUZZI: Cystoid macular edema in the first week after cataract extraction. *Am. J. Ophthal.* 81: 614-615, 1976.
KLEIN, R.M., H.M. KATZIN and L.A. YANNUZZI: The effect of indomethacin pretreatment on aphakic cystoid macular edema. *Am. J. Ophthal.* 87: 487-489, 1979.
KLINE, O.R., Jr.: Visual results and complications of 500 intraocular lens implantations. *Am. Intraoc. Impl. Soc. J.* 4: 184-191, 1978.
KNAPP, A.: Complications of the forceps intracapsular operation for cataract. *Arch. Ophthal.* 16: 770-775, 1936.
KNIGHT, P.M., W.J. LINK and H.E. KAUFMAN: The corneal endothelium, a review of the literature. Irvine, Cal Heyer Schulte Medical Optics Center, 1978.
KNIGHT, P.M. and W.J. LINK: Surface modification of intraocular lenses to reduce corneal endothelial damage. *Am. Intraoc. Impl. Soc. J.* 2: 123-130, 1979.
KNOLLE, G.E., Jr: Bending the platinum clip. *Am. Intraoc. Impl. Soc. J.* 1: 61-63, 1979.
KNOLLE, G.E.: The platina lens: Phacoemulsification extracapsular and intracapsular techniques. In: *Pseudophakia, Current Trends and Concepts.* Ed. by M.L. Kwitko and D.L. Praeger, London/Baltimore: Williams & Wilkins, pp. 165-181, 1980.
KOETTING, R.A.: Progressive addition spectacles over contact lenses in aphakia. *Am. J. Ophthal.* 46: 470-475, 1969.
KOK-VAN ALPHEN, C.C., H.J.M. VÖLKER-DIEBEN and A.J. OTTO: Keratoplastik, cataract extraktion und Kunstlinsen-Implantation in einem Eingriff. *Deutsche Ophthalmologische Gezellschaft.* Ber. 75: 134-136, 1977.
KOK-VAN ALPHEN, C.C., A.J. OTTO and H.J.M. VÖLKER-DIEBEN: Corneal grafting, cataract extraction, lens implantation: Three birds with one stone. *Documenta Ophthalmologica* (Basel). 175: 163-165, 1977.
KOK-VAN ALPHEN C.C. and H.J.M. VÖLKER-DIEBEN: Corneal dystrophy following lens implantation. *Doc. Ophthalmol.* 48(2): 243-250, 1979.'

KOLKER, A.E. and S. BECKER: Epinephrine maculopathy. *Arch. Ophthal.* 79: 552-562, 1968.
KOLLARITS, C.R.: Intraocular irrigating solutions. *Am. J. Ophthal.* 82(4): 594-597, 1976.
KOLLARITS, C.R., J. LITTLE and F.J. KOLLARITS: Calculation of intraocular lens power using the Texas Instruments programmable 59 calculator. *Am. Intraoc. Impl. Soc. J.* 2: 90-98, 1978.
KOLLARITS, F.J., C.R. KOLLARITS and R.T. TORCHIA: A Fortran IV program for intraocular lens power calculation. *Am. Intraoc. Impl. Soc. J.* 4: 330-336, 1979.
KORNBLUETH, W. and G. GOMBOS: The use of intravenous hypertonic urea in cataract extraction. *Am. J. Ophthal.* 54: 753, 1963.
KOTTOW, M. and P. HENDRICKSON: Iris angiography in C.M.E. after cataract extraction. *Arch. Ophthal.* 93, 1975.
KOTTOW, M.H.: *Anterior Segment Fluorescein Angiography.* Baltimore: Williams & Wilkins, 1978.
KOVAL, L.V.: The effect on colour perception of an intraocular lens implantation in aphakia. *Vest. Oftal.* 62: 50-54, 1969.
KRAAS, P.: Die postoperative Refraction nach Binkhorst-Linseneinpflanzung. Thesis, Münster, 1972.
KRAFF, M.C. and H.L. LIEBERMAN: Experience with the large cicular loop medallion lens and a critical comparison with the suture medallion lens: a report of 300 cases. *Ophth. Surg.* 8(3): 89-86, 1977.
KRAFF, M.C., D.R. SANDERS and H.L. LIEBERMAN: Endothelial cell loss and the trauma during intraocular lens implantation—a specular microscopic study. *Am. Intraoc. Impl. Soc. J.* 3: 107-109, 1978.
KRAFF, M.C., D.R. SANDERS and H.L. LIEBERMAN: Determination of Intraocular Lens Power: A comparison with and without Ultrasound. *Ophthal. Surg.* 9(1): 81-84, 1978.
KRAFF, M.C., D.R. SANDERS and H.L. LIEBERMAN: The medallion suture lens: management of complications. *Trans. Am. Ac. Ophthal. & Otol.* 86: 643-654, 1979.
KRAFF, M.C., D.R. SANDERS and H.L. LIEBERMAN: 300 primary anterior chamber lensimplantations: Gonioscopic findings and specular microscopy. *Am. Intraoc. Impl. Soc. J.* 3: 207-209, 1979.
KRASNOV, M.M.: Artificial crystalline fixed to the pararadical area of the iris. *Vest. Oftal.* 82: 46-50, 1969.
KRASNOV, M.M.: Extrapupillary iris lens in aphakia. *Am. J. Ophthal.* 78: 541-543, 1974.
KRASNOV, M.M.: Technique of implantation of extrapupillary iris lens: 8 years of clinical experience. *Brit. J. Ophthal.* 61: 316-321, 1977.
KRATZ, R.P.: Difficulties, complications and management. *Trans. Am. Ac. Ophthal. & Otol.* 78: 18-21, 1974.
KRATZ, R.P.: Technique of phacoemulsification and lens implantation. *Am. Intraoc. Impl. Soc. J.* 2: 15, 1976.
KRATZ, R.P.: Phaco-emulsification and intraocular lenses. *Cont. & Intraoc. Lens Med. J.* 2: 7-9, 1976.
KRATZ, R.: Discussion Aphakia and retinal detachment. In: *Current Concepts in cataract surgery. Selected Proceedings at the Fourth Biennial Cataract Surgery Congress. St. Louis: C.V. Mosby Co., 1976.*
KRATZ, R.P.: Discussions after phacoemulsification with intraocular lens. *Am. Intraoc. Impl. Soc. J.* 3(1): 41-42, 1977.
KRATZ, R.P.: Intraocular lenses: Indications and contra-indications. In: *Controversity in Ophthalmology.* W.B. Saunders Co., 1977, Philadelphia, pp. 279-280.
KRATZ, R.P.: Surgical techniques for placement of intraocular lenses. *International Ophthalmology Clinics.* 18(2): 171-178, 1978.
KRATZ, R.P.: Complications associated with posterior chamber lenses. *Trans. Am. Ac. Ophthal. & Otol.* 86: 659-661, 1979.
KRATZ, R.P.: Current status of 550 Choyce lenses. *Communication,* Am. Intraoc. Impl. Soc. Meeting L.A., March 1978.
KRATZ, R.P., T.R. MAZZOCCO, B. DAVIDSON and W.F. MALONEY: I.O.L. comparison: Binkhorst Choyce and Shearing. *U.S. Intraocular Lens Symposium April 1979* (manuscript).

KRATZ, R.P., T.R. MAZZOCCO and B. DAVIDSON: A report of 756 Shearing posterior chamber intraocular lenses. Communication IV international Charlottenlund Ophthal. Conference, Aug. 1979.

KRATZ, R.P.: The Choyce intraocular lens. Symposium cataracts. *Transactions of the New Orleans Ac. of Ophthal.* St. Louis-Toronto-London: C.V. Mosby Co., pp. 305-309, 1979.

KRATZ, R.P., T.R. MAZZOCCO, B. DAVIDSON and D.M. COLVARD: A comparative analysis of anterior chamber, iris-supported, capsule-fixated, and posterior chamber lenses following cataract extraction by phacoemulsification. *Ophthalmology.* 88(1): 56-58, 1981.

KRAUSE, U., A. TARKKANEN: Histopathology of clinically successful intraocular lens implant. *Acta Ophthalmologica. 58: 56-62, 1980.*

KRIEBIG, W.: Ist die extrakapsuläre Methode der Starausziehung wirklich als veraltet abzulehen? *Klin. Mbl. Augenheilk.* 160: 35-40, 1972.

KRIEGER, A.: Round table discussion on the retina and lensimplantation. *Am. Intraoc. Impl. Soc. Meeting — Los Angeles,* March, 1978.

KRONENTHAL, R.L.: Intraocular degradation of non-absorbable sutures. *Am. Intraoc. Impl. Soc. J.* 3-4: 222-228, 1977.

KRONENTHAL, R.L.: Letter to the Editor. *Am. Intraoc. Impl. Soc. J.* 5: 341, 1979.

KRONFELD, P. and C. DEVNEY: Ein Beitrag zur Kenntnis der Refractionskurve. *Graefes Arch. Ophthal.* 126: 487-501, 1931.

KRONFELD, P.C., C.K. LIN and T.H. LUO: The protein content of re-formed aqueous humour in man. *Am. J. Ophthal.* 24: 264-276, 1941.

KRUPIN, T., A.E. KOLKER and B. BECKER: A comparison of isosorbide and glycerol for cataract surgery. *Am. J. Ophthal.* 69: 737-740, 1970.

KUNZ, E., R. KERN, M.C. OPPONG and J. SCHIPPER: Zum Makulaödem nach Implantation von Binkhorst-Linsen. *Klin. Mbl. Augenheilk.* 176: 690-693, 1980.

KULVIN, S.M., R.C. MAGOON and G.R. MILLER: Surgical treatment of post-pseudophakos membranes. *Ophth. Surg.* 6: 47-53, 1975.

KULVIN, M.A., B. LUSK and T. PETIT: Fungal endophthalmitis following intraocular lens implantation. *Am. J. Ophthal.* 83: 1-8, 1977.

KÖPER, J.: Komplikationen nach Implantation von Vorderkammerlinsen. *Klin. Mbl. Augenheilk.* 140: 639, 1962.

KWITKO, M.L.: Precautions in lens implantation: Eight year follow-up. *Am. J. Ophthal.* 78: 547, 1974.

KWITKO, M.L.: Implantation du cristallin artificiel après l'opération de la cataracte. *L'Information Médicale.* 30: 17, 1975.

KWITKO, M.L.: New lenses for old, a promising method for treating cataracts. *L'information Médicale.* 30: 17, 1975.

KWITKO, M.L.: Intraocular lens: Fixation devices. *Cont. & Intraoc. Lens Med. J.* 2: 12-15, 1976.

KWITKO, M.: *Communication* Internat. Impl. Soc. Meeting, Israël, April 1977.

KWITKO, M.L.: Experience with the Russian made Fyodorov intraocular lens. *Am. Intraoc. Impl. Soc. J.* 1: 32-35, 1978.

KWITKO, M.L.: Secondary lens implantation. *Cont. & Intraoc. Lens Med. J.* 4(2): 56-57, 1978.

KWITKO, M.L.: The platinum clip (platina) intraocular lens. *Trans. Am. Ac. Ophthal. & Otol.* 86: 632-637, 1979.

KWITKO, M.L.: The Fyodorov sputnik intraocular lens. *Trans. Am. Ac. Ophthal. & Otol.* 86: 638-642, 1979.

LAING, R.A., M.M. SANDSTRÖM and H.M. LEIBOWITZ: In vivo photomicrography of the corneal endothelium. *Arch. Ophthal.* 93: 143-145, 1975.

LAING, R.A., M.M. SANDSTRÖM, A.R. BERROSPI and H.M. LEIBOWITZ: Changes in the corneal endothelium as a function of age. *Exp. Eye Research.* 22: 587, 1976.

LAING, R.A., M.M. SANDSTRÖM, A.R. BERROSPI and H.M. LEIBOWITZ: Morphological changes in corneal endothelial cells after penetrating keratoplasty. *Am. J. Ophthal.* 82: 459-464, 1976.

LANDEGGER, G.P. and N. ROTH: Anterior chamber depth and its stability in aphakia. *Am. J. Ophthal.* 65: 706-708, 1968.

LEARY, G.A.: Ultrasonic Assessment of the implant lens required to produce emmetropia after implantation. *Invest. Ophthal.* 10(10): 745-759, 1971.
LECAILLON-THIBON, M.M. and P.A.M. LEONARD: Cataracte traumatique et lentille intraoculaire. *Bull. des Soc. d'Ophthalmologie.* 9-10: 891-893, 1975.
LEE, J.R. and C.H. DOHLMAN: Intraocular lens implantation in combination with keratoplasty. *An. Ophthal.* 513-518, 1977, April.
LEFRANÇOIS, A.: Le syndrome d'Irvine-Gass. *Encyclopédie Medico Chirurgicale.* p. 21250-21251, 1er éd., 5-1976.
LEGRAND, J.: État actuel de la question des lentilles intraoculaires dans la correction des aphakies. *L'année Thérap. et Clin. en Ophtal.* 16: 297-306, 1965.
LEIBOWITZ, H.M. and R.A. LAING: Corneal Endothelium—the effect of air in the anterior chamber. *Arch. Ophth.* 92: 227-230, 1974.
LEONARD, P.A.M.: Cataracte traumatique et lentille intraoculaire. *Bull. Soc. Belge Ophthal.* 159: 701-706, 1971.
LEONARD, P.A.M. and L. EVENS: La vision binoculaire dans l'aphakie unilatérale traumatique. *Bull. Soc. Belge. Ophtal.* 159: 697-700, 1971.
LEONARD, P.A.M.: Lentille intra-oculaire de Binkhorst: indications, contre-indications et problèmes. *Arch. Ophthal.* 37(5): 409-416, 1977.
LETTERS REGARDING METAL LOOP LENSES. *Am. Intraoc. Impl. Soc. J.* 3(1): 63-70, 1977.
LEVENSON, J.E.: Stripping of descemet's membrane. *Am. Intraoc. Impl. Soc. Newsltr.* 1: 37, 1975.
LEVY, P.L., A.M. ROTH and J.L. GANGITANO: Protection of corneal endothelium during intraocular lensimplantation using Polymacon, a new surgical technique. *Trans. Am. Ac. Ophthal. & Otol.* 86: 219-227, 1979.
LIEB, W.A. and III. DU PONT GUERRY: Anterior chamber lenses for refractive correction of unilateral aphakia. *Am. J. Ophthal.* 44: 579-598, 1957.
LIEB, W.A. and III. DU PONT GUERRY: Vorderkammerlinsen zur Korrektion unilateral Aphakien. *Klin. Mbl. Augenheilk.* 132: 465-475, 1958.
LIEB, W.A.: Tissue tolerance of plastic resins: *the Eye, Ear, Nose and Throat Monthly.* 38: 210-215, 1959. *The Eye, Ear, Nose and Throat Monthly.* 38: 303-307+321, 1959.
LIEB, W.A.: Rehabilitation Sehbehinderter durch Haftschale und Vorderkammerlinse. *Klin. Mbl. Augenheilk.* 147: 137, 1965.
LINDSTROM, R.L., C.W. LINDSTROM and W.S. HARRIS: Accuracy of lens implant power determination using A-scan. *Cont. & Intraoc. Lens Med. J.* 3: 61-66, 1979.
LINK, D.: Communication. *Am. Intraoc. Impl. Soc. Meeting Los Angeles* — March 1978.
LINKSZ, A.: Aniseikonia. *Am. J. Ophthal.* 48(4): 441-462, 1959.
LINKSZ, A.: Aniseikonia. With notes on the Jackson-Lancaster controversy. XV Jackson Memorial Lecture. *Trans. Am. Ac. Ophthal. & Otol.* 63: 117-140, 1959.
LINKSZ, A.: Optical complications of aphakia. In: *Complications after Cataract Surgery.* pp. 597-634, Ed. by F.H. Theodore, Boston: Little & Brown, 1964.
LITTLE, J.: Discussion, aphakia and retinal detachment. In: *Current Concepts in Cataract Surgery. Selected Proceedings of the fourth Biennial Cataract Surgery Congress.* St. Louis, C.V. Mosby Co., 1976.
LITTLE, J.H.: Endothelial cell counts following phacoemulsification with and without implants. *Audio Digest Ophthal.* 17(4): 1979.
LOEWENTHAL, L.M.: Comparison of titanium loop and supramid loop lens implants: 100 patients. *Am. Intraoc. Impl. Soc. J.* 3: 104-106, 1978.
LOYD, T. and J.P. GILLS: Deviation from labeled dioptric power for 400 lenses. *Am. Intraoc. Impl. Soc. J.* 3: 229, 1979.
LUBKIN, V., A. LINKSZ and G. CHAMBY: Stereopsis with spectacles in monocular aphakia. *Am. J. Ophthal.* 67: 547-553, 1969.
LUI, S.C. and G.M. KROLMAN: Color perception in pseudophakia. Presented at the International Intraocular Lensimplant Symposium. Singapore, January, 1981.
LYLE, T.K.: The importance of orthoptic investigation before contact lens fitting in unilateral aphakia: a preliminary report. *Trans. Ophthal. Soc.* LXXIII: 387-398, 1953.
LYNCH, S., G.L. WOLF and I. BERLIN: General anaesthesia for cataract surgery: A comparative review of 2217 consecutive cases. *Curr. Researches.* 53: (6): 909-913, 1974.

MAGGI, C.: Binocular vision in unilateral aphakia corrected by the Strampelli lens. *Am. J. Ophthal.* 52: 81-85, 1961.
MAIDA, J.W. and J.H. SHEETS: Intraocular lenses: A review of results and complications Excerpta Medica, Amsterdam-Oxford, p. 1395, 1979.
MAIDA, J.W. and J.H. SHEETS: Intraocular lenses. A review of 1000 consecutive cases. *Cont. & Intraoc. Lens Med. J.* 4(4): 95-101, 1978.
MAIDA, J.W.: The various uses of the lens glide in implant surgery. *Cont. & Intraoc. Lens Med. J.* 6(3): 279-283, 1980.
MAINSTER, M.A.: Spectral transmittance of intraocular lenses and retinal damage from intense light sources. *Am. J. Ophthal.* 85: 167-170, 1978.
MAINSTER, M.A.: Solar retinitis, photic maculopathy and the pseudophakic eye. *Am. Intraoc. Impl. Soc. J.* 4(3): 84-87, 1978.
MAINSTER, M.A.: Corneal endothelial dynamics and intraocular lens implantation. *Am. Intraoc. Impl. Soc. J.* 4(1): 1978.
MALBRAN, E. and R. DODDS: Retinal detachment and aphakia. *Ophthalmologica* (Basel). 147: 361-384, 1964.
MALBRAN, E. and R. DODDS: Retinal detachment and aphakia. *Ophthalmologica* (Basel). 147: 343-360, 1964.
MALONEY, W.F., R.P. KRATZ, T.R. MAZZOCCO and B. DAVIDSON: Posterior chamber intraocular lens power calculation in 441 cases. *Am. Intraoc. Impl. Soc. J.* 4: 349-350, 1979.
MANSCHOT, W.A.: Über die Ebagultige Vertraglichkeit Kunstlicher Augenlinsen bei der Aphakic und deren Verbesserung Mittels Fixation der Linse in der Pupille. *Klin. Mbi. Augenheilk.* 134: 539, 1959.
MANSCHOT, W.A.: Histopathology of eyes containing Binkhorst lenses. *Am. J. Ophthal.* 77: 865-871, 1974.
MANSCHOT, W.A.: Der Fixationsmechanismus der Iridokapsulären Linse. In: *Kunststoff-implantate in der Ophthalmologie.* Ed. by W. Jaeger, Munich. Bergmann Verlag, pp. 104-108, 1978.
MANSCHOT, W.A.: Mechanism of fixation of two-loop iridocapsular lenses. *Am. J. Ophthal.* 85: 565-468, 1978.
MARIA, Y., R. BONNET and P. COCHET: L'intervention de Strampelli. *Clin. Ophthal.* 1: 2-26, 1959.
MARTIN, N.F., W.R. GREEN and L.W. MARTIN: Retinal phlebitis in Irvine-Gass Syndrome. *Am. J. Ophthal.* 83: 377-386, 1977.
MARX, R.: Geschichte der Augenheilkunde in Luebeck. Inauguraldissertation. *Med. Academy Luebeck,* Luebeck 1970.
MASUDA, K., Y. IZAWA and S. MISHIMA: Prostaglandins and uveitis: A preliminary report. *Jap. J. Ophthal.* 17: 166-170, 1973.
MASUDA, K., Y. IZAWA and S. MISHIMA: Prostaglandins and uveitis: A preliminary report. *Jap. J. Ophthal.* 19: 368-375, 1975.
MAUMENEE, A.E.: Postoperative cataract complications. Symposium, Part III. *Trans. Am. Ac. Ophthal. & Otol.* 61: 51, 1957.
MAUMENEE, A.E. and M.F. GOLDBERG: Push-pull cataract aspiration and Franceschetti corepraxy. *Arch. Ophthal.* 74: 72-73, 1965.
MAURER, Y.: Surgery of patients referred of orthoptic examination from the contact lens department with special reference to cases of unilateral aphakia. *Brit. J. Orthop.* 19: 62-79, 1962.
MAURICE, D.M.: Cellular membrane activity in the corneal endothelium of the intact eye. *Experientia.* 24: 1094, 1968.
MAURICE, D.M.: Current concepts in the physiology of the cornea. *Docum. Ophthal. Proc. Series.* 18: 283-292, 1979.
MAWAS, E., F. PARIZOT, F. GUILLAUME and D. RIGNOT: Intérêt de la position proclive pour la prophylaxie de l'issue de vitré dans l'opération de la cataracte. *Bull. des mémoires de la Soc. Franç. d'Ophtal.* 87: 154-158, 1975.
MAWAS, E.: Ideas concerning the problem of lens implants. *Clin. Ophthal.* 4: 75-77, 1976.
MAWAS, E.: La pseudophakie (le point de vue de néo implanteur). *La clinique ophthalmologique — Revue Médicale.* 3: 35-42, 1978.

McCANNEL, M.A.: A retrievable suture for anterior uveal problems. *Ophthal. Surg.* (U.S.A.). 7: 98-103, 1976.
McCAREY, B.E.: Functional and structural changes in the corneal endothelium during in vitro perfusion. *Invest. Ophthal.* 12(6): 410-417, 1973.
McCAREY, B.E., F.M. POLACK and W. MARSHALL: The phacoemulsification procedure. I. The effect of intraocular irrigating solutions on the corneal endothelium. *Invest. Ophthal.* 15(6): 449-457, 1976.
McCLELAND, R.J.: Examination of intraocular lens power and optical quality at surgery. *Am. Intraoc. Impl. Soc. J.* 4(3): 130-131, 1978.
McENERNY, J.K. and G.A. PAYMAN: A new irrigation solution for intraocular surgery: T.C. Earl solution. *Ophthal. Surg.* 9(1): 66-72, 1978.
McINTYRE, D.J.: Coaxial cannula connector system. *Cont. & Intraoc. Lens Med. J.* 2(2): 50-51, 1976.
McINTYRE, D.J.: Extracapsular cataract surgery. *Cont. & Intraoc. Lens Med. J.* 3(3): 51-62, 1977.
McINTYRE, D.J.: Save the endothelium. *Am. Intraoc. Impl. Soc. J.* 1: 51-53, 1978.
McINTYRE, D.J.: The McCannel suture: A bimanual technique. *Am. Intraoc. Impl. Soc. J.* 5(2): 151-154, 1979.
McINTYRE, D.J.: Comparative endothelial biomicroscopy. *Am. Intraoc. Impl. Soc. J.* 4: 346-348, 1979.
McLEMORE, C.S.: Cadillacs, Volkswagens and aphakic corrections. *Arch. Ophthal.* 70: 734-735, 1963.
McLEMORE, C.S.: Aphakic correction from an aphake's point of view. Correspondence. *Arch. Ophthal.* 74: 443, 1965.
McREYNOLDS, W.U. and N.L. SNIDER: The quick, simple measurement of intraocular lens power and lens resolution at surgery. *Am. Intraoc. Impl. Soc. J.* 4(1): 15-17, 1978.
MEESMANN, A.: Über die Einpflanzung von Plexiglaslinsen nach der Starextraktion. *Berl. Med.* 7: 31-32, 1956.
MEHTA, H.: Retro-pupillary implants. *Am. Intraoc. Impl. Soc. J.* 1: 4-8, 1977.
MEHTA, K.R., S.N. SATHE and S.D. KARYEKAR: The new soft intraocular lens implant. *Am. Intraoc. Impl. Soc. J.* 4(4): 200-205, 1978.
MELTZER, D.W.: Sterile hypopyon following intraocular lens surgery. *Arch. Ophthalmol.* 98: 100-104, 1980.
MELTZER, D.W.: Gamma-ray sterilization and its effect on intraocular lenses. *Am. Intraoc. Impl. Soc. J.* 7(2): 126-129, 1981.
MELTZER, D.W., R.C. DREWS and A.S. HAJEK: Millipore filters in opthalmic surgery: A caution concerning their use. *Am. Intraoc. Impl. Soc. J.* 7(2): 143-146, 1981.
MENEZO, J.L., J. FRANCES and AND R. SUAREZ REYNOLDS: Number and shape of tears in aphakic retinal detachment: Its relationship with different surgical techniques of cataract extraction. *Mod. Probl. Ophthal.* 18: 457-463, 1977.
MERTENS, D.A.E., R. ZIVOJNOVIC and G.S. BAARSMA: Retinal detachment and pseudophakos. *Doc. Ophthal.* 48(2): 267-271, 1979.
MIAMI STUDY GROUP: Cystoid macular edema in aphakic and pseudophakic eyes. *Am. J. Ophthal.* 88: 45-48, 1979.
MICHAELIS, M.C.: Statistical summary. *Am. Intraoc. Impl. Soc. J.* 3(1): 43-44, 1977.
MICHELS, R.G., W.R. GREEN, and A.E. MAUMENEE: Cystoid Macular edema following cataract extraction. *Ophthal. Surg.* 2: 217, 1971.
MILLER, D. and C.H. DOHLMAN: Effect of cataract surgery on the cornea. *Trans. Am. Ac. Ophthal. & Otol.* 74: 369-374, 1970.
MILLER, D., P. O'CONNOR and J. WILLIAMS: Use of Na-Hyaluronate during intraocular lens implantation in rabbits. *Ophthal. Surg.* 8(6): 58-61, 1977.
MILLER, D. and R. STEGMANN: Use of Na-Hyaluronate in human IOL implantation. *Manuscript* - 26 jan. 1979 - Annals ophthal. 13: 811, 1981.
MISHIMA, S. and K. MASUDA: *Clinical Implications of Prostaglandins and Synthesis Inhibitors. Symp. on Ocular Therapy.* Ed. by I.H. Leopold and R.P. Burns, New York: Wiley Med. Publ., 10: 1-19, 1977.
MISSOTTEN, L., I. HAUTTEQUIET and J. ROMMEL: Contactlenzen en implantlenzen voor aphakie; een vergelijkende studie. *Sovebeko* 5: 49-61, 1976.

MIYAKE, K.: Prevention of cystoid macular edema after lens extraction by topical indomethacin. (I) *Graefes Arch. Klin. Ophthal.* 203: 81-88, 1977.
MIYAKE, K.: Prevention of cystoid macular edema after lens extraction by topical indomethacin. (II): A control study in bilateral extractions. *Jap. J. Ophthal.* 22: 80-94, 1978.
MIYAKE, K.: Prophylaxis of aphakic cystoid macular edema using topical indomethacin. *Am. Intraoc. Impl. Soc. J.* 4: 174-179, 1978.
MOCHIZUKI, M., M. SAWA and K. MASUDA: Topical indomethacin in intracapsular extraction of senile cataract. *Jap. J. Ophth.* 215-226, 1977.
MOLONEY, G.E.: Letter to the Editor, *Lancet I.* 531, 1958.
MOORE, C.R. and R.T. STELLER: Early recognition and proper treatment of the vip syndrome. *Am. Intraoc. Impl. Soc. J.* 4(3): 114-117, 1978.
MORAX, P.V. and Y. POULIQUEN: Considération sur le décollement de la rétine de l'aphaque. *Annales d'oculistique.* 196: 761-775, 1963.
MOSES, L.: Pupillary block, glaucoma after Choyce lens implantation. *Am. Intraoc. Impl. Soc. J.* 1: 50, 1978.
MOSES, L.: Capsulotomy technique in the presence of an anterior chamber lens. *Am. Intraoc. Impl. Soc. J.* 4: 173, 1978.
MOSES, L.: Ciliochoroidal detachment and pseudophakos implantation. *Am. Intraoc. Impl. Soc. J.* 4(1): 57-59, 1978.
MOSES, L.: Intraocular pressures and visual fields following pseudophakos implantation. *Am. Intraoc. Impl. Soc. J.* 4(2), 1978.
MOSES, L.: Incidences of cystoid macular edema following cataract extraction with pseudophakos implantation: Intracapsular vs. extracapsular vs. phacoemulsification. *Am. Intraoc. Impl. Soc. J.* 2: 17, 1978.
MOSES, L.: Kelman anterior chamber lens, a preliminary report. *Am. Intraoc. Impl. Soc. J.* 1: 54-56, 1978.
MOSES, L.: Cystoid macular edema and retinal detachment following cataract surgery. *Am. Intraoc. Impl. Soc. J.* 4: 326, 1979.
MOSIER, M.A., B. LUSK, T.H. PETTIT, D.H. HOWARD and J. RHODES: Fungal endopthalmitis following intraocular lens implantation. *Am. J. Ophthal.* 83: 1-8, 1977.
MÜNCHOW, W.: Zur Geschichte der intraokularen Korrektur der Aphakie. *Klin. Augenheilk.* 145: 771-777, 1964.

NAGATA, M.: Experience with the cases of Binkhorst irisclip and iridocapsular pseudophakos implantations. *Acta Soc. Ophthal. Jap.* 79: 299-304, 1975.
NAUMANN, G. and R. ORTBAUER: Zur Klinik und Histopathologie nach erfolgreicher Vorderkammerlinseimplantation. *Ber. dtsch. ophth. Gesel.* 70: 63-69, 1969.
NAUMANN, G. and R. ORTBAUER: Histopathology after successful implantation of anterior chamber acrylic lenses. *Surv. Ophthal.* 15: 18-24, 1970.
NEUFELD, A.H., L.M. JAMPOL and M.L. SEARS: Aspirin prevents the disruption of the blood-aqueous barrier in the rabbit eye. *Nature.* 238: 158-159, 1972.
NONNENMACHER, H.: Retinal detachment after cataract extraction. *Klin. Mbl. Augenheil.* 118: 363-369, 1951.
NICHOLLS, J.V.V.: Macular edema in association with cataract extraction. *Am. J. Ophthal.* 37(1): 665-672, 1954.
NIELSEN, J.M.H. and J.P. GILLS: Use of the Choyce lens for IOL replacement. *Am. Intraoc. Impl. Soc. J.* 4(4): 219-221, 1978.
NORDLOHNE, M.E.: *The intraocular implant lens.* Development and results with special reference to the Binkhorst lens. Doctoral Thesis. The Hague, W. Junk, 1975.
NORDLOHNE, M.E.: Dislocation and endothelial corneal dystrophy (E.C.D.) in patients fitted with Binkhorst lens implants, 1958-1972. *Doc. Ophthal. Proceedings Series.* 6: 15-22, 1975.
NORN, M.S.: Vital staining of corneal endothelium in cataract extraction. *Acta Ophthal.* 49: 725-733, 1971.
NORN, M.S.: Pachometric study on the influence of corneal endothelial vital straining. *Acta Ophthal.* 51: 679-686, 1973.
NORN, M.S.: Depth of anterior chamber after cataract extraction. *Brit. J. Ophthal.* 62: 474-477, 1978.
NORTON, A., W. BROWN, M. CARLSON, I.S. PILGER and R.S. RIFFENBURGH: Pathogenesis of aphakic macular edema. *Am. J. Ophthal.* 80: 96-101, 1975.

NORTON, A.: Meeting Am Intraoc. Lens Impl. Soc., Los Angeles, March 1978 (communication).
NORTON, E.W.D.: Retinal detachment in aphakia. *Am. J. Ophthal.* 58: 111-124, 1964.
NORTON, E.W.D.: Management of retinal detachment in patients with intraocular lens (Copeland Model of the Epstein Lens). *Trans. Am. Ac. Ophthal. & Otol.* 81: 135-136, 1976.
NORTON, E.W.D.: Closing Remarks. Symposium: Intraocular lens. *Trans. Am. Ac. Ophthal. & Otol.* 81: 137, 1976.
NORTON, E.W.D. and J.C. JOHNSON: The influence of changing cataract techniques on the ophthalmologist concerned with retinal diseases. *Mod. Probl. Ophthal.* 18: 440-443, 1977.
NOTEBOOM, E.: Über die Optik der Zeiss-Vorderkammerlinse in Verbindung mit dem Auge. *Z. ärztl. Fortbild.* 54: 50-52, 1960.
NOVER, A., P.D. STEINBACH and A. LADWIG: Erfahrungen mit der Implantation von Iris-Clip Linsen. In: *Kunststoffimplantate in der Ophthalmologie.* Ed. by W. Jaeger. Munich: J.F. Bergmann Verlag, pp. 128-131, 1978.
NYGAARD, P. and C.D. BINKHORST: An investigation of post-traumatic lens implants in adults. *Cont. & Intraoc. Lens Med. J.* 4(2): 58-61, 1978.

O'DAY, D.: Fungal endophthalmitis caused by Paecilomyces lilacines after intraocular lens implantation (editorial). *Am. J. Ophthal.* 83: 130-1, 1977.
OGLE, K.N., H.M. BURIAN and R.E. BANNON: On the correction of unilateral aphakia with contact lenses. *Arch. Ophthal.* 59: 639-652, 1958.
OGLESBY, R.B.: Complications of the Copeland implant. *Trans. Am. Ac. Ophthal. & Otol.* 86: 667-671, 1979.
OGUCHI, Y. and A.T.M. VAN BALEN: Prepupillary pseudophakos and iseikonization. *Doc. Ophthalmologica.* 37: 295-306, 1974.
OLMOS, E.Z. and F.H. ROY: Artiphakic refraction. *Cont. & Intraoc. Lens Med. J.* 5(4): 179-181, 1979.
OLMOS, E.Z. and F.H. ROY: Results of over 1000 intraocular lens implants in the last five years. *Cont. & Intraoc. Lens Med. J.* 6(2): 162-170, 1980.
OLSON, R.J., K.S. MORGAN and H. KOLODNER: The Shearing-style intraocular lens and the posterior chamber. *Am. Intraoc. Impl. Soc. J.* 4: 338-345, 1979.
OLSON, R.J. and T.E. SLAPPEY: Corneal endothelial damage induced by intraocular lenses: an in vitro study. *Am. Intraoc. Impl. Soc. J.* 4: 321-323, 1979.
OLSON, R.J., H. KOLODNER and H.E. KAUFMAN: The optical quality of currently manufactured intraocular lenses. *Am. J. Ophthal.* 88: 548-555, 1979.
OLSON, R.J.: Intraocular lens optical quality: Update 1979. *Am. Intraoc. Impl. Soc. J.* 5: 16-17, 1980.
OLSON, T.: Corneal thickness and endothelial damage after intracapsular cataract extraction. *Acta Ophthalmologica.* 58: 424-433, 1980.
OPPONG, M.C., R. KERN, J. SCHIPPER and F. KÄPPELI: Zur Korrektur der traumatish bedingten einseitigen Aphakie bei Kindern und in Erwebsleben stehender Erwachsener mit intraokulären Linsen. *Klin. Mbl. Augenheilk.* 172: 231-234, 1978.
OSHER, M.S.: The simple approach to intraocular lens implantation. *Ophthal. Surg.* 6(3): 32-35, 1975.
OSHER, M.S.: Intraocular lenses: visual results and complications. *Ophthal. Surg.* 7(4): 71-78, 1976.
OSHER, M.S.: Simplified intraocular lens implantation, for residents and the inexperienced implant surgeon. *Cont. & Intraoc. Lens Med. J.* 3(3): 33-35, 1977.
OSHER, M.S.: Technique with Copeland intraocular lenses. *Cont. & Intraoc. Lens Med. J.* 4(3): 111-113, 1978.
ÖSTERLIN, S.: Preludes to retinal detachment in the aphakic eye. *Mod. Probl. Ophthal.* 18: 464-467, 1977.
ÖSTERLIN, S.: On the molecular biology of the vitreous in the aphakic eye. *Acta Ophthalmologica* (Basel). 55: 353-361, 1977.
OZAKI, L.: Permeability of the posterior lens capsule in connection with intraocular lens implant surgery. XXII Concilium Ophthalmologicum Kyoto 1978. *Excerpta Medica, Acta pars II*, Amsterdam-Oxford, pp. 1407-1410, 1979.

PACE-ASCIAK, C. and S. COLE: Inhibitors of prostaglandin catabolism. I. Differential sensitivity of 9 PGDH, 13 PGR and 15-PGDH to concentrations of indomethacin. *Experientia.* 31: 143, 1975.
PARELMAN, A.G.: Monocular aphakia und contralateral pseudophakia. *Ophthal. Surg.* 7(3): 83-88, 1976.
PARELMAN, A.G.: The circular loop intraocular lens. Opht. Surg. 4, 79-91, 1976.
PARELMAN, A.G.: Forceps for transiridectomy safety clip closure of the circular loop intraocular lens. *Cont. & Intraoc. Lens Med. J.* 2: 46, 1976.
PARELMAN, A.G.: Sterile uveitis and intraocular lensimplantation. *Am. Intraoc. Impl. Soc. J.* 4: 301-306, 1979.
PARIZOT, H.: Historique des implants intraoculaires. *La clinique opthalmologique — revue médicale.* 3: 31-34, 1978.
PARK, J.H.: The technique of Park intraocular lens implantation for both intracapsular and extracapsular cataract surgeons. *Am. Intraoc. Impl. Soc. J.* 4(1): 29-31, 1978.
PARRY, T.G.W.: Modification in intraocular acrylic lens surgery. *Brit. J. Ophthal.* 38: 616-618, 1954.
PARRY, T.G.W.: New design in anterior chamber lenses. *Brit. J. Ophthal.* 42: 376-379, 1958.
PASCAL, J.I.: *Studies in visual optics.* St. Louis, C.V. Mosby Co., 1952.
PAUFIQUE, L.: Opération de Ridley technique, complications indications. *Bull. & Mem. Soc. Fr. d'ophtal.* 67: 379-385, 1954.
PEARCE, J.L.: Long-term results of the Binkhorst iris clip lens in senile cataract. *Brit. J. Ophthal.* 56: 319-331, 1972.
PEARCE, J.L.: Survey of 360 eyes with pupillary lenses. Communication to the authors. 1974 (*Manuscript*).
PEARCE, J.L.: Long-term results of the Choyce anterior chamber lens implants. Mk. V, VII, VIII. *Brit. J. Ophthal.* 59: 99-106, 1975.
PEARCE, J.L.: New lightweight sutured posterior chamber lens implant. *Trans. Ophthal. Soc. U.K.* 96: 6-10, 1976.
PEARCE, J.L.: Sixteen months' experience with 140 posterior chamber intraocular lens implants. *Brit. J. Ophthal.* 21: 310-315, 1977.
PEARCE, J.L. and T. GHOSH: Surgical and post-operative problems with Binkhorst II and IV-loop lenses. *Trans. Ophthal. Soc. U.K.* 97: 84-90, 1977.
PEARCE, J.L.: 'The Pearce posterior chamber lens'. *Communication,* Am. Intraoc. Impl. Soc. Meeting L.A., March 1978.
PEARCE, J.L.: Current thoughts on the Pearce posteior chamber lenses. *Manuscript to the authors.* 1979.
PEARCE, J.L.: Pearce-style posterior chamber lenses. *Am. Intraoc. Impl. Soc. J.* 1: 33-36, 1980.
PERCIVAL, S.P.B.: Intraocular versus contact lenses. Results of a three year comparative trial in a presenile age group. *Am. Intraoc. Impl. Soc. J.* 1: 48-49, 1976.
PETIT, T.H., R.J. OLSON, R.Y. FOOS and W.J. MARTIN: Fungal endopthalmitis following intraocular lens implantation. *Arch. Ophthal.* 98: 1025-1039, 1980.
PETIT, T.H.: Communication. *Am. Intraoc. Impl. Soc. Meeting,* Los Angeles, Oct. 1976.
PEYMAN, G.A. and J.E. KOZIOL: Intraocular lens fixation with dacron mesh: Part I. *Opthal. Surg.* 8(2): 58-64, 1977.
PEYMAN, G.A. and J.E. KOZIOL: Intraocular lens fixation with dacron. *Am. Intraoc. Impl. Soc. J.* 4(4): 192-196, 1978.
PEYMAN, G.A., M.A. NYBERG and J.E. KOZIOL: Experimental evaluation of anterior chamber lenses fixated with dacron. *Ophth. Surg.* 9(5): 70-90, 1978.
PEYMAN, G.A. and K. ZWEIG: Dry coating of intraocular lenses with bovine submaxillary mucin. *Am. J. Ophthal.* 87: 561: 566, 1979.
PEYMAN, G.A.: Vitrectomy for the anterior segment surgeon. *Am. Intraoc. Impl. Soc. J.* 1: 4-8, 1979.
PEYMAN, G.A., J.E. KOZIOL and G. NATCHIAR: Dacron fixation of an intraocular posterior chamber lens. *Am. Intraoc. Impl. Soc. J.* 1: 30-32, 1980.
PFOFF, D.S.: Open sky intraocular lens implants in a private and academic setting. *Cont. & Intraoc. Lens Med. J.* 3: 53-60, 1979.
PHILLIPS, L.J. and G.G. SOLTIS: Intraocular lenses and their follow-up in the optometric office. *J. of the Am. Optometric Assoc.* 50(2): 149-161, 1979.

PHILLIPS, C.R.: Gaseous Sterilization. In: *Disinfection, sterilization and preservation.* Ed. by C.A. Lawrence and S.S. Block, Philadelphia: Leo & Febiger, 1968.
PODOS, S.M., B. BECKER and M.A. KASS: Prostaglandin synthesis, inhibition and intraocular pressure. *Invest. Ophtahl.* 12: 426-433, 1973.
POLACK, F.M.: *Corneal Transplantation.* New York: Grune and Stratton, 1977.
POLACK, F.M. and A. SUGAR: The phacoemulsification procedure II. Corneal endothelial changes. *Invest. Ophthal.* 15(8): 458-469, 1976.
POLACK, F.M.: Pathologische Erscheinungen als folge der Einpflanzung intraokularer Linsen. *Klin. Mbl. Augenheilk.* 174: 535-541, 1979.
POLEY, B.: Epidemic of Pseudomonas endophthalmitis associated with contaminated intraocular lenses. Read before the *Am. Intraoc. Impl. Soc. Symposium,* Los Angeles, March, 1978.
POLYCHRONAKOS, D.: Clinical observations on 1000 operations for cataract. *Ophthalmologica.* 144: 375-384, 1962.
POOLE, T.A. and M.A. GALIN: Argon laser photocoagulation of the posterior segment in pseudophakia. *Am. J. Ophthal.* 83: 185-187, 1977.
POOLE, T.A.: Retinal detachment and laser therapy in eyes with intraocular lens implants. *Am. Intraoc. Impl. Soc. J.* 3(1): 46-47, 1977.
POSTLETHWAIT, R.W.: Long-term comparative study of non-absorbable sutures. *Annals of surgery.* 171: 892-898, 1970.
PRAEGER, D.L. and H.A. SCHNEIDER: Corneal thickness measurements following intraocular lens implantation. *Ophthal. Surg.* 8(3): 97-100, 1977.
PRAEGER, D.L.: One man's experience with the Choyce Mark VIII anterior chamber lens. *Am. Intraoc. Impl. Soc. J.* 3: 90-99, 1978.
PRAEGER, D.L.: Posterior chamber pseudophakia. *Cont. & Intraoc. Lens Med. J.* 4(3): 104-110, 1978.
PRAEGER, D.L.: Extracapsular cataract extraction with simultaneous implantation of 300 Copeland iris plane lenses: Five years follow-up — A retrospective study. *Ophthal. Surg.* 10(9): 59-69, 1979.
PRAEGER, D.L.: Indications and contraindications. In: *Pseudophakia, Current Trends and Concepts.* Ed. by M.L. Kwitko and D.L. Praeger. Baltimore-London: Williams & Wilkins, 1980, pp. 43-46, 1980.
PROTKOP, B.S.: Intraocular lenses vs. "routine" cataract extractions — a comparative study. *Cont. & Intraoc. Lens Med. J.* 3(1): 48-52, 1977.
PROTKOP, B.S.: The use of intraocular lens in middle-age cataract patients. *Cont. & Intraoc. Lens Med. J.* 3: 70-73, 1979.

QUIN, L.H. and J.C. PORTER: The removal of tritrated water from the vitreous of the dog. *Trans. Am. Ophthal. Soc. J.* 61: 181-195, 1963.

RAD, G.N., D. BARSOMIAN and J.V. AQUAVELLA: Morphology of corneal Endothelium and Intraocular Lens. *Cont. & Intraoc. Lens Med. J.* 6(2): 154-157, 1980.
RAININ, E.A.: Corneal retraction and intraocular lens implantation. *Annals Ophthal.* 11: 969-970, 1979.
RAVAULT, M.P. and J. MARION: Considérations statistiques sur le décollement de rétine de l'aphake. *Bull. Soc. Ophtal. Franç.* 11: 273-274, 1977.
RAZEMON, P.: Le pronostic de la cataracte traumatique. Doctoral Thesis, Université de Nantes, 1971.
REESE, A.B., I.S. JONES and W.C. COOPER: Macular changes secondary to vitreous traction. *Am. J. Ophthal.* 64: 544-549, 1967.
REESE, W.S., J.R. FINLAY and H. ROMAINE: Reports on the use of the intraocular acrylic lens (Ridley operation). *Trans. Am. Ac. Ophthal. & Otol.* 58: 55-60, 1954.
REESE, W.S. and T.N. HAMDI: Five years' experience with the Ridley operation. *A.M.A. Archives of Ophthal.* 58: 389-391, 1957.
REESE, W.S.: Results in 39 bilateral Ridley intraocular implants. *Brit. J. Ophthal.* 44: 713-717, 1960.
REINHART, W.J. and W.L. ANNABLE: Intraocular lens surgery on a resident's service. *Ophthal. Surg.* 8(3): 156-161, 1977.
RESHMI, C.S. and E.C. KONDROT: Pachymetric evaluation of corneal thickness after cataract extraction and intraocular lens implantation. *Am. Intraoc. Impl. Soc. J.* 2: 17-21, 1976.

RESHMI, C.S. and E.C. KONDROT: Effect of intraocular lensimplant surgery on corneal thickness: Pachymetric evaluation of 100 eyes. In: *XXII concilium Ophthalmologie cours* Kyoto 1978 — acta Pars II ed. by Koichi Shimizu. Excerpta Medica, Amsterdam-Oxford, pp. 1399-1402, 1979.
RESTIVO, M.L.: Contribution to the problem of crystalline lens transplantation. *Am. Ophthal. Clin. Ocul.* 93(11): 1251, 1967.
RICH, A.M., S.D. McPHERSON: Iris response to suture materials. In: *Surgery of the Iris and the Ciliary Body.* Ed. by S. Karger, 1975.
RICH, W.J.: Effect of lid specula and superior rectus traction on intraocular pressure. *Trans. Ophthal. Soc. U.K.* 97: 106-108, 1977.
RICHARD, D.A.: An outline for the testing and subsequent analysis of the resolving power of intraocular lenses. *Am. Intraoc. Impl. Soc. J.* 3-4: 229-231, 1977.
RIDGWAY, A.E.A.: Binocular effects of intraocular lens insertion. *Trans. Ophthal. Soc. U.K.* 79: 96-99: 1977.
RIDGWAY, A.E.A.: Orthopic consequences of Binkhorst lens implantation for unilateral cataract. *Ophthal. Surg.* 8(3): 170-173, 1977.
RIDLEY, F.: Safety requirements for acrylic implants. *Brit. J. Ophthal.* 41: 359-367, 1957.
RIDLEY, H.: Intraocular acrylic lenses. *Trans. Ophthal. Soc. U.K.* 71: 617-621, 1951.
RIDLEY, H.: Further observations on intraocular acrylic lenses in cataract surgery. *J. Int. Coll. Surg.* 18: 825-833, 1952.
RIDLEY, H.: Intraocular acrylic lenses: A recent development in the surgery of cataract. *Brit. J. Ophthal.* 36: 113-122, 1952.
RIDLEY, H.: Further observations on intraocular acrylic lenses. *Trans. Ophthal. Soc. U.K.* 72: 511-514, 1952.
RIDLEY, H.: Demonstration of 4 patients at the joint clinical meeting. *Trans. Ophthal. Soc. U.K.* 72: 669, 1952.
RIDLEY, H.: Further observations on intraocular acrylic lenses in cataract surgery. *Am. J. Ophthal.* 36: 988, 1953.
RIDLEY, H.: Further observations on intraocular acrylic lenses in cataract surgery. *Trans. Am. Ac. Ophthal. & Otol.* 57: 98-106, 1953.
RIDLEY, H.: Further experiences of intraocular acrylic lens surgery. *Brit. J. Ophthal.* 38: 156-162, 1954.
RIDLEY, H.: Late surgical results of use of the intraocular acrylic lens. *J. Int. Coll. Surg.* 26: 335-341, 1956.
RIDLEY, H.: An anterior chamber lenticular implant. *Brit. J. Ophthal.* 41: 355-358, 1957.
RIDLEY, H.: Cataract surgery with particular reference to intraocular lenticular implants of various types. *Trans. Ophthal. Soc. U.K.* 78: 585-592, 1958.
RIDLEY, H.: Intraocular acrylic lenses. *Brit. J. Ophthal.* 44: 705-712, 1960.
RIDLEY, H.: Intraocular acrylic lenses. *An. Inst. Barraquer* III-4: 548-554, 1962.
RIDLEY, H.: Acrylic implants. Current results. *An. Inst. Barraquer* IX-1/2: 143-149, 1969.
RIDLEY, H.: Intraocular acrylic lenses. Improved technique and results. Proceedings of the XXI Intern. Congress. Mexico, 8-14, 1970. Intern. Congr. Series, 222, Amsterdam. *Excerpta Med. Found,* pp. 771-775, 1971.
RIDLEY, H.: The long-term effects of ocular implants. *Proc. Royal Soc. Med. U.K.* 63: 309, 1970.
RIDLEY, H.: The origin and objectives of intraocular lenticular implants. *Trans. Am. Ac. Ophthal. & Otol.* 81: 65-66, 1976.
RIDLEY, H.: In: Abstract meeting Cannes. *Newsletter International Intraocular Implant Club,* nr. 9: Sept. 1979.
RINTELEN, F. and G. SAUBERMANN: Pathohistologische Untersuchungen nach Kunststofflinsen-implantation beim Menschen. *Ophthalmologica* (Basel). 131: 369-373, 1956.
ROBBINS, R. and M.A. GALIN: Effect of osmotic agents on the vitreous body. *Arch. Ophthal.* 82: 694-699, 1969.
ROBBINS, R., M. BLUMENTHAL and M.A. GALIN: Reduction of vitreous weight by ocular massage. *Am. J. Ophthal.* 69: 603-607, 1970.
ROETH, A. DE: Ridley's cataract operation. *Am. J. Ophthal.* 36: 1568-1570, 1953.

ROMMEL, J.: Results in 300 implantations after extracapsular extraction. *Communication French intraoc. Soc. Meeting,* Perpignan Nov. 1977.
ROMMEL, J.: Seven years of experience with Binkhorst lenses. *Communication Intern. Implant Soc. Joint Meeting* Cannes, May 1979.
ROMMEL, J.: Artificial lens decentration. *Communication intern. lens implant symposium* Singapore, Jan. 1981.
ROPER-HALL, M.J.: Intraocular lenticuli. *Brit. J. Ophthal.* 58: 715-717, 1975.
ROPER-HALL, M.J.: The history of intraocular lenses. *Trans. Am. Ac. Ophthal. & Otol.* 81: 67-69, 1976.
ROPER-HALL, M.J.: Traumatic cataract. *Trans. Ophthal. Soc. U.K.* 97: 58-59, 1977.
ROUGIER, M.J.: La correction de l'aphakie unilatérale par les verres de contact et par les lentilles cristalliniennes de Ridley — Étude comparative. *Bull. Mem. Soc. Fr. d'Ophtal.* 67: 391-405, 1954.
ROY, F.H. and E. OLMOS: After-cataract: studies of chemical and radiation inhibition. *Cont. & Intraoc. Lens Med. J.* 5(4): 175-178, 1979.
RUEDEMANN, A.D. Jr.: Quality control. The report of the prosthetic committee of the academy. *Trans. Am. Ac. Ophthal. & Otol.* 81: 132, 1976.
RYCROFT, P.V.: Acrylic lens implants and keratopathy. Perspect. Ophthal. 1: 215-218, Amsterdam. *Excerpta Med. Found,* 1968.

SALZ, J.J. and C.L. JANES: Anterior Chamber Implants, Visual Results, Complications and Gonioscopy Findings. *Cont. & Intraoc. Lens Med. J.* 6(3): 302-309, 1980.
SANDERS, D.R., G.A. PEYMAN, J.K. McENERY and R.V. JANEVICIUS: In vitro evaluation of intraocular infusion fluids: Effects on the lens and cornea. *Ophth. Surg.* 8(5): 63-67, 1977.
SAUBERMANN, G.: Über Resultate nach Kunststofflinseimplantation. *Ophthalmologica* (Basel). 129: 247-252, 1955.
SAUBERMANN, G.: Komplicationen nach Vorderkammerlinseimplantation. *Ophthalmologica* (Basel). 137: 178-182, 1959.
SAUTTER, H. and H. KUNERT: Erfahrungsbericht über unsere ersten 100 Irisclip Linsen. *Ber. Dtsch. Ophthal. Ges.* 75: 47, 123-127, 1978.
SAWA, M. and K. MASUDA: Topical Indomethacin in soft cataract aspiration. *Jap. J. Ophthal.* 20: 514-519, 1976.
SHAFER, D.M.: Retinal detachment after cataract surgery. *Int. Ophthalmol. Clin.* 4: 1091, 1964.
SCHARF, J.: Demonstration einer neuartigen Kunstofflinse zur Korrektur der Aphakie mit Vorstellung operierter Patienten. *Klin. Mbl. Augenheilk.* 128: 233-235, 1956.
SCHARF, J.: Über zweijährige Erfahrungen mit einer Vorderkammerlinse. *Bericht über die Zusammenkunft der Deutschen Ophth. Ges. München.* 59: 222-227, 1957.
SCHEIE, H.G., P.H. MORSE and A. AMINLARI: Incidence of retinal detachment following cataract extraction. *Arch. Ophthal.* 98: 293-295, 1973.
SCHEPENS, C.L. and G.C. BAHN: Examination of the ora serrata. Its importance in retinal detachment. *Arch. Ophthal.* 44: 677-690, 1950.
SCHEPENS, C.L.: Retinal detachment and aphakia. *Arch. Ophthal.* 45: 1-17, 1951.
SCHEPENS, C.L.: Subclinical retinal detachment. *Arch. Ophthal.* 47: 593-606, 1952.
SCHEPENS, C.L.: Fundus changes caused by alterations of the vitreous body. *Am. J. Ophthal.* 39: 631-633, 1955.
SCHIFERLI, R.: Theoretisch praktische Abhandlung über den grauen Starr. Gabler, Jena und Leipzig: 1797, cited by Münchow, 1964.
SCHILLINGER, R.J., V. SHEARER and O.R. LEVY: Animal experiments with a new type of intraocular acrylic lens. *Arch. Ophthal.* 59: 423-434, 1958.
SCHIMEK, R.A., J.C. COOKSEY, M. LANDRENEAU and J.B. STEIGNER: The recovery phase after ocular hypotension induced by compression. *Arch. Ophthal.* 85: 288-294, 1971.
SCHIMMELPFENNIG, B., F. BIGAR, R. WITMER and R. HÜRZELER: Endothelial changes in human donor corneas. *Graefes Arch. Klin. Ophthal.* 200-210, 1976.
SCHMITT, H. and W. DODEN: Mikroskopische und Bakteriologische Untersuchungen an Kunststoff-fäden nach längerer Verweildauer im Hornhautgewebe. *Klin. Mbl. Augenheilk.* 161: 654-658, 1972.

SCHNEIDER, H.A. and D.L. PRAEGER: Corneal thickness measurements following intraocular lens implantation. *Am. Intraoc. Impl. Soc. J.* 1: 36-38, 1977.
SCHOTT, K.: Ergebnisse und Erfahrungen bei der Implantation intraocularer Linsen. *Manuscript read before the German Ophth. Soc. Meeting, Heidelberg, Sept. 1977.*
SCHOTT, K.: Ergebnisse und Erfahrungen bei der Implantation intraocularer Linsen. In: Kunststoffimplantate in der Ophthalmologie. Ed. by W. Jaeger, Münich J.F., Bergmann Verlag, 1978.
SCHRECK, E.: Vorderkammerlinsen zur Behandlung der Aphakic and hoher Ametropien. *59 Ber. Deutsch, Ophth. Gesell.*, Heidelberg, p. 212, 1955.
SCHRECK, E.: Über ältere und neuere Möglichkeiten zum Ersatz der menschlichen Linse. *Münch. Med. Wschr.* 98: 401-404, 1956.
SCHRECK, E.: Erfahrungen mit Vorderkammerlinsen. *Klin. Mbl. Augenheilk.* 129: 112-113, 1956.
SCHRECK, E.: Besteck zur Implantation von Vorderkammerlinsen. *Med. Techn.* 77: 68, 1957.
SCHRECK, E.: Linsenimplantation nach Staroperation. In: *Augenheilkunde in Klinik und Praxis.* Ed. by W. Rohrschneider, Stuttgart: Enke Verlag, pp. 151-163, 1958.
SCHRECK, E.: Erfahrungen mit über 150 Vorderkammerlinsen eines eigenen Models. *Acta Conc. Ophthal. Belgica.* 2: 1609-1704, 1959.
SCHULTZ, R.D., H.F. EDELHAUSER, D.L. VAN HORN and R.A. HYNDIUK: Bullous Keratopathy: Hazards of intraocular irrigating solutions and epinephrine in cataract surgery. In: *Current Concepts in Cataract Surgery.* Ed. by J. Emery St. Louis, C.V. Mosby Co., 1976.
SCHWERTASSEK, K.: Studien über der Mikroskopische Struktur von Polyamid-6-Fasern. *Faserforschung und Textiltechnik.* 11: 125-129, 1960.
SCHWERTASSEK, K. and J. DVORAK: Beitrag zum Studium des Abbaues von Synthesefaserstoffen im lebenden Organismus. *Faserforschung und Textiltechnik.* 21: 78-83, 1970.
SCOTT, K., R.M. BURDE and S.R. WALTMAN: Minimizing corneal endothelial damage due to intraocular lens contact. *Invest. Ophthal. Visual Sci.* 16(11): 1053-1056, 1977.
SEARLE, J.F. and J. THOMSITT: Anaesthesia for cataract surgery: A preliminary communication. *Trans. Ophthal. Soc. U.K.* 97: 109-111, 1977.
SETÄLÄ, K. and A. VANNAS: Endothelial cells in the glaucomatocyclitic crisis. *Adv. Ophth.* 36: 218-224, 1978.
SETÄLÄ, K.: Corneal endothelial cell density in iridocyclitis. *Acta Ophthal.* 57: 277-286, 1979.
SETIAWAN-ONG, H.D.: Intra und postoperative Komplikationen bei der Linseneinpflanzung nach Binkhorst. Therapie und Prophylaxe. *Versammlung des Vereins Rhein. — Westf. Augenärtze.* 125: 54-67, 1972.
SETIAWAN-ONG, H.D., M.U. DARDENNE and U. LIPPERT: Über eine neue Apparatur zur dosierten bimanuellen Irrigations-Aspirations-Technik für weiche und mittelweiche Katarakte. *Klin. Mbl. Augenheilk.* 160: 490-496, 1972.
SEVERIN, D.: Erfahrungen mit der Iris-Clip-Linse nach Binkhorst. *Klin. Mbl. Augenheilk.* 159: 711, 1971.
SEVERIN, S.L.: The Severin posterior chamber lens for intracapsular and extracapsular cataract surgery. *Cont. & Intraoc. Lens Med. J.* 6(3): 291-294, 1980.
SHAFER, D.M.: Retinal detachment after phacoemulsification. *Trans. Am. Ac. Ophthal. & Otol.* 78: 28-30, 1974.
SHAKIB, M. and J.G. CUNHA-VAZ: Studies on the permeability of the blood-retinal barrier. IV. Junctional Complexes of the retinal and their role in the permeability of the blood-retinal barrier. *Exptl. Eye Res.* 5: 229-234, 1966.
SHAMMAS, H.J.F. and C.F. MILKIE: Cystoid macular edema following the implantation of anterior chamber lenses. *Am. Intraoc. Impl. Soc. J.* 3: 87, 1978.
SHAMMAS, H.J.F. and C.F. MILKIE: Secondary lens implantation in aphakia: Visual results and complications. *Am. Intraoc. Impl. Soc. J.* 4: 180-183, 1978.
SHAMMAS, H.J.F. and C.F. MILKIE: Primary vs. secondary insertion of anterior chamber lenses. *Am. Intraoc. Impl. Soc. J.* 2: 141-149, 1979.
SHAPLAND, C.D.: Retinal detachment in aphakia. *Trans. Ophthal. Soc. U.K.* 54: 176-196, 1934.

SHEARING, S.P.: A practical posterior chamber lens. *Cont. & Intraoc. Lens Med. J.* 4(3): 114-119, 1978.
SHEARING, S.P.: Complications of the Shearing posterior chamber intraocular lens. *Cont. & Intraoc. Lens Med. J.* 5(2): 64-74, 1979.
SHEARING, S.P.: The histroy of ciliary fixated intraocular lenses. *Cont. & Intraoc. Lens Med. J.* 6(3): 295-302, 1980.
SHEETS, J.H.: *Bridge over Trouble Waters.* Publ. by J.H. Sheets, 1975.
SHEETS, J.H.: A comparable study of intraocular lens cases and cataract removal without lens implantation. *Cont. & Intraoc. Lens Med. J.* 3(4): 34-38, 1977.
SHEETS, J.H.: Lens glide in implant surgery. *Arch. Ophthal.* 96: 145-146, 1978.
SHEPARD, D.D.: Analysis of 275 Intraocular Lens Implantations. *Read before. Int. I.O.L. Club, Paris.* June 1, 1974.
SHEPARD, D.D.: Intraocular lens advances: repositioning of subluxated lenses, treatment of flat anterior chamber and pre-operative vitreous pressure reduction. *Am. Intraoc. Impl. Soc. J.* 2: 7, 1976.
SHEPARD, D.D.: *The intraocular lens instruction manual.* Santa Maria, Calif. 1976 and 1977.
SHEPARD, D.D.: Indications for intraocular lens removal. *Ophthal. Surg.* 8(3): 144-148, 1977.
SHEPARD, D.D.: Intraocular lens implantation: Analysis of 500 consecutive cases. *Ophthal. Surg.* 8(3): 57-63, 1977.
SHEPARD, D.D.: The dangers of metal-loop intraocular lenses. *Ophthal. Surg.* 8(5): 93-95, 1977.
SHEPARD, D.D.: Retinal detachment with intraocular lenses. *Am. Intraoc. Lens Med. J.* 2: 55, 1978.
SHEPARD, D.D.: Round table discussion on Anterior chamber lenses: *Communication,* Am. Intraoc. Impl. Soc. Meeting, March 1978.
SHEPARD, D.D. The fate of eyes from which intraocular lenses have been removed. *Ophthal. Surg.* 10(12), 1979.
SHEPARD, D.D.: The 'toxic lens' sydrome. *Cont. & Intraoc. Lens Med. J.* 8(2): 158-161, 1980.
SHOCK, J.P.: Alternative techniques phacofragmentation phacocryolysis and irrigation of cataracts. *Trans. Am. Ac. Ophthal. & Otol.* 78: 22-27, 1974.
SHOLITON, D.B., W.J. REINHART and K.E. FRANK: Indomethacin as a means of preventing cystoid macular edema following intracapsular cataract extraction. *Am. Intraoc. Impl. Soc. J.* 2: 137-140, 1979.
SHUSTERMAN, M. and J.P. HARSHMAN: Experiences with the Ridley plastic lens insertion after cataract extraction. *Trans. Canad. Ophthal. Soc.* 9: 108-115, 1958.
SIMCOE, C.W.: Simplified extracapsular extraction. *Am. Intraoc. Impl. Soc. J.* 3-4: 194-198, 1977.
SIMCOE, C.W.: Iris suture fixation of intraocular lenses. *Am. Intraoc. Impl. Soc. J.* 3-4: 217-221, 1977.
SIMCOE, C.W.: Simplified extracapsular extraction and new techniques in lensimplantation. *Cont. & Intraoc. Lens Med. J.* 3-4: 217-221, 1977.
SIMCOE, C.W.: An ounce of prevention. *Am. Intraoc. Impl. Soc. J.* 1: 39-44, 1978.
SIMCOE, C.W.: Simplified extracapsular cataract extraction. *Am. Intraoc. Impl. Soc. J.* 2: 154-155, 1979.
SIMCOE, C.W.: Retaining devices for protection of corneal endothelium. *Am. Intraoc. Impl. Soc. J.* 3: 234-236, 1979.
SIMCOE, C.W.: New instruments: Forceps removal of nucleus. *Cont. & Intraoc. Lens Med. J.* 1: 62-63, 1980.
SIMCOE, C.W.: Capsular discission behind posterior chamber lens. *Cont. & Intraoc. Lens Med. J.* 1: 60-61, 1980.
SIMEL, P.L.: Anticoagulation, intraocular bleeding and pupillary paralysis following Choyce intraocular lens implantation. *Am. Intraoc. Impl. Soc. J.* 3: 117-119, 1978.
SINSKEY, R.M. and W. CAIN Jr.: The posterior capsule and phacoemulsification. *Am. Intraoc. Impl. Soc. J.* 4: 206-207, 1978.
SINSKEY, R.M.: Letter. in: Consultation section. Ed. by D.D. Shepard. *Am. Intraoc. Impl. Soc. J.* 5: 358, 1979.

SLOANE, A.E.: Perspectives in management of aphakia after 40 years. *Opth. Surg.* 8(4): 75-77, 1977.
SMITH, J.A. and D.R. ANDERSON: Effect of the intraocular lens on intraocular pressure. *Arch. Ophthal.* 94: 1291-1294, 1976.
SMITH, R.: Histopathological studies of eyes enucleated after failure of intraocular acrylic lens operations. *Brit. J. Ophthal.* 40: 473-479, 1956.
SNIDER, N.L. and W.U. McREYNOLDS: Results and complications of our first 500 implantations. *Am. Intraoc. Impl. Soc. J.* 3(1): 10-13, 1977.
SNYDER, D.L. and D.D. SHEPARD: Intraocular lens implants widen surgery's scope. *Calif. Optom.* 1: 16-18, 1975.
SNYDER, W.B., I. BERNSTEIN, D. FULLER, W.L. HUTTON and A. VAISER: Retinal detachment and pseudophakia. *Trans. Am. Ac. Ophthal. & Otol.* 86: 229-241, 1979.
SOCH, D.: The intraocular lens miracle or manace. *Cont. & Intraoc. Lens Med. J.* 4(2): 70-75, 1978.
SOLL, D.B. and R.A. YOHEY: Aphakic myodisc lenses. In: *Current Concepts in Cataract Surgery.* Ed. by J.M. Emery and D. Paton, St. Louis: C.V. Mosby Co., pp. 409-411, 1974.
SORSBY, A.: Measurement of the optical components of the globe. *Mod. Trends in Ophthal.* 4: 30-33, 1967.
SORSBY, A.: Epidemiology of refraction. *Intern. Ophthalmological Clinics.* 11: 1-18, 1971.
SPALTER, H.F.: Retinal detachment in pseudophakia. In: *Pseudophakia: Current Trends and Concepts.* Ed. by M.L. Kwitko and D.L. Praeger. London, Baltimore: Williams & Wilkins, 1980, pp. 357-365.
SPERLING, S.: Human corneal endothelium in organ culture: The influence of temperature and medium of incubation. *Acta Ophthalmologica.* 57: 269-275, 1979.
STAATZ, W.D., D.L. VAN HORN, H.F. EDELHAUSER and R.D. SCHULTZ: Effects of phenylephrine on bovine corneal endothelium in culture. *Ophth. Res.* 12: 244-251, 1980.
STARK, W.J., L.W. HIRST, R.C. SNIP and A.E. MAUMENEE: A two-year trial of intraocular lenses at the Wilmer Institute. *Am. J. Ophthal.* 84(6): 769-774, 1977.
STARK, W.J.: Wet-pack versus dry-pack lenses. *Am. Intraoc. Impl. Soc. J.* 4(4): 213, 1978.
STARK, W.J., G.P. KRACHNER, C.L. COWAN, H.R. TAYLOR, L.W. HIRST, R.T. OYAKAWA and A.E. MAUMENEE: Extended wear contact lenses and intraocular lenses for aphakic correction. *Am. J. Ophthal.* 88: 535-542, 1979.
STARK, W.J.: Sterilizing with ethylene oxide. *Highlights of Ophthal.* B.F. Boyd. *Monthly Letter* 7(2), 1979.
STEIGER, R.M., H.R. BÖHRINGER and C. WUNDERLY: Quantitative und elektrophoretische Untersuchungen am neugebildeten Kammerwasser normaler menschlicher Augen. *Klin. Mbl. Augenheilk.* 126: 490-492, 1955.
STEIN, H.A.: Question and Answers on intraocular lenses. *Cont. & Intraoc. Lens Med. J.* 2(1): 64-67, 1977.
STENSTRÖM, S.: Untersuchungen über die Variation und Kovariation der optischen Elemente des menschlichen Auges. *Acta Ophthal. suppl. XXVI.* 59: 1946 (Kbh).
STENSTRÖM, S.: Variations and correlations of the optical components of the eye. In: *Modern Trends in Ophthalmology.* London: Butterworth and Co., Vol. II, 87-102, 1948.
STOCKER, F.W., M.T. MATTON-VAN LEUVEN and N. GEORGIADE: Influence of alpha-chymtrypsin on endothelial corneal dystrophy. *Trans. Am. Ophth. Soc.* 60: 202-212, 1962.
STRAATSMA, B.R.: Introduction and classification of intraocular lenses. *Am. Intraoc. Impl. Soc. Newsletter.* 1: 38-40, 1975.
STRAATSMA, B.R.: Lattice degeneration of the retina. In: *Periphere Retina.* Ed. by W. Jaeger, Munich: Bergmann-Verlag, 1977.
STRAMPELLI, B.: Soppotabilità di lenti acriliche in camera anteriore nella afachia a Nei Vizi di Refrazione. *Atti Soc. Oftal. Lombarda.* 8: 292-302, 1953. *An. Ottal.* 80: 75-82, 1954.
STRAMPELLI, B.: Due anni di esperienza con le lenti camerulari. *Atti Soc. Oftal. Ital.* 15: 427-433, 1955.

STRAMPELLI, B.: Fissazione di lenti camerulari mediante filo di supramid. *Atti Soc. Oftal. Ital.* 17: 669-682, 1957.

STRAMPELLI, B.: Complications de l'opération de Strampelli. *L'année thérap. Clin. Ophthal.* 9: 349-370, 1958.

STRAMPELLI, B.: Les lentilles camérulaires après six années d'expérience. *Acta Conc. Ophthal. Belgica II: 1692-1698, 1958.*

STRAMPELLI, B.: Anterior Chamber Lenses. *Arch. Ophthal.* 66: 12-17, 1961.

STRAMPELLI, B.: Anterior chamber lenses. In: *Modern Advances in Cataract Surgery.* Ed. by R.M. Fasanella, Philadelphia & Montreal: J.B. Lippincott Co., 1963.

STRAMPELLI, B.: L'évolution des lentilles plastiques de chambre antérieure. Dernières acquisitions techniques. *An. Inst. Barraquer.* 111-4: 519-530, 1962.

STRAMPELLI, B., W. MARCHI and A. VALVO: Lentine in camera anteriore con fissazione esterna (10 anni di esperienza clinica). *Ann. Ottal.* 94: 9-42, 1968.

STROBEL, J. and K.W. JACOBI: Zur Brechkraft der intraocularen Linsen. *Ber. Dtsch. Ophthal. Ges.* 75: 153, 1978.

STUBBS, G.M.: The pupillary lens: Some postoperative complications. *Trans. of the Ophthal. Soc. of Australia.* 26: 106-109, 1967.

STUBBS, G.M.: Corneal dystrophy and the intraocular lens. *Am. Intraoc. Impl. Soc. J.* 1: 39-40, 1977.

SUGAR, A., E.C. FETHEROLF and L.K. LIN: Endothelial cell loss from intraocular lens insertion. *Ophthalmology.* 85: 394-399, 1978.

SUGAR, J., J. BURNETT and S.L. FORSTOT: Scanning electron microscopy of intraocular lens and endothelial cell interaction. *Am. J. Ophthal.* 86: 157-161, 1978.

SUGAR, J., J. MITCHELSON and M. KRAFF: The effect of phacoemulsification on corneal endothelial cell density. *Arch. Ophthal.* 96: 446-448, 1978.

SUGAR, J., J. MITCHELSON and M. KRAFF: Endothelial trauma and cell loss from intraocular lens insertion. *Arch. Ophthal.* 96: 449-450, 1978.

SVENDSON, E., H. RINDORF and G. WULFF: Raychem's 10 MEV Linac Establishment at Glostrup. *Leaflet.* Nov. 1975.

TAIEB, A.: Des mémoires de Casanova à l'opération de Ridley. *Arch. Ophthal.* (Paris) 15: 501-503, 1955.

TASSMAN, W. and W.H. ANNESLEY Jr.: Retinal detachment in Prosthetophakia. *Arch. Ophthal.* 75: 179-188, 1966.

TAYLOR, D.M., L.A. DALBURG, R.T. CONSENTINO and R.O. HOWARD: Intraocular lenses: One hundred consecutive cases of intracapsular cataract extraction with Copeland iris plane lens implantation. *Ophthal. Surg.* 6: 13-30, 1975.

TAYLOR, D.M.: Keratoplasty and intraocular lenses. *Opthal. Surg.* 7: 31-42, 1976.

TAYLOR, D.M.: Keratoplasty and intraocular lenses: follow-up study. *Ophthal. Surg.* 8(2): 49-57, 1977.

TAYLOR, D.M., L.A. DALBURG, R.T. CONSENTINO and A. KHALIQ: Intraocular lenses: 500 consecutive intracapsular cataract extractions with 500 intracapsular extractions — observations and comments. *Opthal. Surg.* 9(1): 29-55, 1978.

TAYLOR, D.M. and A.L. STERN: Long-term follow-up of 43 intraocular lenses in eyes with primary glaucoma. *Am. Intraoc. Impl. Soc. J.* 4: 313-315, 1979.

TAYLOR, D.M., A. KHALIQ and R. MAXWELL: Keratoplasty and intraocular lenses: Current status. *Trans. Am. Ac. Ophthal. & Otol.* 86: 242-248, 1979.

TENNANT, J.L.: *A lens for all seasons.* Dallas, Texas, 1976.

TENNANT, J.L.: Is cystoid macular edema reversible by oral indocin, yes or no? In: *Current Concepts in Cataract Surgery.* Ed. by J.M. Emery and D. Paton. St. Louis: C.V. Mosby Co., 1976.

TENNANT, J.L.: Results of primary and secondary implants using Choyce Mark VIII lenses. *Ophthal. Surg.* 8(3): 54-55, 1977.

THEOBALD, G.D.: In regard to the Ridley implant. *Am. J. Ophthal.* 36: 1471, 1953.

THEODORE, F.H., Ed. *Complications after Cataract Surgery*, Boston: Little and Brown, 1964.

THIJSSEN, J.M. and A.J. OTTO: Echo-diagnostiek, toepassing in de oogheelkunde. *Ned. T. Geneesk.* 115(26): 1117-1118, 1971.

THIJSSEN, J.M.: The emmetropic and the iseikonic implant lens: computer calculation of the refractive power and its accuracy. *Ophthalmologica* (Basel). 171: 467-486, 1975.

THYGESEN, J., P. REERSTED, H. FLEDELIUS and L. CORYDON: Corneal astigmatism after cataract extraction — a comparison of corneal and corneoscleral incisions. *Acta Ophthalmologica.* 57: 243-250, 1979.
THOMAS, J.V., E.S. GRAGOUDAS, N.P. BLAIR and J.V. LAPUS: Correlation of epinephrine use and macular edema in aphakic glaucomatous eyes. *Arch. Ophthal.* 96: 625-628, 1978.
THOMAS, R.M., Jr.: Intracapsular or extracapsular? *Am. Intraoc. Impl. Soc. News ltr.* 1: 45, 1975.
TJAN, T.T.: Ultrasonic diagnosis of ocular pathology: Its significance for cataract surgery with and without IOL implantation. *Am. Intraoc. Impl. Soc. J.* 1: 15-22, 1978.
TOLENTINO, F.I. and C.L. SCHEPENS: Edema of posterior poole after cataract extraction. *Arch. Ophthal.* 74: 781-786, 1965.
TRAGAKIS, M., I. ECONOMIDIS, P. ATHANASSIADES and S. POLLALIS: Corneal thickness after cataract surgery. *Trans. Ophth. Soc. U.K.* 97: 114-116, 1977.
TREMOULET, O.: Angiographie fluorescéinique du segment antérieur chez les porteurs de cristallins artificiels. *La clinique opthalmologique — revue médicale.* 3: 53-56, 1978.
TROUTMAN, R.C.: Artiphakia and aniseikonia. *Trans. Am. Ophthal. Soc. J.* 60: 590-658, 1962.
TROUTMAN, R.C.: Correction of unilateral aphakia: The use of intraocular lens implants. *Arch. Ophtahl.* 68: 861-869, 1962.
TROUTMAN, R.C.: Artiphakia and aniseikonia. *Am. J. Ophthal.* 56: 602-639, 1963.
TROUTMAN, R.C., J.N. GOLDMAN, R.D. BINKHORST, D.E. WILLARD and A.C. CLAHANE: Anterior chamber depht in aphakia. *Trans. Am. Ophthal. Soc.* 61: 385-396, 1963.
TROUTMAN, R.C.: Intraocular lenses in aphakia: A letter to the editor. *Am. J. Ophthal.* 68: 1125-1126, 1969.
TROUTMAN, R.C. and H. HIRSCHMANN: Intraocular lens implants, more popular, still controversial. *Med. World News.* 20-21, Sept. 13, 1974.
TROUTMAN, R.C.: Why deep wound closure? In: *Current Concepts in Cataract Surgery.* Ed. by J.M. Emery and D. Paton, St. Louis: C.V. Mosby Co., 1974.
TROUTMAN, R.C.Intraocular lenses for the correction of aphakia. *Contact lens.* 1(1-2): 109-114, 1975.
TROUTMAN, R.C.: The weightless intraocular lens. *Opthal. Surg.* 8(3): 153-155, 1977.
TROUTMAN, R.C.: The intraocular lens — boon or bomb? In: *Controversy in Opthalmology*, pp. 281-286, 1977.

URRETS-ZAVALIA, A. Jr.: *Le décollement de la rétine.* Paris: Masson & Co., 1968.
VALERIO, M.: Considerazioni sull'introduzione in camera anterior della lentina do Strampelli negli occhi afachici. *Atti Soc. Oftal. Lombarda, N.S.* 11: 183-187, 1956.
VAN BALEN, A.T.M.: De implantatie van pseudophakoi volgens Binkhorst bij eenzijdige traumatische cataract. *Ned. T. Geneesk.* 114: 1883-1884, 1970.
VAN BALEN, A.T.M.: Binkhorst's method of implantation of pseudophakoi in unilateral traumatic cataract. *Opthalmologica.* 165: 490-494, 1972.
VAN BALEN, A.T.M.: Four years experience with Binkhorst lens implantation. *Am. J. Ophthal.* 75(5): 755-763, 1973. *Trans. Ophthal. Soc. U.K.* 92: 839-841, 1972.
VAN BALEN, A.T.M.: First international symposium on artificial lens implantation. *Documenta Opth. Proc. Series 6.* The Hague. Junk Publ., 1974.
VAN BALEN, A.T.M.: The implantation of artificial lenses in traumatic cataract in children. *Doc. Ophth. Proc. Series.* 6: 1-4, 1975.
VAN DER HEIJDE, G.L.: A monogram for calculating the power the prepupillary lens in the aphakic eye. *Bibl. Ophthal.* 83: 273-275, 1975.
VAN DER HEIJDE, G.L.: The optical correction of unilateral aphakia. *Trans. Am. Ac. Ophthal. & Otol.* 81: 80-88, 1976.
VAN DER HEIJDE, G.L. and J.S. STILMA: Biometrie und Aphakie. *Klin. Mbl. Augenheilk.* 169: 289-293, 1976.
VANE, J.R.: Inhibition of prostaglandin synthesis as a mechanism of action of aspirinlike drugs. *Nature New Biology.* 231: 232-235, 1971.
VAN HORN, D.: L., H.F. EDELHAUSER, T.M. AABERG and H.L. PEDERSON: In vivo effects of air and sulfur hexafluoride gas on rabbit corneal endothelium. *Invest. Ophthal.* 11(12): 1028-1036, 1972.

VAN HORN, D.L., P.D. RICHARD, O. SCHULTZ and J. DEBRUIN: Endothelial survival in corneal tissue stored in M-K. *Am. J. Ophthal.* 80: 642-647, 1975.
VANNAS, A., K. SETÄLÄ and P. RUUSUVAARA: Endothelial cells in capsular glaucoma. *Acta Ophthalmologica.* 55: 951-958, 1977.
VAN RIJ, G.: Suture loosening and γ-sterilization of 10.0 nylon. *Doc. Ophthal.* 48(2): 303-307, 1979.
VANYSEK, J., J. ISERLE, J. SVERAK and J. ALTMAN: Implantation of an acrylic lens for correction of aphakia. *Scripta med.* 30: 301-307, 1957.
VERGNE, J.L.: Correction de l'aphaquie unilatérale chez les malades de plus de 40 ans. *La Clinique opthalmologique — revue médicale 3.* 23-26, 1978.
VIT, H. and F. TODTER: Ergebnisse nach Einpflanzung von Vorderkammerlinsen. *Ophthalmologica.* 157: 76-82, 1969.
VOGT, A.: *Lehrbuch und Atlas der Spaltlampenmikroskopie des lebenden Auges.* Part I: Technik und Methodik Hornhaut und Vorderkammer. Berlin: Julius Springer Verlag, 1930.
VOIGT, G.J. and W. BÖKE: Verhalten der Hornhaut nach Implantation intraokularer Linsen durch kornealen Starschnitt. In: *Kunststoffimplantate in der Ophthalmologie.* Ed. W. Jaeger, Munich: J.F. Bergmann Verlag, pp. 137-138, 1978.
VÖLKER-DIEBEN, H.J.M., C.C. KOK-VAN ALPHEN and E.R. BARTHEN: Iatrogenic endothelial damage during cataract extraction. *Doc. Ophthalmologica.* 46(2): 207-213, 1979.

WAITZMAN, M.B.: Topical indomethacin in treatment and prevention of intraocular inflammation with special reference to lens extraction and cystoid macular edema. *An. Ophthal.* 11: 489-491, 1979.
WEEKERS, R., Y. DELMARCELLE, J. LUYCKX-BACUS and J.F. WEEKERS: L'échographie en opthalmologie. *Arch. Ophthal.* (Paris). 29(11): 839-848, 1969.
WEEKERS, J.F. and J. LUYCKX-BACUS: Utilisation de l'ultrasonographie dans le diagnostic de différentes affections oculaires. *Arch. Ophthal.* 27(7): 671-682, 1967.
WEGNER, W.: Lentilles intraoculaires de la chambre antérieure. Observations tardives. *An. Inst. Barraquer.* 111-4: 573-584, 1962.
WEINSTOCK, F.J.: The effect of intraocular lenses on intraocular pressure. *Cont. & Intraoc. Lens Med. J.* 3(4): 40-42, 1977.
WELCH, R.B. and J.C. COOPER: Macular edema: papiledema and optic atrophy after cataract extraction. *Arch. of Ophthal.* 59: 665-675, 1958.
WELCH, R.B., A.E. MAUMENEE and H.E. WAHLEN: Peripheral posterior segment inflammation, vitreous opacities and edema of the posterior pole. *Arch. Ophthal.* 64: 540-549, 1960.
WELSH, R.C.: Contact lenses in aphakia. *Int. Ophthal. Clin.* 1/2: 401-440, 1961.
WELSH, R.C.: The roving ring scotoma with its jack-in-the-box phenomenon of strong plus (aphakic) spectacle lenses. *Am. J. Ophthal.* 51: 1277-1281, 1961.
WELSH, R.C.: Roving ring scotoma: Letter to the editor and reply from P. Boeder. *Arch. Ophthal.* 69: 685-687, 1963.
WELSH, R.C.: Ring scotoma. Letter to the editor. *Arch. Ophthal.* 70: 139, 1963.
WELSH, R.C.: Experimental simulation of aphakia. *Brit. J. Ophthal.* 49: 84-86, 1965.
WELSH, R.C.: Newer design of aphakic spectacle eyeglasses. *Trans. Am. Ac. Ophthal. & Otol.* 86: 380-388, 1979.
WERNER, D. and M. KABACK: Pseudophakic pupillary block glaucoma. *Brit. J. Ophthal.* 61: 329-333, 1977.
WEST, C.E., C.R., FITZGERALD and J.H. SEWELL: Cystoid Macular edema following aphakic keratoplasty. *Am. J. Ophthal.* 75: 77-81, 1973.
WIBAUT, F.: Über die Emmetropisation und den Ursprong der Sphärischen Refractionsanomalien. *Graefes Arch. Klin. Ophthal.* 116: 596-612, 1926.
WILLENSKY, J.F.: *Intraocular Lenses.* New York: Appleton-Century-Crofts, 1977.
WILKINSON, C.P., L.S. ANDERSON and J.H. LITTLE: Retinal detachment following phacoemulsification. *Am. Ac. Ophthal. & Otol.* 85, 1978.
WILKINSON, C.P.: Retinal detachment after phacoemulsification. *Am. J. Ophthal.* 87: 628-632, 1979.
WILLIAMSON, D.E.: The use of 8-0 Dexon and 8-0 Vicryl in out-patient cataract (IOL) implant surgery. *Cont. & Intraoc. Lens Med. J.* 4(3): 47-48, 1977.

WILLIAMSON, D.E.: Two hundred consecutive outpatient cataract-intraocular lens implant operations. *Ophthal. Surg.* 8(1): 29-34, 1977.
WILLIAMSON, D.E.: The use of Davis and Gek's 9-0 monofilament polyglycolic acid suture in outpatient cataract implant surgery. *Cont. & Intraoc. Lens Med. J.* 5(3): 81-90, 1979.
WINSLOW, R.L., B.C. TAYLOR and W.S. HARRIS: A one-Year follow-up of cystoid macular edema following intraocular lens implantation. *Am. Ac. Ophthal. & Otol.* 85, 1978.
WISE, J.: Treatment of retinal detachment after phacoemulsification. In: *Current Concepts in Cataract Surgery.* Ed. by J.M. Emery and D. Paton, St. Louis. C.V. Mosby Co., 1974.
WITMER, R.: Retinal detachment in aphakia. *An. Inst. Barraquer.* 10: 412-417, 1972.
WITMER, R. and C. REME: Experimental iris suture in rabbits and monkeys. In: *Surgery of the Iris and the Ciliary Body.* Basel: S. Karger, 1975.
WOLFF, E.: *The Anatomy of the Eye and Orbit,* 3rd. ed. p. 375, 1950.
WOLLENSAK, J.: Matières plastiques et lentilles artificielles. *An. Inst. Barraquer.* 111-4: 543-547, 1962.
WOLLENSAK, J.: Chemische Einflüsse bei Keratopathia post Implantationen (Von Vorderkammerlinsen). *Ber. 62. Zus. dtsch. Ophthal. Ges. Heidelberg.* 1959: 246-226, 1978.
WOOD, W.J. and A.E. MAUMENEE: Corneal thickness after cataract surgery. *Trans. Am. Ac. Ophthal. & Otol.* 79: 631-634, 1975.
WOODS, A.C.: The adjustment to aphakia. *Am. J. Ophthal.* 35: 118-122, 1952.
WORST, J.G.F.: Over fixatie van de „Binkhost lens". *Ned. T. Geneesk.* 114: 489, 1970.
WORST, J.G.F., H.H.H. LUDWIG and R.G. MASSARO: Binkhorst's artificial lens. *Ophthalmology.* 222: 776-780, 1970.
WORST, J.G.F.: L'implantation d'un cristallin artificiel. *Bull. et Mem. Soc. Fr. d'ophtal.* 84: 547-562, 1971.
WORST, J.F. and R.G. MASSARO: The introduction of an artificial lens to the eye using Binkhorst's technique. *Ophthalmologica.* 164: 387-391, 1972.
WORST, J.G.F.: Biotoxicität des Kammerwassers. *Klin. Mbl. Augenheilk.* 167: 367-384, 1975.
WORST, J.G.F.: The Bursa intravitrealis premacularis. In: *New developments in Ophthalmology: Doc. Ophthal. Proceedings Series,* Nijmegen, 13-16 oct. 1975, pp. 275-279.
WORST, J.G.F.: Special indications for the artificial lens. *Ophthalmologica* (Basel). 171: 57-66, 1975.
WORST, J.G.F.: Iris suture for artificial lens fixation — Perlon vs. stainless steel. *Trans. Am. Ac. Ophthal. & Otol.* 81: 102-104, 1976.
WORST, J.G.F.: Complications, complication factors and adverse conditions in lens implantation surgery. *Trans. Am. Ac. Ophthal.* 81: 105-117, 1976.
WORST, J.G.F.: Extracapsular surgery and lensimplantation. *Ophthal. Surg.* 8(3): 33-35, 1977.
WORST, J.G.F., C.D. MOSSELMAN and H.H.H. LUDWIG: The artificial lens — Experience with 2000 lens implantations. *Am. Intraoc. Impl. Soc. J.* 1: 14-19, 1977.
WORST, J.G.F.: Complications, complicating factors and adverse conditions in lensimplantation surgery: part I. *Am. Intraoc. Impl. Soc. J.* 2: 20-27, 1977.
WORST, J.G.F.: Extracapsular surgery in lens implantation: part II. *Am. Intraoc. Impl. Soc. J.* 2: 102-104, 1977.
WORST, J.G.F.: Extracapsular surgery in lens implantation: part II. *Am. Intraoc. Impl. Soc. J.* 3(3-4): 166-169, 1977.
WORST, J.G.F.: Extracapsular surgery in lensimplantation (Binkhorst lecture): Part IV: Some anatomical and pathophysiological implications. *Am. Intraoc. Impl. Soc. J.* 4(1): 7-14, 1978.
WORST, J.G.F.: A procedure for slitlamp endothelioscopy with a lens implant. *Am. Intraoc. Impl. Soc. J.* 2: 150, 1979.
WORST, J.M.F.: Interview by B. Boyd. *Highlights of Ophthalmology.* 15: 309-324, 1978-1979.
WORST, J.G.F.: Communication Dutch Ophth. Soc. Meeting, Breda, March 1980.

WORTHEN, D.M.: The role of the university in teaching the correction of aphakia. *Cont. & Intraoc. Lens Med. J.* 2(3): 41-47, 1976.

YAMANAKA, A.: Les propriétés physiques et chimiques des lentilles intraoculaires. Read before the French and Internat. Impl. Club. Meeting Perpignan. Nov. 1977.

YAMANAKA, A., T. MATSUMOTO, K. NAKAMAE, Y. KANAJI, H. GOTO and M. KITAYAMA: Physical and chemical analysis of intraocular lens materials. *Am. Intraoc. Impl. Soc. J.* 5: 131, 1979.

YANNUZZI, L.A., R.M. KLEIN, R.H. WALLYN, N. COHEN and I. KATZ: Ineffectiveness of indomethacin in the treatment of chronic cystoid macular edema. *Am. J. Ophthal.* 84: 517-519, 1977.

YANNUZI, L.A. and R.H. WALLYN: Cystoid macular edema: A controlled treatment study utilizing indomethacin. In: *Current Concepts in Cataract Surgery — Selected Proceedings of the Fourth Biennial Cat. Surg. Congress.* St. Louis: C.V. mosby Co., p. 313, 1976.

YTTEBORG, J. and C.H. DOHLMAN: Corneal edema and intraocular pressure. *Arch. Ophthal.* 74: 477-484, 1965.

ZIMMERMAN, T.J., N. GRAVENSTEIN, A. SUGAR and H.E. KAUFMAN: Aspirin stabilization of the blood aqueous barrier in the human eye. *Am. J. Ophthal.* 79: 817-819, 1975.

ZOBIAN, E.J. and J.W. BEEM: Letter to the editor. *Am. Intraoc. Impl. Soc. J.* 3: 235, 1977.

Authors' address:

Dr. Paul LEONARD
Lange Leemstraat, 128
2000 Antwerpen
BELGIUM

Dr. Jos ROMMEL
Grote Markt, 28
8800 Roeselare
BELGIUM

(T3187) by Ceuterick s.a.
Brusselse straat 153 B 3000-Leuven
A. Struyf Oude Baan 353 B 3000-Leuven

GPSR Compliance

The European Union's (EU) General Product Safety Regulation (GPSR) is a set of rules that requires consumer products to be safe and our obligations to ensure this.

If you have any concerns about our products, you can contact us on ProductSafety@springernature.com

In case Publisher is established outside the EU, the EU authorized representative is:

Springer Nature Customer Service Center GmbH
Europaplatz 3
69115 Heidelberg, Germany

Batch number: 10607220

Printed by Printforce, the Netherlands